The Nervous System: A Cellular and Molecular Approach

The Nervous System: A Cellular and Molecular Approach

Edited by Charles Carter

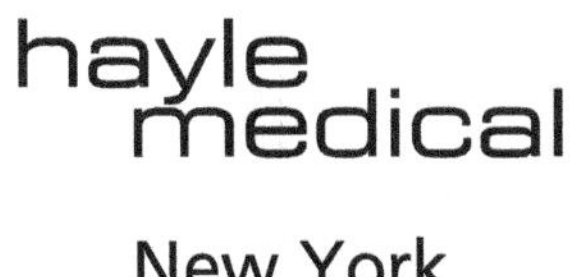

New York

Hayle Medical,
750 Third Avenue, 9th Floor,
New York, NY 10017, USA

Visit us on the World Wide Web at:
www.haylemedical.com

ISBN: 978-1-63241-676-6

Cataloging-in-Publication Data

The nervous system : a cellular and molecular approach / edited by Charles Carter.
p. cm.
Includes bibliographical references and index.
ISBN 978-1-63241-676-6
1. Nervous system. 2. Molecular neurobiology. 3. Nerves--Cytology.
I. Carter, Charles.
QP361 .N47 2019
612.8--dc23

Table of Contents

Preface

The nervous system is an important system of the human body that coordinates its action by transmitting signals from one part of the body to another. It can be divided into the central and the peripheral nervous system. It consists of the brain, spinal cord and the nerves of the body. At the cellular level, the fundamental mechanism is that of the neuron, which transmits signals through axons that trigger the activation of neurotransmitters, which are then released at synapses. This signaling process involves a complicated molecular machinery, which allows the rapid electrical or chemical transmission of signals. Cells that receive a synaptic signal will be excited, inhibited or modulated. The organization of neural pathways, neural circuits and neural networks together build a functioning nervous system. Any abnormality in nervous function can manifest due to a genetic defect, infection, trauma, toxicity, or due to aging. This book provides comprehensive insights into the cellular and molecular basis of the working of the nervous system. It presents researches and studies performed by experts across the globe. It will serve as a reference to a broad spectrum of readers.

The researches compiled throughout the book are authentic and of high quality, combining several disciplines and from very diverse regions from around the world. Drawing on the contributions of many researchers from diverse countries, the book's objective is to provide the readers with the latest achievements in the area of research. This book will surely be a source of knowledge to all interested and researching the field.

In the end, I would like to express my deep sense of gratitude to all the authors for meeting the set deadlines in completing and submitting their research chapters. I would also like to thank the publisher for the support offered to us throughout the course of the book. Finally, I extend my sincere thanks to my family for being a constant source of inspiration and encouragement.

Editor

1

The novel cannabinoid receptor GPR55 mediates anxiolytic-like effects in the medial orbital cortex of mice with acute stress

Qi-xin Shi[1†], Liu-kun Yang[1†], Wen-long Shi[2], Lu Wang[1], Shi-meng Zhou[1], Shao-yu Guan[1], Ming-gao Zhao[1] and Qi Yang[1,3*]

Abstract

The G protein-coupled receptor 55 (GPR55) is a novel cannabinoid receptor, whose exact role in anxiety remains unknown. The present study was conducted to explore the possible mechanisms by which GPR55 regulates anxiety and to evaluate the effectiveness of O-1602 in the treatment of anxiety-like symptoms. Mice were exposed to two types of acute stressors: restraint and forced swimming. Anxiety behavior was evaluated using the elevated plus maze and the open field test. We found that O-1602 alleviated anxiety-like behavior in acutely stressed mice. We used lentiviral shRNA to selectively knockdown GPR55 in the medial orbital cortex and found that knockdown of GPR55 abolished the anxiolytic effect of O-1602. We also used Y-27632, a specific inhibitor of ROCK, and U73122, an inhibitor of PLC, and found that both inhibitors attenuated the effectiveness of O-1602. Western blot analysis revealed that O-1602 downregulated the expression of GluA1 and GluN2A in mice. Taken together, these results suggest that GPR55 plays an important role in anxiety and O-1602 may have therapeutic potential in treating anxiety-like symptoms.

Keywords: GPR55, O-1602, Medial orbital cortex, Stress, Anxiety

Introduction

Depression and anxiety are the most prevalent neurological and psychiatric disorders affecting millions of people worldwide, with an estimated prevalence rate of 10–20% [1], and a tendency to increase. Stress is defined as any threat or perceived threat that disturbs an organism's ability to maintain homeostasis. Although activation of stress response is initially adaptive, exposure to prolonged stress poses a significant risk for the development of numerous psychiatric disorders, including memory deficits [2], posttraumatic stress disorder [3, 4], and major depression [5, 6].

The endocannabinoid system is a neuromodulatory system that has been implicated in a wide range of physiological and pathological brain functions [7]. Clinical and animal studies consistently support the notion that the endocannabinoid system plays a central role in emotional homeostasis, stress responsiveness, energy balance, and cognitive function, whereas deregulation of the endocannabinoid signaling has been associated with neuropsychiatric conditions, such as depression, anxiety disorders, and schizophrenia [8, 9].

Recently, another G protein-coupled receptor, GPR55, was identified as a novel cannabinoid (CB) receptor owing to its high affinity for cannabinoid ligands, such as Δ^9-tetrahydrocannabinol, 2-arachidonoylglycerol, anandamide, and rimonabant, independent of the CB_1 and CB_2 receptors (CB_1R and CB_2R) [10–13]. GPR55 was first identified in the human brain and liver [10]. The GPR55 gene has a widespread expression in the brain including the striatum, hippocampus, forebrain, cortex, and cerebellum [14].

* Correspondence: yangqifmmu@126.com
†Equal contributors
[1]Department of Pharmacology, School of Pharmacy, Fourth Military Medical University, Xi'an, China
[3]Department of Neurobiology and Collaborative Innovation Center for Brain Science, Fourth Military Medical University, Xi'an, China
Full list of author information is available at the end of the article

Unlike the classical CB_1R and CB_2R signaling pathways, GPR55 is coupled to $G\alpha_{12/13}$ [13, 15] and $G\alpha_q$ proteins [16], and signals through ras homolog gene family member A (RhoA), Rho-associated protein kinase (ROCK), and phospholipase C (PLC) pathways. Increased intracellular Ca^{2+} triggers the activation of RhoA, Rac, and cdc42, which in turn induces the phosphorylation of extracellular-regulated protein kinase (ERK) [16–18]. Activation of GPR55 was reported to have regulatory roles in the central nervous system. For example, GPR55 regulates growth cone morphology and axon growth in the retina during development [19]. GPR55 knockout mice failed to develop mechanical hyperalgesia associated with inflammatory and neuropathic pain [20]. However, the exact role of GPR55 in the modulation of anxiety is unknown [21].

In the present study, the effects of GPR55 agonist and antagonist on stress-induced anxiety-like behaviors were evaluated. We first determined the expression level of GPR55 in emotion-related regions of the brain after chronic stress. Next, a panel of behavioral tests was used to examine the effect of GPR55 activation on anxiety-like symptoms. Lentiviral shRNA-mediated knockdown of GPR55 was used to confirm the effect of GPR55. Finally, we investigated the downstream pathway of GPR55 by using signal transduction antagonists. Our study results clarified the role of GPR55 in stress-induced mood disorders, and suggested that GPR55 may serve as a potential therapeutic target for the treatment of clinical anxiety or depression.

Results

Expression and distribution of GPR55 receptor in the cortex of chronic stress mice

Chronic stress has been associated with impaired endocannabinoid system in the cortex of mice [22]. Through immunofluorescence staining, we observed that GPR55 was highly expressed in the MO cortex (Fig. 1a). Although CRS exposure did not alter the mRNA level of GPR55 (Fig. 1b), western blot analysis indicated that GPR55 expression significantly reduced after CRS exposure for 21 consecutive days (Fig. 1c). Downregulation of GPR55 expression in the MO cortex of CRS mice raises the possibility that GPR55 influences the development of anxiety, possibly acting as a compensatory response after stress.

Effects of GPR55 agonist and antagonist in mice subjected to acute restraint stress

To investigate the influence and role of GPR55 in anxiety/depression-like behaviors, we used the acute restraint model. We intraperitoneally injected the GPR55 agonist O-1602 (10 mg/kg, 0.2 ml) into mice to induce anxiolytic effects. After 3 h, the mice were subjected to EPM and OFT. In the EPM test, acutely stressed mice treated with O-1602 spent more time in the open arms, although the number of entries into the open arms did not change significantly as compared to that reported for the vehicle group (Fig. 2a). To confirm the action of O-1602, the selective GPR55 antagonist CID16020046 (10 mg/kg, 0.2 ml) was simultaneously used with O-1602

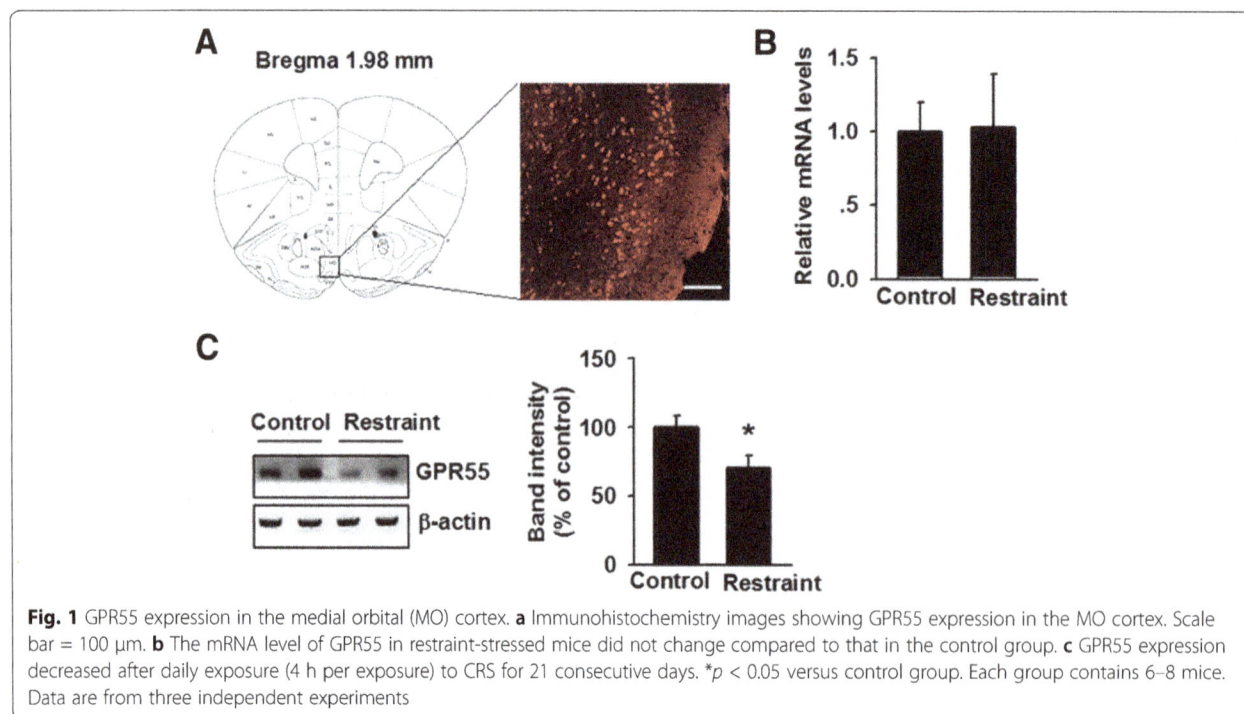

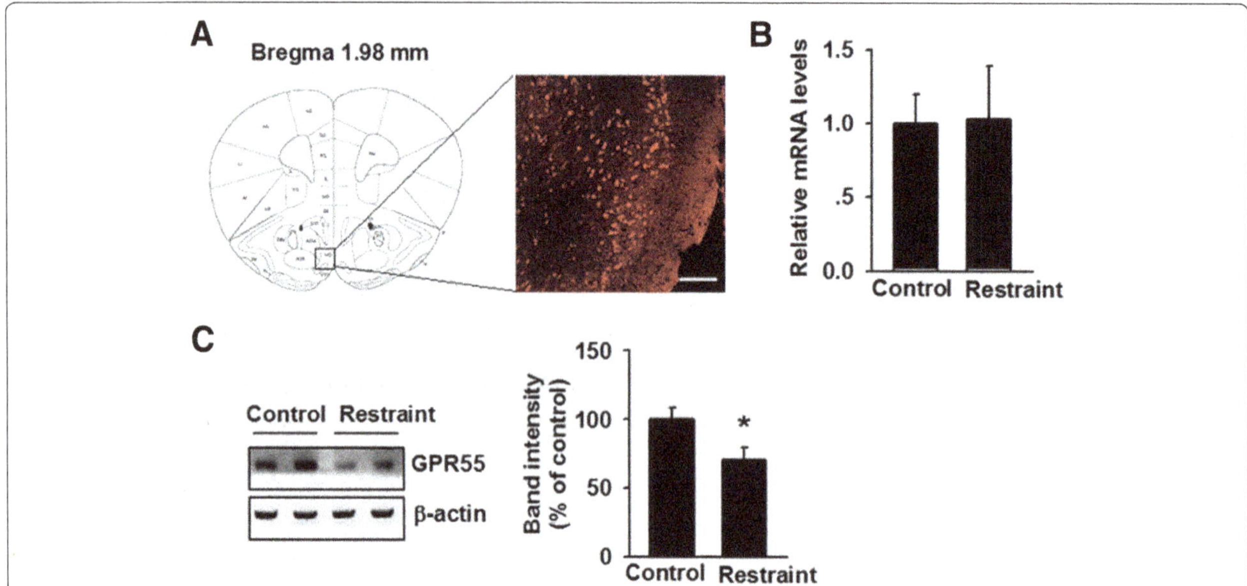

Fig. 1 GPR55 expression in the medial orbital (MO) cortex. **a** Immunohistochemistry images showing GPR55 expression in the MO cortex. Scale bar = 100 μm. **b** The mRNA level of GPR55 in restraint-stressed mice did not change compared to that in the control group. **c** GPR55 expression decreased after daily exposure (4 h per exposure) to CRS for 21 consecutive days. *$p < 0.05$ versus control group. Each group contains 6–8 mice. Data are from three independent experiments

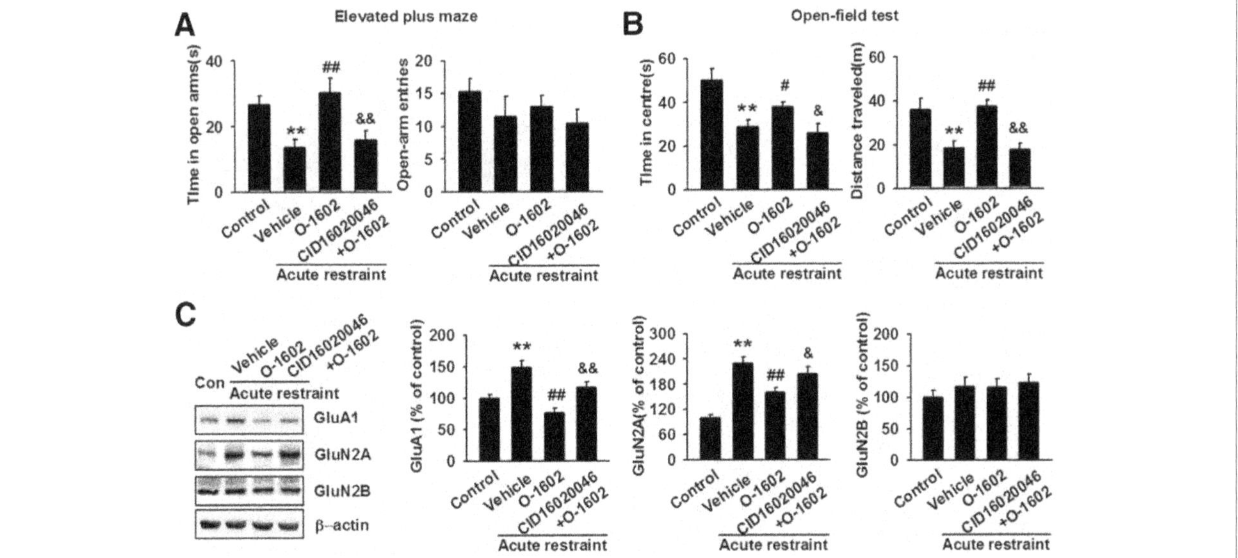

Fig. 2 Intraperitoneal injection of O-1602 reverses acute restrain stress-induced anxiety-like behavior. **a** In the EPM, administration of O-1602 increased the time spent in the open arms compared to the vehicle group. O-1602 had no effect on the number of entries in the open arms. Treatment with CID16020046 and O-1602 decreased the time spent in the open arms and had no significant effect on the entries in the open arms compared to the O-1602 group. $^{**}p < 0.01$ versus control group; $^{\#\#}p < 0.01$ versus vehicle group; $^{\&\&}p < 0.01$ versus O-1602 group. **b** In the OFT, O-1602 treatment increased the time spent in the central area slightly and the total distance traveled significantly compared to the vehicle group. CID16020046 and O-1602 treatmentdecreased the total time spent in the central area and the total distance traveled as compared to the O-1602 group. $^{*}p < 0.05$, $^{**}p < 0.01$ versus control group; $^{\#}p < 0.05$, $^{\#\#}p < 0.01$ versus vehicle group; $^{\&}p < 0.05$, $^{\&\&}p < 0.01$ versus O-1602 group. **c** Intraperitoneal injection of O-1602 reversed stress-induced expression of GluA1 and GluN2A, while GluN2B were unchanged. CID16020046 and O-1602 treatment abolished O-1602-mediated decrease in GluA1 and GluN2A expression. The expression of GluN2B were unchanged. $^{**}p < 0.01$ versus control group; $^{\#\#}p < 0.01$ versus vehicle group; $^{\&}p < 0.05$, $^{\&\&}p < 0.01$ versus O-1602 group. Each group contains 6–8 mice. Data are from three independent experiments

to mice exposed to acute restraint stress. Compared to the O-1602-treated group, simultaneous injection of CID16020046 and O-1602 significantly decreased the duration in the open arms of the EPM, while the frequency in the open arms had no significant changes (Fig. 2a). Results from the OFT showed that the time of O-1602 treatment spent in the central area increased slightly, whereas the total distance traveled increased significantly as compared to the vehicle group (Fig. 2b). Meanwhile, compared to the O-1602-treated group, CID16020046 and O-1602 treatment slightly decreased the time spent in the central area of the OFT and significantly decreased the total distance traveled (Fig. 2b). In addition, we tested the expression levels of several glutamate receptors, because a lot of studies suggested the glutamate receptors have a strong association with anxiety. Western blot analysis showed that intraperitoneal injection of O-1602 prevented acute stress-induced increase in GluA1 and GluN2A expression, but not in GluN2B (Fig. 2c). Simultaneous injection administration of CID16020046 and O-1602 abolished O-1602-mediated decrease in GluA1 and GluN2A expression. The expressions of GluN2B were not changed in the MO cortex of stressed mice exposed to CID16020046 and O-1602 treatment (Fig. 2c). Overall, these results suggest that GPR55 play an important role in anxiety/depression-like behaviors and activation of GPR55 can reverse anxiety/depression-like behaviors after acute stress.

Effects of GPR55 agonist and antagonist in mice exposed to forced swimming stress

In order to confirm the importance of GPR55 in acute stress, the forced swimming model was used. In the EPM test, stressed mice injected with O-1602 increased the number of entries into the open arms significantly, although the time into the open arms did not change significantly as compared to the vehicle group (Fig. 3a). Meanwhile, simultaneous injection of CID16020046 and O-1602 significantly decreased the frequency in the open arms of the EPM as compared to that reported for the O-1602 group, while the duration in the open arms had no significant changes (Fig. 3a). In addition, compared to the vehicle group, the O-1602 group increased the time spent in the central area significantly in the OFT, whereas the total distance traveled did not change (Fig. 3b). CID16020046 and O-1602 group significantly decreased the time spent in the central area of the OFT as compared to the O-1602 group and had no effect on the total distance traveled (Fig. 3b). Western blot analysis showed O-1602 treatment prevented stress-induced increase in GluA1 and GluN2A expression in the MO

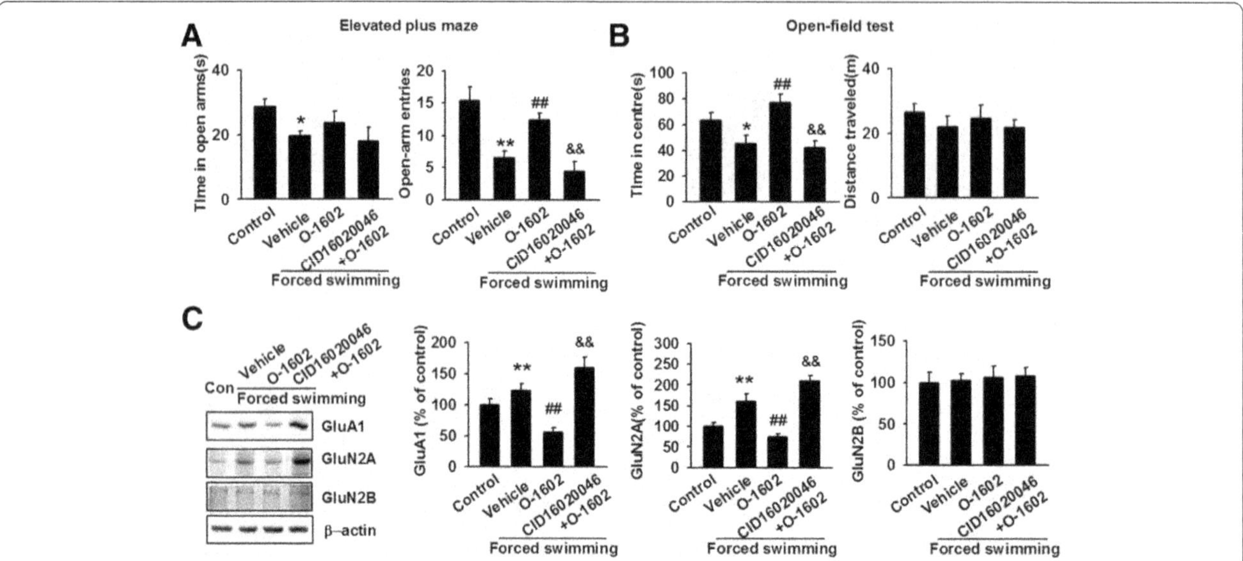

Fig. 3 Intraperitoneal injection of O-1602 reverses forced swimming-induced anxiety-like behavior. **a** In the EPM, administration of O-1602 increased the number of entries in the open arms and the time into the open arms did not change significantly as compared to the vehicle group. CID16020046 and O-1602 decreased the frequency in the open arms and had no significant changes on the duration in the open arms as compared to the O-1602 group. $^{*}p < 0.05$, $^{**}p < 0.01$ versus control group; $^{\#\#}p < 0.01$ versus vehicle group; $^{\&\&}p < 0.01$ versus O-1602 group. **b** In the OFT, administration of O-1602 significantly increased the time spent in the central area and had no effect on the total distance traveled. CID16020046 and O-1602 treatment decreased the time spent in the central area, while it had no significant effect on the total distance traveled. $^{*}p < 0.05$ versus control group; $^{\#\#}p < 0.01$ vehicle group; $^{\&\&}p < 0.01$ versus O-1602 group. **c** Administration of O-1602 reversed stress-induced expression of GluA1 and GluN2A, but not GluN2B. CID16020046 and O-1602 treatment abolished O-1602-mediated decrease in GluA1 and GluN2A expression, while had no effect on the expression of GluN2B. $^{**}p < 0.01$ versus control group; $^{\#\#}p < 0.01$ versus vehicle group; && $p < 0.01$ versus O-1602 group. Each group contains 6–8 mice. Data are from three independent experiments

cortex of mice, while the expression of GluN2B was unchanged (Fig. 3c). Simultaneous injection of CID16020046 and O-1602 abolished O-1602-mediated decrease in GluA1 and GluN2A expression in the MO cortex, while the expression of GluN2B had no significant changes (Fig. 3c). Overall, these results further confirm that GPR55 is involved in anxiolytic response and that pharmacological enhancement of GPR55 function can reverse anxiety/depression-like behaviors after acute stress.

Role of GPR55 activation in O-1602-mediated anxiolytic effects

Previous studies have associated CB_1R and CB_2R with anxiety/depression-like behaviors [23, 24]. In order to exclude the possible involvement of CB_1R and CB_2R in O-1602-mediated anxiolytic effect, a lentiviral shRNA specific for GPR55 was constructed and stereotaxically microinjected into the MO cortex of mice at a concentration of 10^9 TU/ml. After 7 days of infection, cells were labeled green by GFP (Fig. 4a). Western blot analysis confirmed the efficiency of knockdown, which resulted in a 62.7 ± 4.1% reduction in the GPR55 protein band intensity (Fig. 4b). In the EPM, O-1602 with negtive shRNA increased the time in the open arms and the number of entries into the open arms significantly, but the increase was reversed by O-1602 with GPR55 shRNA (Fig. 4c). Results from the OFT showed that the O-1602 with negtive shRNA increased the time spent in the central area and the total distance traveled. However, O-1602 with GPR55 shRNA prevented the behavioral improvement mediated by O-1602 with negtive shRNA (Fig. 4d). Moreover, O-1602 with negtive shRNA decreased the expression of GluA1 and GluN2A, but GluN2B did not decrease. O-1602 with GPR55 shRNA abolished the decrease in GluA1 and GluN2A expression, although no change in the expression of GluN2B was observed (Fig. 4e). These observations show that GPR55 plays an important role in the development of anxiety/depression-like behaviors.

Possible signaling pathways involved in O-1602-induced anxiolytic effect

The downstream signaling cascade by which GPR55 agonist initiates its effect was investigated using selective PLC inhibitor U73122 and RhoA/ROCK inhibitor Y-27632. Simultaneous injection of U73122 (10 mg/kg, 0.2 ml) and O-1602 significantly decreased the duration and frequency in the open arms of the EPM as compared to O-1602 treatment alone (Fig. 5a). In the OFT, the time spent in the central area and the total distance traveled also significantly decreased (Fig. 5b). Meanwhile, simultaneous injection of Y-27632 (30 mg/kg, 0.15 ml) and O-1602 slightly

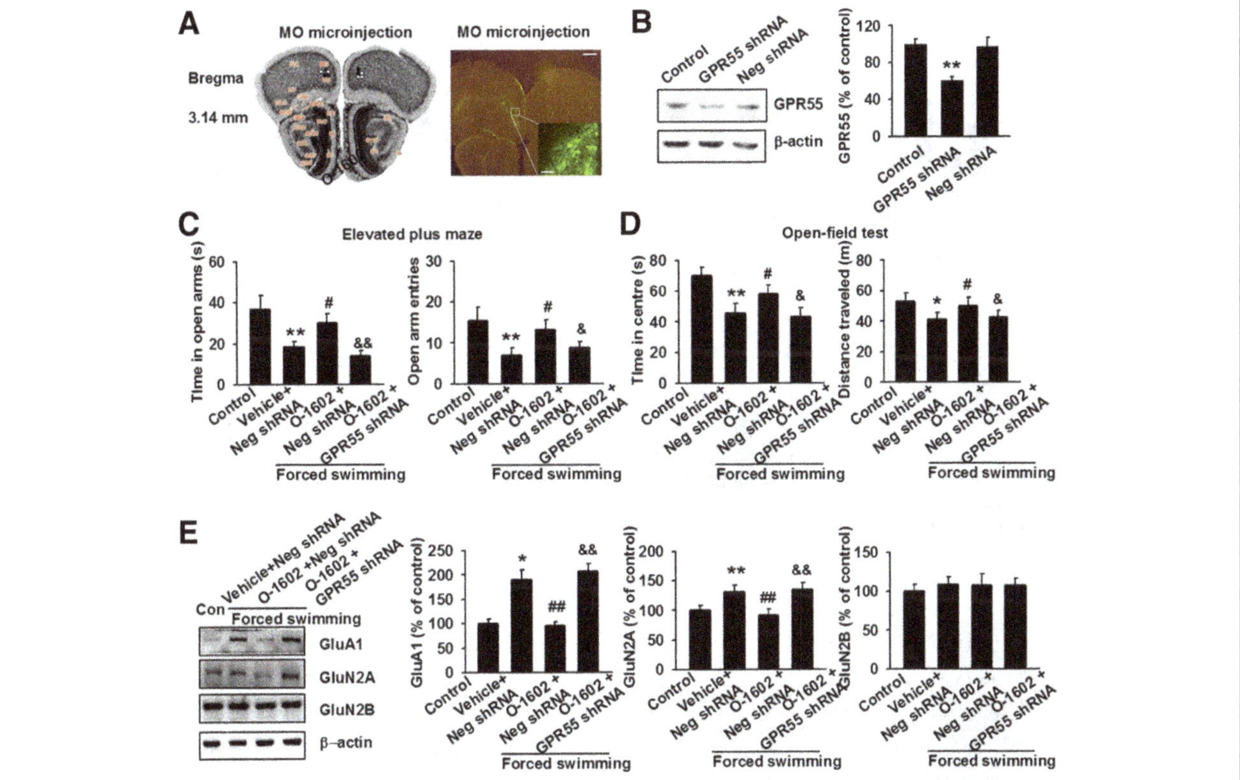

Fig. 4 GPR55 knockdown abolished O-1602-mediated anxiolytic effects. **a** Immunohistochemistry image showing the GPR55 shRNA infected cells (GFP positive) in the MO cortex (Scale bar, 500 um; insert: scale bar, 100 um). **b** Western blot image showing the expression of GPR55 in GPR55 knockdown (GPR55 shRNA-injected group) in the MO cortex as compared to negative shRNA-injected group. $^{**}p < 0.01$ versus control group; **c** In the EPM, O-1602 with negtive shRNA increased the duration and frequency in the open arms. O-1602 with GPR55 shRNA abolished the increase on duration and frequency in the open arms. $^{**}p < 0.01$ versus control group; $^{\#}p < 0.05$ versus vehicle + negative shRNA group; $^{\&}p < 0.05$, $^{\&\&}p < 0.01$ versus O-1602 + negative shRNA group. **d** In the OFT, O-1602 with negtive shRNA increased the time in the center area and the total distance traveled. O-1602 with GPR55 shRNA reversed the effect on time in the center area and the total distance traveled. $^{*}p < 0.05$, $^{**}p < 0.01$ versus control group; $^{\#}p < 0.05$ versus vehicle + negative shRNA group; $^{\&}p < 0.05$versus O-1602 + negative shRNA group. **e** O-1602 with negtive shRNA decreased the expression of GluA1 and GluN2A, but GluN2B did not decrease. O-1602 with GPR55 shRNA abolished the decrease in GluA1 and GluN2A expression, although knockdown did not affect the expression of GluN2B. $^{*}p < 0.05$, $^{**}p < 0.01$ versus control group; $^{\#\#}p < 0.01$ versus vehicle group; $^{\&\&}p < 0.01$ versus O-1602 + negative shRNA group. Each group contains 6–8 mice. Data are from three independent experiments

decreased the duration and frequency in the open arms of the EPM, as well as the time spent in the central area and the total distance traveled in the OFT (Fig. 5a and b). Overall, although both Y-27632 and U73122 reversed the anxiolytic effects of O-1602, the reversal effect of U73122 is more effective than that of Y-27632. Immunoblot analysis showed that both Y-27632 and U73122 abolished O-1602-mediated decrease in GluA1 and GluN2A expression in the MO cortex, while the expression of GluN2B increased slightly but did not reach statistical significance (Fig. 5c). Next, we investigated the effects of Y-27632 and U73122 on AKT and ERK phosphorylation. Both inhibitors reduced p-ERK (Fig. 5e) but had no effect on total AKT and AKT phosphorylation at both Thr308 and Ser473 (Fig. 5d). These results show that both PLC-PKC and RhoA-ROCK pathways are involved in GPR55 activation, leading to ERK phosphorylation.

Discussion

The orphan G-protein coupled receptor, GPR55, is described as an atypical cannabinoid receptor that can be activated by lysophosphatidylinositols and certain synthetic or endogenous cannabinoid molecules [13]. Therefore, the GPR55 receptor plays an important role in the pharmacological actions of cannabinoids. However, the exact role of the GPR55 receptor in the central nervous system, especially in anxiety, warrants further investigation. In the present study, we focused on the role of GPR55 activation in modulating anxiolytic-like effects.

Previous studies have shown that GPR55 mRNA/protein is expressed in several brain areas such as the hippocampus, hypothalamus, frontal cortex, and cerebellum [25]. We found that GPR55 was expressed in the MO cortex, which is considered an important region that

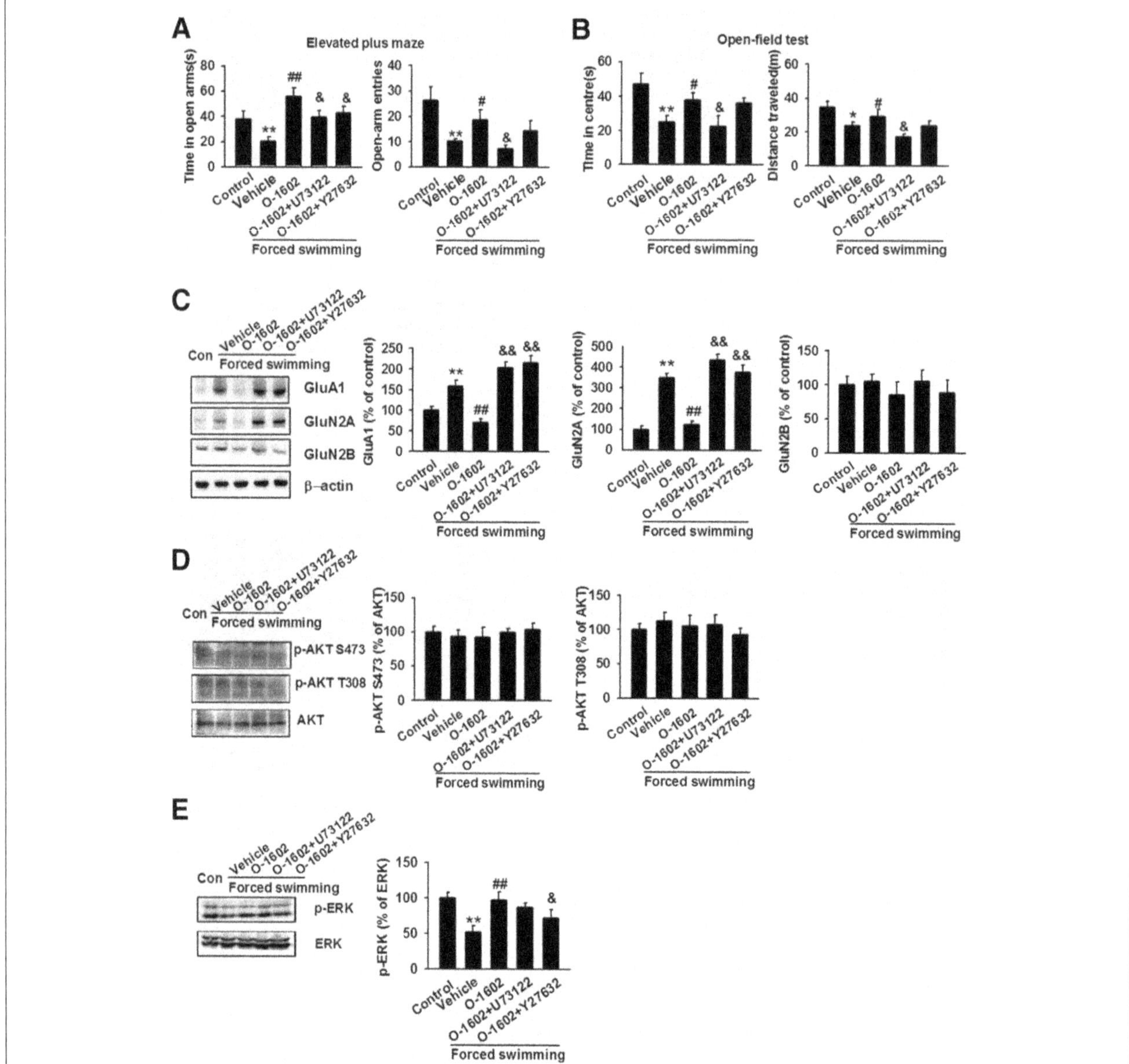

Fig. 5 Administration of Y-27632 and U73122 abolished the effect of O-1602. **a** In the EPM test, co-administration of Y-27632 or U73122 with O-1602 decreased the time spent and the number of entries in the open arms. $^{**}p < 0.01$ versus control group; $^{\#}p < 0.05$, $^{\#\#}p < 0.01$ versus vehicle group; $^{\&}p < 0.05$ versus O-1602-treated group. **b** In the OFT, co-administration of Y-27632 or U73122 with O-1602 decreased the time in the central area and the total distance traveled. $^{*}p < 0.05$, $^{**}p < 0.01$ versus control group; $^{\#}p < 0.05$ versus vehicle group; $^{\&}p < 0.05$ versus O-1602-treated group. **c** Administration of Y-27632 or U73122 reversed O-1602-induced expression of GluA1, GluN2A, and GluN2B. $^{*}p < 0.05$, $^{**}p < 0.01$ versus control group; $^{\#\#}p < 0.01$ versus vehicle group; $^{\&}p < 0.05$, $^{\&\&}p < 0.01$ versus O-1602 group. **d** Administration of Y-27632 or U73122 had no effect on the phosphorylation of AKT at S473 and T308. **e** Administration of Y-27632 and U73122 decreased O-1602-induced expression of p-ERK. $^{**}p < 0.01$ versus control group; $^{\#\#}p < 0.01$ versus vehicle group; $^{\&}p < 0.05$ versus O-1602 group. Each group contains 6–8 mice. Data are from three independent experiments

controls mood and cognitive functions [26]. MO cortex is strongly connected to the hippocampus and associated areas of the cingulate, retrosplenial, and entorhinal cortices, anterior thalamus, and septal diagonal band [27]. It has been suggested that the MO cortex is involved in the process of decision-making. Activity in the MO cortex was also detected when suppressing negative emotions, especially in approach-avoidance situations [28]. Chronic stress is a risk factor for the development of mood disorders [29], and can also disrupt the MEK/ERK signaling in the MO cortex [30]. In this study, we used a 21-day restraining protocol to induce chronic stress. With this protocol, we observed a significant decrease in the protein expression of GPR55 in the MO cortex, although GPR55 mRNA level remained unchanged. To our knowledge, this is the first study reporting the role of GPR55 in the development of anxiety/depression.

In a previous study in which the GPR55 agonist O-1602 was used, it was shown that activation of GPR55 relieved anxiety-like behaviors in normal rats [21]. However, it is unknown whether similar anxiolytic effects can be observed in stress-induced mice and the role GPR55 plays under these pathological conditions. Therefore, we used two kinds of acute stress models, restraint and forced swimming, to induce anxiety-like behaviors, which were measured via EPM and OFT. Restraint has been widely characterized as an acute stressor as it is a simple experimental procedure with high reproducibility [31, 32], while forced swimming was adopted as a stressor because its neurochemical and hormonal aspects satisfy the stress criteria in this study [33, 34]. In our study, both restraint and forced swimming decreased the time spent in the open arms and central area, and increased GluA1 expression in the MO cortex of mice. These changes were reversed by the GPR55 agonist O-1602, and the GPR55 antagonist CID16020046 were able to abolish O-1602-mediated anxiolytic effect. Our results are consistent with the known anxiolytic effects of O-1602 mediated through GPR55 activation, as determined previously by behavioral tests [21].

We also investigated the involvement of glutamate receptors during stress-induced anxiety. A large number of clinical and preclinical studies have demonstrated the important role of glutamate in the pathophysiology of anxiety disorders [35–38]. Likewise, findings from animal studies have established a strong association between anxiety and glutamate receptors [39–41]. Ionotropic glutamate receptors include the α-amino-3-hydroxy-5-methyl-4-isoxazolepropionic acid (AMPA) and *N*-Methyl-D-aspartic acid (NMDA) receptors, such as GluA1, GluA2, GluN2A, and GluN2B, which play crucial roles in regulating synaptic neurotransmission and plasticity [42]. Our study indicated that acute stress results in increased baseline expression of GluA1 and GluN2A in the MO cortex, with no alterations in GluN2B expression. A related study also showed negative correlation between the time spent in the open arms of the EPM and the protein levels of glutamate receptors [43]. In addition, several studies have shown that the AMPA and NMDA receptor antagonists are effective anxiolytics over a wide range of animal models of anxiety [44–46]. These results may indirectly support our findings that anxiety-like behavior is related to reduced GluA1 and GluN2A levels in the MO cortex. In addition, we demonstrated that stress-induced suppression of glutamate receptor expression could be reversed by O-1602 treatment. To date, there are no reports implicating the role of glutamate receptors in GPR55 activity, and a previous study only demonstrated that GPR55 co-localized with the synaptic vesicle protein vesicular glutamate transporter 1 in the stratum radiatum [14]. Thus, we are the first group to establish the relationship between glutamate receptors and GPR55-mediated anxiolytic effects.

In accordance with the diverse and complex pharmacology of GPR55, the current literature regarding the downstream signaling of the receptor is equally disparate. There is growing evidence that GPR55 couples to $G\alpha_{13}$, $G\alpha_{12}$, or $G\alpha_q$ in the GTPγS assay [13, 15, 16], but not to $G\alpha_{i/o}$ protein, which is coupled to CB_1R and CB_2R [47, 48]. We hypothesized that GPR55 activation triggers the activation two separate downstream signaling cascades, namely the $G\alpha_{12/13}$-RhoA-ROCK and $G\alpha_q$-PLC-PKC pathways, both of which have been shown to play important physiological roles in other G protein-coupled receptors [49, 50]. Our results indicated that some anxiolytic effects induced by O-1602 in the acute stress model can be attenuated by Y-27632, a specific inhibitor of ROCK, and U73122, an inhibitor of PLC. Thus, activation of GPR55 links the RhoA-ROCK and PLC-PKC pathways to the development of mood disorders, evident by alteration of the expression of glutamate receptors.

Although involvement of the mitogen-activated protein kinase (MAPK) signaling, elevation of calcium levels, and expression of transcription factors initiated by GPR55 activation have been reported in various papers, the converging pathway is the activation of MAPK, which results in the phosphorylation of ERK [51]. ERK plays a crucial role in regulating mood-related phenotypes and participates in the antidepressant response in various brain regions [52–54]. Mice exposed to CRS exhibited depressive-like behavior along with reduced MAPK/ERK signaling in the MO cortex and dorsal endopiriform nuclei of the prefrontal cortex [30]. Although altered ERK signaling in the cortex of mice with anxiety/depression has been documented, it is unclear whether GPR55 plays any modulatory role. In the current study, phosphorylation of ERK markedly decreased in the MO cortex of acute stress-induced mouse brains, and this reduction was blocked in O-1602-treated mice, which corresponded with the lack of anxiety-like behavioral responses. In contrast, phosphorylation of AKT was not altered. All of these observations suggest that GPR55 activation induces ERK signaling which mediates O-1602-induced anxiolytic effects. However, we cannot rule out the possible involvement of other signaling pathways, such as p38, NFAT, and Rac [15, 17, 18].

Interestingly, GPR55 knockout mice were reported to have similar anxiety-like behaviors as wild-type mice [55]. This inconsistent result may be due to the compensatory increase in homologous superfamily after genetic deletion. Nevertheless, results obtained for the O-1602-treated mice we used are consistent with its known activity on GPR55 [21, 56]. However, recent studies have suggested targets other than GPR55 for O-1602. For example, it was reported that O-1602 also has affinity for GPR18 receptors [56]. Although other studies have attempted to determine the specificity of O-1602 for GPR55 by using the GPR55 antagonist ML193 [21, 57], the question regarding its specificity still remains. Because ML193 may also antagonize CB_1R or GPR35 at higher doses [58], we used lentiviral shRNA to selectively knockdown GPR55 in the MO cortex by stereotactic microinjection. We found that GPR55 knockdown abolished the anxiolytic effect of O-1602. Therefore, our work confirms the specific role of GPR55 in the modulation of anxiety.

Taken together, the present findings show that O-1602 ameliorated anxiety-like symptoms and reversed stress-induced suppression of glutamate receptor expression through GPR55 activation. These data support the notion that GPR55 is a neurobiological target in anxiety- and stress-related disorders. Future studies may reveal whether GPR55 shows anxiolytic effect in other models of stress-induced anxiety, such as predator scent stress or chronic unpredictable stress.

Methods

Animals

Adult male C57BL mice (6–8 weeks of age) were used in all experiments, and were obtained from the Laboratory Animal Center of the Fourth Military Medical University (FMMU). The animals were housed in plastic boxes in groups of six with food and water available ad libitum in a colony room with controlled temperature (24 ± 2 °C), humidity (50–60%), and a light cycle from 8:00 A.M. to 8:00 P.M. under laminar airflow. The mice were given commercial chow diets and allowed to adapt to laboratory conditions for at least 1 week before the start of experiments. All animal protocols were approved by the Fourth Military Medical University Animal Care and Use Committee.

Drug

All drugs used in this study were purchased from Tocris Bioscience (Missouri, USA). The GPR55 agonist O-1602 and the selective GPR55 antagonist CID16020046 were dissolved in 10% dimethyl sulfoxide (DMSO) at a concentration of 1 mg/ml. Y-27632 was dissolved in distilled water at a concentration of 4 mg/ml. U73122 was dissolved in a mixture of Tween-20: DMSO: normal saline (1: 49: 50 ratio) at a concentration of 1 mg/ml. All drugs were stored at −20 °C. The drugs were given immediately after acute stress in mice. We intraperitoneally injected the O-1602, CID16020046 and Y-27632 into mice. The U73122 was given by intragastric administration.

Immunohistochemistry

Mice were anesthetized with pentobarbital sodium and perfused with sterile saline, followed by 4% paraformaldehyde. The brain was post-fixed in 4% paraformaldehyde for 6 h at 4 °C, and then transferred to 20% sucrose for 48 h. A coronal section including the medial orbital (MO) cortex was cut using a microtome-cryostat (Leica, Heidelberg, Germany) and processed for immunostaining. After blocking with normal goat serum containing 0.1% Triton X-100 for 30 min, sections were incubated overnight with rabbit anti-GPR55 (1:200; Abcam, Cambridge, MA; ab203663) primary antibody at 4 °C. Subsequently, the sections were rinsed with PBS three times and then incubated with Cy3-conjugated anti-rabbit secondary antibody (1:200; Boster Bio-Technology, Wuhan, China). Sections were visualized using a FV1000 confocal laser microscope (Olympus, Tokyo, Japan).

Chronic restraint stress (CRS)

Mice were restrained with restrainers constructed of clear plastic tubes (height: 5 cm, width: 5.5 cm, length: 22 cm) without physical compression or pain, 4 h daily for 21 consecutive days [59]. Mice were deprived of food and water during restraint.

Acute stress

Restraint *(Model 1)* and forced swimming *(Model 2)* are two types of stressors used extensively to induce anxiety [60, 61]. In the acute stress model, mice were subjected to either restraint or forced swimming. After acute stress, the mice were placed in plastic boxes with food and water available ad libitum without restraint. Mice were housed in the same experimental room during the stress period. After 24 h, the mice were subjected to two behavioral tests: open field test (OFT) and elevated plus maze (EPM).

Restraint (model 1)

In the restraint model, mice were restrained with restrainers constructed of clear plastic tubes (height: 5 cm, width: 5.5 cm, length: 22 cm) without physical compression or pain, 4 h daily for 2 consecutive days.

Forced swimming (model 2)

In the forced swimming experiment, mice were individually placed in an open cylindrical container (diameter: 10 cm, height: 25 cm) containing 20 cm of water at 20 ± 1 °C for 15 min. This depth forced the mice to swim without allowing their tails to touch the bottom of the container. Mice were forced to swim 15 min daily for 2 consecutive days. At the end of each session, the mice were removed from the water, and immediately and gently wiped dry.

Elevated plus maze (EPM)

The apparatus was made of grey plastic and consisted of two opposing open arms (25 × 8 × 0.5 cm) and two closed arms (25 × 8 × 12 cm) that extended from a common central platform (8 × 8 cm). The apparatus was elevated to a height of 50 cm above the floor. Mice were allowed to habituate in the testing room for 2 days before the test, and were pretreated with gentle handling twice per day to minimize nervousness. Mice were adapted to apparatus for the 3 min before the experiment. For each test, individual animals were placed in the center square, facing an open arm, and allowed to move freely for 5 min. Mice were videotaped using a camera fixed above the maze and analyzed using a video tracking system. Open and closed arm entries (all four paws in an arm) were scored by an experienced observer. The number of entries and time spent in each arm were recorded. After each test, the EPM was carefully cleaned with 75% ethanol and allowed to dry.

Open-field test (OFT)

The open field consisted of a square arena (30 × 30 × 30 cm^3) with clear Plexiglas walls and floor placed inside an isolation chamber with dim illumination and a fan. Mice were placed in the center of the box and allowed to adjust to the environment for 10 min. Mice were videotaped using a camera fixed above the floor and analyzed with a video tracking system. The "center" field is defined as the central area (15 × 15 cm^2) of the open field, one-fourth of the total area. Each subject was placed in the center of the open field, and its activity was measured for 5 min.

Western blot analysis

After behavioral testing, all mice were anesthetized with an overdose of pentobarbital sodium, and then decapitated. The MO cortex tissue was chopped into small pieces and homogenized in ice-cold RIPA lysis buffer containing 1× protease inhibitor cocktail. Equal amounts of protein were resolved using 9% sodium dodecyl sulfate-polyacrylamide electrophoresis (SDS-PAGE) gel and transferred to a nitrocellulose membrane. The membrane was then incubated with primary antibodies overnight at 4 °C. The following antibodies were used: anti-GPR55 (1:200; Abcam, ab203663), anti-GluA1 (1:1000; Abcam, ab31232), anti-GluN2A (1:1000; Abcam, ab133265), anti-GluN2B (1:400; Millipore, Billerica, MA; MAB5780), anti-β-actin (1:10,000; Sigma, St Louis, MO; A5316), anti-ERK (1:1000; ZSGB-BIO, Beijing, China; L2115), anti-p-ERK (1:1000; ZSGB-BIO, J2114), anti-AKT (1:1000; Cell Signaling, Danvers, MA; 4691), anti-p-AKT (Thr308) (1:1000; Cell Signaling, 13,038), and anti-p-AKT (Ser473) (1:1000; Cell Signaling, 9271). The membranes were incubated with horseradish peroxidase-conjugated secondary antibodies (anti-rabbit/anti-mouse IgG for the primary antibodies), and bands were visualized using enhanced chemiluminescence (ECL, GE Healthcare Pharmacia). Densitometric analysis of Western blots was conducted using a ChemiDoc XRS (Bio-Rad, Hercules, CA, USA) and quantified using Quantity One version 4.1.0 (Bio-Rad). Band intensity of target proteins was expressed as percentage relative to the control.

RNA preparation and RT-qPCR

Total RNA was extracted from cultured neurons and prefrontal cortex using the RNeasy mini kit (Qiagen, Valencia, CA). Reverse transcription-polymerase chain reaction (RT-PCR) was performed on 1 μg of RNA using the PrimeScript RT reagent kit with gDNA Eraser (TaKaRa Biotechnology, Dalian, China) to generate cDNA. Following synthesis, the cDNA and primers were mixed with 2× SYBR Premix Ex TaqII (TaKaRa Biotechnology, Dalian, China), and quantitative real-time PCR was performed using the ABI PRISM 7500 Sequence Detection System (Applied Biosystems, Warrington, UK). The following primer sequences were used: 5′-AGGCTATCTTCAC CAAGCAGCAC-3′ (forward) and 5′-TGGTTCAGCTG TCTGCCATTTC-3′ (reverse) for *gpr55*, and 5′-TGTG TCCGTCGTGGATCTGA-3′ (forward) and 5′- TTGCT GTTGAAGTCGCAGGAG-3′ (reverse) for *gapdh*, which served as the internal control. The relative amounts of mRNA were calculated using the comparative threshold cycle method. The thermal cycling conditions were as follows: 95 °C for 30 s, followed by 40 cycles of 95 °C for 5 s, and 60 °C for 34 s.

Intracerebral shRNA lentivirus infusion

Mice were anesthetized using intraperitoneal injection of pentobarbital sodium (30 mg/kg). The GPR55 shRNA lentivirus (10^9 TU/ml) was stereotaxically microinjected into the MO (3.14 mm anterior to bregma, ± 0.1 mm lateral to midline, and 2.5 mm ventral to bregma) at a rate of 0.2 μl/min for 5 min, resulting in a dose of 1 μl of lentivirus. GPR55 lentiviral vectors with a green fluorescent protein (GFP) tag were constructed by Genepharma (Shanghai, China). To generate the GPR55 shRNA, a target sequence was designed against mouse GPR55: 5′-AGATCTTTGGCTTC CTCCTTCCCAT-3′. After microinjection, the hole was sealed with bone wax, and the wound was sutured. The mice were used for subsequent experiments 1 week after surgery.

Statistical analysis

The data were expressed as mean ± standard error of the mean (SEM). Statistical comparisons were performed via analysis of variance (ANOVA). If the ANOVA was significant, post hoc comparisons were conducted using Tukey's test. In all cases, $p < 0.05$ was considered statistically significant.

Abbreviations
AMPA: α-amino-3-hydroxy-5-methyl-4-isoxazolepropionic acid; ANOVA: Analysis of variance; CB: Cannabinoid; CRS: Chronic restraint stress; DMSO: Dimethyl sulfoxide; ECL: Enhanced chemiluminescence; EPM: Elevated plus maze; ERK: Extracellular-regulated protein kinase; GFP: Green fluorescent protein; GPR55: G protein-coupled receptor 55; MAPK: Mitogen-activated protein kinase1; MO: Medial orbital; NMDA: N-Methyl-D-aspartic acid; OFT: Open field test; PLC: Phospholipase C; RhoA: Ras homolog gene family member A; ROCK: Rho-associated protein kinase; RT-PCR: Reverse transcription-polymerase chain reaction; SDS-PAGE: Sodium dodecyl sulfate-polyacrylamide electrophoresis; SEM: Standard error of the mean

Acknowledgements
We thank Sheng-Xi Wu for suggestions and helpful discussion.

Funding
This work was supported by the Military Medical Science and Technology Youth Training Project of China Grant Number 14QNP095 (to Q.Y.), and National Postdoctoral Program for Innovative Talents Grant Number BX20160025 (to Q.Y.).

Authors' contributions
QY conceived and designed the study. MG-Z assisted in designing the study. QX-S, LK-Y, and WL-S performed the experiments. LW, SM-Z, and SY-G analyzed the data. QX-S and QY wrote the manuscrpt, and MG-Z proofread it. All authors read and approved the final manuscript.

Competing interest
The authors declare that they have no competing interest.

Author details
[1]Department of Pharmacology, School of Pharmacy, Fourth Military Medical University, Xi'an, China. [2]Department of Pharmacy, The 155th Central Hospital of PLA, Kaifeng, China. [3]Department of Neurobiology and Collaborative Innovation Center for Brain Science, Fourth Military Medical University, Xi'an, China.

Reference
1. Kisely S, Alichniewicz KK, Black EB, Siskind D, Spurling G, Toombs M. The prevalence of depression and anxiety disorders in indigenous people of the Americas: a systematic review and meta-analysis. J Psychiatr Res. 2017;84:137–52.
2. Bhagya V, Srikumar BN, Veena J, Shankaranarayana Rao BS. Short-term exposure to enriched environment rescues chronic stress-induced impaired hippocampal synaptic plasticity, anxiety, and memory deficits. J Neurosci Res. 2016.
3. Breslau N, Chilcoat HD, Kessler RC, Davis GC. Previous exposure to trauma and PTSD effects of subsequent trauma: results from the Detroit area survey of trauma. Am J Psychiatry. 1999;156(6):902–7.
4. Briere J, Agee E, Dietrich A. Cumulative trauma and current posttraumatic stress disorder status in general population and inmate samples. Psychol Trauma. 2016;8(4):439–46.
5. Kendler KS, Karkowski LM, Prescott CA. Causal relationship between stressful life events and the onset of major depression. Am J Psychiatry. 1999;156(6):837–41.
6. Risch N, Herrell R, Lehner T, Liang KY, Eaves L, Hoh J, Griem A, Kovacs M, Ott J, Merikangas KR. Interaction between the serotonin transporter gene (5-HTTLPR), stressful life events, and risk of depression: a meta-analysis. JAMA. 2009;301(23):2462–71.
7. Marco EM, Laviola G. The endocannabinoid system in the regulation of emotions throughout lifespan: a discussion on therapeutic perspectives. J Psychopharmacol. 2012;26(1):150–63.
8. Marco EM, Garcia-Gutierrez MS, Bermudez-Silva FJ, Moreira FA, Guimaraes F, Manzanares J, Viveros MP. Endocannabinoid system and psychiatry: in search of a neurobiological basis for detrimental and potential therapeutic effects. Front Behav Neurosci. 2011;5:63.
9. Di Marzo V, Petrosino S. Endocannabinoids and the regulation of their levels in health and disease. Curr Opin Lipidol. 2007;18(2):129–40.
10. Sawzdargo M, Nguyen T, Lee DK, Lynch KR, Cheng R, Heng HH, George SR, O'Dowd BF. Identification and cloning of three novel human G protein-coupled receptor genes GPR52, PsiGPR53 and GPR55: GPR55 is extensively expressed in human brain. Brain Res Mol Brain Res. 1999;64(2):193–8.
11. Begg M, Pacher P, Batkai S, Osei-Hyiaman D, Offertaler L, Mo FM, Liu J, Kunos G. Evidence for novel cannabinoid receptors. Pharmacol Ther. 2005;106(2):133–45.
12. Pertwee RG. GPR55: a new member of the cannabinoid receptor clan? Br J Pharmacol. 2007;152(7):984–6.
13. Ryberg E, Larsson N, Sjogren S, Hjorth S, Hermansson NO, Leonova J, Elebring T, Nilsson K, Drmota T, Greasley PJ. The orphan receptor GPR55 is a novel cannabinoid receptor. Br J Pharmacol. 2007;152(7):1092–101.
14. Sylantyev S, Jensen TP, Ross RA, Rusakov DA. Cannabinoid- and lysophosphatidylinositol-sensitive receptor GPR55 boosts neurotransmitter release at central synapses. Proc Natl Acad Sci U S A. 2013;110(13):5193–8.
15. Henstridge CM, Balenga NA, Ford LA, Ross RA, Waldhoer M, Irving AJ. The GPR55 ligand L-alpha-lysophosphatidylinositol promotes RhoA-dependent Ca2+ signaling and NFAT activation. FASEB J. 2009;23(1):183–93.
16. Lauckner JE, Jensen JB, Chen HY, Lu HC, Hille B, Mackie K. GPR55 is a cannabinoid receptor that increases intracellular calcium and inhibits M current. Proc Natl Acad Sci U S A. 2008;105(7):2699–704.
17. Henstridge CM, Balenga NA, Schroder R, Kargl JK, Platzer W, Martini L, Arthur S, Penman J, Whistler JL, Kostenis E, et al. GPR55 ligands promote receptor coupling to multiple signalling pathways. Br J Pharmacol. 2010;160(3):604–14.
18. Oka S, Kimura S, Toshida T, Ota R, Yamashita A, Sugiura T. Lysophosphatidylinositol induces rapid phosphorylation of p38 mitogen-activated protein kinase and activating transcription factor 2 in HEK293 cells expressing GPR55 and IM-9 lymphoblastoid cells. J Biochem. 2010;147(5):671–8.
19. Cherif H, Argaw A, Cecyre B, Bouchard A, Gagnon J, Javadi P, Desgent S, Mackie K, Bouchard JF. Role of GPR55 during axon growth and target Innervation. eNeuro. 2015;2(5):0011–15.
20. Staton PC, Hatcher JP, Walker DJ, Morrison AD, Shapland EM, Hughes JP, Chong E, Mander PK, Green PJ, Billinton A, et al. The putative cannabinoid receptor GPR55 plays a role in mechanical hyperalgesia associated with inflammatory and neuropathic pain. Pain. 2008;139(1):225–36.
21. Rahimi A, Hajizadeh Moghaddam A, Roohbakhsh A. Central administration of GPR55 receptor agonist and antagonist modulates anxiety-related behaviors in rats. Fundam Clin Pharmacol. 2015;29(2):185–90.
22. Hu W, Zhang M, Czeh B, Zhang W, Flugge G. Chronic restraint stress impairs endocannabinoid mediated suppression of GABAergic signaling in the hippocampus of adult male rats. Brain Res Bull. 2011;85(6):374–9.
23. O'Shea M, Singh ME, McGregor IS, Mallet PE. Chronic cannabinoid exposure produces lasting memory impairment and increased anxiety in adolescent but not adult rats. J Psychopharmacol. 2004;18(4):502–8.
24. Kupferschmidt DA, Newman AE, Boonstra R, Erb S. Antagonism of cannabinoid 1 receptors reverses the anxiety-like behavior induced by central injections of corticotropin-releasing factor and cocaine withdrawal. Neuroscience. 2012;204:125–33.
25. Marichal-Cancino BA, Fajardo-Valdez A, Ruiz-Contreras AE, Mendez-Diaz M, Prospero-Garcia O. Advances in the physiology of GPR55 in the central nervous system. Curr Neuropharmacol. 2016;
26. Kringelbach ML. The human orbitofrontal cortex: linking reward to hedonic experience. Nat Rev Neurosci. 2005;6(9):691–702.
27. Elliott R, Dolan RJ, Frith CD. Dissociable functions in the medial and lateral orbitofrontal cortex: evidence from human neuroimaging studies. Cereb Cortex. 2000;10(3):308–17.

28. Meshi D, Biele G, Korn CW, Heekeren HR. How expert advice influences decision making. PLoS One. 2012;7(11):e49748.
29. Ader R, Cohen N. Psychoneuroimmunology: conditioning and stress. Annu Rev Psychol. 1993;44:53–85.
30. Leem YH, Yoon SS, Kim YH, Jo SA. Disrupted MEK/ERK signaling in the medial orbital cortex and dorsal endopiriform nuclei of the prefrontal cortex in a chronic restraint stress mouse model of depression. Neurosci Lett. 2014;580:163–8.
31. Malisch JL, deWolski K, Meek TH, Acosta W, Middleton KM, Crino OL, Garland T Jr. Acute restraint stress alters wheel-running behavior immediately following stress and up to 20 hours later in house mice. Physiol Biochem Zool. 2016;89(6):546–52.
32. Thakare VN, Dhakane VD, Patel BM. Attenuation of acute restraint stress-induced depressive like behavior and hippocampal alterations with protocatechuic acid treatment in mice. Metab Brain Dis. 2016;
33. Jodar L, Takahashi M, Kaneto H. Effects of footshock-, psychological- and forced swimming-stress on the learning and memory processes: involvement of opioidergic pathways. Jpn J Pharmacol. 1995;67(2):143–7.
34. Schneider AM, Simson PE. NAN-190 potentiates the impairment of retention produced by swim stress. Pharmacol Biochem Behav. 2007;87(1):73–80.
35. Barbosa Neto JB, Tiba PA, Faturi CB, de Castro-Neto EF, da Graca N-MM, de Jesus MJ, de Mello MF, Suchecki D. Stress during development alters anxiety-like behavior and hippocampal neurotransmission in male and female rats. Neuropharmacology. 2012;62(1):518–26.
36. Herlenius E, Lagercrantz H. Development of neurotransmitter systems during critical periods. Exp Neurol. 2004;190(Suppl 1):S8–21.
37. McQuillen PS, Ferriero DM. Selective vulnerability in the developing central nervous system. Pediatr Neurol. 2004;30(4):227–35.
38. Van den Hove DL, Kenis G, Brass A, Opstelten R, Rutten BP, Bruschettini M, Blanco CE, Lesch KP, Steinbusch HW, Prickaerts J. Vulnerability versus resilience to prenatal stress in male and female rats; implications from gene expression profiles in the hippocampus and frontal cortex. Eur Neuropsychopharmacol. 2013;23(10):1226–46.
39. Amiel JM, Mathew SJ. Glutamate and anxiety disorders. Curr Psychiatry Rep. 2007;9(4):278–83.
40. Aroniadou-Anderjaska V, Pidoplichko VI, Figueiredo TH, Almeida-Suhett CP, Prager EM, Braga MF. Presynaptic facilitation of glutamate release in the basolateral amygdala: a mechanism for the anxiogenic and seizurogenic function of GluK1 receptors. Neuroscience. 2012;221:157–69.
41. Cortese BM, Phan KL. The role of glutamate in anxiety and related disorders. CNS Spectr. 2005;10(10):820–30.
42. Popoli M, Yan Z, McEwen BS, Sanacora G. The stressed synapse: the impact of stress and glucocorticoids on glutamate transmission. Nat Rev Neurosci. 2011;13(1):22–37.
43. Wang Y, Ma Y, Cheng W, Jiang H, Zhang X, Li M, Ren J, Zhang X, Li X. Sexual differences in long-term effects of prenatal chronic mild stress on anxiety-like behavior and stress-induced regional glutamate receptor expression in rat offspring. Int J Dev Neurosci. 2015;41:80–91.
44. Shimizu K, Kurosawa N, Seki K. The role of the AMPA receptor and 5-HT(3) receptor on aggressive behavior and depressive-like symptoms in chronic social isolation-reared mice. Physiol Behav. 2016;153:70–83.
45. Inta D, Filipovic D, Lima-Ojeda JM, Dormann C, Pfeiffer N, Gasparini F, Gass P. The mGlu5 receptor antagonist MPEP activates specific stress-related brain regions and lacks neurotoxic effects of the NMDA receptor antagonist MK-801: significance for the use as anxiolytic/antidepressant drug. Neuropharmacology. 2012;62(5–6):2034–9.
46. Chojnacka-Wojcik E, Klodzinska A, Pilc A. Glutamate receptor ligands as anxiolytics. Curr Opin Investig Drugs. 2001;2(8):1112–9.
47. Howlett AC, Barth F, Bonner TI, Cabral G, Casellas P, Devane WA, Felder CC, Herkenham M, Mackie K, Martin BR, et al. International Union of Pharmacology. XXVII. Classification of cannabinoid receptors. Pharmacol Rev. 2002;54(2):161–202.
48. Pertwee R G Cannabinoid pharmacology: the first 66 years. Br J Pharmacol. 2006; v Suppl 1: S163-S171.
49. Luttrell DK, Luttrell LM. Signaling in time and space: G protein-coupled receptors and mitogen-activated protein kinases. Assay Drug Dev Technol. 2003;1(2):327–38.
50. Rozengurt E. Mitogenic signaling pathways induced by G protein-coupled receptors. J Cell Physiol. 2007;213(3):589–602.
51. Lefkowitz RJ, Shenoy SK. Transduction of receptor signals by beta-arrestins. Science. 2005;308(5721):512–7.
52. Novaes LS, Dos Santos NB, Batalhote RF, Malta MB, Camarini R, Scavone C, Munhoz CD. Environmental enrichment protects against stress-induced anxiety: role of glucocorticoid receptor, ERK, and CREB signaling in the basolateral amygdala. Neuropharmacology. 2017;113(Pt A):457–66.
53. Di Benedetto B, Kuhn R, Nothdurfter C, Rein T, Wurst W, Rupprecht R. N-desalkylquetiapine activates ERK1/2 to induce GDNF release in C6 glioma cells: a putative cellular mechanism for quetiapine as antidepressant. Neuropharmacology. 2012;62(1):209–16.
54. Einat H, Yuan P, Gould TD, Li J, Du J, Zhang L, Manji HK, Chen G. The role of the extracellular signal-regulated kinase signaling pathway in mood modulation. J Neurosci. 2003;23(19):7311–6.
55. Wu CS, Chen H, Sun H, Zhu J, Jew CP, Wager-Miller J, Straiker A, Spencer C, Bradshaw H, Mackie K, et al. GPR55, a G-protein coupled receptor for lysophosphatidylinositol, plays a role in motor coordination. PLoS One. 2013;8(4):e60314.
56. Ashton JC. The atypical cannabinoid O-1602: targets, actions, and the central nervous system. Cent Nerv Syst Agents Med Chem. 2012;12(3):233–9.
57. Console-Bram L, Brailoiu E, Brailoiu GC, Sharir H, Abood ME. Activation of GPR18 by cannabinoid compounds: a tale of biased agonism. Br J Pharmacol. 2014;171(16):3908–17.
58. Kotsikorou E, Sharir H, Shore DM, Hurst DP, Lynch DL, Madrigal KE, Heynen-Genel S, Milan LB, Chung TD, Seltzman HH, et al. Identification of the GPR55 antagonist binding site using a novel set of high-potency GPR55 selective ligands. Biochemistry. 2013;52(52):9456–69.
59. Chiba S, Numakawa T, Ninomiya M, Richards MC, Wakabayashi C, Kunugi H. Chronic restraint stress causes anxiety- and depression-like behaviors, downregulates glucocorticoid receptor expression, and attenuates glutamate release induced by brain-derived neurotrophic factor in the prefrontal cortex. Prog Neuro-Psychopharmacol Biol Psychiatry. 2012;39(1):112–9.
60. Smith JS, Schindler AG, Martinelli E, Gustin RM, Bruchas MR, Chavkin C. Stress-induced activation of the dynorphin/kappa-opioid receptor system in the amygdala potentiates nicotine conditioned place preference. J Neurosci. 2012;32(4):1488–95.
61. Patki G, Li L, Allam F, Solanki N, Dao AT, Alkadhi K, Salim S. Moderate treadmill exercise rescues anxiety and depression-like behavior as well as memory impairment in a rat model of posttraumatic stress disorder. Physiol Behav. 2014;130:47–53.

2

GABAergic deficits and schizophrenia-like behaviors in a mouse model carrying patient-derived neuroligin-2 R215H mutation

Dong-Yun Jiang[1], Zheng Wu[1], Cody Tieu Forsyth[1], Yi Hu[1], Siu-Pok Yee[2] and Gong Chen[1*]

Abstract

Schizophrenia (SCZ) is a severe mental disorder characterized by delusion, hallucination, and cognitive deficits. We have previously identified from schizophrenia patients a loss-of-function mutation $Arg^{215} \rightarrow His^{215}$ (R215H) of *neuroligin 2* (*NLGN2*) gene, which encodes a cell adhesion molecule critical for GABAergic synapse formation and function. Here, we generated a novel transgenic mouse line with neuroligin-2 (NL2) R215H mutation. The single point mutation caused a significant loss of NL2 protein in vivo, reduced GABAergic transmission, and impaired hippocampal activation. Importantly, R215H KI mice displayed anxiety-like behavior, impaired pre-pulse inhibition (PPI), cognition deficits and abnormal stress responses, recapitulating several key aspects of schizophrenia-like behaviors. Our results demonstrate a significant impact of a single point mutation NL2 R215H on brain functions, providing a novel animal model for the study of schizophrenia and neuropsychiatric disorders.

Keywords: Schizophrenia, GABA, Neuroligin-2, Mouse model, Mutation

Introduction

Schizophrenia (SCZ) is a chronic neuropsychiatric disorder caused by both genetic and environmental factors. It is featured by long-standing delusion and hallucination (psychosis), and cognitive deficits [17, 27, 39]. SCZ is a highly heritable disorder [55] with a complex genetic basis. Recent genomic studies identified a number of genetic variants associated with SCZ, including a group of variants resided in the genes encoding synaptic adhesion molecules that promoting synaptic development and function such as *IGSF9B*, and *NLGN4X* [52].

Neuroligins (NLGNs) are a family of synaptic adhesion molecules highly expressed in the brain and are ligands for another group of cell adhesion molecules neurexins (NRXNs) [26]. There are five neuroligin genes (neuroligin-1, – 2, – 3, – 4, and – 5) in humans and four in mice (neuroligin 1–4). Neuroligin-1, – 2, and – 3 are close homologs between human and mice. Neuroligin-1 and neuroligin-2 differentially locate to excitatory and inhibitory synapses and are critical for the excitatory and inhibitory synapse formation and function, respectively [9, 12, 35, 44, 51, 53, 59]. Neuroligin-3 locates at both type of synapses and contributes to both neurotransmission [7, 14, 57]. In recent years, genetic variants of neuroligin-1, neuroligin-3 and neuroligin-4 have been identified in autism patients [28, 43]. Mutations in proteins interacting with neuroligins such as Neurexin1, SHANK and MDGA have also been associated with autism and schizophrenia patients [6, 13, 31, 32]. Genetic mouse models based on these findings recapitulate several aspects of patient symptoms, providing an entry point for the mechanistic study and drug development on psychiatric disorders [2, 10, 14, 15, 29, 46, 50, 54, 57, 66].

We have previously reported several novel mutations of *NLGN2* from schizophrenia patients [56]. Among the NL2 mutants, we found that the R215H mutant protein was retained in the endoplasmic reticulum (ER) and could not be transported to the cell membrane, resulting in a failure to interact with presynaptic neurexin and a loss of function in GABAergic synapse assembly [56]. Based on these studies, we have now generated a transgenic mouse

* Correspondence: gongchen@psu.edu
[1]Department of Biology, Huck Institutes of Life Sciences, Pennsylvania State University, University Park, PA 16802, USA
Full list of author information is available at the end of the article

line carrying the same NL2 R215H mutation to test its functional consequence in vivo. We demonstrate that the R215H knock-in (KI) mice show severe GABAergic deficits and display not only anxiety-like behavior seen in global NL2 KO mice [1, 3, 61], but also impaired pre-pulse inhibition, cognitive deficits, and abnormal stress responses which are not reported in global NL2 KO mice. Our results suggest that a single-point mutation R215H of NL2 can result in significant GABAergic deficits and contribute to SCZ-like behaviors. This newly generated NL2 R215H KI mouse may provide a useful animal model for the studies of neuropsychiatric disorders including SCZ.

Results

Generation of neuroligin-2 R215H mutant mice

Following our original discovery of a loss-of-function mutation R215H of NL2 in SCZ patients [56], we generated the NL2 R215H mutant mice by introducing the same R215H mutation into the exon 4 of *Nlgn2* gene in the mouse genome via homologous recombination (Fig. 1a). NL2 R215H heterozygotes were mated to obtain wild type (WT), heterozygotes (referred here as Het mice), and homozygotes (referred here as KI mice) (Additional file 1: Figure S1a). Sequencing analysis confirmed the R215H mutation in the NL2 KI mice (Additional file 1: Figure S1b). Mice carrying R215H mutation were born at a normal Mendelian rate (Male mice: WT = 26.5%, Het = 52.9%, KI = 20.6%; Female mice: WT = 24.1%, Het = 52.8%, KI = 23.1%). Both R215H Het and KI mice were viable and fertile and did not exhibit premature mortality. During development, we observed a reduction of body weight in R215H KI mice comparing to R215H Het and WT mice in large litters (litter size > 6, Additional file 1: Figure S2a-b), but this phenomenon is not significant in small litters (litter size < 5, Additional file 1: Figure S2c). Body length and tail length is not significantly different between genotypes (Additional file 1: Figure S2d-g). The mouse colony was maintained on a hybrid genetic background to avoid the artificial phenotype contributed by other homozygous genetic variants in a homozygous inbred background.

Reduction of neuroligin-2 protein level in NL2 R215H KI mice

After obtaining the NL2 R215H Het and KI mice, we first analyzed the NL2 protein expression level in the brain. We found that as early as postnatal 2 days, NL2 already showed substantial expression in the WT mice (Fig. 1b, top row). In NL2 R215H Het mice, the NL2 protein level was about half of the WT mice; whereas in R215H KI mice, the NL2 level was very low comparing to the WT level, but with a clear band of lower molecular weight representing non-glycosylated immature NL2 R215H protein [56, 65]. Such immature band of NL2 R215H protein persisted at adult stage in the KI mice, and was observed in a variety of brain regions (Fig. 1b, and quantified in Fig. 1c). In contrast, NL2 KO mice showed a complete absence of NL2 without any immature band at all (Fig. 1b, top row). Such difference of NL2 protein level between our KI mice and previous KO mice may underlie their functional difference reported later. To test whether NL2 R215H mutation affects the expression of other NL family members, we examined the protein level of NL1 and NL3 in both NL2 R215H Het and KI mice but found no significant changes (Additional file 1: Figure S3).

To investigate the localization of NL2 R215H proteins inside the brain, we performed immunohistochemistry with NL2-specific antibodies and found a significant reduction of NL2 puncta in R215H Het mice and almost absence of NL2 puncta in homozygous R215H KI mice (Fig. 1d-f). In WT mouse brains, NL2 formed numerous postsynaptic puncta on cell soma and dendrites opposing presynaptic vGAT puncta (Fig. 1d-f, puncta density 15.0 ± 0.9 per 100 μm^2, puncta size = 0.27 ± 0.01 μm^2). The number and size of NL2 puncta were significantly reduced in the NL2 R215H Het mouse brains (Fig. 1d-f, puncta density, 9.4 ± 1.6 per 100 μm^2, $p < 0.01$, puncta size, 0.21± 0.02 μm^2, $p = 0.02$). Interestingly, in the homozygous NL2 R215H KI mouse brains, only faint NL2 signal was observed inside cell soma (Fig. 1d, right columns, Additional file 1: Figure S4) and not colocalized with vGAT, further suggesting that the NL2 R215H proteins could not be transported to the cell membrane [56]. To get a clear understanding of the physiological role of NL2 R215H mutation in vivo, we focused our studies on the homozygous NL2 R215H KI mice in this study.

Reduced GABAergic synapse density in NL2 R215H KI mice

NL2 has been reported to form complex with gephyrin and collybistin at postsynaptic sites to recruit $GABA_A$ receptors [47]. Consistent with a substantial reduction of NL2 puncta in the KI mice, we detected a remarkable decrease of postsynaptic $GABA_A$ receptor γ2 subunit and the scaffold protein gephyrin around cell soma in hippocampal regions (Fig. 2a). Quantitative analysis revealed that both the puncta number and size of postsynaptic γ2 subunit and gephyrin decreased significantly in homozygous R215H KI mice (Fig. 2b-e), consistent with previous findings in NL2 KO mice [1, 19, 30, 47]. In addition to postsynaptic changes, we also examined presynaptic marker vGAT (vesicular GABA transporter) and parvalbumin (PV) positive GABAergic neurons that are reported to be associated with SCZ patients [37]. Immunohistochemistry analysis revealed that the number of PV neurons was not changed in the hippocampal

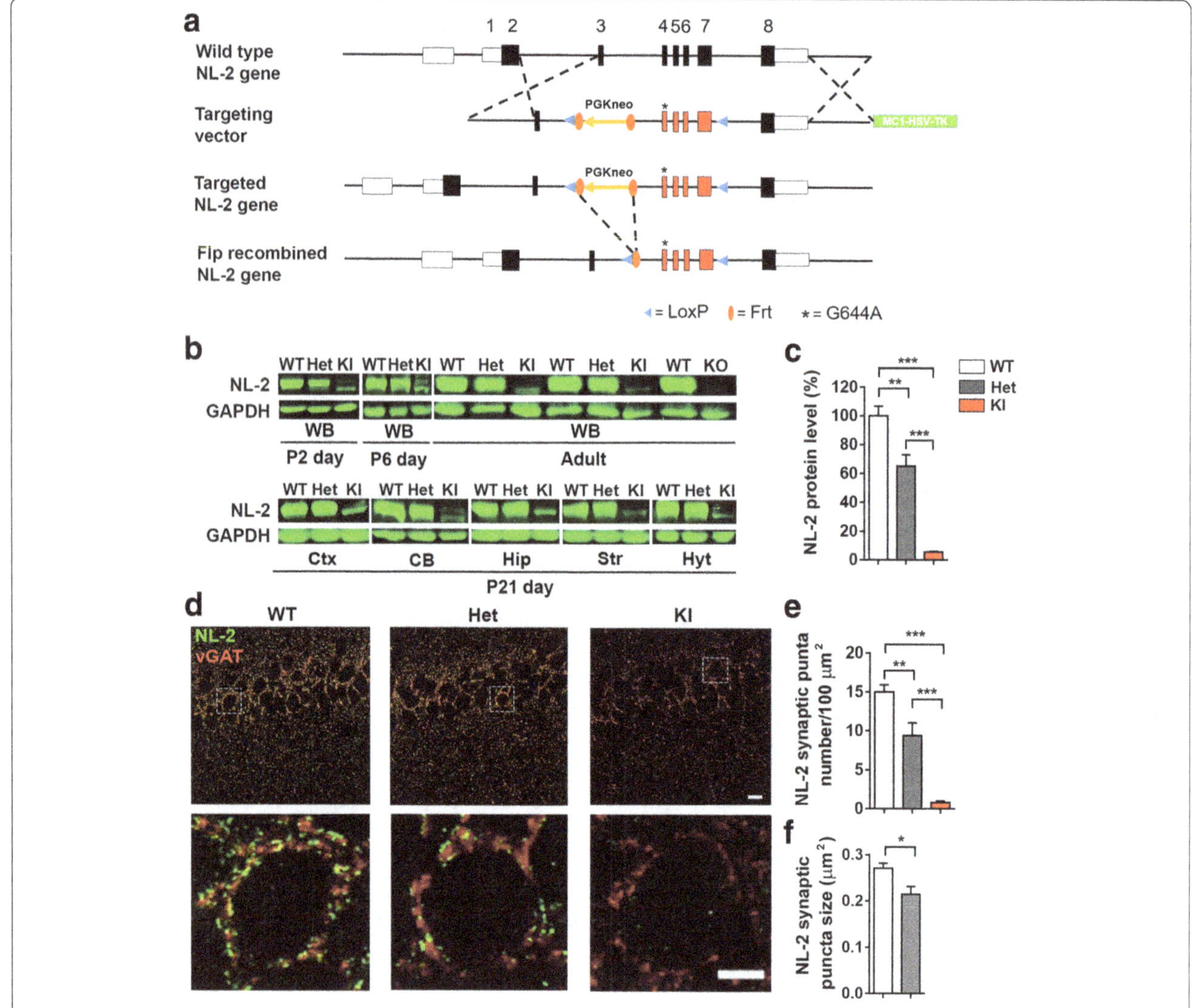

Fig. 1 Generation and characterization of NL2 R215H mice. **a** A simplified diagram of NL2 R215H homologous recombination strategy. **b** Representative Western blot of NL2 protein expression at postnatal 2 days, 6 days, 21 days, and adult stage of WT, NL2 R215H Het, and NL2 R215H KI mice. GAPDH was used as internal control. **c** Quantification of NL2 protein expression level in littermates. WT, $n = 6$ mice, Het, $n = 5$ mice, and KI, $n = 6$ mice. One-way ANOVA with post-hoc Tukey multi-comparison test was used for statistical analysis. **d** Representative images of NL2 postsynaptic puncta in WT, NL2 R215H Het and NL2 R215H KI mice. Images were taken at hippocampal CA1 region. Upper row scale bar = 10 μm. Bottom row scale bar = 5 μm. **e**, **f** Quantification of NL2 puncta number and size. Nine brain slices from 3 mice for each genotype were used for analysis. One-way ANOVA with post-hoc Tukey multi-comparison test was used for statistical analysis in (**e**). Student's *t*-test was used for statistical analysis in (**f**). Data were shown as Mean ± SEM, $*P < 0.05$, $**P < 0.01$, $***P < 0.001$

area of the KI mice (Fig. 3a-d). However, both PV and vGAT puncta number and size were significantly reduced in the dentate granule cells (Fig. 3e-i), as well as in the CA1/CA3 pyramidal cells in the KI mice (Additional file 1: Figure S5a-j). Consistently, we observed a reduction of PV and vGAT protein level in the hippocampal tissue of KI mice (Additional file 1: Figure S6a-b). In contrast, the excitatory presynaptic marker vGluT1 was not altered in R215H KI mice (Additional file 1: Figure S6c-e). These results suggest that NL2 R215H mutation impaired both pre- and post-synaptic GABAergic components.

Impaired GABAergic neurotransmission in NL2 R215H KI mice

We next investigated the function of inhibitory neurotransmission in the R215H KI mice. Whole-cell patch-clamp recordings were performed on dentate granule cells in acute brain slices of adult WT and homozygous R215H KI mice. We found that both the frequency and amplitude of miniature inhibitory postsynaptic currents (mIPSCs) were significantly decreased in the granule cells of R215H KI mice (Fig. 4a-d; Frequency: WT = 8.28 ± 2.21 Hz, KI = 3.98 ± 0.78 Hz, $p = 0.041$; Median amplitude: WT = 41.3 ± 2.9 pA, KI = 32.7 ± 1.8 pA, $p = 0.019$; Student's *t*-test). In contrast,

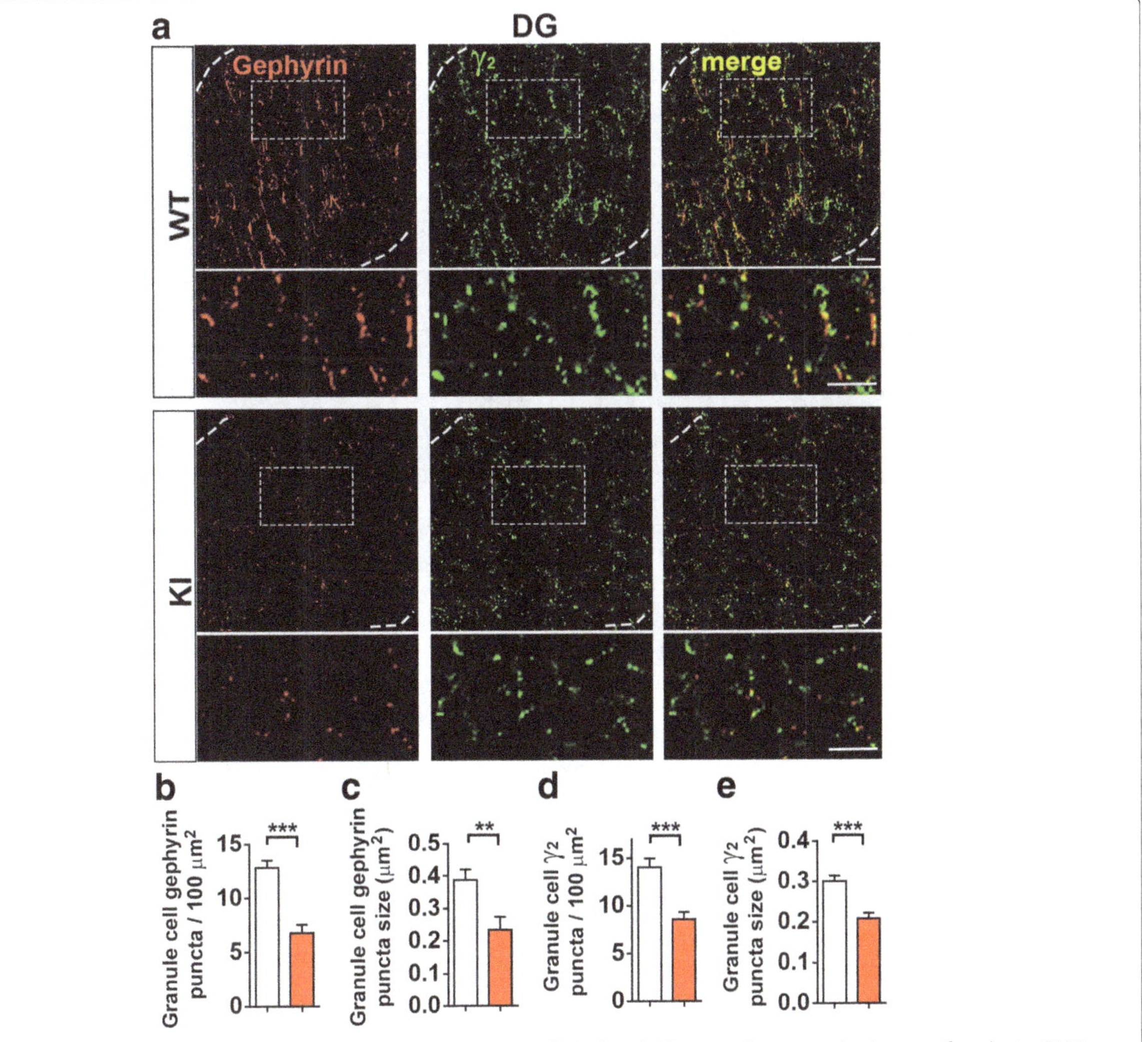

Fig. 2 Reduced GABAergic postsynaptic components in the hippocampus of NL2 R215H KI mice. **a** Representative images of gephyrin, $GABA_A$ receptor γ2 subunit and merged immunostaining in the granule cell layer of WT and R215H KI mice. **b, c** Quantification of gephyrin puncta number and size at granule cell soma region. **d, e** Quantification of γ2 puncta number and size at the same region as gephyrin. WT = 9 slices from 3 mice, R215H KI = 12 slices from 3 mice. Scale bar = 10 μm. Student's *t*-test was used for analysis and data were shown as Mean ± SEM, $^*P < 0.05$, $^{**}P < 0.01$, $^{***}P < 0.001$

there was no significant change of miniature excitatory postsynaptic currents (mEPSCs) in the dentate granule cells of R215H KI mice compared to WT mice (Fig. 4e-h). The kinetics of both mIPSCs and mEPSCs were not altered (Additional file 1: Figure S7). These Results indicate that NL2 R215H mutation is primarily affecting inhibitory neurotransmission.

Behavioral deficits in NL2 R215H KI mice

The significant reduction of inhibitory neurotransmission in the NL2 R215H mutant mice prompted us to further investigate whether such severe GABAergic deficits will result in any behavioral deficits. We first performed open field test (10 min). We found that the KI mice spent significantly less time in the center region, although the total distance traveled was similar to the WT mice (Fig. 5a-d). Consistently, in the elevated plus maze test, the KI mice spent much less time in the open arm compared to the WT mice, while the total travel distance was also similar between the KI and WT mice (Fig. 5e-h). These results suggest that the R215H KI mice display an increased level of anxiety while their locomotion activity is relatively normal.

We next examined in R215H KI mice the acoustic startle response and pre-pulse inhibition, a standard test for the sensory motor gating function often assessed in schizophrenia patients [5]. R215H KI mice showed a significant reduction in the startle response when stimulated at 100–120 dB (Fig. 5i). Furthermore, the pre-pulse inhibition was significantly impaired in the KI mice

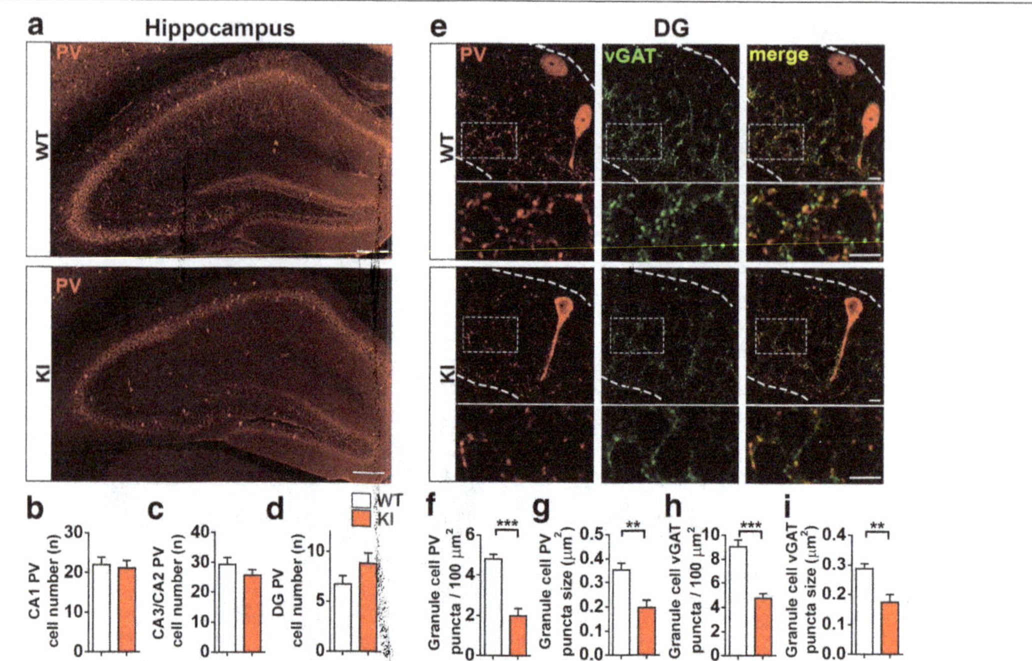

Fig. 3 Reduced GABAergic presynaptic components in the hippocampus of NL2 R215H KI mice. **a** Representative images of PV staining at the hippocampus in WT and R215H KI mice. Scale bar = 200 μm. **b-d** Quantification of PV-positive neurons at DG, CA2/3, and CA1 region. WT, $n = 14$ slices / 5 mice; KI, $n = 14$ slices / 5 mice. **e** Representative images of PV, vGAT and merged immunostaining in the granule cell layer of WT and R215H KI mice. **f, g** Quantification of PV puncta number and size that targeted to the granule cell layer. **h, i** Quantification of vGAT puncta number and size that targeted to the same region. WT = 12 slices / 5 mice, R215H KI = 12 slices / 5 mice. Scale bar = 10 μm. Student's *t* test was used for analysis and data were shown as Mean ± SEM, $^{*}P < 0.05$, $^{**}P < 0.01$, $^{***}P < 0.001$

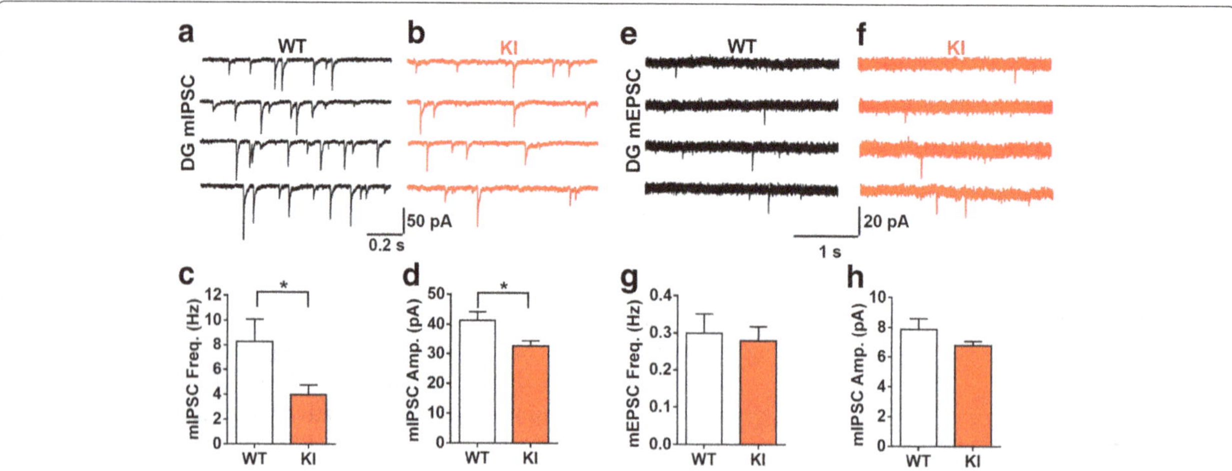

Fig. 4 NL2 R215H KI mice have decreased inhibitory synaptic transmission at the hippocampal region. **a, b** Representative traces of miniature inhibitory postsynaptic currents (mIPSCs) recorded from DG granule cells in hippocampal slices of WT (black) and R215H KI (red) mice. WT, $n = 14$ cells / 4 mice; R215H KI, $n = 18$ cells / 4 mice. **c, d** Quantification of the mIPSC frequency and amplitude (Student's *t*-test). **e, f** Representative traces of miniature excitatory postsynaptic currents (mEPSCs) in the DG region of hippocampal slices from WT (black) and R215H KI (red) mice. WT, $n = 11$ cells / 4 mice; KI, $n = 12$ cells / 3 mice. **g, h** Quantification of the mEPSC frequency and amplitude (Student's *t*-test). Data represent mean ± SEM; $^{*}P < 0.05$, $^{**}P < 0.01$, $^{***}P < 0.001$

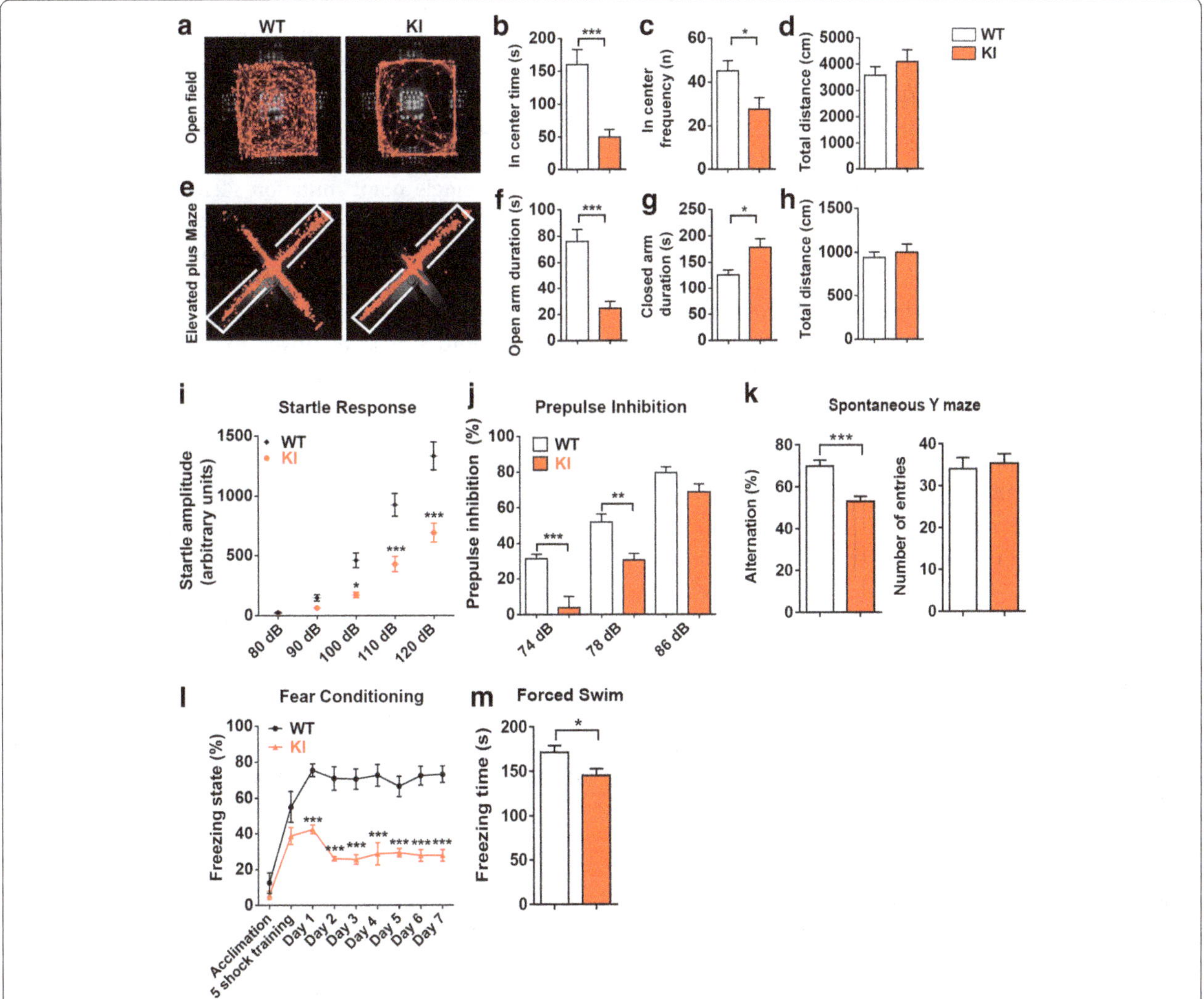

Fig. 5 NL2 R215H KI mice display schizophrenia-like behaviors. **a** Representative running track of WT and R215H KI mice (male) in an open field within 10 min duration. **b** The center time of WT and KI mice spent in the open field. **c** The frequency of WT and KI mice entering the center zone of the open field. **d** The total distance of WT and KI mice traveled in the open field test. **e** Representative running track of WT and R215H KI mice (male) in elevated plus maze for 5 min. White line indicates closed-arms. **f** The quantified time spent in the open-arms of WT and KI mice. **g** The time spent in the closed-arms of WT and KI mice. (**h**) The total distance traveled in the elevated plus maze test. **a**-**h** WT mice $n = 11$, KI mice $n = 12$,; Student's *t*-test was used for analysis. **i** Startle response of WT and R215H KI mice (male) toward 80, 90, 100, 110, and 120 dB sound pulses. **j** The percentage of pre-pulse inhibition (PPI) to a pre-pulse of 74 dB, 78 dB, and 86 dB. WT mice $n = 12$, KI mice $n = 9$. Two-way ANOVA with Sidak's multiple comparison test was used for analysis. **k** Spontaneous Y maze test. WT mice $n = 10$, KI mice $n = 12$, Student's *t*-test. **l** Contextual fear conditioning test. R215H KI mice exhibit significant reduction of freezing time when placed back in the test chamber after 1–7 days of shock training (Two-way ANOVA with Sidak's multiple comparison test, genotype $F_{(1, 99)} = 172.7$, $P < 0.0001$, WT $n = 8$, KI $n = 5$). **m** Forced swim test. Freezing time were analyzed. WT mice $n = 23$, KI mice $n = 16$, Student's *t*-test. Data represent mean ± SEM; $^{*}P < 0.05$, $^{**}P < 0.01$, $^{***}P < 0.001$

compared to the WT mice (Fig. 5j). Together, these deficits of R215H KI mice suggest that this new transgenic mouse model may recapitulate symptoms of schizophrenia patients.

To further characterize the R215H KI mice, we investigated their cognitive functions by spontaneous Y maze and contextual fear conditioning test. In the Y maze test, we found that R215H KI mice displayed a significant reduction of spontaneous alternation compared to the WT mice (Fig. 5k), indicating a working memory dysfunction. In the contextual fear conditioning test, while the KI mice were capable to associate the conditioning chamber with foot-shock in the initial training, indicated by an increase of freezing state after foot-shock, they failed to retain the fear context memory in the following days when tested (Fig. 5l), indicating an impaired hippocampal dependent cognitive function. Furthermore, we performed forced swim test to investigate whether R215H KI mice have any depression-like behavior, because certain SCZ patients display depression symptom. Interestingly, we observed a reduction of freezing time in KI mice when performing the forced swim test (Fig. 5m), consistent with our observation below that the KI mice show hyperactivity induced by acute stress. The behavioral data shown above was all obtained from male mice, and the female mice were also tested and exhibited the same trend (Additional file 1: Figure S8).

Impaired hippocampal activation toward acute stress in NL2 R215H KI mice

Schizophrenia is associated with abnormal response to stress [60]. Stress is known to activate the hypothalamic-pituitary-adrenal axis (HPA axis) and induce the hormone release of corticosterone (CORT) into circulation [34, 41]. To investigate the stress response of R215H KI mice, we put the WT and R215H KI mice into restraining tubes for 1 hour as an acute stress test. We found that R215H KI mice struggled much more intensively for a long time and excreted much more than the WT mice during the restraining test. After restraining, KI mice were more dirty and stinky than the WT mice (Fig. 6a). In accordance, R215H KI mice showed a much higher level of CORT (384 ± 53 ng/ml) after restraining compared to the WT mice (215 ± 20 ng/ml). The baseline level of CORT was similar between WT (49 ± 4 ng/ml) and KI mice (36 ± 4 ng/ml) (Fig. 6b; $p = 0.0035$ after restraint, Two way ANOVA followed with Sidak's post hoc test). These results suggest that R215H KI mice have hyperactive HPA response toward stress.

Following the activation of HPA axis, hippocampus will be activated as a negative feedback regulator and control the CORT level within normal range [23, 58]. To examine the hippocampal activation in R215H KI mice following the acute stress, we used a naïve cohort of mice to perform the restraining test again. R215H KI and WT mice were subjected to restraint for half an hour and then sacrificed after 2 h. Hippocampal activation was examined by assessing the expression level of an immediate early gene cFos [42, 48]. At the baseline level, very few cFos-positive neurons were detected in the hippocampal regions in both WT and KI mice (Fig. 6c, top row). After stress, we observed a significant increase of cFos-positive cells in the DG and CA2/3 regions of the hippocampus in WT mice (Fig. 6c, bottom left). In contrast, the R215H KI mice showed much reduced cFos-positive cells in the same regions of hippocampus (Fig. 6c, bottom right). This is better illustrated in the enlarged images showing the CA2/3 and DG regions of WT mice (Fig. 6d, top row) and KI mice (Fig. 6d, bottom row). Quantitative analysis confirmed the reduction of cFos-positive cells in both CA2/3 (Fig. 6e) and DG (Fig. 6f) regions in the KI mice. These results suggest that NL2 R215H KI mice had impaired hippocampal activation during acute stress.

Discussion

In the present study, we generated a unique mouse model carrying a single point mutation R215H of *NLGN2* gene that was originally identified from human schizophrenia patients. The NL2 R215H KI mice have impaired GABAergic synapse development, reduced inhibitory synaptic transmission, and decreased hippocampal activation in response to stress. Moreover, the R215H KI mice display anxiety-like behavior, impaired pre-pulse inhibition, cognitive deficits and abnormal stress response, partially recapitulating some of the core symptoms of schizophrenia patients. These results suggest that this newly generated R215H KI mouse line may provide a unique animal model for studying molecular mechanisms underlying schizophrenia and related neuropsychiatric disorders.

GABAergic and behavioral deficits in NL2 R215H KI mice

NL2 plays important roles in regulating perisomatic GABAergic synapse development, phasic GABAergic transmission, and neural excitability [1, 3, 9, 19, 24, 25, 30, 40, 47, 59, 61]. Consistent with our previous in vitro studies, the current in vivo work demonstrates that R215H mutation disrupts GABAergic synapse development. Functionally, NL2 R215H mutation caused a reduction of both frequency and amplitude of inhibitory neurotransmission. These results suggest that the R215H KI mice display more GABAergic deficits than the reported NL2 KO mice [1, 9, 19, 30, 47], which might explain why our KI mice display more behavioral deficits than the NL2 KO mice, such as PPI impairment, cognitive deficits, and abnormal stress response. Coincidentally, previous studies reported that NL3 R451C KI mouse also displayed stronger phenotypes than the NL3 KO mice [14, 16, 57, 64]. These evidences suggest that genetic mouse models based on mutations identified from patients may be more suitable than the germline KO mouse models for studying pathological mechanisms of human diseases, because of less compensation from other genes in KI mice than in KO mice.

Behaviorally, NL2 R215H KI mice display an anxiety phenotype, which may be the result of decreased GABAergic inhibition [3, 11, 63]. Interestingly, R215H KI mice also show impaired startle responses and deficits in pre-pulse inhibition (PPI). Previous study in rats has reported that disturbance of PV neuron development in the hippocampal DG region may cause reduction of PPI [21]. A recent study also demonstrates that specific inhibition of PV neurons in the ventral hippocampus results in a reduction of both startle response and PPI [45]. Consistent with these findings, we demonstrate here that our R215H KI mice display a

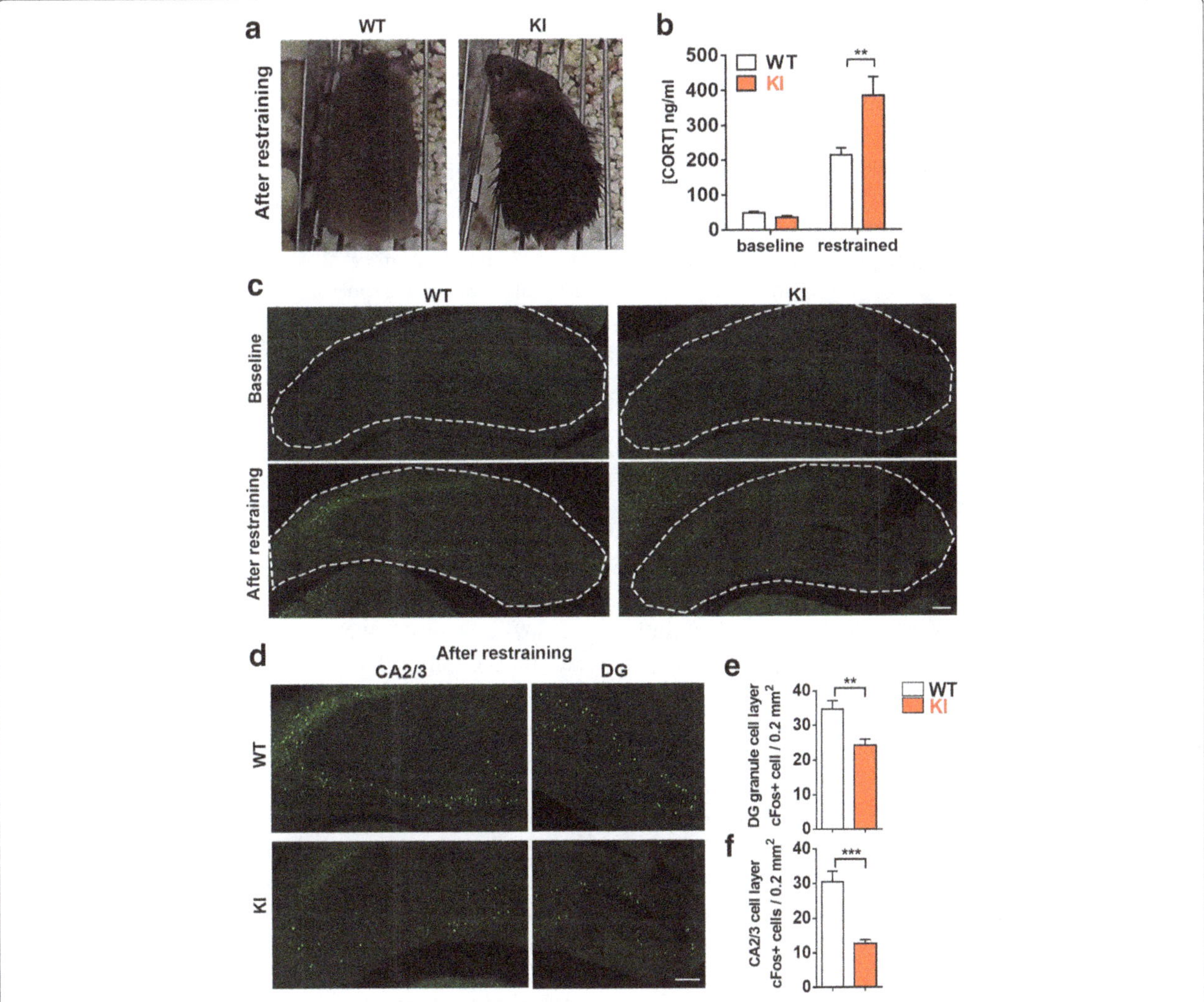

Fig. 6 Hippocampal neurons have impaired activation toward acute stress in NL2 R215H KI mice. **a** Typical appearance of WT and KI mice after restraining. **b** Quantified corticosteroid level of WT and KI mice at the baseline level and after 1 h restraining. 4 to 8 mice were used for each genotype at each condition, age 4 to 6 months. Two-way ANOVA with Sidak's multiple comparison test was used for analysis. **c** Upper row: representative images of baseline cFos immunoreactivity of WT and R215H KI hippocampus; bottom row: cFos immunoreactivity of WT and R215H KI hippocampus after restraining. **d** enlarged DG and CA2/3 region of WT and R215H mice after restraining. **e** Quantification of cFos-positive cells at DG granule cell layers. **f** Quantification of cFos positive cells at CA2/3 pyramidal cell layers. WT: $n = 16$ brain slices / 4 mice; R215H KI: $n = 20$ brain slices / 5 mice; scale bar = 200 μm. Student's t-test was used for analysis. Data represent mean ± SEM; $*P < 0.05$, $**P < 0.01$, $***P < 0.001$

significant reduction of PV innervation in the hippocampus, which may underlie the deficits of PPI. In contrast, the NL2 KO mice lack PPI deficit, which might be related to an insufficient loss of PV innervation at hippocampal regions [61]. Besides PV neurons, CCK (cholecystokinin) neurons are another type of inhibitory neurons mainly innervate CA1/2/3 pyramidal cells and DG proximal dendrites. CCK neurons can release GABA to act on $GABA_A$ receptor α2 subunits that are known to mediate anxiolytic effect, or release CCK to act on CCK2 receptors and induce anxiogenic effect [18]. It would be important to further investigate the expression and functional alteration of CCK neurons in our R215H KI mice in future studies.

Surprisingly, our former collaborator Dr. Chia-Hsiang Chen's group recently reported that their NL2 R215H KI mice displayed an increased pre-pulse inhibition phenotype [8]. However, because the startle response of their KI mice was not reported, it makes the data difficult to compare with ours. Additionally, they reported that their KI mice didn't express NL2 and resembled global NL2 KO mice, but they did not present the actual comparison with NL2 KO mice. In contrast, our R215H KI mice are clearly different from the NL2 KO mice, because our KI mice showed small amount of NL2 expression, particularly during early developmental stages. The low expression level of NL2 in our R215H KI mice distinguishes our KI mice from the NL2 KO mice, which showed completely absent expression of NL2 in our Western blot analysis. Furthermore, our R215H KI mice also showed clear GABAergic deficits as expected, but it is unknown whether their KI mice have any GABAergic deficits or not [8].

Another interesting observation is that the R215H KI mice are hyperactive after acute stress and are associated with impaired hippocampal activation. It has been reported that robust neuron activation requires low background activity before stimulus [33, 49]. However, due to the reduction of GABAergic inhibition in our R215H KI mice, the background activity of hippocampal neurons may be chronically elevated, which will dampen further activation of the hippocampus by external stimulation [40]. The impaired activation of hippocampal neurons in R215H KI mice may contribute to the abnormal stress response we observed, as hippocampus acts like a "brake" during acute stress to prevent HPA axis from over activation [22]. Besides hippocampus, sensitized HPA-axis involves brain regions such as hypothalamus and amygdala. Loss of NL2 in these areas could directly affect their GABAergic transmission and releasing of corticosteroids into the circulation, which is worth of further investigation as well.

NL2 R215H mutation and schizophrenia

It is well documented that schizophrenia patient's show impaired pre-pulse inhibition as an abnormal sensorimotor gating deficit [5, 20]. Many patients also have emotional symptoms such as anxiety and depression [39]. Additionally, patients are hypersensitive toward stress and certain patients have been found with altered HPA axis function [4]. Intriguingly, R215H KI mice recapitulated these SCZ-like behaviors, suggesting a potential role of NL2 R215H in the development of schizophrenia symptoms. Furthermore, reduction of PV expression and PV-positive synapses is a prominent phenotype observed in SCZ patients [36–38, 62]. The R215H mutation KI mice also show a significant reduction of PV innervation, consistent with the pathogenic deficit of SCZ patients. These GABAergic deficits, together with cognition and PPI deficits manifested in the KI mice, support the hypothesis that GABA dysfunction makes an important contribution to the cognitive and attention deficits of SCZ. Taken together, NLGN2 R215H single point mutation has a significant impact on GABAergic synapse development and the pathogenesis of neuropsychiatric disorders. Our newly generated NL2 R215H KI mice may provide a useful mouse model for the study of molecular mechanisms and drug development of neuropsychiatric disorders including schizophrenia.

Methods

NL2 R215H knock-in mice

The NL2 R215H knock-in mice were generated by homologous recombination in embryonic stem cells by Dr. Siu-Pok Yee's team at the University of Connecticut Health Center. NL2 KO mice were purchased from Jackson Laboratory (stock# 008139). The detailed procedures are described in the Additional file 1.

All the experimental mice were group housed (2–3 mice per cage) in home cages and lived at a constant 25 °C in a 12 h light/dark cycle. Mice were given ad libitum access to food and water. Littermate or age and gender matched mice were used for experiments. All animal care and experiments followed the Penn State University IACUC protocol and NIH guidelines.

Biochemical measurements

Protein levels were quantified using total brain homogenates from 3 groups of adult male littermates- WT, heterozygous and homozygous. The western blot system used was the standard Bio-Rad mini protein electrophoresis system and the procedure followed the system manual. LiCOR Odyssey Clx was used for protein signal detection. The antibodies used were Rb anti-Neuroligin 2 (1:1000, SYSY 129202), Rb anti-GAPDH (1:10000, Sigma G9545), and Gt anti-Rb 800 (1:15000, P/N 925-32210, P/N 925-32211). Detailed procedures are described in the Additional file 1.

Immunohistochemistry, image acquisition, and image analysis

Mouse brain slices were prepared at 20–40 μM and reacted with the primary antibodies Rb anti-Neuroligin 2 (1:1000, SYSY129203), Ms. anti-Parvalbumin (1:1000, MAB1572), GP anti-vGAT (1:1000, SYSY 131004), Gephyrin (1:1000, SYSY 147011), GABAaR γ2 (1:1000 SYSY 224003), and c-Fos (1:5000 Sigma F7799). The fluorescent secondary antibodies used were Gt anti-Rb 488, Gt anti-Ms Cy3, and Gt anti-GP 647. Images were taken with the Olympus FV1000 confocal microscope. The number of neurons and the density and size of synaptic puncta were analyzed with the NIH ImageJ software (NIH, Bethesda, MD, USA). A detailed description of the experimental procedures is in the Additional file 1.

Slice electrophysiology

Horizontal acute hippocampal slices were used for whole-cell patch clamp recordings. Miniature inhibitory or excitatory postsynaptic currents (mIPSCs or mEPSCs) were pharmacologically isolated by including DNQX and APV or picrotoxin together with tetrodotoxin in artificial cerebrospinal fluid. Details are in the Additional file 1.

Behavioral tests

Overview

The mice for behavior tests were group housed by genotype. All tests were performed during 1 pm to 6 pm. Four cohorts of mice were used: First cohort of mice was first tested for open field, elevated plus maze, and Y maze at 2–3 months old, and then tested for the startle response and pre-pulse inhibition at 3.5 months old. Second cohort of mice was used for contextual fear conditioning test at 2–3 months old. Third cohort of mice was used for restraining and corticosteroid serum level test at 4–6 months old. Fourth cohort of mice was tested for forced swim at 3 months old. The open field test and elevated maze data were analyzed by Noldus Ethovision XT 8.0 software. Y maze and forced swim tests were analyzed with the researcher blind to genotype. Detailed procedures are in Additional file 1.

Abbreviations

APV: D(–)-2-Amino-5-phosphonopentanoic acid; CORT: Corticosterone; DG: Dentate gyrus; DNQX: 6,7-dinitroquinoxaline-2,3-dione; ER: Endoplasmic reticulum; HPA: Hypothalamic-pituitary-adrenal axis; KI: Knock in; KO: Knock out; mEPSC: Miniature excitatory postsynaptic current; mIPSC: Miniature inhibitory postsynaptic current; NL-2: Neuroligin-2; NLGN: Neuroligin; NRXN: Neurexin; PPI: Pre-pulse inhibition; PV: Parvalbumin; SCZ: Schizophrenia; vGAT: Vesicular GABA transporter; WT: Wild type

Acknowledgements

We would like to thank Dr. Thomas Fuchs for providing advices on behavioral tests, Yuting Bai for providing initial genotyping support. We thank all members from Chen lab for thoughtful suggestions.

Funding

This study is supported by grants from NIH (MH092740 and MH083911) and Charles H. "Skip" Smith Brain Repair Endowment Fund to G. C.

Authors' contributions

DYJ performed most of the experiments and wrote the draft manuscript. GC supervised the entire work and revised the manuscript. CF performed forced swim test and measured body weight. CF and YH helped genotyping and Western blot. ZW helped electrophysiology recordings. SPY generated the NL-2 R215H transgenic mice as a paid service. All authors read and approved the final manuscript.

Competing interests

The authors declare that they have no competing interests.

Author details

[1]Department of Biology, Huck Institutes of Life Sciences, Pennsylvania State University, University Park, PA 16802, USA. [2]Department of Cell Biology, University of Connecticut Health center, Farmington, CT 06030, USA.

References

1. Babaev O, Botta P, Meyer E, Muller C, Ehrenreich H, Brose N, Luthi A, Krueger-Burg D. Neuroligin 2 deletion alters inhibitory synapse function and anxiety-associated neuronal activation in the amygdala. Neuropharmacology. 2016;100:56–65.
2. Baudouin SJ, Gaudias J, Gerharz S, Hatstatt L, Zhou K, Punnakkal P, Tanaka KF, Spooren W, Hen R, De Zeeuw CI, et al. Shared synaptic pathophysiology in syndromic and nonsyndromic rodent models of autism. Science. 2012; 338:128–32.
3. Blundell J, Tabuchi K, Bolliger MF, Blaiss CA, Brose N, Liu X, Sudhof TC, Powell CM. Increased anxiety-like behavior in mice lacking the inhibitory synapse cell adhesion molecule neuroligin 2. Genes Brain Behav. 2009;8: 114–26.
4. Bradley AJ, Dinan TG. Review: a systematic review of hypothalamic-pituitary-adrenal axis function in schizophrenia: implications for mortality. J Psychopharmacol. 2010;24:91–118.
5. Braff DL, Grillon C, Geyer MA. Gating and habituation of the startle reflex in schizophrenic patients. Arch Gen Psychiatry. 1992;49:206–15.
6. Bucan M, Abrahams BS, Wang K, Glessner JT, Herman EI, Sonnenblick LI, Alvarez Retuerto AI, Imielinski M, Hadley D, Bradfield JP, et al. Genome-wide analyses of exonic copy number variants in a family-based study point to novel autism susceptibility genes. PLoS Genet. 2009;5:e1000536.
7. Budreck EC, Scheiffele P. Neuroligin-3 is a neuronal adhesion protein at GABAergic and glutamatergic synapses. Eur J Neurosci. 2007;26:1738–48.
8. Chen CH, Lee PW, Liao HM, Chang PK. Neuroligin 2 R215H mutant mice manifest anxiety, increased prepulse inhibition, and impaired spatial learning and memory. Front Psychiatry. 2017;8:257.
9. Chubykin AA, Atasoy D, Etherton MR, Brose N, Kavalali ET, Gibson JR, Sudhof TC. Activity-dependent validation of excitatory versus inhibitory synapses by neuroligin-1 versus neuroligin-2. Neuron. 2007;54:919–31.
10. Connor SA, Ammendrup-Johnsen I, Chan AW, Kishimoto Y, Murayama C, Kurihara N, Tada A, Ge Y, Lu H, Yan R, et al. Altered cortical dynamics and cognitive function upon haploinsufficiency of the autism-linked excitatory synaptic suppressor MDGA2. Neuron. 2016;91:1052–68.
11. Dalvi A, Rodgers RJ. GABAergic influences on plus-maze behaviour in mice. Psychopharmacol. 1996;128:380–97.
12. Dong N, Qi J, Chen G. Molecular reconstitution of functional GABAergic synapses with expression of neuroligin-2 and GABAA receptors. Mol Cell Neurosci. 2007;35:14–23.
13. Durand CM, Betancur C, Boeckers TM, Bockmann J, Chaste P, Fauchereau F, Nygren G, Rastam M, Gillberg IC, Anckarsater H, et al. Mutations in the gene encoding the synaptic scaffolding protein SHANK3 are associated with autism spectrum disorders. Nat Genet. 2007;39:25–7.
14. Etherton M, Foldy C, Sharma M, Tabuchi K, Liu X, Shamloo M, Malenka RC, Sudhof TC. Autism-linked neuroligin-3 R451C mutation differentially alters hippocampal and cortical synaptic function. Proc Natl Acad Sci U S A. 2011; 108:13764–9.
15. Etherton MR, Blaiss CA, Powell CM, Sudhof TC. Mouse neurexin-1alpha deletion causes correlated electrophysiological and behavioral changes consistent with cognitive impairments. Proc Natl Acad Sci U S A. 2009;106: 17998–8003.
16. Foldy C, Malenka RC, Sudhof TC. Autism-associated neuroligin-3 mutations commonly disrupt tonic endocannabinoid signaling. Neuron. 2013;78:498–509.
17. Freedman R. Schizophrenia. N Engl J Med. 2003;349:1738–49.
18. Freund TF, Katona I. Perisomatic inhibition. Neuron. 2007;56:33.
19. Gibson JR, Huber KM, Sudhof TC. Neuroligin-2 deletion selectively decreases inhibitory synaptic transmission originating from fast-spiking but not from somatostatin-positive interneurons. J Neurosci. 2009;29:13883–97.
20. Grillon C, Ameli R, Charney DS, Krystal J, Braff D. Startle gating deficits occur across prepulse intensities in schizophrenic patients. Biol Psychiatry. 1992;32: 939–43.
21. Guo N, Yoshizaki K, Kimura R, Suto F, Yanagawa Y, Osumi N. A sensitive period for GABAergic interneurons in the dentate gyrus in modulating sensorimotor gating. J Neurosci. 2013;33:6691–704.
22. Hariri AR. Looking inside the disordered brain: an introduction to the functional neuroanatomy of psychopathology. Sunderland: Sinauer Associates, Inc.; 2015.

23. Herman JP, McKlveen JM, Solomon MB, Carvalho-Netto E, Myers B. Neural regulation of the stress response: glucocorticoid feedback mechanisms. Braz J Med Biol Res. 2012;45:292–8.
24. Hines RM, Wu L, Hines DJ, Steenland H, Mansour S, Dahlhaus R, Singaraja RR, Cao X, Sammler E, Hormuzdi SG, et al. Synaptic imbalance, stereotypies, and impaired social interactions in mice with altered neuroligin 2 expression. J Neurosci. 2008;28:6055–67.
25. Hoon M, Bauer G, Fritschy JM, Moser T, Falkenburger BH, Varoqueaux F. Neuroligin 2 controls the maturation of GABAergic synapses and information processing in the retina. J Neurosci. 2009;29:8039–50.
26. Ichtchenko K, Hata Y, Nguyen T, Ullrich B, Missler M, Moomaw C, Sudhof TC. Neuroligin 1: a splice site-specific ligand for beta-neurexins. Cell. 1995;81:435–43.
27. Insel TR. Rethinking schizophrenia. Nature. 2010;468:187–93.
28. Jamain S, Quach H, Betancur C, Rastam M, Colineaux C, Gillberg IC, Soderstrom H, Giros B, Leboyer M, Gillberg C, et al. Mutations of the X-linked genes encoding neuroligins NLGN3 and NLGN4 are associated with autism. Nat Genet. 2003;34:27–9.
29. Jamain S, Radyushkin K, Hammerschmidt K, Granon S, Boretius S, Varoqueaux F, Ramanantsoa N, Gallego J, Ronnenberg A, Winter D, et al. Reduced social interaction and ultrasonic communication in a mouse model of monogenic heritable autism. Proc Natl Acad Sci U S A. 2008;105:1710–5.
30. Jedlicka P, Hoon M, Papadopoulos T, Vlachos A, Winkels R, Poulopoulos A, Betz H, Deller T, Brose N, Varoqueaux F, et al. Increased dentate gyrus excitability in neuroligin-2-deficient mice in vivo. Cereb Cortex. 2010;21:357–67.
31. Kim HG, Kishikawa S, Higgins AW, Seong IS, Donovan DJ, Shen Y, Lally E, Weiss LA, Najm J, Kutsche K, et al. Disruption of neurexin 1 associated with autism spectrum disorder. Am J Hum Genet. 2008;82:199–207.
32. Kirov G, Gumus D, Chen W, Norton N. Comparative genome hybridization suggests a role for NRXN1 and APBA2 in schizophrenia. Hum Mol Genet. 2008;17(3):458–65.
33. Koistinaho J, Hicks KJ, Sagar SM. Tetrodotoxin enhances light-induced c-fos gene expression in the rabbit retina. Brain Res Mol Brain Res. 1993;17:179–83.
34. Koob GF. Corticotropin-releasing factor, norepinephrine, and stress. Biol Psychiatry. 1999;46:1167–80.
35. Levinson JN, Chery N, Huang K, Wong TP, Gerrow K, Kang R, Prange O, Wang YT, El-Husseini A. Neuroligins mediate excitatory and inhibitory synapse formation: involvement of PSD-95 and neurexin-1beta in neuroligin-induced synaptic specificity. J Biol Chem. 2005;280:17312–9.
36. Lewis DA, Cruz DA, Melchitzky DS, Pierri JN. Lamina-specific deficits in parvalbumin-immunoreactive varicosities in the prefrontal cortex of subjects with schizophrenia: evidence for fewer projections from the thalamus. Am J Psychiatry. 2001;158:1411–22.
37. Lewis DA, Curley AA, Glausier JR, Volk DW. Cortical parvalbumin interneurons and cognitive dysfunction in schizophrenia. Trends Neurosci. 2012;35:57–67.
38. Lewis DA, Hashimoto T, Volk DW. Cortical inhibitory neurons and schizophrenia. Nat Rev Neurosci. 2005;6:312–24.
39. Lewis DA, Lieberman JA. Catching up on schizophrenia: natural history and neurobiology. Neuron. 2000;28:325.
40. Liang J, Xu W, Hsu YT, Yee AX, Chen L, Sudhof TC. Conditional neuroligin-2 knockout in adult medial prefrontal cortex links chronic changes in synaptic inhibition to cognitive impairments. Mol Psychiatry. 2015;20:850–9.
41. McGill BE, Bundle SF, Yaylaoglu MB, Carson JP, Thaller C, Zoghbi HY. Enhanced anxiety and stress-induced corticosterone release are associated with increased Crh expression in a mouse model of Rett syndrome. Proc Natl Acad Sci U S A. 2006;103:18267–72.
42. Morgan JI, Cohen DR, Hempstead JL, Curran T. Mapping patterns of c-fos expression in the central nervous system after seizure. Science. 1987;237:192–7.
43. Nakanishi M, Nomura J, Ji X, Tamada K, Arai T, Takahashi E, Bućan M, Takumi T. Functional significance of rare neuroligin 1 variants found in autism. PLoS Genet. 2017;13:e1007035.
44. Nam CI, Chen L. Postsynaptic assembly induced by neurexin-neuroligin interaction and neurotransmitter. Proc Natl Acad Sci U S A. 2005;102:6137–42.
45. Nguyen R, Morrissey MD, Mahadevan V, Cajanding JD, Woodin MA, Yeomans JS, Takehara-Nishiuchi K, Kim JC. Parvalbumin and GAD65 interneuron inhibition in the ventral hippocampus induces distinct behavioral deficits relevant to schizophrenia. J Neurosci. 2014;34:14948–60.
46. Peça J, Feliciano C, Ting JT, Wang W, Wells MF, Venkatraman TN, Lascola CD, Fu Z, Feng G. Shank3 mutant mice display autistic-like behaviours and striatal dysfunction. Nature. 2011;472:437–42.
47. Poulopoulos A, Aramuni G, Meyer G, Soykan T, Hoon M, Papadopoulos T, Zhang M, Paarmann I, Fuchs C, Harvey K, et al. Neuroligin 2 drives postsynaptic assembly at perisomatic inhibitory synapses through gephyrin and collybistin. Neuron. 2009;63:628–42.
48. Ramirez S, Liu X, Lin PA, Suh J, Pignatelli M, Redondo RL, Ryan TJ, Tonegawa S. Creating a false memory in the hippocampus. Science. 2013;341:387–91.
49. Rao VR, Pintchovski SA, Chin J, Peebles CL, Mitra S, Finkbeiner S. AMPA receptors regulate transcription of the plasticity-related immediate-early gene Arc. Nat Neurosci. 2006;9:887–95.
50. Rothwell PE, Fuccillo MV, Maxeiner S, Hayton SJ, Gokce O, Lim BK, Fowler SC, Malenka RC, Sudhof TC. Autism-associated neuroligin-3 mutations commonly impair striatal circuits to boost repetitive behaviors. Cell. 2014; 158:198–212.
51. Scheiffele P, Fan J, Choih J, Fetter R, Serafini T. Neuroligin expressed in nonneuronal cells triggers presynaptic development in contacting axons. Cell. 2000;101:657–69.
52. Schizophrenia Working Group of the Psychiatric Genomics, C. Biological insights from 108 schizophrenia-associated genetic loci. Nature. 2014;511:421–7.
53. Song JY, Ichtchenko K, Sudhof TC, Brose N. Neuroligin 1 is a postsynaptic cell-adhesion molecule of excitatory synapses. Proc Natl Acad Sci U S A. 1999;96:1100–5.
54. Südhof TC. Neuroligins and neurexins link synaptic function to cognitive disease. Nature. 2008;455:903–11.
55. Sullivan PF, Kendler KS, Neale MC. Schizophrenia as a complex trait: evidence from a meta-analysis of twin studies. Arch Gen Psychiatry. 2003;60:1187–92.
56. Sun C, Cheng MC, Qin R, Liao DL, Chen TT, Koong FJ, Chen G, Chen CH. Identification and functional characterization of rare mutations of the neuroligin-2 gene (NLGN2) associated with schizophrenia. Hum Mol Genet. 2011;20:3042–51.
57. Tabuchi K, Blundell J, Etherton MR, Hammer RE, Liu X, Powell CM, Sudhof TC. A neuroligin-3 mutation implicated in autism increases inhibitory synaptic transmission in mice. Science. 2007;318:71–6.
58. Ulrich-Lai YM, Herman JP. Neural regulation of endocrine and autonomic stress responses. Nat Rev Neurosci. 2009;10:397–409.
59. Varoqueaux F, Jamain S, Brose N. Neuroligin 2 is exclusively localized to inhibitory synapses. Eur J Cell Biol. 2004;83:449–56.
60. Walker EF, Diforio D. Schizophrenia: a neural diathesis-stress model. Psychol Rev. 1997;104:667–85.
61. Wohr M, Silverman JL, Scattoni ML, Turner SM, Harris MJ, Saxena R, Crawley JN. Developmental delays and reduced pup ultrasonic vocalizations but normal sociability in mice lacking the postsynaptic cell adhesion protein neuroligin2. Behav Brain Res. 2013;251:50–64.
62. Woo TU, Whitehead RE, Melchitzky DS, Lewis DA. A subclass of prefrontal gamma-aminobutyric acid axon terminals are selectively altered in schizophrenia. Proc Natl Acad Sci U S A. 1998;95:5341–6.
63. Zarrindast M, Rostami P, Sadeghi-Hariri M. GABA(A) but not GABA(B) receptor stimulation induces antianxiety profile in rats. Pharmacol Biochem Behav. 2001;69:9–15.
64. Zhang B, Seigneur E, Wei P, Gokce O, Morgan J, Sudhof TC. Developmental plasticity shapes synaptic phenotypes of autism-associated neuroligin-3 mutations in the calyx of Held. Mol Psychiatry. 2017;22:1483–91.
65. Zhang C, Milunsky JM, Newton S, Ko J, Zhao G, Maher TA, Tager-Flusberg H, Bolliger MF, Carter AS, Boucard AA, et al. A neuroligin-4 missense mutation associated with autism impairs neuroligin-4 folding and endoplasmic reticulum export. J Neurosci. 2009;29:10843–54.
66. Zhou Y, Kaiser T, Monteiro P, Zhang X, Van der Goes MS, Wang D, Barak B, Zeng M, Li C, Lu C, et al. Mice with Shank3 mutations associated with ASD and schizophrenia display both shared and distinct defects. Neuron. 2016; 89:147–62.

3

Characterization of excitatory synaptic transmission in the anterior cingulate cortex of adult tree shrew

Xu-Hui Li[1], Qian Song[1], Qi-Yu Chen[1], Jing-Shan Lu[1], Tao Chen[1,2] and Min Zhuo[1,3*]

Abstract

The tree shrew, as a primate-like animal model, has been used for studying high brain functions such as social emotion and spatial learning memory. However, little is known about the excitatory synaptic transmission in cortical brain areas of the tree shrew. In the present study, we have characterized the excitatory synaptic transmission and intrinsic properties of pyramidal neurons in the anterior cingulate cortex (ACC) of the adult tree shrew, a key cortical region for pain perception and emotion. We found that glutamate is the major excitatory transmitter for fast synaptic transmission. Excitatory synaptic responses induced by local stimulation were mediated by AMPA and kainate (KA) receptors. As compared with mice, AMPA and KA receptor mediated responses were significantly greater. Interestingly, the frequency of spontaneous excitatory postsynaptic currents (sEPSCs) and miniature excitatory postsynaptic currents (mEPSCs) in tree shrews was significantly less than that of mice. Moreover, both the ratio of paired-pulse facilitation (PPF) and the time of 50% decay for fast blockade of NMDA receptor mediated EPSCs were greater in the tree shrew. Finally, tree shrew neurons showed higher initial firing frequency and neuronal excitability with a cell type-specific manner in the ACC. Our studies provide the first report of the basal synaptic transmission in the ACC of adult tree shrew.

Keywords: Tree shrew, Glutamate, Calcium signals, Excitatory synaptic transmission, Intrinsic properties, Anterior cingulate cortex

Introduction

The tree shrew has a well-developed brain and central nervous system. Cumulative evidence has shown that the tree shrew is an ideal animal model for brain diseases of humans. Molecular phylogeny and whole genome sequencing analysis studies suggest that tree shrew has a close affinity to primates [1–4]. Tree shrews have higher brain-to-body mass ratio and more developed pyramidal neuron compared with rodents [5]. Particularly, some information involved in cognitive impairment during aging, such as the amyloid accumulation and somatostatin degeneration, is missing in the mice and rats but can be found in monkeys and tree shrews [6, 7].

Both animal and human studies have consistently demonstrated that the anterior cingulate cortex (ACC) plays important roles in many major brain functions such as awareness, emotion, memory, and pain [8–15]. However, there is limited information of synaptic transmission and plasticity in cortical areas obtained from primate models. Therefore, the tree shrew will be a valuable primate-like animal for the mechanism of cortical synaptic transmission and plasticity, especially in the ACC.

Glutamate is the major excitatory neurotransmitter for synaptic transmission in the central nervous system. Glutamatergic synaptic transmission is mainly mediated by three kinds of gate ionotropic receptors, α-amino-3-hydroxy-5-methyl-4-isoxazole-propionic acid (AMPA), kainate (KA) and N-methyl-D-aspartate (NMDA) receptors [8, 13, 16–18]. Integrative experimental approaches including genetic, biochemical, electrophysiological and pharmacological methods demonstrate that AMPA, KA

* Correspondence: min.zhuo@utoronto.ca
[1]Center for Neuron and Disease, Frontier Institutes of Science and Technology, Xi'an Jiaotong University, Xi'an 710049, China
[3]Department of Physiology, Faculty of Medicine, University of Toronto, Medical Science Building, Room #3342, 1 King's College Circle, Toronto, ON M5S 1A8, Canada
Full list of author information is available at the end of the article

and NMDA receptors are required for distinct physiological functions and pathological conditions in the ACC, including chronic pain, fear memory, anxiety and aversion [8, 10, 15, 19–23]. However, since previous investigations are mainly focused on glutamatergic synaptic transmission in rodents, less information is known about the synaptic transmission in the ACC of primates. Using tree shrews as a primate model, our recent studies have found that both the volume of the ACC and the sizes of cell bodies in the ACC pyramidal neurons of the tree shrew are larger than those in the mouse and rat. Furthermore, there are more apical/basal dendritic branches and apical dendritic spines of the ACC pyramidal neurons in tree shrews compared with rodents [5]. However, it is not known whether the basic excitatory synaptic transmission and intrinsic properties of pyramidal neurons in the ACC of tree shrews are different from those in rodents.

In the present study, by combing whole-cell patch recording, pharmacology blocking, and two-photon calcium imaging observation, we investigated the composition characteristics of basal synaptic transmission in the ACC pyramidal neurons of tree shrew. Using mice as a control, we found the AMPA and KA receptor mediated postsynaptic responses were enlarged, but the presynaptic glutamate release probabilities were lower in tree shrews. The global calcium signals and intrinsic neuronal excitability of pyramidal neurons were also found higher in tree shrews. Our studies provide the first report for the basic electrophysiological characteristics of glutamatergic synaptic transmission and neuronal properties in the ACC pyramidal neurons of tree shrews.

Methods

Animals

Experiments were performed with adult male tree shrews (10–12 months old) and male C57BL/6 mice (6–8 weeks old). Tree shrews were purchased from Kunming Institute of Zoology in China. All tree shrews and mice were maintained on a 12 h light/dark cycle with food and water provided ad libitum. Animal care, as well as all experiments, was conducted in accordance with the European Community guidelines for the use of experimental animals (86/609/EEC). All performed research protocols were approved by the Ethics Committee of Xi'an Jiaotong University.

Brain slice preparation

Coronal brain slices (300 μm) at the level of the ACC were prepared using standard methods [22, 24–26]. Adult tree shrews and mice were anesthetized with 1–2% isoflurane. The whole brain was quickly removed from the skull and submerged in the oxygenated (95% O_2 and 5% CO_2), ice cold cutting artificial cerebrospinal fluid (ACSF) containing the following (in mM): 252 sucrose, 2.5 KCl, 6 $MgSO_4$, 0.5 $CaCl_2$, 25 $NaHCO_3$, 1.2 NaH_2PO_4 and 10 glucose, pH 7.3–7.4. After cooling in the ACSF for a short time, the whole brain was trimmed for an appropriate part to glue onto the ice-cold stage of a vibrating tissue slicer (VT1200S, Leica). Slices were transferred to a submerged recovery chamber containing oxygenated (95% O_2 and 5% CO_2) ACSF (in mM): 124 NaCl, 4.4 KCl, 2 $CaCl_2$, 1 $MgSO_4$, 25 $NaHCO_3$, 1 NaH_2PO_4, and 10 glucose at room temperature for recording at least 1 h later.

Whole cell patch-clamp recording

Whole cell recordings were performed in a recording chamber on the stage of a BX51W1 (Olympus) microscope equipped with infrared differential interference contrast (DIC) optics for visualization. EPSCs were recorded from layer II/III neurons with an Axon 200B amplifier (Molecular Devices), and the stimulations were delivered by a bipolar tungsten stimulating electrode placed in layer V/VI of the ACC. The recording pipettes (3–5 MΩ) were filled with a solution containing (in mM) 145 K-gluconate, 5 NaCl, 1 $MgCl_2$, 0.2 EGTA, 10 HEPES, 2 Mg-ATP, 0.1 Na^3-GTP (adjusted to pH 7.2 with KOH, 290 mOsmol). AMPA and kainate receptor mediated EPSCs were induced by repetitive stimulations at 0.02 Hz, and neurons were voltage clamped at −60 mV in the presence of AP5 (50 μM) for AMPA currents and both AP5 and GIKI 53655 (100 μM) for KA currents. NMDA receptor mediated EPSCs were pharmacologically isolated in Mg^{2+}-free ACSF containing CNQX (20 μM) and glycine (1 μM), and neurons were voltage-clamped at −20 to −30 mV and induced by repetitive stimulations at 0.05 Hz. The patch electrode internal solution (in mM) 112 Cs-Gluconate, 5 TEA-Cl, 3.7 NaCl, 0.2 EGTA, 10 HEPES, 2 Mg-ATP, 0.1 Na^3-GTP and 5 QX-314 (adjusted to PH 7.2 with CsOH, 290 mOsmol) were used for recording NMDA receptor mediated EPSCs and AMPA, KA, NMDA receptors mediated I-V curves. For miniature EPSCs (mEPSCs) recording, TTX (1 μM) was added in the perfusion solution. The current-clamp configuration was used recording action potentials (APs) for a single spike (current injection of 100 pA/5 ms) and five spikes at 5, 10, 20, and 50 Hz (current injection five times of 100 pA/5 ms at different frequencies). Picrotoxin (100 μM) was always present to block $GABA_A$ receptor mediated inhibitory synaptic currents in all experiments. Access resistance was 15–30 MΩ and monitored throughout the experiment. Data were discarded if access resistance changed 15% during an experiment. Data were filtered at 1 kHz, and digitized at 10 kHz using the digidata 1440A.

To identify the morphological properties of the pyramidal cells in the tree shrew, 0.5% biocytin was added into the recording solution for the labeled patched neurons. After recording, the brain slices containing biocytin labeled cells were immediately fixed with 4% paraformaldehyde in 0.1 M PB (pH 7.4, containing saturation picric acid) for 4 h at room temperature. Then the slices were transferred to 30% sucrose overnight at 4 °C temperature. After thoroughly washing with PBS, all slices were immunostained with FITC conjugated avidin (1:200, Jackson) for 2 h at room temperature. The immunofluorescence labeled neurons were imaged with a confocal microscope (Fluoview FV1000, Olympus, Tokyo, Japan) using the appropriate filter for FITC. Each section was imaged through the depth scan and collapsed stack using z projection generated a two-dimensional reconstruction of the labeled neurons. The photomicrograph was assembled by the software of Adobe Photoshope. Only brightness and contrast were adjusted.

Two-photon calcium imaging

In vitro calcium imaging was performed using a two-photon laser scanning microscope (Olympus FV1000-MPE system, BX61WI microscope) based on a pulsed Ti-sapphire laser (MaiTai HP DeepSee, 690–1040 nm wavelength, 2.5 W average power, 100 fs pulse width, 80 MHz repetition rate; New Port Spectra-Physics, Santa Clara, CA, USA). The laser was focused through a × 40 water-immersion objective lens (LUMPLFL/IR40XW, N.A.: 0.8, Olympus, Tokyo, Japan) and the average power was set to <15 mW (measured under the objective). Neurons were filled with indicators via the patch pipette for 20–30 min to allow diffusion of the dye into the cells. Fluorescent imaging of Cal-520 K^+ salt (200 μM) and Alexa594 K^+ salt (20 μM) were separated into green and red channels by a dichroic mirror and emission filters (Chroma, Bellows Falls, VT, USA), and detected by a pair of photomultiplier tubes (Hamamatsu, Shizuoka, Japan) at 800 nm. To obtain time series of fluorescent signals from global soma images, images were collected with the following parameters [26–29]: 512 × 512 pixel images, digital zoom 3× with ×40 objective (N.A. 0.8), 2-μs pixel dwell time, 50 ms/frame for frame scan model with different recording times for different recording frames. Bidirectional scanning and line-scanning models were used to increase scan speed. Each

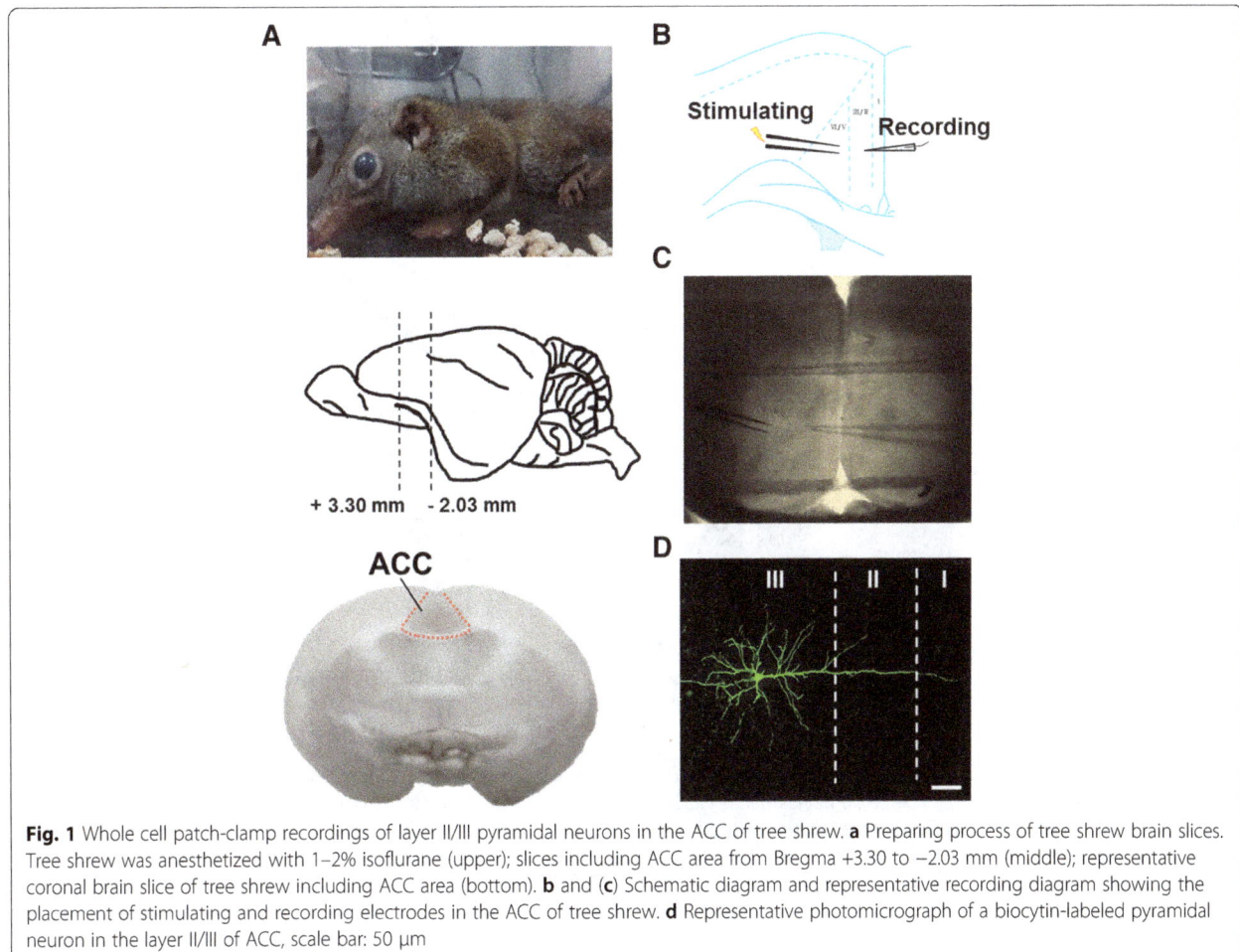

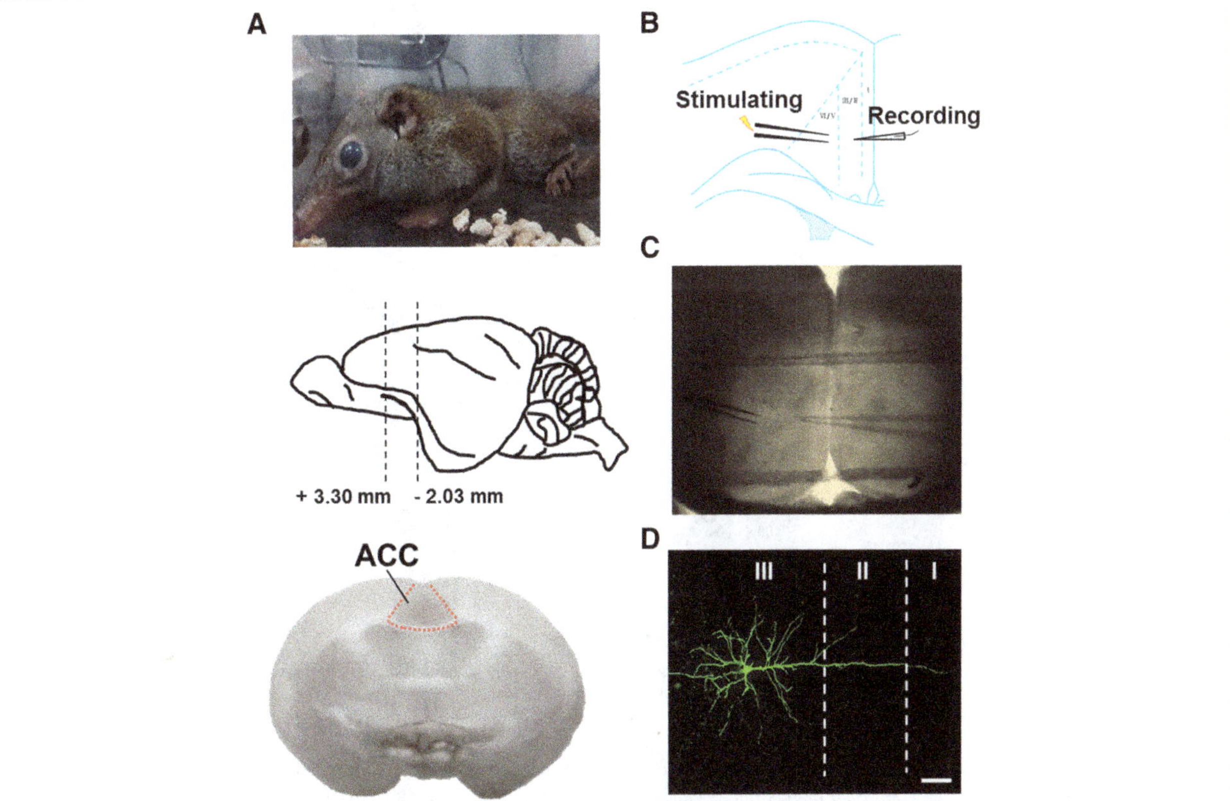

Fig. 1 Whole cell patch-clamp recordings of layer II/III pyramidal neurons in the ACC of tree shrew. **a** Preparing process of tree shrew brain slices. Tree shrew was anesthetized with 1–2% isoflurane (upper); slices including ACC area from Bregma +3.30 to −2.03 mm (middle); representative coronal brain slice of tree shrew including ACC area (bottom). **b** and (**c**) Schematic diagram and representative recording diagram showing the placement of stimulating and recording electrodes in the ACC of tree shrew. **d** Representative photomicrograph of a biocytin-labeled pyramidal neuron in the layer II/III of ACC, scale bar: 50 μm

trial was repeated at least 3 times and the mean value was collected. Fluorescence changes were quantified as increases in green fluorescence from the baseline of $\Delta F/F = (F-F_0)/F_0$.

Drugs

The chemicals and drugs used in this study were as follows: all the chemicals and drugs used in this study were obtained from Sigma (St. Louis, MO, USA), except for CNQX (20 μM), which was purchased from Tocris Cookson (Bristol, UK). All experiments were conducted in the presence of picrotoxin (100 μM) to block $GABA_A$ receptor mediated inhibitory synaptic currents. Drugs were prepared as stock solutions for frozen aliquots at −20 °C. All these drugs were diluted from the stock solution to the final desired concentration in the ACSF before being applied to the perfusion solution.

Data analysis

Data were collected and analyzed with Clampex 10.3 and Clampfit 10.3 software (Molecular Devices). The data were presented as means ± SEM. Statistical analysis of differences were tested by unpaired and paired two-tailed Student's t-test, one-way ANOVA or two-way ANOVA (Student-Newmann-Keuls or Tukey test was used for post-hoc comparisons). In all cases, * $P < 0.05$ was considered statistically significant.

Results

Glutamate mediated excitatory synaptic transmission in the tree shrew

To explore the excitatory synaptic transmission in the ACC of the tree shrew, whole cell patch-clamp recordings were performed on pyramidal neurons in layer II/III of the ACC. In this research, there were 32 male tree shrews used in the experiments, totally. Local electrical stimulation was delivered by a bipolar stimulation electrode placed in layer V/VI of the ACC (Fig. 1b and c). Neurons in layer II/III were selected since our previous studies showed that neurons from this area receive sensory information inputs from the periphery, and play important roles in ACC related functions [8, 10, 23]. In order to characterize morphological properties of the

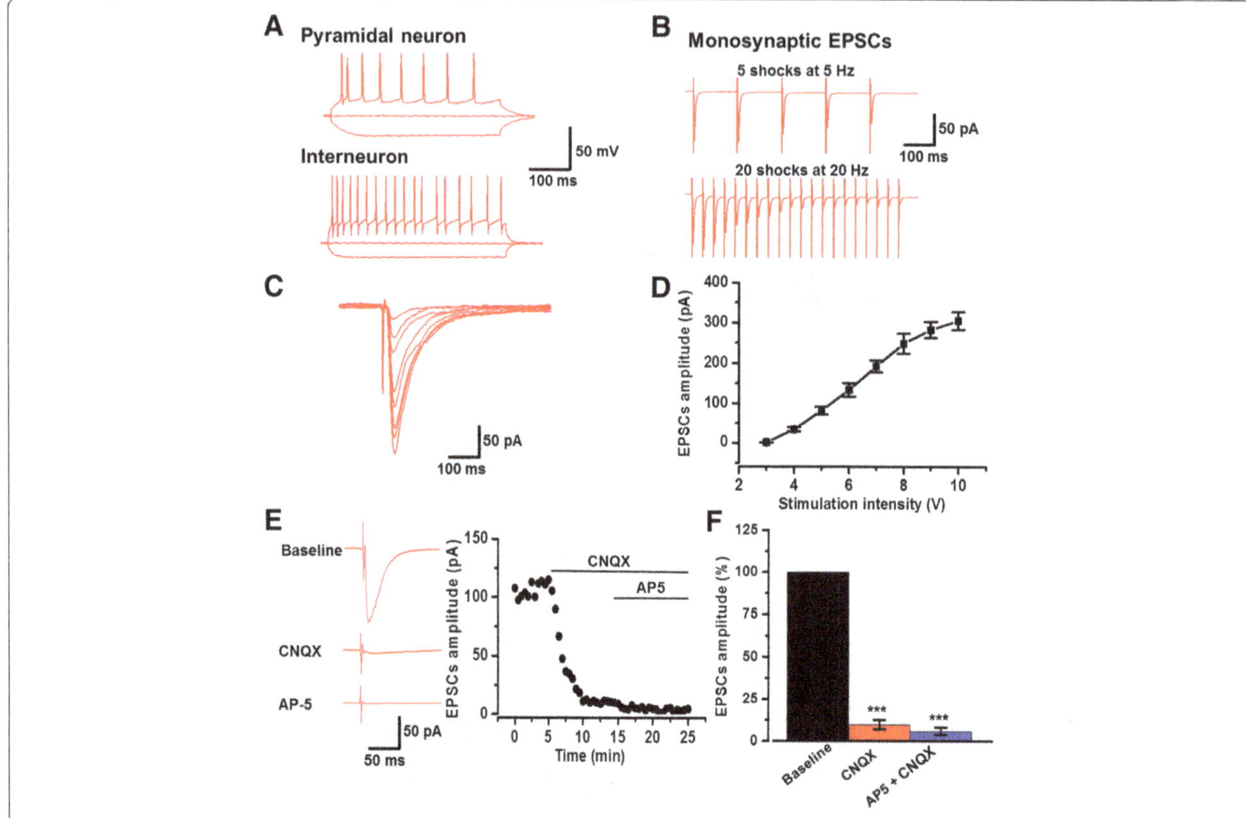

Fig. 2 Glutamatergic neuron mediated EPSCs in the tree shrew. **a** Identification of pyramidal neuron (upper) and interneuron (bottom) by injection of step currents (−50, 0, and 50 pA). **b** Monosynaptic EPSCs induced by 5 shocks at 5 Hz (upper) and 20 shocks at 20 Hz (bottom). **c** and (**d**) Sample traces and pooled data showed the input-output relationship of basal EPSCs in the ACC of tree shrew ($n = 7$ neurons/3 tree shrews). **e** EPSCs were recorded in the presence of picrotoxin (100 μM). After the perfusion of CNQX (20 μM) 10 min, a small residual current remained that could be totally blocked by CNQX and AP5 (50 μM) together. Sample traces (left) and sample time course points (right) showed the EPSCs in the presence of CNQX and AP5. **d** Statistical results showed that the percentage of EPSCs in the presence of CNQX and AP5 ($n = 8$ neurons/4 tree shrews). ***$P < 0.001$, error bars indicated SEM

ACC neurons, we labeled the neurons with biocytin during recording. As expected, we found that all pyramidal neurons had mass basal dendrites and a prominent apical dendrite. Basal dendrites were mainly located at same layer and surrounded the soma. Apical dendrite ascended toward the layer I with many branches (Fig. 1d).

The pyramidal neuron of the ACC in the tree shrew was identified by injecting depolarizing currents which induced repetitive action potentials, with the firing pattern differing from interneurons (Fig. 2a) [30, 31]. Monosynaptic synaptic inputs were tested by delivering 5 shocks at 5 Hz and 20 shocks at 20 Hz (Fig. 2b). These synaptic responses followed the repetitive stimuli without failure in the presence of picrotoxin (100 μM), suggesting that they are monosynaptic in nature. To examine synaptic responses, we recorded the input (stimulation intensity)-output (EPSC amplitude) (I-O curves) relationship of excitatory postsynaptic currents (EPSCs) in the ACC neurons. We found the amplitudes of these EPSCs increased with a stimulation density dependent manner (Fig. 2c and d) ($n = 7$ neurons/3 tree shrews).

To test whether the excitatory synaptic transmission is mediated by glutamate, we bath applied an AMPA/Kainate (KA) receptor antagonist 6-cyano-7-nitroquinoxaline-2, 3-dione (CNQX, 20 μM). EPSCs were rapidly and largely reduced by CNQX. Small residual EPSCs persisted in the presence of CNQX 10 min after perfusion. These EPSCs were blocked by following application of NMDA receptor antagonist D-2-amino-5-phosphonopentanoic acid (AP5, 50 μM) (Baseline: −138.4 ± 8.5 pA; CNQX: -11.2 ± 2.0 pA, 8.1 ± 1.5% of baseline; AP5: −6.8 ± 1.4 pA, 4.9 ± 1.0% of baseline; $n = 8$ neurons/4 tree

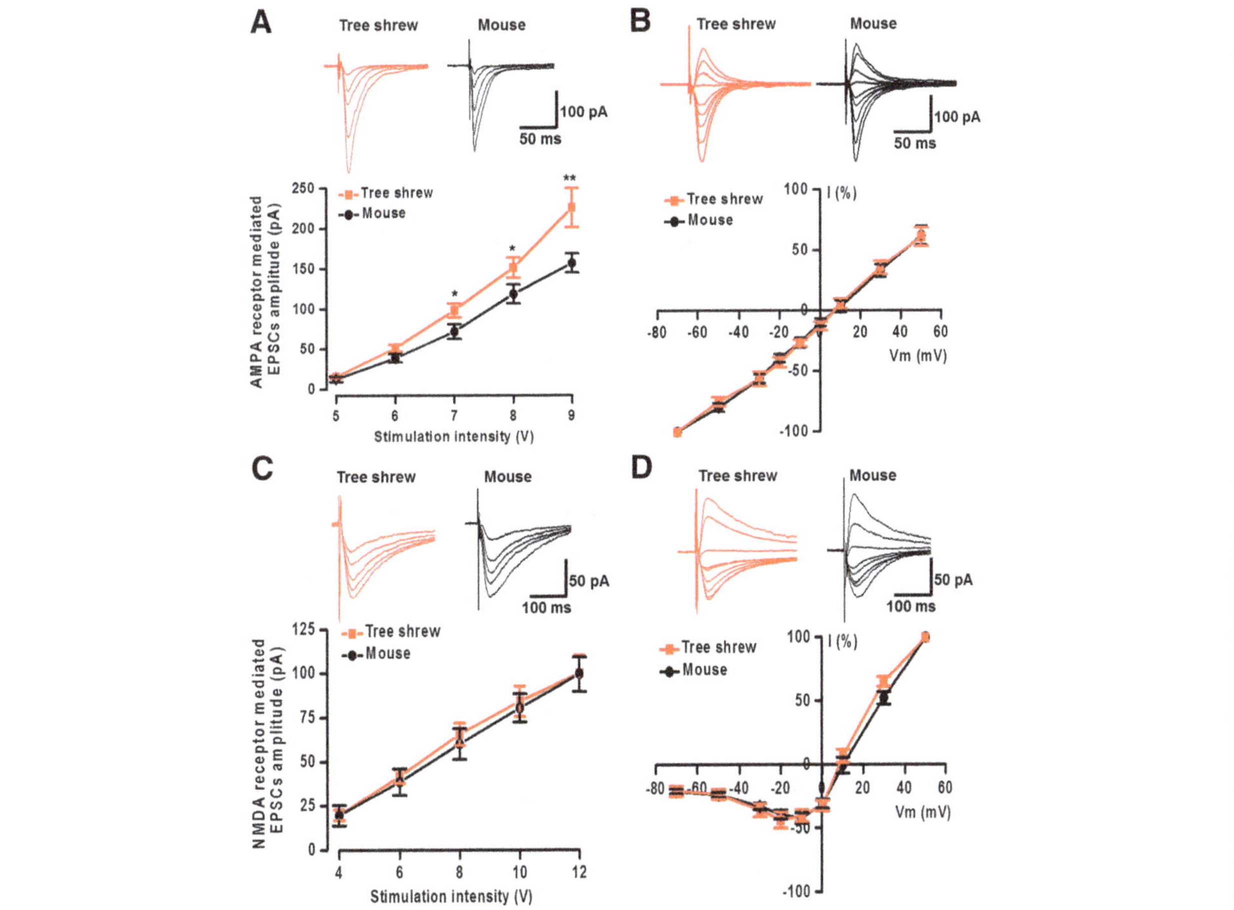

Fig. 3 The characteristics of AMPA and NMDA receptor mediated EPSCs in the tree shrew. **a** Representative traces and pooled data showed the input-output curve of AMPA receptor mediated EPSCs were shifted to the left in tree shrew ($n = 13$ neurons/6 tree shrews) compared with in mouse ($n = 17$ neurons/6 mice). **b** AMPA receptor mediated I-V curves were not different in the ACC neurons between tree shrew and mouse (n = 8 neurons/4 tree shrews and 11 neurons/5 mice). **c** NMDA receptor mediated input-output curves in tree shrew and mouse were not different (n = 8 neurons/4 tree shrews and n = 13 neurons/4 mice). **d** NMDA receptor mediated I-V curves in tree shrew and mouse were not different between in tree shrew and mouse (n = 7 neurons/3 tree shrews and $n = 10$ neurons/4 mice). $^{*}P < 0.05$, $^{**}P < 0.01$, error bars indicated SEM

shrews; Fig. 2e and f). These results indicate that, as with the rodents, glutamate is the major excitatory synaptic transmitter in the ACC pyramidal neurons of the tree shrew and the post-synaptic responses are mainly mediated by AMPA/KA receptors, but less mediated by NMDA receptor.

The AMPA and NMDA receptor mediated EPSCs in the tree shrew

To investigate the properties of AMPA and NMDA receptor-mediated responses in tree shrews, the input-output responses (I-O curves) and current-voltage curves (I-V curves) were recorded in ACC neurons. Picrotoxin (100 μM) and AP5 (50 μM) were bath applied for recording AMPA receptor mediated EPSCs. As shown in Fig. 3a, we found that AMPA receptor mediated I-O curve was shifted to the left in tree shrew (*n* = 13 neurons/6 tree shrews) compared with mouse (*n* = 17 neurons/6 mice; $F_{(1, 151)} = 8.24$, $P < 0.01$, two-way ANOVA), indicating that the basal excitatory responses are potentiated in tree shrew. However, the I-V curves (−70 to +50 mV) were not different between tree shrew and mouse (*n* = 8 neurons/4 tree shrews and *n* = 11 neurons/5 mice; $F_{(1, 141)} = 0.13$, $P = 0.72$, two-way ANOVA) (Fig. 3b).

We then tested the NMDA receptor mediated responses in the tree shrew, by investigating the I-O curves and I-V curves in the presence of picrotoxin (100 μM) and CNQX (20 μM). As the results shown in Fig. 3c, NMDA receptor mediated I-O curves were not different between tree shrew and mouse (n = 8 neurons/4 tree shrews and *n* = 13 neurons/4 mice, $F_{(1, 95)} = 0.26$, $P = 0.61$, two-way ANOVA). Furthermore, the I-V curves were also not different between tree shrew and mouse (*n* = 7 neurons/3 tree shrews and *n* = 10 neurons/4 mice, $F_{(1, 127)} = 0.49$, $P = 0.48$, two-way ANOVA) (Fig. 3d). Our results suggest that the basal NMDA receptor mediated responses are not different in tree shrew and mouse.

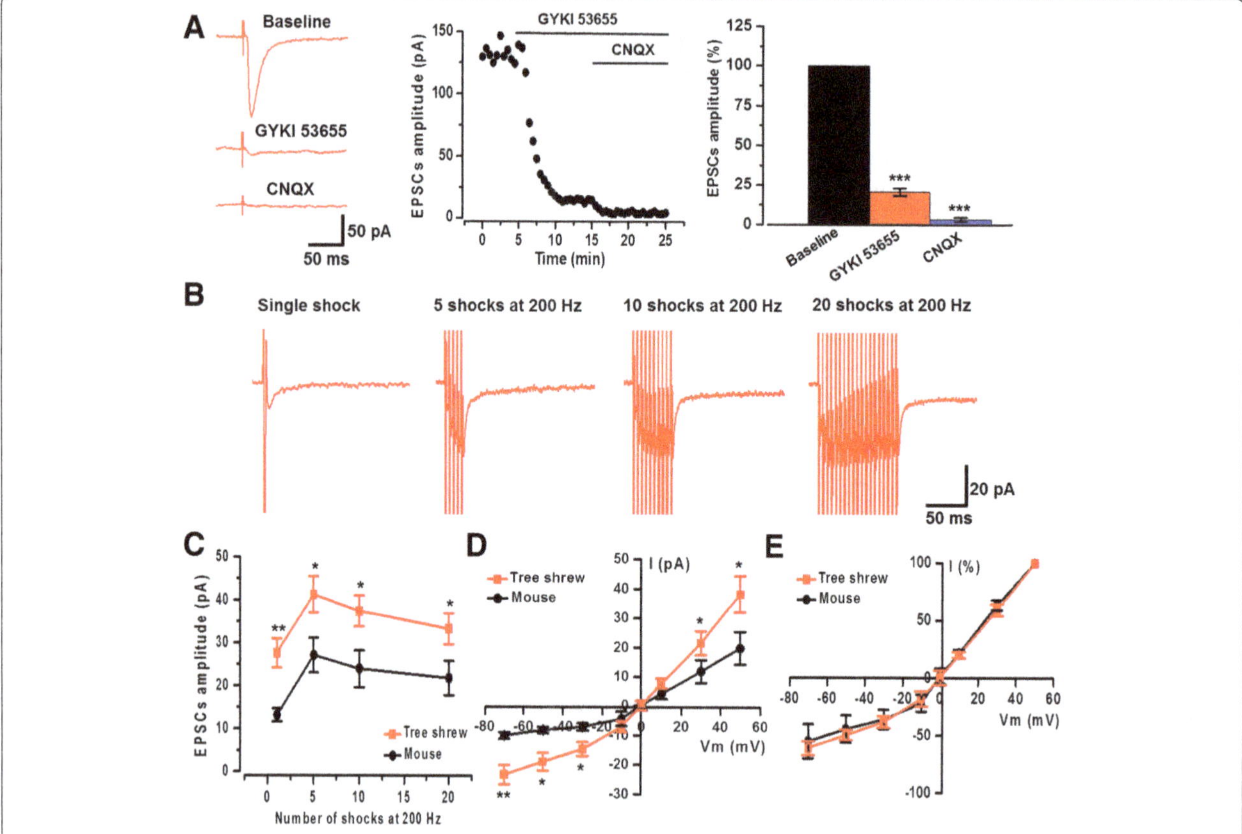

Fig. 4 Kainate receptor mediated EPSCs in the tree shrew. **a** In the presence of picrotoxin (100 μM) and AP5 (50 μM), KA receptor mediated EPSCs could be observed after application of GYKI 53655 (100 μM) and then blocked by CNQX (20 μM). Sample traces (left), sample time course points (middle), and statistical results (right) showed that the EPSCs in the presence of GYKI 53655 and CNQX (*n* = 6 neurons/3 tree shrews). **b** Representative traces of KA receptor mediated EPSCs obtained after application of different number of stimuli (1, 5, 10 and 20 shocks) at 200 Hz. **c** Statistical results showed that the peak amplitude of the KA EPSCs in tree shrew was larger than those in mouse by repetitive stimulations (200 Hz) (*n* = 11 neurons/4 tree shrews and *n* = 9 neurons/3 mice). Note that 5 shocks induced a saturated current. The amplitude (**d**) and the percentage (**e**) of current-voltage relationship (I-V curves from −70 to +50 mV) for KA receptor mediated EPSCs in tree shrew and mouse (n = 10 neurons/4 tree shrews; n = 7 neurons/3 mice). *$P < 0.05$, **$P < 0.01$, error bars indicated SEM

KA receptor mediated EPSCs in the tree shrew

In addition to AMPA receptors, KA receptors have been found to play roles in synaptic transmission in the ACC [17, 18, 23, 32]. We then examined whether KA receptors contribute to synaptic responses in the ACC neuron of tree shrew (Fig. 4). After recording a steady basal EPSCs in the presence of picrotoxin (100 μM) and AP5 (50 μM), a potent AMPA receptor antagonist GYKI 53655 (100 μM) was bath applied to isolate KA receptor mediated EPSCs. As shown in Fig. 4a, GYKI 53655 rapidly and rigorously reduced the basal EPSCs in the ACC of tree shrew. The small residual EPSCs were then blocked by following application of CNQX. As calculated, KA receptors contributed 19.4 ± 2.2% of the AMPA/KA currents (AMPA/KA EPSCs: −148.8 ± 12.7 pA; KA EPSCs: -28.8 ± 3.3 pA, $n = 6$ neurons/3 tree shrews). These results suggest that KA receptors mediate a relatively small component of the excitatory non-NMDA receptor mediated synaptic transmission in the ACC of tree shrew.

Previous studies have been shown that brief repetitive impulse trains increased KA receptor mediated EPSCs [17, 18]. To determine the summarized amplitude of KA receptor mediated EPSCs, repetitive stimuli were applied for 1, 5, 10 and 20 shocks at 200 Hz in the presence of GYKI 53655 in the ACC of tree shrew. As shown in Fig. 4b and c, the amplitudes of KA receptor mediated EPSCs were accumulated with five repetitive stimuli (−41.3 ± 4.2 pA by 5 shocks, −37.5 ± 3.6 pA by 10 shocks, and −33.4 ± 3.6 pA by 20 shocks compared with −27.6 ± 3.4 pA by single stimulation, $n = 11$ neurons/4 tree shrews, $P < 0.05$; Fig. 4c). However, the amplitudes were not further increased with more number of shocks (10–20), suggesting a saturation of the KA EPSCs. Interestingly, we found the KA receptor mediated EPSCs were significantly larger in tree shrew compared with mouse (n = 11 neurons/4 tree shrews; $n = 9$ neurons/3 mice; $F_{(1,\ 71)} = 18.80$, $P < 0.01$, two-way ANOVA) (Fig. 4c).

Next we wanted to study the further characteristics of the current-voltage (*I-V*) relationship in KA receptor mediated EPSCs. The *I-V* curve of KA receptor can reflect the calcium permeability and the subunit composition of channels [17, 18, 33]. KA EPSCs were induced by single shock in the presence of GYKI 53655. When recorded at various holding potentials ranging from −70

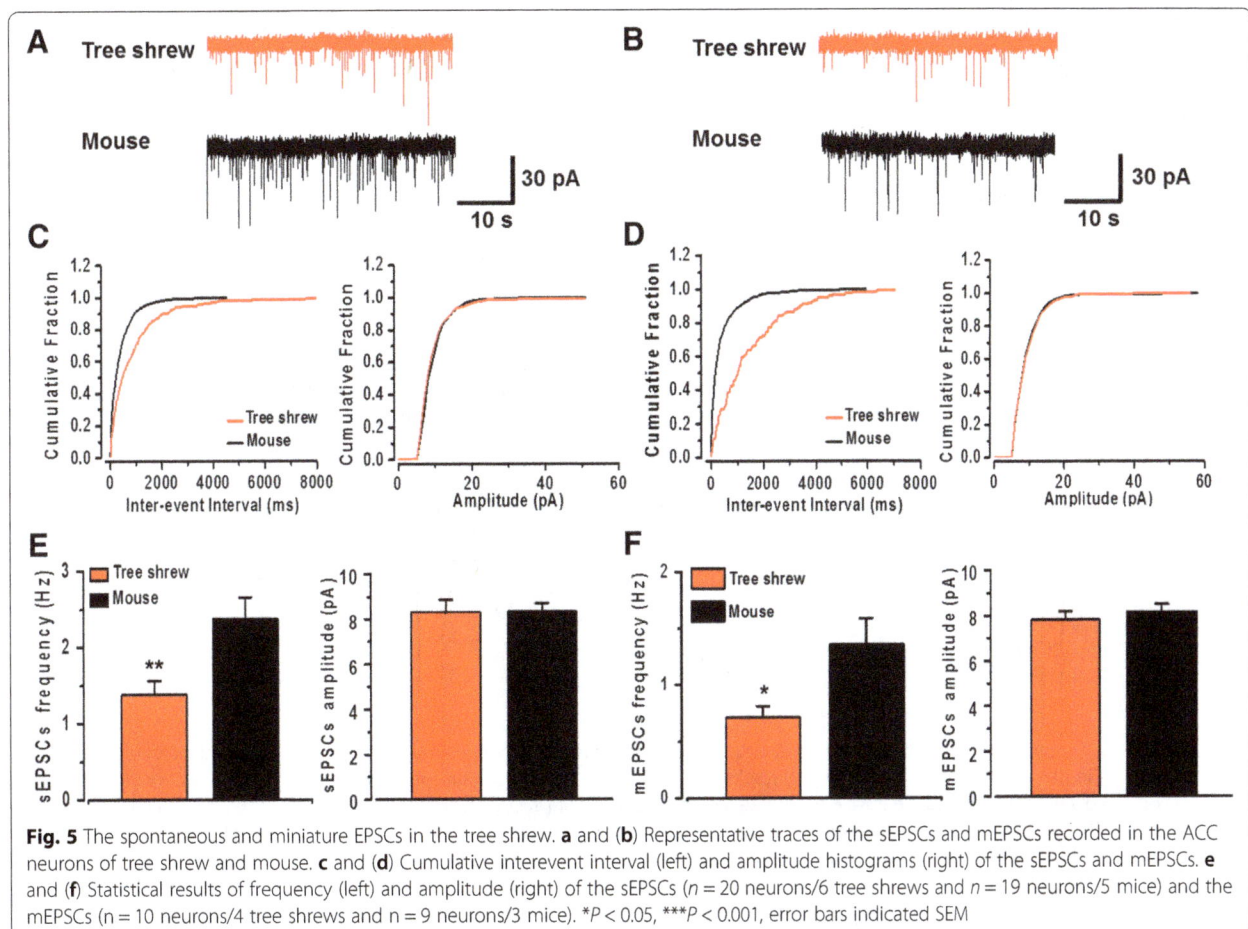

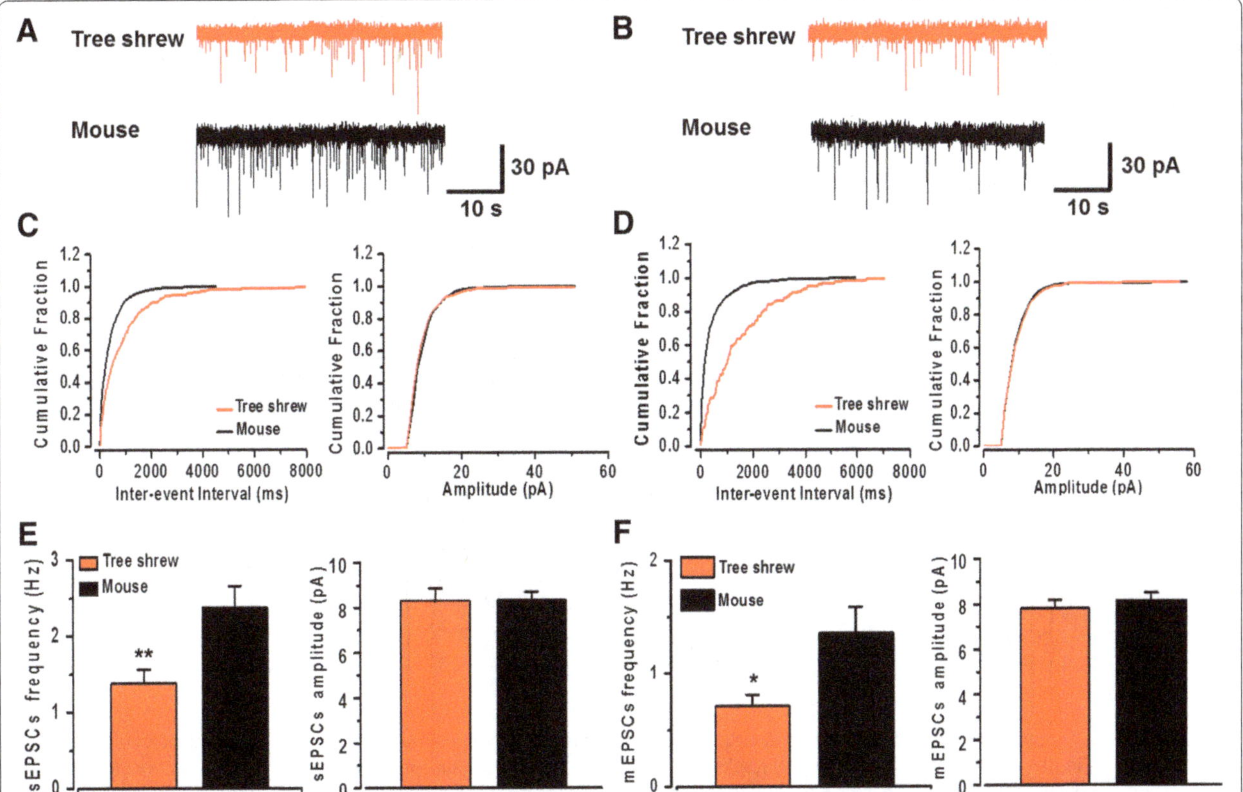

Fig. 5 The spontaneous and miniature EPSCs in the tree shrew. **a** and (**b**) Representative traces of the sEPSCs and mEPSCs recorded in the ACC neurons of tree shrew and mouse. **c** and (**d**) Cumulative interevent interval (left) and amplitude histograms (right) of the sEPSCs and mEPSCs. **e** and (**f**) Statistical results of frequency (left) and amplitude (right) of the sEPSCs ($n = 20$ neurons/6 tree shrews and $n = 19$ neurons/5 mice) and the mEPSCs (n = 10 neurons/4 tree shrews and n = 9 neurons/3 mice). *$P < 0.05$, ***$P < 0.001$, error bars indicated SEM

to 50 mV, KA EPSCs reversed at a potential of −0.12 ± 3.3 mV (n = 10 neurons/4 tree shrews, Fig. 4d). The mean rectification index of the KA EPSCs (ratio of estimated conductance at +40 and −60 mV) was 1.67 ± 0.17. In some cases, there were few neurons shown lower rectification index (0.93 ± 0.07, n = 3 neurons in total 10 neurons), indicating they have smaller outward currents of KA EPSCs. The *I-V* curves of the amplitude of KA EPSCs showed both stronger inward currents and outward currents in the ACC neuron of tree shrew than that of mouse (n = 10 neurons/4 tree shrews and n = 7 neurons/3 mice; $F_{(1, 112)} = 6.07$, $P < 0.05$, two-way ANOVA) (Fig. 4d). The I-V curves of the percentage of KA EPSCs were not different in the ACC neuron between tree shrew and mouse (n = 10 neurons/4 tree shrews and n = 7 neurons/3 mice, $F_{(1, 112)} = 0.14$, P = 0.70, two-way ANOVA) (Fig. 4e).

Presynaptic glutamate release probability in the tree shrew

To determine the presynaptic glutamate release probability in tree shrew, the spontaneous EPSCs (sEPSCs) and miniature EPSCs (mEPSCs) were recorded in the ACC neurons (Fig. 5). We found that the frequencies of sEPSCs (tree shrew: 1.38 ± 0.18 Hz, n = 20 neurons/6 tree shrews; mouse: 2.37 ± 0.29 Hz, n = 19 neurons/5 mice, $P < 0.01$) and mEPSCs (tree shrew: 0.71 ± 0.10 Hz, n = 10 neurons/4 tree shrews; mouse: 1.36 ± 0.23 Hz, n = 9 neurons/3 mice, $P < 0.05$) were lower in tree shrew compared with mouse. However, the amplitudes of sEPSCs (tree shrew: 8.31 ± 0.56 pA, n = 20 neurons/6 tree shrews; mouse: 8.35 ± 0.37 pA, n = 19 neurons/5 mice, $P > 0.05$) and mEPSCs (tree shrew: 7.82 ± 0.37 pA, n = 10 neurons/4 tree shrews; mouse: 8.16 ± 0.35 pA, n = 9 neurons/3 mice, $P > 0.05$) (Fig. 5) were no different. These results indicate that the presynaptic glutamate release probability is smaller in the ACC of tree shrew.

Spontaneous and action potential related presynaptic glutamate release may come from different vesicle pools and reflect different physiological functions [34]. By testing the ratio of paired-pulse facilitation (PPF), we measured whether the electrical evoked presynaptic glutamate release is also reduced. PPF is a transient form of plasticity that is normally used to measure the presynaptic function [31]. As the results shown in Fig. 6a and b, the PPF ratios, recorded at the intervals of 35, 50, 75, 100, and 150 ms, were significantly greater in tree shrew (n = 27 neurons/6 tree shrews) compared with mouse (n = 22 neurons/6 mice) ($F_{(1, 227)} = 9.78$, $P < 0.01$, two-way ANOVA).

The blocking rate of NMDA receptor mediated responses by (+)-5-methyl-10,11-dihydro-5*H*-dibenzo-[*a,d*]cyclohepten-5,10-imine maleate (MK-801), a non-competitive NMDA receptor antagonist with activity-dependent manner, has been widely reported to estimate the glutamate release probability [31, 35, 36]. As shown

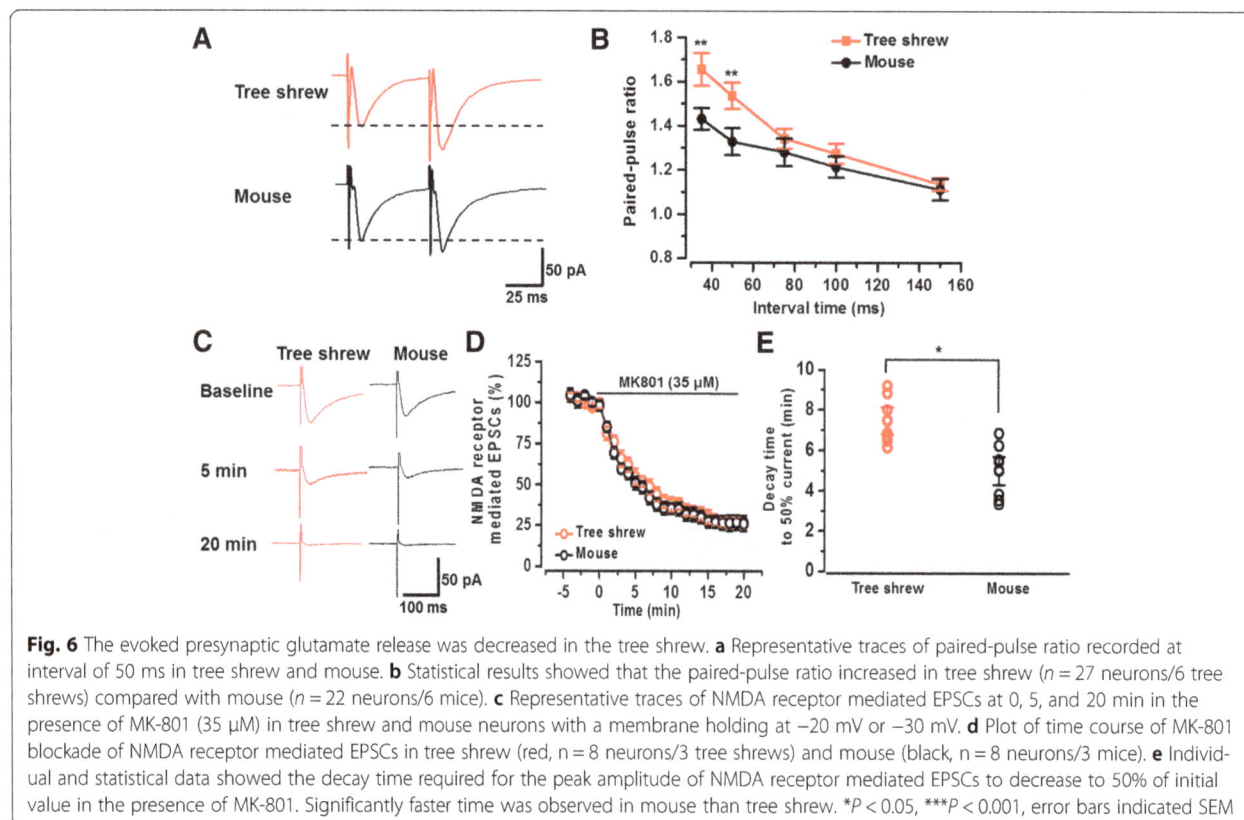

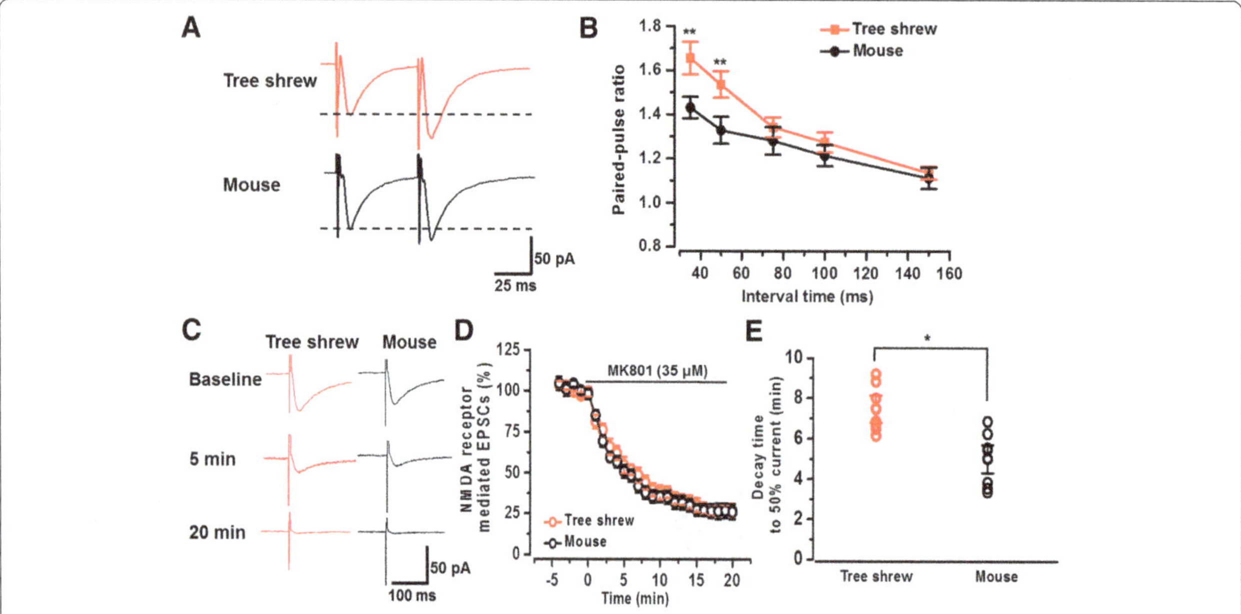

Fig. 6 The evoked presynaptic glutamate release was decreased in the tree shrew. **a** Representative traces of paired-pulse ratio recorded at interval of 50 ms in tree shrew and mouse. **b** Statistical results showed that the paired-pulse ratio increased in tree shrew (n = 27 neurons/6 tree shrews) compared with mouse (n = 22 neurons/6 mice). **c** Representative traces of NMDA receptor mediated EPSCs at 0, 5, and 20 min in the presence of MK-801 (35 μM) in tree shrew and mouse neurons with a membrane holding at −20 mV or −30 mV. **d** Plot of time course of MK-801 blockade of NMDA receptor mediated EPSCs in tree shrew (red, n = 8 neurons/3 tree shrews) and mouse (black, n = 8 neurons/3 mice). **e** Individual and statistical data showed the decay time required for the peak amplitude of NMDA receptor mediated EPSCs to decrease to 50% of initial value in the presence of MK-801. Significantly faster time was observed in mouse than tree shrew. *$P < 0.05$, ***$P < 0.001$, error bars indicated SEM

in Fig. 6c-e, NMDA receptor mediated EPSCs were recorded in the presence of CNQX (20 μM) and picrotoxin (100 μM) at 0.1 Hz with a membrane holding at −20 or −30 mV. MK-801 (35 μM) was perfused after obtaining stable NMDA receptor mediated EPSCs. We found that MK-801 progressively blocked and completely inhibited the NMDA EPSCs in 25 min. The blocking rate of the inhibition of NMDA EPSCs by MK-801 in tree shrew was considerably slower than that of the mouse (Fig. 6d). We compared the decay time from peak to 50% value of initial amplitude of NMDA EPSCs and found the decay time in tree shrew was significantly slower than in mouse (tree shrew: 7.47 ± 0.67 min, $n = 8$ neurons/3 tree shrews; mouse: 4.97 ± 0.69 min, n = 8 neurons/3 mice, $P < 0.05$). Taken together, these results indicate that the rate of presynaptic glutamate release in the ACC of tree shrews is slower as compared with that in mice.

Stimulation intensity and frequency dependent global calcium signals in the tree shrew

Calcium signaling is critical for synaptic transmission and plasticity in the ACC [10, 26]. In the present study, by combining whole-cell patch recording and two-photon Ca^{2+} imaging observation, we recorded the global Ca^{2+} signals in the ACC pyramidal neurons of tree shrew. After 30 min diffusion of Alexa594 and Cal-520, the neuronal morphology was well labeled (Fig. 7a). Action potentials (APs) could be induced by injecting depolarizing currents into the soma of cells through the patch pipette. We found that global calcium transients were obviously observed when APs occurred (Fig. 7b). We then studied the Ca^{2+} signal responses for different stimulus intensities and frequencies in tree shrew neurons. The ΔF/F values of Ca^{2+} signals were both increased with intensities (10 to 100 pA) and frequencies (five APs at 5, 10, 20, and 50 Hz) dependent manners. Interesting, we found the Ca^{2+} signals were significantly larger in tree shrew than mouse (intensity: $F_{(1, 63)} = 4.25$, $P < 0.05$, $n = 6$ neurons/3 tree shrews and $n = 7$ neurons/3 mice; frequency: $F_{(1, 36)} = 8.92$, $P < 0.01$, $n = 5$ neurons/3 tree shrews and 5 neurons/3 mice; two-way ANOVA) (Fig. 7c and d).

Intrinsic properties of the pyramidal neuron in the ACC of tree shrew

Our previous studies have shown that the intrinsic electrophysiological properties of the ACC pyramidal

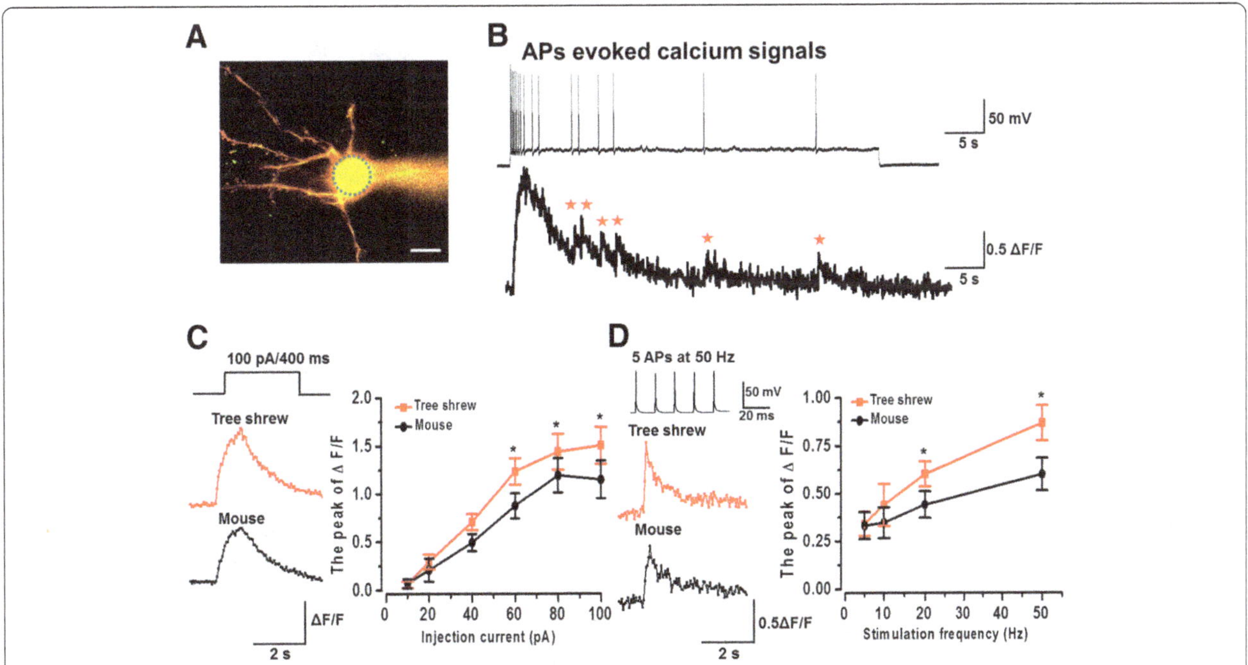

Fig. 7 The global calcium signals in the ACC neurons of tree shrew. **a** Representative two-photon fluorescent photomicrograph of a patched pyramidal neuron loaded by Alexa 594 and Cal-520 in the ACC of tree shrew. Blue dashed circle indicated the scanned area on soma. **b** Injection of currents induced action potentials (APs) and related Ca^{2+} signals. Upper: representative traces of APs evoked by injection of 40 pA (50 s) current; Bottom: related waveforms of fluorescence changes (ΔF/F) of global calcium signals. **c** Calcium signals were increased in a stimulation ntensity dependent manner in tree shrew and mouse. Left: representative waveforms of fluorescence changes (ΔF/F) of Ca^{2+} signals evoked by injection of 100 pA (400 ms) current in tree shrew and mouse. Right: statistical data of stimulation intensity dependent Ca^{2+} signals in tree shrew (n = 6 neurons/3 tree shrews) and mouse (n = 7 neurons/3 mice). **d** Calcium signals were increased in a frequency dependent manner in tree shrew and mouse. Left: representative waveforms of fluorescence changes (ΔF/F) of Ca^{2+} signals evoked by five APs at 50 Hz in tree shrew and mouse. Right: statistical data of frequency dependent Ca^{2+} signals in tree shrew ($n = 5$ neurons/3 tree shrews) and mouse (n = 5 neurons/3 mice). Ca^{2+} signals (ΔF/F) were normalized to control values. *$P < 0.05$, error bars indicated SEM

neurons in mice are important characteristics for neuronal excitability and can undergo dynamic changes according to sensory information inputs [37, 38]. We then examined the intrinsic properties of the ACC pyramidal neurons in tree shrews. As shown in Table 1, tree shrew neurons ($n = 65$ neurons/22 tree shrews) showed a larger membrane capacitance (Cm) (tree shrew: 131.48 ± 6.22 pF; mouse: 107.68 ± 4.90 pF; $P < 0.05$), smaller membrane resistance (Rm) (tree shrew: 263.56 ± 12.37 MΩ; mouse: 324.07 ± 31.52 MΩ; $P < 0.05$) and faster charge-discharge time (Tau) (tree shrew: 4.02 ± 0.14 ms; mouse: 4.92 ± 0.38 ms; $P < 0.01$), suggesting that the tree shrew pyramidal cells have a larger membrane surface and higher electrical responses capability. By analyzing single AP at the threshold, we found the half width (tree shrew: 1.25 ± 0.02 ms; mouse: 1.37 ± 0.04 ms; $P < 0.01$) and decay time (tree shrew: 1.09 ± 0.04 ms; mouse: 1.36 ± 0.08 ms; $P < 0.01$) were smaller in tree shrews than mice. The decay slope (tree shrew: −78.65 ± 2.72 mV/ms; mouse: −60.41 ± 4.69 mV/ms; $P < 0.001$) was larger in tree shrews as well. These results indicate that the spike of pyramidal cell is more narrow and sharp in tree shrews than mice. However, although the resting membrane potential (RMP) and the threshold membrane potential ($V_{threshold}$) were not different, the rheobase (the minimum current required to evoke an AP) was higher in tree shrews compared to mice. Taken together, the present results suggest that, although a stronger current input is needed to initiate the spike (maybe due to the larger surface membrane and capacitance), pyramidal cells in tree shrews will spike more intensely than in mice. The hypothesis were further confirmed after injection of increased step current, in which the spike number of tree shrew neurons was not different with mouse neurons in face of weak inputs, but was significantly larger in face of stronger inputs ($n = 12$ neurons/4 tree shrews and $n = 15$ neurons/5 mice; $F_{(1, 217)} = 38.94$, $P < 0.001$, two-way ANOVA) (Fig. 8a).

Table 1 Summary of basal electrophysiological properties of pyramidal neurons in the ACC of tree shrew

	Tree shrew (n = 22)	Mouse (n = 17)	*t*-Test
Number of neurons	$n = 65$	$n = 60$	
Cm (pF)	131.48 ± 6.22	107.68 ± 4.90	$P < 0.05$
Rm (MΩ)	263.56 ± 12.37	324.07 ± 31.52	$P < 0.05$
Tau (ms)	4.02 ± 0.14	4.92 ± 0.38	$P < 0.01$
RMP (mV)	−71.46 ± 0.68	−70.36 ± 1.34	
$V_{threshold}$ (mV)	−42.73 ± 0.87	−43.86 ± 0.85	
Rheobase (pA)	27.23 ± 1.91	17.60 ± 1.42	$P < 0.01$
Peak amplitude (mV)	98.47 ± 1.15	101.19 ± 1.51	
Time of peak (ms)	222.35 ± 8.51	233.60 ± 12.19	
Area (mV.ms)	124.30 ± 2.91	131.84 ± 4.39	
Half-width (ms)	1.25 ± 0.02	1.37 ± 0.04	$P < 0.01$
Rise time (ms)	0.63 ± 0.01	0.64 ± 0.02	
Rise slope (mV/ms)	130.85 ± 2.57	132.33 ± 3.39	
Decay time (ms)	1.09 ± 0.04	1.36 ± 0.08	$P < 0.01$
Decay slope (mV/ms)	−78.65 ± 2.72	−60.41 ± 4.69	$P < 0.001$
AHP peak (mV)	−9.67 ± 1.07	−7.75 ± 1.14	
ADP peak (mV)	9.05 ± 0.61	7.08 ± 1.36	

Values are means ± SEM
RMP Resting membrane potential, *AHP* Afterhyperpolarization, *ADP* Afterdepolarization

According to the action potential firing pattern, the pyramidal cells are classified into three groups: the regular spiking (RS) (AHP without ADP), intermediate (IM) (AHPs with ADP), and intrinsic bursting (IB) (the ADP will trigger bursting spikes) neurons. In our previous studies, IM and IB cells showed the higher membrane excitability than RS cell, and the population distribution of them were increased in neuropathic pain mice [38]. IB cells showed significantly greater firing frequencies than RS and IM cells after peripheral noxious pinch stimuli. In the present study, we found the ratio of IM and IB cells were higher, and RS cells were smaller in tree shrews than in mice (tree shrew: RS 6.1%, IM 55.4%, IB 38.5%, total $n = 65$ neurons/22 tree shrews; mouse: RS 36.7%, IM 43.3%, IB 20.0%, total $n = 60$ neurons/17 mice) (Fig. 8b and Table 1). For the morphological properties, we observed that all three kinds of neurons showed abundant basal dendrites and a prominent apical dendrite. Specifically, the apical dendrites of IB neuron sent forth mass branches which formed apical tufts. Taken together, these results further suggest that pyramidal cells in tree shrews are more active.

Discussion

Cortical synaptic transmission and plasticity are critical for sensory and cognitive processes in mammals. However, there is limited information about cortical synaptic transmission and plasticity obtained from primate animal models. Recent cumulative evidence has shown that the tree shrew is a potentially useful primate-like animal model for human brain diseases [1–4]. In the present study, we investigated the excitatory synaptic transmission and intrinsic properties of pyramidal neurons in the ACC of adult tree shrews. We found that glutamate is the major excitatory transmitter for fast synaptic transmission. Both AMPA and KA receptors contribute to postsynaptic responses. As compared with excitatory responses recorded in mouse ACC, ACC in the tree shew show stronger excitatory transmission.

Postsynaptic transmission in the tree shrew

Glutamatergic synaptic transmission plays important roles in both physiological and pathological conditions to play important roles in the ACC [9, 10]. In the

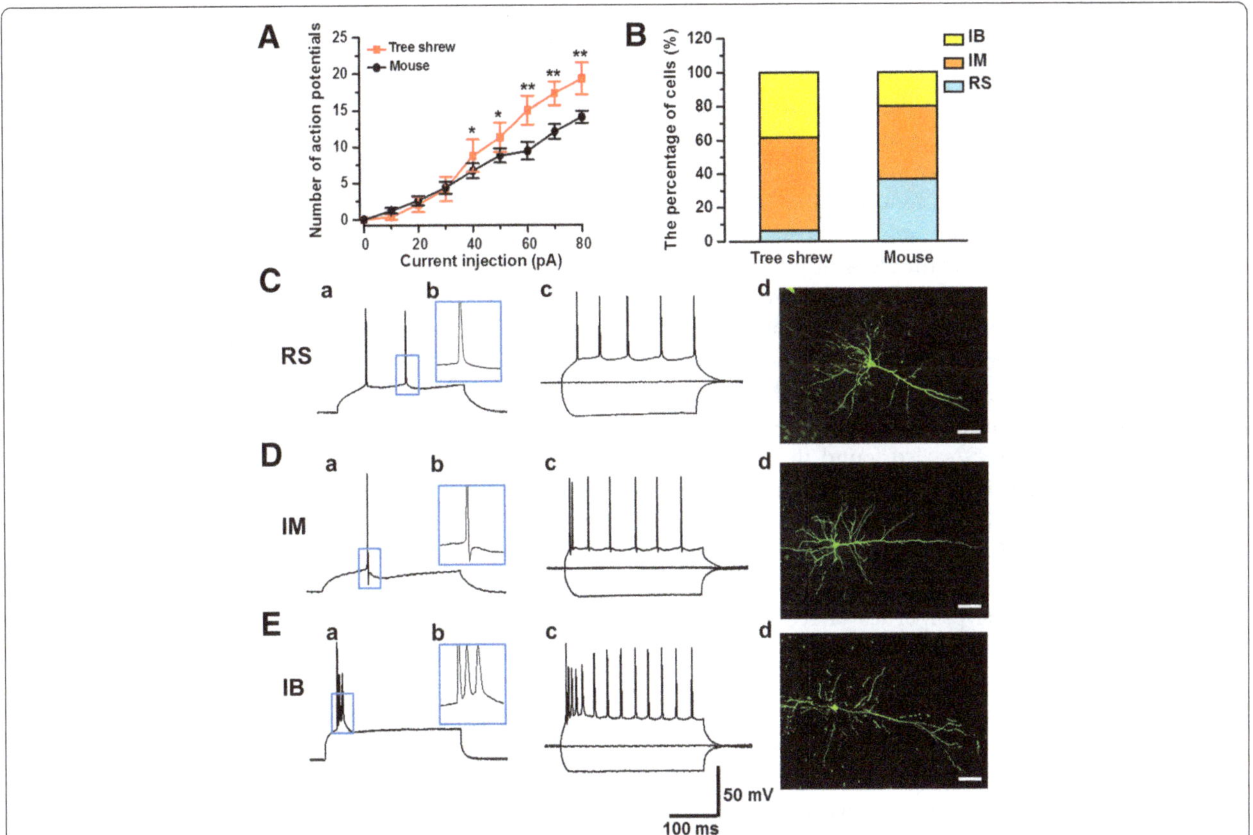

Fig. 8 Morphological and intrinsic properties of pyramidal neurons in the ACC of tree shrew. **a** Averaged action potential numbers induced by step currents injection (400 ms, 10 pA per step) showed that the spike numbers of tree shrew neurons ($n = 12$ neurons/4 tree shrews) was larger than compared with mouse ($n = 15$ neurons/5 mice). **b** The percentage of three kinds of pyramidal neurons in tree shrew: regular spike (RS), intermediate (IM) and intrinsic bursting (IB) neurons ($n = 65$ neurons/22 tree shrews; $n = 60$ neurons/17 mice). **c-e** Electrophysiological and morphological properties of three kinds of pyramidal neurons in the ACC of tree shrew. A single current-clamp trace for the first spike induced by a series of intracellular current pulses (400 ms, 5 pA per step) (a). The blue frame in image (a) was enlarged in image (b). Superimposed current-clamp traces evoked by the current injections of −50, 0, +50 pA (c). Representative biocytin labeled profiles of recording pyramidal neurons as visualized with confocal laser scanning microscopy (d), scale bar: 50 μm

current study, we found that AMPA receptor mediated responses were greater in tree shrews as compared with mice. However, there is no difference of NMDA receptor mediated EPSCs between tree shew and mouse ACC. This finding suggests that postsynaptic AMPA receptors are more effective in response to glutamate in tree shrew synapses. Future studies are clearly needed to explore a molecular basis for such difference.

Postsynaptic KA receptors contribute to fast synaptic responses in pain related cortical areas [17, 18, 39]. Here, we also detected a small fast excitatory synaptic response that is also mediated by KA receptors in the ACC of the tree shrew. Similar to AMPA receptor mediated responses, KA receptor mediated EPSCs are significantly greater than that in mouse ACC.

Presynaptic transmitter release in the tree shrew

Both presynaptic and postsynaptic glutamate transmissions contribute to synaptic plasticity in the ACC [31, 35, 40]. In the present studies, we found that the frequencies of spontaneous/miniature EPSCs were smaller in tree shrews, suggesting that spontaneous release of glutamate in tree shrews is different from that of rodents. Furthermore, the ratio of PPF and the decay time for fast blockade of NMDA receptor mediated EPSCs are greater in tree shrews, which further indicate that presynaptic release of glutamate and plasticity may be different. It is interesting to note that enhanced postsynaptic responses and reduced spontaneous release of glutamate are features of tree shrew synapses in the ACC.

Postsynaptic calcium signals and intrinsic properties of pyramidal neurons

Calcium signals are thought to be critical for synaptic transmission and plasticity in the ACC [9, 10, 13, 41]. By using two-photon Ca^{2+} imaging observation, our recent studies have characterized the properties of postsynaptic calcium signals in the pyramidal neurons of ACC in mice. We also reveal the dynamic change of Ca^{2+} ion in the induction phase of LTP in the ACC of mice [26]. In the current study, by using a similar method, we found that action potentials evoke significant Ca^{2+} signals in the ACC neurons of tree shrews and that the summation of calcium signals induced by repetitive stimulation is larger in tree shrew neurons as compared with mouse ACC.

We also identified three main types of pyramidal cells (RS, IM, and IB) in the ACC of adult tree shrews, which are similar with cell types reported in mouse ACC [37, 38]. We found that there are a higher proportion of IB and IM cells in tree shrews as compared with mice. This result indicates that neurons in the ACC are likely more excitable in tree shrews. We also found that tree shrew neurons showed higher initial firing frequency and neuronal excitability in the ACC. These results support the notion that the ACC of tree shrews are better developed on a functional level, which is similar with the suggestion about morphological properties of ACC neuron in tree shrew in our previous studies [5].

Physiological and pathological implications

Animal models have been useful for the investigation of different physiological and pathological mechanisms of brain diseases. Cumulative studies have consistently indicated that ACC and related cortical areas play vital roles in many brain functions, including pain perception, fear memory, and anxiety [10, 19, 21]. Although human imaging studies provide strong evidence for ACC, the information on molecular and cellular mechanism in primate brain is generally lacking. The present study of tree shrew ACC provides a possible link between rodent ACCs and the human brain. We believe that the study of tree shrew brains, including the ACC area, will greatly improve our understanding of human brain mechanisms at molecular and synaptic levels, and help us to design better medicines and treatment for patients with different brain disorders in the future.

Abbreviations

ACC: anterior cingulate cortex; ACs: adenylyl cyclases; ACSF: artificial cerebrospinal fluid; ADP: afterdepolarization; AHP: afterhyperpolarization;; AMPA: α-amino-3-hydroxy-5-methyl-4-isoxazole-propionic acid; AP5: D-2-amino-5-phosphonopentanoic acid; CNQX: 6-cyano-7-nitroquinoxaline-2, 3-dione; eEPSCs: evoked excitatory postsynaptic currents; KA: kainate; LTP: long-term potentiation; mEPSCs: miniature excitatory postsynaptic currents; NMDA: N-methyl-D-aspartic acid; PPF: paired-pulse facilitation; RMP: resting membrane potential; sEPSCs: spontaneous excitatory postsynaptic currents

Acknowledgements

We would like to thank Melissa Lepp for the help with English editing.

Funding

This work was supported by grants from the Canadian Institute for Health Research (CIHR) Michael Smith Chair in Neurosciences and Mental Health, Canada Research Chair, CIHR operating grant (MOP-124807) and project grant (PJT-148648), Azrieli Neurodevelopmental Research Program and Brain Canada, awarded to M. Z. and National Natural Science Foundation of China (31,371,126 and 81,671,095) to T. C.

Authors' contributions

XHL, TC and MZ designed the experiments. XHL, QS, QYC, and JSL performed experiments and analyzed data; XHL, TC and MZ drafted the manuscript and finished the final vision of the manuscript. All authors read and approved the final manuscript.

Competing interests

The authors declare that they have no competing interests.

Author details

[1]Center for Neuron and Disease, Frontier Institutes of Science and Technology, Xi'an Jiaotong University, Xi'an 710049, China. [2]Department of Anatomy & K.K. Leung Brain Research Center, Fourth Military Medical University, Xi'an, ShaanXi 710032, China. [3]Department of Physiology, Faculty of Medicine, University of Toronto, Medical Science Building, Room #3342, 1 King's College Circle, Toronto, ON M5S 1A8, Canada.

References

1. Xu L, Chen SY, Nie WH, Jiang XL, Yao YG. Evaluating the phylogenetic position of Chinese tree shrew (Tupaia Belangeri Chinensis) based on complete mitochondrial genome: implication for using tree shrew as an alternative experimental animal to primates in biomedical research. J Genet Genomics. 2012;39:131–7. doi:10.1016/j.jgg.2012.02.003.
2. Fan Y, Huang ZY, Cao CC, Chen CS, Chen YX, Fan DD, He J, Hou HL, Hu L, Hu XT, et al. Genome of the Chinese tree shrew. Nat Commun. 2013;4:1426. doi:10.1038/ncomms2416.
3. Zhou X, Sun F, Xu S, Yang G, Li M. The position of tree shrews in the mammalian tree: comparing multi-gene analyses with phylogenomic results leaves monophyly of Euarchonta doubtful. Integrative Zoology. 2015;10: 186–98. doi:10.1111/1749-4877.12116.
4. Tucholski J, Pinner AL, Simmons MS, Meador-Woodruff JH. Evolutionarily conserved pattern of AMPA receptor subunit glycosylation in mammalian frontal cortex. PLoS One. 2014;9:e94255. doi:10.1371/journal.pone.0094255.
5. Lu JS, Yue F, Liu X, Chen T, Zhuo M. Characterization of the anterior cingulate cortex in adult tree shrew. Mol Pain. 2016;12:1744806916684515. doi:10.1177/1744806916684515.
6. Yamashita A, Fuchs E, Taira M, Yamamoto T, Hayashi M. Somatostatin-immunoreactive senile plaque-like structures in the frontal cortex and nucleus accumbens of aged tree shrews and Japanese macaques. J Med Primatol. 2012;41:147–57. doi:10.1111/j.1600-0684.2012.00540.x.
7. Yamashita A, Fuchs E, Taira M, Hayashi M. Amyloid beta (Abeta) protein- and amyloid precursor protein (APP)-immunoreactive structures in the brains of aged tree shrews. Current Aging Sci. 2010;3:230–8.
8. Zhuo M. Ionotropic glutamate receptors contribute to pain transmission and chronic pain. Neuropharmacology. 2017;112:228–34. doi:10.1016/j.neuropharm.2016.08.014.
9. Zhuo M. Neural mechanisms underlying anxiety-chronic pain interactions. Trends Neurosci. 2016;39:136–45. doi:10.1016/j.tins.2016.01.006.

10. Bliss TV, Collingridge GL, Kaang BK, Zhuo M. Synaptic plasticity in the anterior cingulate cortex in acute and chronic pain. Nat Rev Neurosci. 2016; 17:485–96. doi:10.1038/nrn.2016.68.
11. Zhuo M. Long-term potentiation in the anterior cingulate cortex and chronic pain. Philos Trans R Soc Lond A. 2014;369:20130146. doi:10.1098/rstb.2013.0146.
12. Bushnell MC, Ceko M, Low LA. Cognitive and emotional control of pain and its disruption in chronic pain. Nat Rev Neurosci. 2013;14:502–11. doi:10.1038/nrn3516.
13. Zhuo M. Cortical excitation and chronic pain. Trends Neurosci. 2008;31:199–207. doi:10.1016/j.tins.2008.01.003.
14. Vogt BA. Pain and emotion interactions in subregions of the cingulate gyrus. Nat Rev Neurosci. 2005;6:533–44. doi:10.1038/nrn1704.
15. Johansen JP, Fields HL. Glutamatergic activation of anterior cingulate cortex produces an aversive teaching signal. Nat Neurosci. 2004;7:398–403. doi:10.1038/nn1207.
16. Zhuo M. Contribution of synaptic plasticity in the insular cortex to chronic pain. Neuroscience. 2016;338:220–9. doi:10.1016/j.neuroscience.2016.08.014.
17. Koga K, Sim SE, Chen T, Wu LJ, Kaang BK, Zhuo M. Kainate receptor-mediated synaptic transmissions in the adult rodent insular cortex. J Neurophysiol. 2012;108:1988–98. doi:10.1152/jn.00453.2012.
18. Wu LJ, Zhao MG, Toyoda H, Ko SW, Zhuo M. Kainate receptor-mediated synaptic transmission in the adult anterior cingulate cortex. J Neurophysiol. 2005;94:1805–13. doi:10.1152/jn.00091.2005.
19. Zhao MG, Toyoda H, Lee YS, Wu LJ, Ko SW, Zhang XH, Jia Y, Shum F, Xu H, Li BM, et al. Roles of NMDA NR2B subtype receptor in prefrontal long-term potentiation and contextual fear memory. Neuron. 2005;47:859–72. doi:10.1016/j.neuron.2005.08.014.
20. Li XY, Ko HG, Chen T, Descalzi G, Koga K, Wang H, Kim SS, Shang Y, Kwak C, Park SW, et al. Alleviating neuropathic pain hypersensitivity by inhibiting PKMzeta in the anterior cingulate cortex. Science. 2010;330:1400–4. https://doi.org/10.1126/science.1191792.
21. Koga K, Descalzi G, Chen T, Ko HG, Lu J, Li S, Son J, Kim T, Kwak C, Huganir RL, et al. Coexistence of two forms of LTP in ACC provides a synaptic mechanism for the interactions between anxiety and chronic pain. Neuron. 2015;85:377–89. doi:10.1016/j.neuron.2014.12.021.
22. Song Q, Zheng HW, Li XH, Huganir RL, Kuner T, Zhuo M, Chen T. Selective phosphorylation of AMPA receptor contributes to the network of long-term potentiation in the anterior cingulate cortex. J Neurosci. 2017; doi:10.1523/JNEUROSCI.0925-17.2017.
23. Zhuo M. Cortical kainate receptors and behavioral anxiety. Mol Brain. 2017; 10:16. https://doi.org/10.1186/s13041-017-0297-8.
24. Chen T, Koga K, Descalzi G, Qiu S, Wang J, Zhang LS, Zhang ZJ, He XB, Qin X, Xu FQ, et al. Postsynaptic potentiation of corticospinal projecting neurons in the anterior cingulate cortex after nerve injury. Mol Pain. 2014;10:33. doi:10.1186/1744-8069-10-33.
25. Yamanaka M, Tian Z, Darvish-Ghane S, Zhuo M. Pre-LTP requires extracellular signal-regulated kinase in the ACC. Mol Pain. 2016;12 doi:10.1177/1744806916647373.
26. Li XH, Song Q, Chen T, Zhuo M. Characterization of postsynaptic calcium signals in the pyramidal neurons of anterior cingulate cortex. Mol Pain. 2017;13:1744806917719847. doi:10.1177/1744806917719847.
27. Tada M, Takeuchi A, Hashizume M, Kitamura K, Kano M. A highly sensitive fluorescent indicator dye for calcium imaging of neural activity in vitro and in vivo. Eur J Neurosci. 2014;39:1720–8. doi:10.1111/ejn.12476.
28. Araya R, Vogels TP, Yuste R. Activity-dependent dendritic spine neck changes are correlated with synaptic strength. Proc Natl Acad Sci U S A. 2014;111:E2895–904. doi:10.1073/pnas.1321869111.
29. Camire O, Topolnik L. Dendritic calcium nonlinearities switch the direction of synaptic plasticity in fast-spiking interneurons. J Neurosci. 2014;34:3864–77. doi:10.1523/JNEUROSCI.2253-13.2014.
30. Tsvetkov E, Shin RM, Bolshakov VY. Glutamate uptake determines pathway specificity of long-term potentiation in the neural circuitry of fear conditioning. Neuron. 2004;41:139–51.
31. Xu H, Wu LJ, Wang H, Zhang X, Vadakkan KI, Kim SS, Steenland HW, Zhuo M. Presynaptic and postsynaptic amplifications of neuropathic pain in the anterior cingulate cortex. J Neurosci. 2008;28:7445–53. doi:10.1523/JNEUROSCI.1812-08.2008.
32. Wu LJ, Ko SW, Zhuo M. Kainate receptors and pain: from dorsal root ganglion to the anterior cingulate cortex. Curr Pharm Des. 2007;13:1597–605.
33. Ruano D, Lambolez B, Rossier J, Paternain AV, Lerma J. Kainate receptor subunits expressed in single cultured hippocampal neurons: molecular and functional variants by RNA editing. Neuron. 1995;14:1009–17.
34. Kavalali ET. The mechanisms and functions of spontaneous neurotransmitter release. Nat Rev Neurosci. 2015;16:5–16. doi:10.1038/nrn3875.
35. Zhao MG, Ko SW, Wu LJ, Toyoda H, Xu H, Quan J, Li J, Jia Y, Ren M, Xu ZC, Zhuo M. Enhanced presynaptic neurotransmitter release in the anterior cingulate cortex of mice with chronic pain. J Neurosci. 2006;26:8923–30. doi:10.1523/JNEUROSCI.2103-06.2006.
36. Weisskopf MG, Nicoll RA. Presynaptic changes during mossy fibre LTP revealed by NMDA receptor-mediated synaptic responses. Nature. 1995;376:256–9. doi:10.1038/376256a0.
37. Koga K, Li X, Chen T, Steenland HW, Descalzi G, Zhuo M. In vivo whole-cell patch-clamp recording of sensory synaptic responses of cingulate pyramidal neurons to noxious mechanical stimuli in adult mice. Mol Pain. 2010;6:62. doi:10.1186/1744-8069-6-62.
38. Cao XY, Xu H, Wu LJ, Li XY, Chen T, Zhuo M. Characterization of intrinsic properties of cingulate pyramidal neurons in adult mice after nerve injury. Mol Pain. 2009;5:73. https://doi.org/10.1186/1744-8069-5-73.
39. Kerchner GA, Wang GD, Qiu CS, Huettner JE, Zhuo M. Direct presynaptic regulation of GABA/glycine release by kainate receptors in the dorsal horn: an ionotropic mechanism. Neuron. 2001;32:477–88.
40. Chen T, Wang W, Dong YL, Zhang MM, Wang J, Koga K, Liao YH, Li JL, Budisantoso T, Shigemoto R, et al. Postsynaptic insertion of AMPA receptor onto cortical pyramidal neurons in the anterior cingulate cortex after peripheral nerve injury. Mol Brain. 2014;7:76. doi:10.1186/s13041-014-0076-8.
41. Kang SJ, Liu MG, Shi TY, Zhao MG, Kaang BK, Zhuo M. N-type voltage gated calcium channels mediate excitatory synaptic transmission in the anterior cingulate cortex of adult mice. Mol Pain. 2013;9:58. doi:10.1186/1744-8069-9-58.

4

Foxg1 deletion impairs the development of the epithalamus

Bin Liu[1], Kaixing Zhou[1], Xiaojing Wu[1] and Chunjie Zhao[1,2*]

Abstract

The epithalamus, which is dorsal to the thalamus, consists of the habenula, pineal gland and third ventricle choroid plexus and plays important roles in the stress response and sleep–wake cycle in vertebrates. During development, the epithalamus arises from the most dorsal part of prosomere 2. However, the mechanism underlying epithalamic development remains largely unknown. *Foxg1* is critical for the development of the telencephalon, but its role in diencephalic development has been under-investigated. Patients suffering from FOXG1-related disorders exhibit severe anxiety, sleep disturbance and choroid plexus cysts, indicating that *Foxg1* likely plays a role in epithalamic development. In this study, we identified the specific expression of *Foxg1* in the developing epithalamus. Using a "self-deletion" approach, we found that the habenula significantly expanded and included an increased number of habenular subtype neurons. The innervations, particularly the habenular commissure, were severely impaired. Meanwhile, the *Foxg1* mutants exhibited a reduced pineal gland and more branched choroid plexus. After ablation of *Foxg1* no obvious changes in Shh and Fgf signalling were observed, suggesting that *Foxg1* regulates the development of the epithalamus without the involvement of Shh and Fgfs. Our findings provide new insights into the regulation of the development of the epithalamus.

Keywords: Epithalamus, Habenula, Pineal gland, Choroid plexus, FOXG1-related disorders, Sleep disturbance, *Fgf15*

Introduction

The epithalamus, which consists of the habenula, pineal gland, and third ventricle choroid plexus (3^{rd}Chp), is involved in many functions, including motor control, the sleep–wake cycle and stress responses [1–3]. The habenula is highly conserved in vertebrates and acts as a critical node connecting the forebrain to the midbrain and hindbrain by receiving inputs from the limbic system and the basal ganglia and projecting to the monoaminergic nuclei [4, 5]. The pineal gland is critical for the regulation of circadian rhythms due to its production of melatonin [6], and the choroid plexus synthesizes cerebrospinal fluid (CSF) and many growth factors, including fibroblasts and insulin-like and platelet-derived growth factors, and plays important roles, such as providing a route for nutrients and removing by-products of metabolism [7, 8]. Dysfunction of the epithalamus has been reported to be related to mood disorders, such as major depression, and schizophrenia and sleeping disorders [2, 9–12]. However, knowledge regarding the developmental process of the epithalamus is limited.

During early development, the progenitor domain in the diencephalon is divided into three prosomeres (p), i.e., p1, p2, and p3, along the anterior-posterior axis [13, 14]. P1 and p3 give rise to the pretectum and prethalamus, respectively. The most dorsal region of p2 produces the epithalamus, and the other part generates the thalamus. In the presumptive epithalamic progenitor domain, the most anterior area containing the roof plate develops into the 3^{rd}Chp, while the adjacent part generates the habenular commissure, paired habenulas and pineal gland. Previously, a member of the fibroblast growth factor (Fgf) family, *Fgf8*, has been reported to regulate the development of the habenula and pineal gland in a dose-dependent manner [15]. In zebrafish, Fgf signalling also controls the specification of the pineal complex [16]. However, the molecular and cellular mechanisms underlying the development of the epithalamus still remain largely unknown.

* Correspondence: zhaocj@seu.edu.cn
[1]Key Laboratory of Developmental Genes and Human Diseases, MOE, School of Medicine, Southeast University, Nanjing 210009, People's Republic of China
[2]Depression Center, Institute for Brain Disorders, Beijing 100069, China

Foxg1 encodes a winged-helix transcriptional repressor and has been reported to play critical roles during telencephalic development [17–20]. Patients with mutations in *FOXG1* have been reported to suffer from mental retardation, poor social interactions and severe anxiety [21]. Notably, severe sleep disturbance, deformation of the third ventricle and choroid plexus cysts have also been reported [22, 23]. Thus, *Foxg1* may also be involved in the regulation of epithalamic development. In the present study, we found that a disruption of *Foxg1* leads to an impaired epithalamus with an expanded habenula, a smaller pineal gland and an extremely complicated choroid plexus. Various subtypes of neurons in the habenula exhibited a remarkable increase in number with impaired innervations. Furthermore, ablation of *Foxg1* led to the abnormal sub-regionalization of the epithalamic progenitor domain. Our data provide novel perspectives regarding the development of the epithalamus.

Methods

Animals

Foxg1-Cre (*Foxg1* $^{tm1(cre)Skm}$) [24] mouse line was purchased from the Jackson laboratory (US, *Foxg1-Cre* stock: 006084). The *Foxg1*$^{fl/fl}$ line was obtained as previously described [19, 25]. The *Fzd10-EGFP* transgenic line was generated using standard methods (unpublished data). *Foxg1* disruption was achieved by an intercross of *Foxg1-cre* or crossing *Foxg1-cre* with *Foxg1*$^{fl/+}$. Both *Foxg1*$^{cre\text{-}cre}$ *and Foxg1-cre;Foxg1*$^{fl/+}$ were considered mutants, and their wild-type littermates and *Foxg1*$^{fl/+}$ were considered controls. All animals were maintained on an outbred CD1 genetic background and were housed in the animal facility of the Southeast University. All experimental procedures followed the guidelines approved by Southeast University. To stage the embryos, the mice were mated in the afternoon. The day the vaginal plug was found at noon was considered embryonic day 0.5 (E0.5), and the day of birth was considered postnatal day 0 (P0).

Tissue processing and Nissl staining

Embryonic brains were directly dissected in cold phosphate buffered saline (PBS) and immediately transferred to 4% paraformaldehyde (PFA, Sigma-Aldrich, 441,244, US) overnight at 4 °C. The brains from P0 were perfused and then post-fixed at 4 °C for 12–16 h. The brains were then cryoprotected in 30% sucrose and embedded in OCT. Coronal sections (8–12 μm thick) were obtained using a Leica cryostat (CM 3050S) and stored at − 70 °C until use. The Nissl staining was performed according to standard protocols.

In situ hybridization

E12.5 brains were dissected, immediately transferred to 500 μL of TRI Reagent (Sigma-Aldrich, T9424, US) and processed for total RNA isolation according to the manufacturer's instructions. After purification using the RNeasyPlus Mini Kit (QIAGEN, 74,106, DE), the RNA concentration was measured using an Agilent 2100 Bioanalyser (Agilent Technologies, Palo Alto, CA). In total, 2 μg of purified total RNA was used as the template to synthesize cDNA using the PrimeScript ™ RT Master Mix (Takara, RR036A, CN). The cDNA was then used as the template to amplify DNA fragments by PCR for the probe synthesis. The PCR products were inserted into the pBlueScript vector by T4 ligation polymerase (Takara, 2040A, CN). The probes were synthesized using the Digoxigenin-labelling Mix (Roche, 11,277,073,910, DE) and T3 RNA polymerase (Roche, 11,031,171,001, DE) or T7 RNA polymerase (Roche, 10,881,175,001, DE). The in situ hybridization was performed as previously described [26, 27].

Immunofluorescence

Immunofluorescence was performed as previously described [19]. The primary antibodies and dilutions were as follows: anti-Calretinin (Millipore, AB5054, 1:500); anti-Calbindin (Millipore, AB1778, 1:250); anti-Foxg1 (Abcam, ab18259, 1:1000); anti-GFP (Abcam, ab13970, 1:1000); anti-L1 (Millipore, MAB5272, 1:500); anti-Pax6 (BioLegend, 901,301, 1:1000); and anti-Vglut2 (Millipore, MAB5504, 1:500). The secondary antibodies used were Alexa Fluro 488 donkey anti-chicken (Jackson Lab, 703–545-155, 1:500), Alexa Fluor 488 donkey anti-rabbit (Life, A21206, 1:500), Alexa Fluor 546 donkey anti-rabbit (Life, A10040, 1:500), Alexa Fluro 647 donkey anti-rabbit (Life, A31573, 1:500), Alexa Fluor 488 donkey anti-rat (Life, A21208, 1:500), CF 633 donkey anti-rat (Sigma-Aldrich, SAB4600133, 1:500) and Alexa Fluro 647 donkey anti-mouse (Invitrogen, A21236, 1:500).

Statistical analysis and cell counting

The measurements for the volumetric analyses were performed using every tenth 8 μm coronal section stained with anti-Calretinin. The regions of the habenula were measured using ImageJ software as previously described [28, 29]. The volumes (V) were calculated as $V = \Sigma A \times i \times d$, according to Cavalieri's principle, where A represents the sum of the areas in the habenula, I represents the intervals between the sections, and d represents the thickness of the sections. The measurements for analysis of the thickness of habenular commissure were performed using every third 10 μm coronal section by the immunofluorescence of L1. The thickness at the midline area were measured by ImageJ software and calculated by the average. Cells of each distinct cell type in the sub-nuclei of the habenula were counted, and the numbers of CR^+, CB^+, $Tac1^+$ and $Pax6^+$ cells were counted in every tenth 8 μm coronal section from each side of the habenula and summed to obtain the total number. We considered every strong Tac1$^+$ staining dot as a single cell under high magnification views. Very weak staining was not taken into account. Both controls and mutants were counted under the same criterion. The area of Brn3a$^+$ cells in the medial habenula was measured by ImageJ software in every third 10 μm coronal section from one side of the habenula and averaged to obtain the mean area per section. All experiments were performed using at least three different litters, and the data were statistically analysed using GraphPad Prism software. Two-tailed Student's t-test was performed to analyse the statistical significance at $p < 0.05$ (*), $p < 0.01$(**) and $p < 0.001$(***).

Quantitative real time polymerase chain reaction (qRT-PCR)

qRT-PCR was carried out according to the protocols as previously described [19]. The dorsal part of E12.5 diencephalon at least from three different litters were used. The specific primers for *Fgf15* is: 5′-GAGGAAGC CAGAAGGTATGAAG-3′ and 5′-GGCAAGCTAAGA TCCCATGA- 3′.

Results

Foxg1 is specifically expressed in the developing dorsal diencephalon, and ablation of *Foxg1* leads to an impaired epithalamus

The forkhead box transcription factor *Foxg1* has been reported to be critical for telencephalic development [17]. However, the function of *Foxg1* in the diencephalon has been under-investigated. Considering the symptoms, including poor sleep patterns, emotional disorders and choroid plexus cysts, observed in patients suffering from FOXG1 syndrome [21–23], we suspect that *Foxg1* plays an important role in the developing diencephalon. Previously, the forced overexpression of *Foxg1* in chicks has been shown to downregulate *Otx2* in the alar plate of the diencephalon, indicating that *Foxg1* likely plays a role in diencephalic development [30]. In this study, we first analysed the expression of *Foxg1* in detail using in situ hybridization. As shown in Fig. 1a, at E12.5, although extremely strong staining was detected in the developing telencephalon, *Foxg1* was also found to be weakly expressed in the progenitors in the third ventricular zone (3rdVZ) and their postmitotic derivatives. This expression pattern was confirmed by immunostaining with anti-Foxg1 (Fig. 1b, arrow). Strong staining was particularly detected at the dorsal-most region of the diencephalon, which was presumably the epithalamus area from which the habenula, pineal gland and 3rdChp arise (Fig. 1a, b). As development proceeded, the expression level of *Foxg1* gradually increased with stronger expression in the medial habenula (MHb) and weaker expression in the lateral habenula (LHb) at E18.5 (Fig. 1d, e). Previously, a new *Foxg1-IRES-Cre* line that faithfully recapitulates the endogenous *Foxg1* expression also exhibited Cre-medicated recombination in the developing epithalamus [31], which is consistent with our observations. Collectively, *Foxg1* is specifically expressed in the developing diencephalon, particularly in the dorsal part of the 3rdVZ, strongly supporting that *Foxg1* plays a role in the development of the epithalamus.

Subsequently, we adopted the "self-deletion" approach by crossing *Foxg1-Cre* with *Foxg1$^{fl/fl}$* to obtain compound homozygous *Foxg1$^{cre/fl}$* mice [32]. Both *Foxg1$^{cre/fl}$* and *Foxg1$^{cre/cre}$* were considered *Foxg1*-phenotypical null mutants and in this study, all results were obtained in comparable levels from serial sections of the habenula. As shown in Fig. 1c and f, the expression of *Foxg1* in the dorsal diencephalon were effectively eliminated in the mutants at E12.5 and E18.5. We first analysed the changes of the epithalamus during early development. Previously, *Brn3a* (also called *Pou4f1*) has been reported to be strongly expressed in postmitotic neurons in the MHb and weakly expressed in the LHb and critical for the development of the habenula [33]. At the stages of E12.5 and E14.5, in situ staining of *Brn3a* showed the habenula was slightly enlarged and expanded dorsal-laterally after *Foxg1* deletion (Fig. 1g, g'; h, h'). This is confirmed by Nissl staining as well (Fig. 1i, i'). At E18.5, the habenula visualized by Nissl staining expanded much more than that of observed in E12.5 and E14.5. The third ventricle was found to be significantly enlarged which could be a result of the changes caused in the lateral ventricle due to the decrease in the size of the cortex as previously reported [34, 35] (Fig. 1j, j'). However, the pineal gland was smaller (Fig. 1k, k'). Interestingly, the 3rdChp were more branched in *Foxg1* mutants compared to the controls (Fig. 1k, k', asterisk). To further confirm these abnormalities, we performed in situ hybridization for *Frizzled10* (*Fzd10*), one of the Wnt receptors, specifically expressed in the MHb progenitors and postmitotic neurons [36]. As shown in Fig. 1l-l', Fzd10$^+$ region was enlarged. We also generated a *Fzd10-EGFP* transgenic mouse line in which EGFP faithfully reflected the endogenous Fzd10 expression (unpublished data). As shown in Fig. 1m-m', the MHb appeared to expand to the lateral side, resulting in an irregular shape, and the habenular commissure was lengthened and became thinner. A smaller pineal gland was also observed, which is consistent with the observations using Nissl staining. Finally, we evaluated the volume of the habenula and found that it was relative increased by approximately 12% in mutants (Fig. 1n). Collectively, the disruption of *Foxg1* caused an impaired epithalamus.

Increased numbers of epithalamic progenitors and habenular subtype neurons

To further investigate the cause of the enlarged habenula following the *Foxg1* deletion, we examined the progenitor

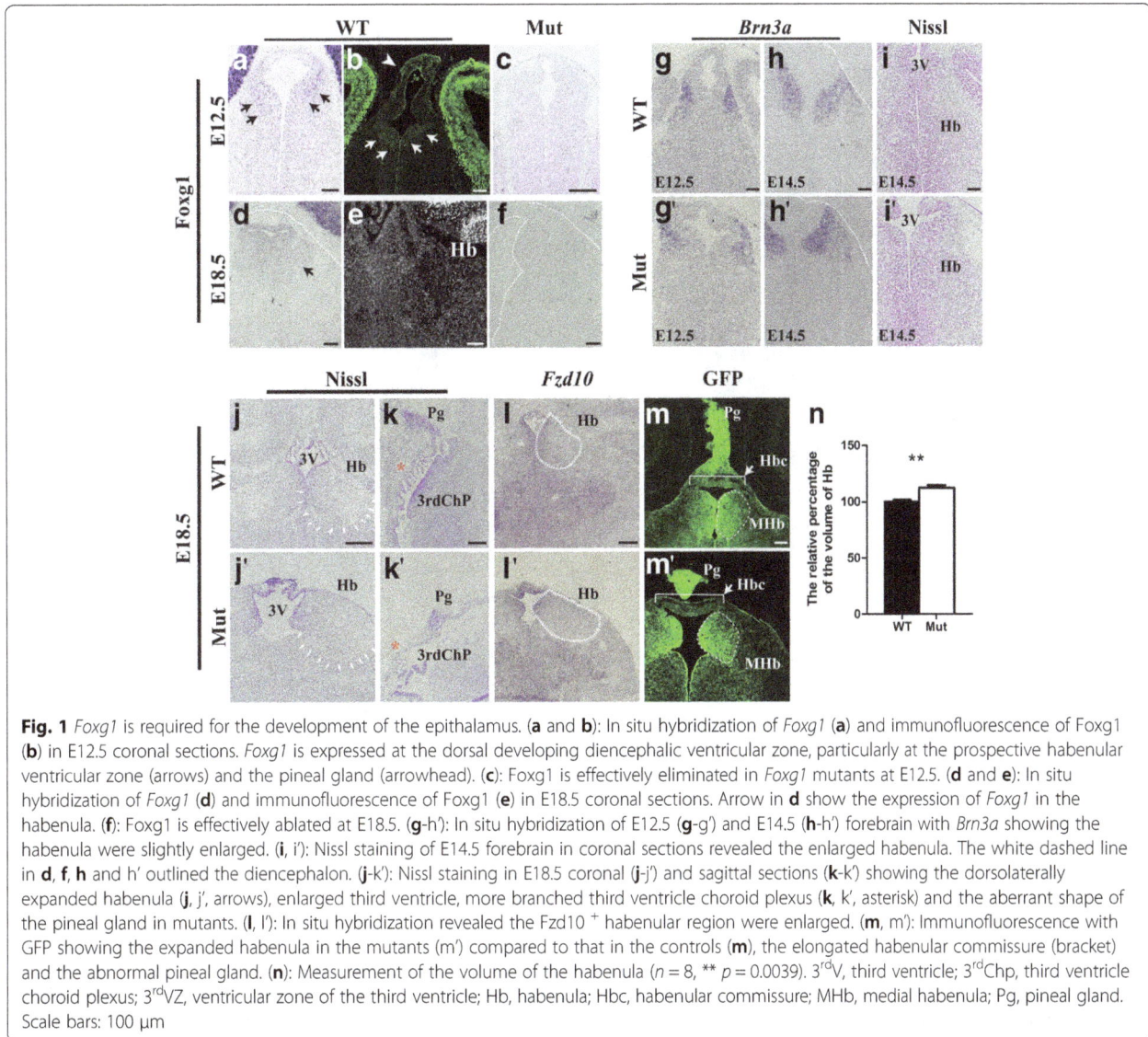

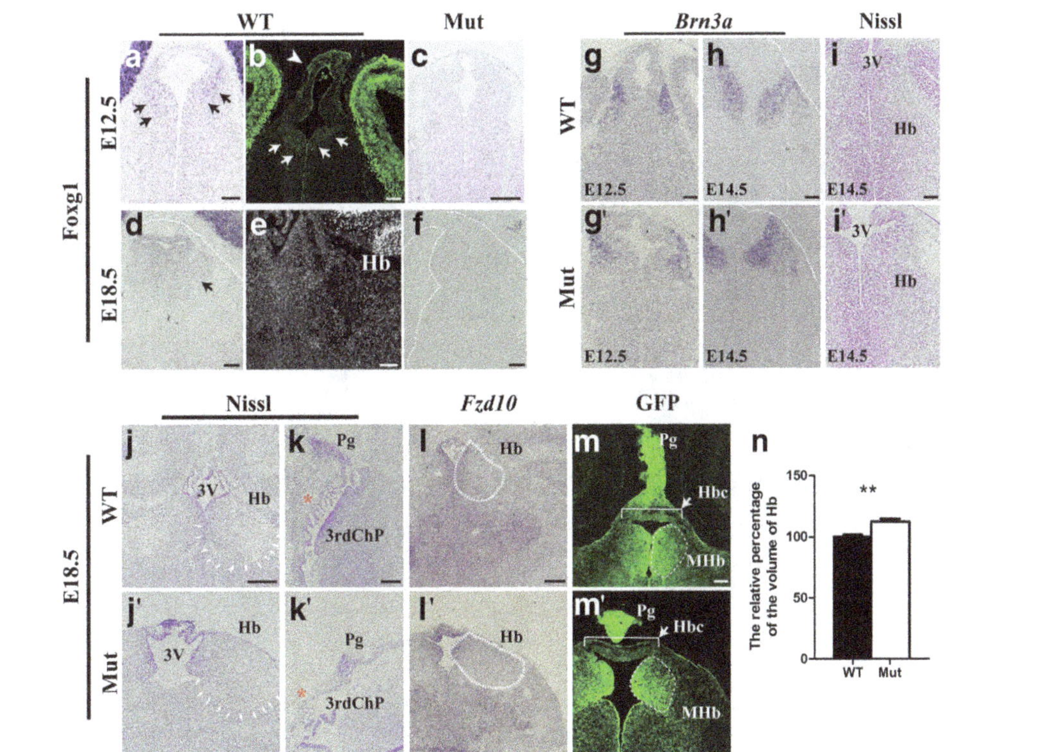

Fig. 1 *Foxg1* is required for the development of the epithalamus. (**a** and **b**): In situ hybridization of *Foxg1* (**a**) and immunofluorescence of Foxg1 (**b**) in E12.5 coronal sections. *Foxg1* is expressed at the dorsal developing diencephalic ventricular zone, particularly at the prospective habenular ventricular zone (arrows) and the pineal gland (arrowhead). (**c**): Foxg1 is effectively eliminated in *Foxg1* mutants at E12.5. (**d** and **e**): In situ hybridization of *Foxg1* (**d**) and immunofluorescence of Foxg1 (**e**) in E18.5 coronal sections. Arrow in **d** show the expression of *Foxg1* in the habenula. (**f**): Foxg1 is effectively ablated at E18.5. (**g**-h'): In situ hybridization of E12.5 (**g**-g') and E14.5 (**h**-h') forebrain with *Brn3a* showing the habenula were slightly enlarged. (**i**, i'): Nissl staining of E14.5 forebrain in coronal sections revealed the enlarged habenula. The white dashed line in **d**, **f**, **h** and h' outlined the diencephalon. (**j**-k'): Nissl staining in E18.5 coronal (**j**-j') and sagittal sections (**k**-k') showing the dorsolaterally expanded habenula (**j**, j', arrows), enlarged third ventricle, more branched third ventricle choroid plexus (**k**, k', asterisk) and the aberrant shape of the pineal gland in mutants. (**l**, l'): In situ hybridization revealed the Fzd10 $^+$ habenular region were enlarged. (**m**, m'): Immunofluorescence with GFP showing the expanded habenula in the mutants (m') compared to that in the controls (**m**), the elongated habenular commissure (bracket) and the abnormal pineal gland. (**n**): Measurement of the volume of the habenula ($n = 8$, ** $p = 0.0039$). 3^{rd}V, third ventricle; 3^{rd}Chp, third ventricle choroid plexus; 3^{rd}VZ, ventricular zone of the third ventricle; Hb, habenula; Hbc, habenular commissure; MHb, medial habenula; Pg, pineal gland. Scale bars: 100 μm

pool at E18.5. In the controls, Pax6 was expressed in the dorsal 3^{rd}VZ, and its expression was particularly intense in the epithalamic progenitors. A portion of the Pax6$^+$ progenitor cells was also dispersed within the dorsal MHb (dMHb) (Fig. 2a, dotted line) and the lateral division of the LHb (LHbL) (Fig. 2a, yellow arrowhead). In the mutants, the epithalamic VZ seemed thicker than that in the controls, and more Pax6$^+$ cells were scattered in the dMHb and LHbL; the total number of Pax6$^+$ cells was significantly increased by approximately 37% (Fig. 2a, a', i), demonstrating that disruption of *Foxg1* results in an increased number of progenitors in the developing epithalamus. Then, we examined the alterations in several subtypes of habenular neurons. *Calretinin* (*CR*) and *Calbindin* (*CB*) are two members of the EF-hand family of calcium-binding proteins that are required for the differentiation of early generated thalamic neurons [37]. Here, we found that CR$^+$ neurons were mainly populated in the dMHb and LHbL, which are the similar regions in which the Pax6$^+$ progenitors were located; additionally, the CR$^+$ neurons were distributed in the central part of the medial division of the LHb (LHbMC). The total number of CR$^+$ cells in the habenula was remarkably increased by approximately 33%, a 42% increase in the dMHb and a 22% increase in the LHbL were observed (Fig. 2b, b'; j). The CB $^+$ neurons were mainly detected in the boundary between the MHb and the LHb. In the mutants, the number of CB $^+$ neurons was also significantly increased by approximately 78%, and more CB$^+$ neurons were scattered in the LHb (Fig. 2c, c'; k). In situ staining showed Brn3a$^+$ areas in both the mutant MHb and LHb were expanded (Fig. 2d, d'). We measured the Brn3a$^+$ area at the central level of the MHb and found there was approximate 51% increase in mutants (Fig. 2l).

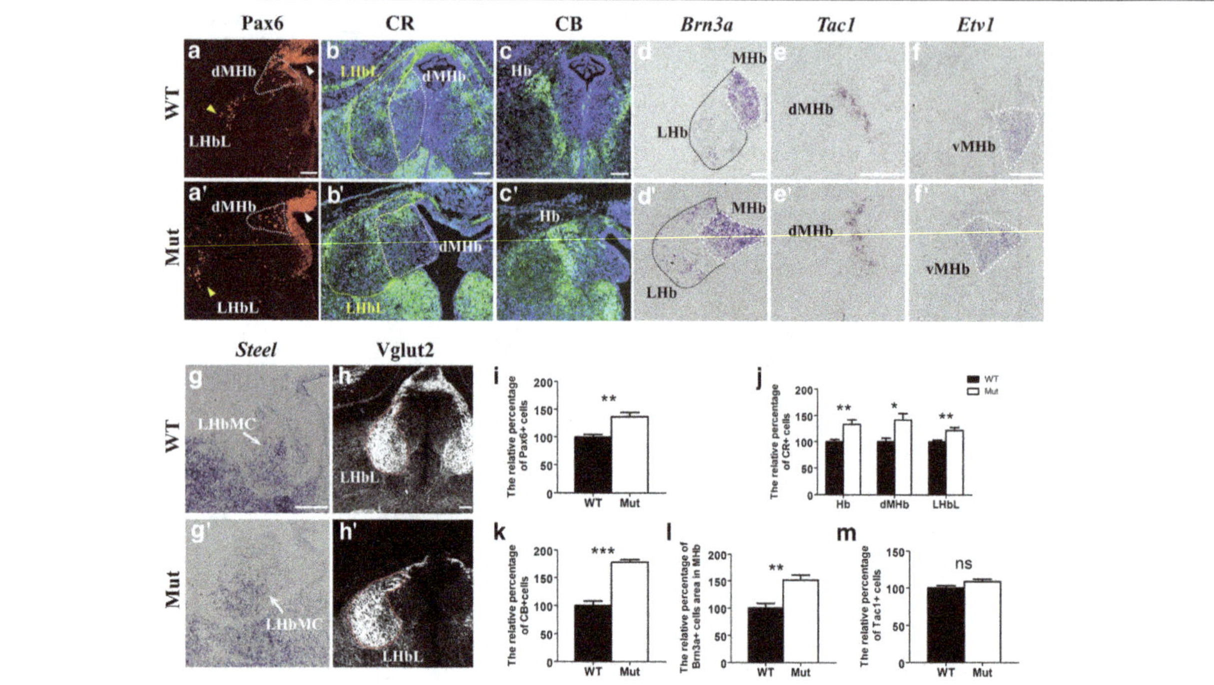

Fig. 2 Abnormal development of the habenular subtype neurons. (**a**-a'): Immunofluorescence of anti-Pax6. Pax6$^+$ progenitors in the epithalamic VZ (white arrowhead) were remarkably increased compared to those in the controls, and more Pax6$^+$ cells were scattered in the dMHb (dotted line) and LHbL (yellow arrowhead). (**b**-b'): Increased number of CR$^+$ subtype neurons in the dMHb (white dotted line) and LHbL (yellow dotted line). (**c**, c'): Increased numbers of CB$^+$ subtype neurons in the habenula. (**d**, d'): In situ hybridization showing *Brn3a* strongly expressed in postmitotic neurons in the MHb (white dotted line) and weakly expressed in the LHb (black dotted line), and both stained areas were expanded with irregular morphologies in the *Foxg1* mutants. (**e**-f'): Substance P-ergic neurons in the dMHb showing *Tac1* in situ hybridization and Etv1$^+$ glutamatergic neurons in the vMHb. (**g**-h'): Enlarged LHbMC and LHbL. (**i**-**m**): Quantitative analysis of the numbers of Pax6$^+$ progenitors (**i**, $n = 6$, $^{**}p = 0.002$), CR$^+$ neurons (**j**, n = 6, Hb, $^{**}p = 0.0085$; dMHb, $^{*}p = 0.0148$; LHbL, $^{**}p = 0.0069$), CB$^+$ neurons (**k**, n = 6, $^{***}p < 0.0001$), and Tac1$^+$ neurons (**m**, n = 8, $p = 0.067$). (**l**) Quantitative analysis of Brn3a$^+$ area in coronal section crossing the midmost level of the habenula (**l**, $n = 4$, $^{**}p = 0.0063$). The data are presented as the mean ± S.E.M. Hb, habenula; MHb, medial habenula; dMHb, dorsal medial habenula; vMHb, ventral medial habenula; LHb, lateral habenula; LHbL, lateral division of the lateral habenula; LHbMC, central part of the medial division of the lateral habenula. Scale bars: 100 μm

We further analysed the changes in several other neuronal subtypes in the MHb and LHb. The dMHb has been previously shown to contain a group of neurons that release the neuropeptide substance P, and the ventral part of the MHb (vMHb) contains glutamatergic neurons [5, 38]. According to the in situ staining of *Tachykinin1* (*Tac1*), which acts as a precursor of substance P, the number of substance P-ergic neurons was comparable to that in the controls (Fig. 2e, e'; m). However, *Etv1*, which is a member of the ETS family of transcription factors, was specifically expressed in a partition of the habenular glutamatergic neurons [33], which was significantly enlarged (Fig. 2f, f'). Regarding the LHb subdivisions, we examined the LHbMC and LHbL. As visualized by the staining of *Steel*, the ligand for the receptor tyrosine kinase c-kit and type 2 vesicular glutamate transporter (*Vglut2*), the mutant Steel$^+$ LHbMC and Vglut2$^+$ LHbL expanded more broadly than the controls. However, the expression level of Steel seemed less compared with the controls (Fig. 2g-h'). Collectively, the disruption of *Foxg1* led to an increased number of progenitors in the developing epithalamic VZ, which may ultimately result in defects in subtype neurons in both the MHb and LHb.

Impaired habenular innervations after *Foxg1* deletion

Due to the remarkable structural alteration in the mutant epithalamus, we investigated the changes in the innervations. Immunostaining of anti-L1, which is a neural cell adhesion molecule, was performed. As shown in Fig. 3a-a', the stria medullaris (SM), which project forebrain inputs to the habenula [39], were dramatically impaired, which may also be a consequence of the severely impaired telencephalon in the mutants. The habenular commissure, which conveys information between the paired habenulas, was much thinner than that in the controls, although it could cross the midline (Fig. 3b, b'). The control processes were well fasciculated and projected dorsally across the midline. However, the mutant processes were poorly fasciculated and significantly decreased. The decrease was consistent throughout the rostro-caudal axis when observed in serial

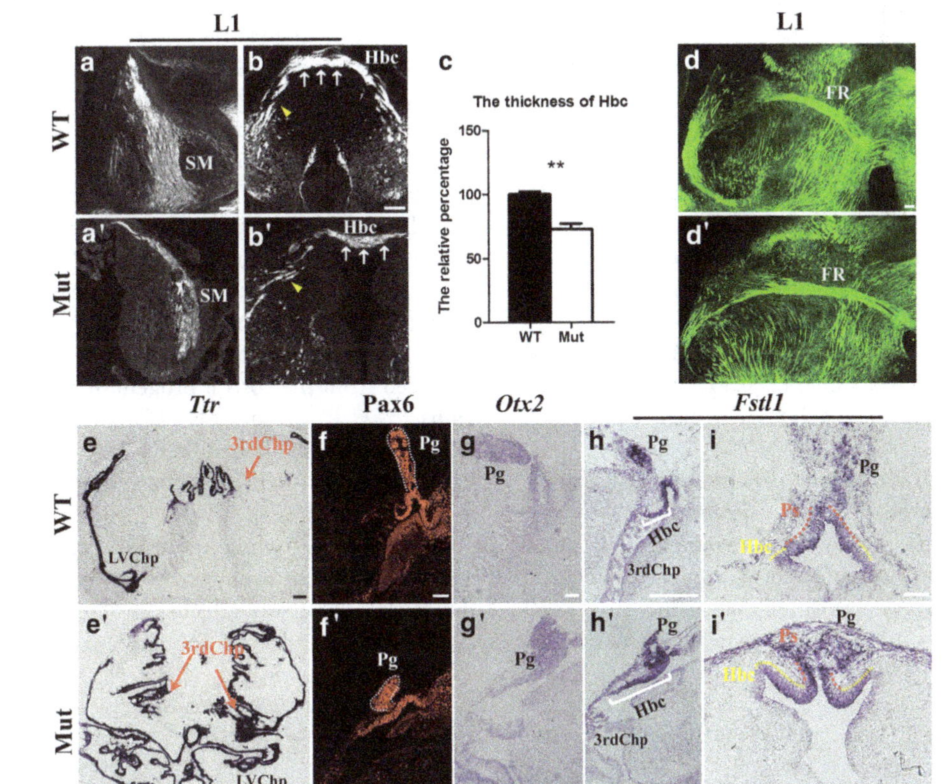

Fig. 3 Disrupted habenular innervations and abnormal diencephalic Chp and pineal gland. (**a**-b'): Immunofluorescence of L1 showing a reduced SM and habenular commissure (arrows in **b** and b'). Arrowhead indicates poorly fasciculated projections in the mutants compared with those in the controls. (**c**): Quantitative analysis of thickness of the habenular commissure at the midline area ($n = 4$, $^{**}p = 0.0015$). (**d**, **d**'): less fasciculated FR and slightly changed projection angle. (**e**, e'): In situ hybridization of *Ttr* showing a more branched choroid plexus in the mutants. (**f**-i'): Immunofluorescence with Pax6 (**f**, f') and in situ hybridisation of *Otx2* (**g**, g') and *Fstl1* (**h**-**i**') revealing an aberrant pineal gland, a shortened pineal stalk, which links the pineal gland to the habenula (**i**, i', red broken line), and a lengthened Hbc area (**h**, h', bracket; **i**, i', yellow broken line). SM, stria medullaris; 3rdChp, third ventricle choroid plexus; LVChp, lateral ventricle choroid plexus; FR, fasciculus retroflexus; Hb, habenula; Hbc, habenular commissure; IPN, interpeduncular nucleus; Pg, pineal gland; Ps, pineal stalk. Scale bars: 100 μm (scale bar in **g** and g': 400 μm)

sections. We then analysed the thickness of habenular commissure in the midline area and found it was reduced by approximate 28% in *Foxg1* mutants (Fig. 3c). The dramatically decreased habenular commissure was also detected by immunostaining with anti-CR and Vglut2 at E18.5 as shown in Fig. 2b, b'; h, and h'. Despite the increased numbers of neuron subtypes, the severely decreased habenular commissure indicates that neuronal differentiation may be affected by the *Foxg1* deletion as well.

Interestingly, the fasciculus retroflexus (FR), through which the habenula projects to the interpeduncular nucleus (IPN) of the midbrain [39, 40], appeared to project correctly, although it was less fasciculated and its projecting angle was slightly changed, which may be due to the irregular morphology of the habenula (Fig. 3d, d'). Thus, *Foxg1* is essential for the development of habenular innervations, particularly the habenular commissure.

Reduced pineal gland and extremely complicated Chp after *Foxg1* deletion

During development, both the pineal gland and the 3rdChp, along with the habenula, arise from the dorsal region of p2, which is the presumptive epithalamic domain. In addition to the habenula, the pineal gland and 3rdChp were also impaired in *Foxg1* null mutants. According to the in situ hybridization of *Ttr*, the 3rdChp and lateral ventricle Chp displayed extremely complicated morphologies compared to those in the controls (Fig. 3e, e') and, to a certain extent, reflected the Chp cyst in FOXG1 patients. Meanwhile, the size of the pineal gland was reduced viewed by immunostaining of Pax6 (Fig. 3f, f'). Previous studies have shown that misregulation of *Foxg1* in chick prosencephalon causes the downregulation of *Otx2*, which is required for the development of the pineal gland and Chp [30, 41, 42]. However, here, we found that in the absence of *Foxg1*, the expression level of *Otx2* in the pineal gland appears normal (Fig. 3g, g'), indicating that *Otx2* is not involved in the *Foxg1*-regulated development of the pineal gland in mice. We observed strong expression of Follistatin-like 1 (Fstl1), which is a secreted glycoprotein that functions as an antagonist of BMP signalling in the developing pineal gland [43, 44]. As shown in Fig. 3h-i', at E18.5 in the controls, *Fstl1* was densely expressed in a distinct cell population in the pineal gland, pineal stalk, and habenula commissure. However, in the mutants, the Fstl1$^+$cells were not well organized, and the Fstl1$^+$ pineal stalk was remarkably shortened with a lengthened habenula commissure. In summary, *Foxg1* may be essential for the regional identities of the dorsal part of p2.

Early sub-regionalization of the presumptive epithalamic domain was disrupted after *Foxg1* deletion

To further examine whether the regionalization of the epithalamic domain was affected by the loss of *Foxg1*, in situ hybridization was performed during the early developmental stage at E12.5. As shown in Fig. 4a-a", the high-level expression of the homeodomain gene *Dbx1* normally demarcates the habenular progenitor region [45]. In the absence of *Foxg1*, the Dbx1$^+$ domain was obviously expanded and shifted dorsolaterally (Fig. 4b-b"). The whole-mount in situ hybridization further confirmed the expansion of *Dbx1* in *Foxg1* mutants (Fig. 4a''' and b'''). *Ngn2*, which is a member of the proneural bHLH transcription factor family, has been shown to be widely expressed in the habenular VZ, caudal progenitor domain of the thalamus (pTH-C), and key diencephalic organizer zona limitans intrathalamica (ZLI) which is located at the interval between p2 and p3, but specifically excluded from the rostral progenitor domain of the thalamus (pTH-R) in controls [46] (Fig. 4c-c"). In the mutants, the Ngn2$^+$ habenular VZ was expanded, while ZLI, pTH-C and pTH-R appeared comparable to those in the controls (Fig. 4d-d"). The similar results were obtained by the whole-mount hybridization (Fig. 4c''' and d'''). Next, we examined whether the primordium of the pineal gland was affected by the in situ staining of *Fzd10* and found that the mutant pineal recess was

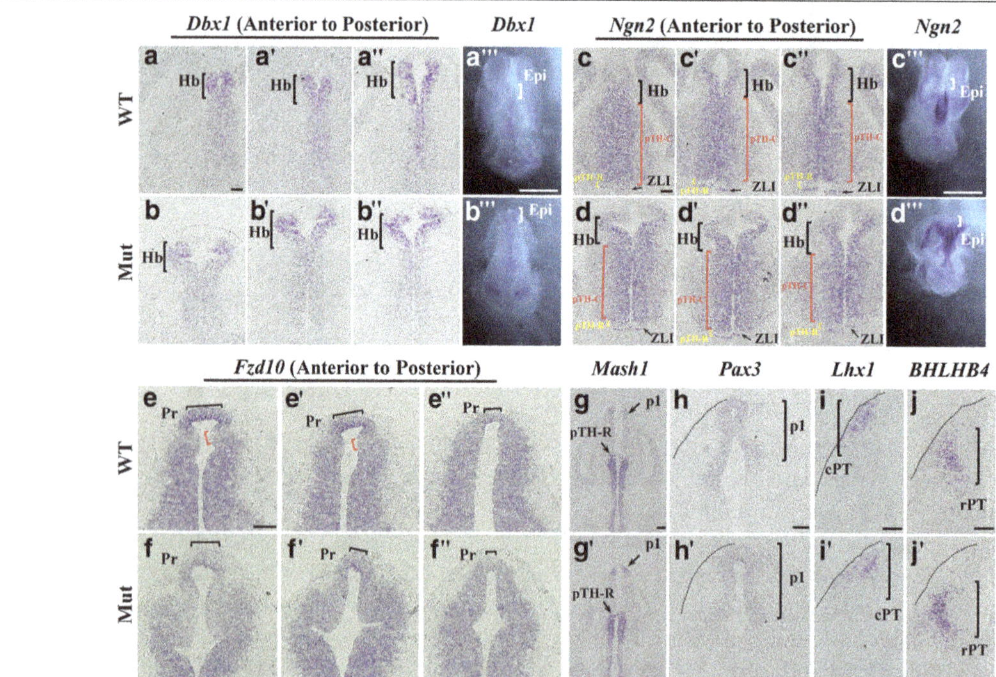

Fig. 4 *Foxg1* is required for early epithalamic sub-regionalization. (**a**-**b**"): In situ hybridization of *Dbx1* showing that the habenular progenitor region (bracket) was obviously expanded and shifted dorsolaterally after *Foxg1* deletion. (**a**''', **b**''') Whole-mount in situ hybridization for *Dbx1* at E12.5 The bracket indicates the epithalamus. (**c**-**d**"): Expanded Ngn2$^+$ habenular VZ (black bracket) but normal pTH-C (red bracket), pTH-R (yellow bracket) and ZLI (arrow) in the mutants. (**c**''', **d**'''): Whole-mount in situ hybridization for *Ngn2* at E12.5. The bracket indicates the epithalamus. (**e**-**f**"): Smaller pineal recess (black bracket) shown by in situ staining of *Fzd10*. The red bracket marked the *Fzd10^{weak}* strip between the pineal recess and the habenular ventricle zone. (**g**-g'): In situ hybridization of *Mash1* showing normal pTH-R (arrow) and ZLI. (**h**-**j**'): No obvious changes in the patterning of p1 were revealed by the in situ staining with *Pax3*, which labels the pretectal VZ (**h**, h'); *Lhx1*, which labels the mantle zone of the caudal pretectum (**i**, i'); and *BHLHB4*, which labels the mantle zone of the rostral pretectum (**j**, **j**'). The black dashed line in **h**-**j**' outlined the diencephalon. Epi, epithalamus; Hb, habenula; pTH-C, caudal progenitor domain of the thalamus; pTH-R, rostral progenitor domain of the thalamus; Pr, pineal recess; p1, prosomere 1; cPT, caudal pretectum; rPT, rostral pretectum; ZLI, zona limitans intrathalamica. Scale bars: 100 μm (scale bar in **a**''', **b**''', **c**''' and **d**''': 2 mm; **g** and g': 200 μm)

obviously smaller than that in the control (Fig. 4e-f"). Thus, sub-regionalization in the developing epithalamus was severely impaired.

To further investigate whether *Foxg1* affects pTH-C, pTH-R and ZLI, in situ hybridization of *Mash1* was also performed. As shown in Fig. 4g-g', *Mash1* was strongly expressed in pTH-R and p3 but specifically excluded from the ZLI [46]. There were no differences to be detected between the control and the mutant, consistent with that viewed by in situ hybridization of *Ngn2* (Fig. 4c-d"). We further analysed the patterning of p1 by *Pax3*, which labels the pretectal VZ [47]; LIM-homeodomain transcription factor 1 (*Lhx1*), which is a commonly used marker of the mantle zone of the caudal pretectum [48]. *BHLHB4*, which is a member of the basic helix-loop-helix (bHLH) family; and a specific marker for the mantle zone of the rostral pretectum [49]. No obvious alterations were observed (Fig. 4h-j'). Collectively, *Foxg1* is required for the sub-regionalization of the presumptive epithalamic domain but has no effects on the other parts of p2 and p1 during early diencephalic development.

Shh and Fgf signalling were not affected during the development of the epithalamus

Multiple signals, including fibroblast growth factor (Fgfs) are expressed in the dorsal midline of the diencephalon [15] and coordinate with Shh, which is secreted from the ZLI and basal plate, to establish regional identity in the developing diencephalon [50, 51]. *Fgf8* has been reported to be involved in the patterning of the p2 region. In *Fgf8* hypomorphic mice, the pineal gland and habenula are lost or reduced, exhibiting dose-dependent changes [15]. *Fgf15*, which is another member of the Fgf family, has been shown to act as a downstream target of *Shh* that regulates the development of the diencephalon [52]. Using in situ hybridization, we explored whether Fgf signalling is involved in the regulation of *Foxg1* in the sub-regionalization of the epithalamic domain. As shown in Fig. 5a, at E12.5, *Fgf15* was expressed in the future habenula and thalamic VZ with no detectable expression in the developing pineal gland and 3[rd]Chp in the controls; the transcription level of *Fgf15* in the mutant presumptive habenula was comparable to that of controls, no significant changes were observed in p2 (Fig. 5a, a', arrowhead). The same result was obtained using whole-mount hybridization and qRT-PCR (Fig. 5b, b'; c). No detectable changes were observed in *Fgf8* either along the AP axis (Fig. 5d-d"; e-e"). Therefore, *Fgf15*, as well as *Fgf8*, were not involved in the *Foxg1*-mediated regulation of the development of the epithalamus. Previously *Wnt3a* has been reported to be expressed in the dorsal p2 and *Wnt8b* is expressed in the prethalamus [15].

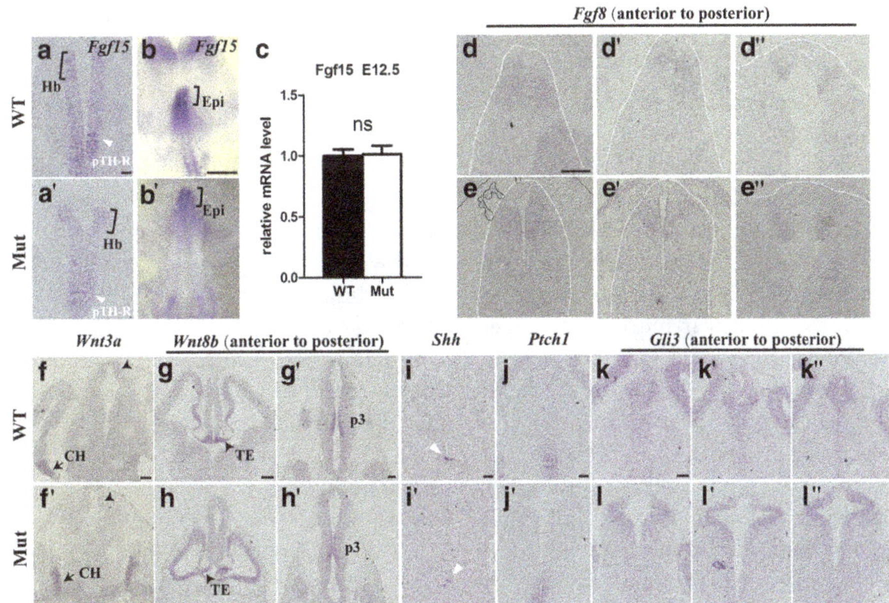

Fig. 5 Shh and Fgf signalling were not affected in the epithalamic development. (**a**-a'): Transcription level of *Fgf15* in the presumptive habenula (bracket) was not obviously affected in the mutants, no changes were observed in the region of pTH-R (arrowhead) in p2. (**b**-b'): The whole mount in situ from E12.5 embryos also showing a comparable transcription level in the epithalamus (bracket). **c**: Relative mRNA levels of *Fgf15* ($n = 4$, $p = 0.898$). (**d**-**e**"): No obvious differences in *Fgf8* were observed in the *Foxg1* mutants. The white dashed line outlined the diencephalon. (**f**-**h**'): Staining of *Wnt3a* in dorsal P2 and *Wnt8b* in TE and P3 in mutants were comparable to that of controls. Arrows in **f** and f' indicate the cortical hem, arrowheads in **g** and **h** indicate the thalamic eminence. (**i**-**l**"): The activity of the Shh signalling pathway appeared normal in the mutants. The white arrow in **i** and i' indicates the ZLI. CH, cortical hem; Epi, epithalamus; Hb, habenula; IPN, interpeduncular nucleus; TE, thalamic eminence; ZLI, zona limitans intrathalamica. Scale bars: 100 μm (scale bar in **b** and b': 1 mm, **g**-**h**': 200 μm)

Foxg1 has been shown to suppress Wnt function in the developing telencephalon [15, 53]. To explore whether *Foxg1* regulate the development of epithaluams through Wnt signalling, we then examined *Wnt3a* and *Wnt8b*; however, no obvious alteration were detected either (Fig. 5f-h').

Shh, which is secreted by the ZLI, is critical for the development of the diencephalon [50, 54–56]. The ventral ^{high}-dorsal^{low} gradient of Shh specifies the diencephalic regional identity [57]. Therefore, we examined whether Shh signalling contributes to the epithalamic defects. At E12.5, in the *Foxg1* mutants, the expression of *Shh* in the ZLI was comparable to that in the controls (Fig. 5i, i'). We then examined the activity of the Shh signalling pathway as reflected by *Ptch1* [58]. No obvious differences were detected (Fig. 5j, j'). Meanwhile, the level of *Gli3*, which is a member of the Glioma-associated oncogene (*Gli*) family that has been reported to inhibit Shh signalling [59], also appeared normal in the epithalamic VZ (Fig. 5k-k"; l-l"). Collectively, *Foxg1* may regulate the development of the epithalamus independently of Shh signalling.

Discussion

Foxg1 has been reported to be critical for telencephalic development [17, 19]. However, its role in the development of the diencephalon remains unclear. Individuals with FOXG1 syndrome exhibit a disturbed sleep pattern, Chp cysts and emotional disorders [21–23], suggesting that *Foxg1* likely plays a role in epithalamic development. In this study, we demonstrate that *Foxg1* is essential for the development of the epithalamus. The disruption of *Foxg1* leads to an extremely complicated Chp, a reduced pineal gland and an enlarged habenula. Moreover, we demonstrate that *Foxg1* may be required for the regional specification of the epithalamic progenitor domain independently of Shh and Fgf signalling. Our findings shed light on the molecular mechanism underlying the subdivision of the epithalamic domain.

Previously, the function of *Foxg1* was under-investigated in the developing diencephalon. In this study, we identified specific expression of *Foxg1* in the dorsal part of p2 from which the epithalamus derives and further elucidated its function during epithalamic development. The habenula has been reported to be closely related to emotional disorders and has recently attracted increasing attention [2, 9, 10]. By receiving inputs from the limbic system and basal ganglia and projecting to monoaminergic nuclei, the habenula acts as a node that connects the forebrain to the brainstem [39]. Here, we found that the disruption of *Foxg1* results in an enlarged habenula with an increased number of subtype habenular neurons. The loss of *Foxg1* also caused differentiation defects in habenular neurons, which led to impaired habenular innervations and ultimately resulted in abnormal information conveyance among the forebrain, brainstem and paired habenula, which may account for the emotional disorders observed in patients with *FOXG1* mutations. To the best of our knowledge, this is the first report illustrating that *Foxg1* regulates the development of the epithalamus.

During development, the most dorsal domain of p2 gives rise to the epithalamus, which consists of 3rdChp, pineal gland, habenular commissure and habenula. However, the mechanism by which the sub-regional identities are established is unknown. Multiple signals, including Fgfs have been found to be specifically expressed in the dorsal region of p2 and involved in the development of the epithalamus [15, 60, 61]. Previous studies have shown that the pineal gland and habenula are lost or reduced in *Fgf8* hypomorphic mice, which exhibit dosage-dependent changes in the epithalamus [15]. Previously, we have reported a strong expression of *Fstl1* in the pineal gland [43]. In this study, we have detected *Fstl1* is also expressed in the habenular commissure. The remarkably shorten pineal stalk with the lengthened habenular commissure observed in the *Foxg1* mutants indicate *Fstl1* may be required for the development of the pineal gland and the habenular commissure. Further study is needed to elucidate its function. Shh is secreted from the ZLI and basal plate, and by coordinating with signals from the dorsal region, *Shh* is critical for the regionalization of the diencephalon [45, 50, 51]. *Fgf15* has been identified as a downstream target of *Shh* that suppresses cell proliferation and promotes differentiation in the developing telencephalon [62]. In this study, we did not detect obvious changes in Shh and Fgf signalling in our mutants. The mutant ZLI was comparable to that in the controls, and the activity of the Shh signalling pathway, as shown by *Ptch1* and *Gli3,* appeared normal, suggesting that the regulation of *Foxg1* during epithalamic development is independent of Shh and Fgf signallings. Further studies are required to determine the downstream targets of *Foxg1* during the development of the epithalamus.

Conclusions

In the present study, we have identified a specific expression of *Foxg1* in the developing epithalamus and further found that disruption of *Foxg1* resulted in an impaired epithalamus with an expanded habenula, a reduced pineal gland and more branched choroid plexus. No obvious changes in Shh and Fgf signaling were detected in *Foxg1* mutants, indicating that *Foxg1* may regulates the development of the epithalamus independent of Shh and Fgfs. Our findings provide new insights into the regulation of the development of the epithalamus. Further study is required to elucidate the molecular mechanism.

Abbreviations

3rdChp: Third ventricle choroid plexus; 3^{rd}V: Third ventricle; 3^{rd}VZ: Ventricular zone of the third ventricle; CH: Cortical hem; cPT: Caudal pretectum; dMHb: Dorsal medial habenula; FR: Fasciculus retroflexus; Hb: Habenula; Hbc: Habenular commissure; IPN: Interpeduncular nucleus; LHb: Lateral habenula; LHbL: Lateral division of the lateral habenula; LHbMC: Central part of the medial division of the lateral habenula; MHb: Medial habenula; p: Prosomere; Pg: Pineal gland; Pr: Pineal recess; Ps: Pineal stalk; pTH-C: Caudal progenitor domain of the thalamus; pTH-R: Rostral progenitor domain of the thalamus; rPT: Rostral pretectum; SM: Stria medullaris; TE: Thalamic eminence; vMHb: Ventral medial habenula; ZLI: Zona limitans intrathalamica

Acknowledgements

We would like to thank Mr. Yiquan Wei and Ms. Li Liu for their assistance with the laboratory and animal care, Xiaochun Gu and other members of the laboratory for discussions.

Funding

This study was supported by grant 2016YFA0501001 from the Ministry of Science and Technology of China and grants 91232301 and 31471041 from the National Natural Science Foundation of China to C.Z. and 31500844 from the National Natural Science Foundation of China to X.W.

Authors' contributions

Designed the study: BL and CZ. Conducted the experiments: BL. Analysed and interpreted the data: BL, CZ, XW and KZ. Prepared the manuscript: BL and CZ. All authors read and approved the final manuscript.

Competing interests

The authors declare that they have no competing interests.

References

1. Andres KH, von During M, Veh RW. Subnuclear organization of the rat habenular complexes. J Comp Neurol. 1999;407(1):130–50.
2. Lecourtier L, Neijt HC, Kelly PH. Habenula lesions cause impaired cognitive performance in rats: implications for schizophrenia. Eur J Neurosci. 2004;19(9):2551–60.
3. Mathuru AS, Jesuthasan S. The medial habenula as a regulator of anxiety in adult zebrafish. Front Neural circuits. 2013;7:99.
4. Klemm WR. Habenular and interpeduncularis nuclei: shared components in multiple-function networks. Med Sci Monit. 2004;10(11):RA261–73.
5. Lecourtier L, Kelly PH. A conductor hidden in the orchestra? Role of the habenular complex in monoamine transmission and cognition. Neurosci Biobehav Rev. 2007;31(5):658–72.
6. Klein DC, Bailey MJ, Carter DA, Kim JS, Shi Q, Ho AK, Chik CL, Gaildrat P, Morin F, Ganguly S, et al. Pineal function: impact of microarray analysis. Mol Cell Endocrinol. 2010;314(2):170–83.
7. Lehtinen MK, Zappaterra MW, Chen X, Yang YJ, Hill AD, Lun M, Maynard T, Gonzalez D, Kim S, Ye P, et al. The cerebrospinal fluid provides a proliferative niche for neural progenitor cells. Neuron. 2011;69(5):893–905.
8. Currle DS, Cheng X, Hsu CM, Monuki ES. Direct and indirect roles of CNS dorsal midline cells in choroid plexus epithelia formation. Development. 2005;132(15):3549–59.
9. Li B, Piriz J, Mirrione M, Chung C, Proulx CD, Schulz D, Henn F, Malinow R. Synaptic potentiation onto habenula neurons in the learned helplessness model of depression. Nature. 2011;470(7335):535–9.
10. Li K, Zhou T, Liao L, Yang Z, Wong C, Henn F, Malinow R, Yates JR 3rd, Hu H. betaCaMKII in lateral habenula mediates core symptoms of depression. Science. 2013;341(6149):1016–20.
11. Valjakka A, Vartiainen J, Tuomisto L, Tuomisto JT, Olkkonen H, Airaksinen MM. The fasciculus retroflexus controls the integrity of REM sleep by supporting the generation of hippocampal theta rhythm and rapid eye movements in rats. Brain Res Bull. 1998;47(2):171–84.
12. Wu W, Cui L, Fu Y, Tian Q, Liu L, Zhang X, Du N, Chen Y, Qiu Z, Song Y, et al. Sleep and cognitive abnormalities in acute minor thalamic infarction. Neurosci Bull. 2016;32(4):341–8.
13. Puelles L, Rubenstein JL. Expression patterns of homeobox and other putative regulatory genes in the embryonic mouse forebrain suggest a neuromeric organization. Trends Neurosci. 1993;16(11):472–9.
14. Puelles L, Rubenstein JL. Forebrain gene expression domains and the evolving prosomeric model. Trends Neurosci. 2003;26(9):469–76.
15. Martinez-Ferre A, Martinez S. The development of the thalamic motor learning area is regulated by Fgf8 expression. J Neurosci. 2009;29(42):13389–400.
16. Clanton JA, Hope KD, Gamse JT. Fgf signaling governs cell fate in the zebrafish pineal complex. Development. 2012;140(2):323–32.
17. Xuan S, Baptista CA, Balas G, Tao W, Soares VC, Lai E. Winged helix transcription factor BF-1 is essential for the development of the cerebral hemispheres. Neuron. 1995;14(6):1141–52.
18. Pratt T, Quinn JC, Simpson TI, West JD, Mason JO, Price DJ. Disruption of early events in thalamocortical tract formation in mice lacking the transcription factors Pax6 or Foxg1. J Neurosci. 2002;22(19):8523–31.
19. Tian C, Gong Y, Yang Y, Shen W, Wang K, Liu J, Xu B, Zhao J, Zhao C. Foxg1 has an essential role in postnatal development of the dentate gyrus. J Neurosci. 2012;32(9):2931–49.
20. Yang Y, Shen W, Ni Y, Su Y, Yang Z, Zhao C. Impaired interneuron development after Foxg1 disruption. Cereb Cortex. 2017;27(1):793–808.
21. Kortum F, Das S, Flindt M, Morris-Rosendahl DJ, Stefanova I, Goldstein A, Horn D, Klopocki E, Kluger G, Martin P, et al. The core FOXG1 syndrome phenotype consists of postnatal microcephaly, severe mental retardation, absent language, dyskinesia, and corpus callosum hypogenesis. J Med Genet. 2011;48(6):396–406.
22. Brunetti-Pierri N, Paciorkowski AR, Ciccone R, Della Mina E, Bonaglia MC, Borgatti R, Schaaf CP, Sutton VR, Xia Z, Jelluma N, et al. Duplications of FOXG1 in 14q12 are associated with developmental epilepsy, mental retardation, and severe speech impairment. Eur J Human Genet. 2011;19(1):102–7.
23. Allou L, Lambert L, Amsallem D, Bieth E, Edery P, Destree A, Rivier F, Amor D, Thompson E, Nicholl J, et al. 14q12 and severe Rett-like phenotypes: new clinical insights and physical mapping of FOXG1-regulatory elements. Eur J Human Genet. 2012;20(12):1216–23.
24. Hebert JM, McConnell SK. Targeting of cre to the Foxg1 (BF-1) locus mediates loxP recombination in the telencephalon and other developing head structures. Dev Biol. 2000;222(2):296–306.
25. Gu X, Yan Y, Li H, He D, Pleasure SJ, Zhao C. Characterization of the Frizzled10-CreER transgenic mouse: an inducible Cre line for the study of Cajal-Retzius cell development. Genesis. 2009;47(3):210–6.
26. Zhao C, Guan W, Pleasure SJ. A transgenic marker mouse line labels Cajal-Retzius cells from the cortical hem and thalamocortical axons. Brain Res. 2006;1077(1):48–53.
27. Correia KM, Conlon RA. Whole-mount in situ hybridization to mouse embryos. Methods. 2001;23(4):335–8.
28. Ansorg A, Witte OW, Urbach A. Age-dependent kinetics of dentate gyrus neurogenesis in the absence of cyclin D2. BMC Neurosci. 2012;13:46.
29. Noguchi H, Murao N, Kimura A, Matsuda T, Namihira M, Nakashima K. DNA Methyltransferase 1 is indispensable for development of the Hippocampal dentate Gyrus. J Neurosci. 2016;36(22):6050–68.
30. Aguiar DP, Sghari S, Creuzet S. The facial neural crest controls fore- and midbrain patterning by regulating Foxg1 expression through Smad1 activity. Development. 2014;141(12):2494–505.
31. Kawaguchi D, Sahara S, Zembrzycki A, O'Leary DDM. Generation and analysis of an improved Foxg1-IRES-Cre driver mouse line. Dev Biol. 2016;412(1):139–47.
32. Li K, Zhang J, Li JY. Gbx2 plays an essential but transient role in the formation of thalamic nuclei. PLoS One. 2012;7(10):e47111.

33. Quina LA, Wang S, Ng L, Turner EE. Brn3a and Nurr1 mediate a gene regulatory pathway for habenula development. J Neurosci. 2009;29(45):14309–22.
34. Rash BG, Grove EA. Shh and Gli3 regulate formation of the telencephalic-diencephalic junction and suppress an isthmus-like signaling source in the forebrain. Dev Biol. 2011;359(2):242–50.
35. Bulchand S, Grove EA, Porter FD, Tole S. LIM-homeodomain gene Lhx2 regulates the formation of the cortical hem. Mech Dev. 2001;100(2):165–75.
36. Yan Y, Li Y, Hu C, Gu X, Liu J, Hu YA, Yang Y, Wei Y, Zhao C. Expression of Frizzled10 in mouse central nervous system. Gene Expr Patterns. 2009;9(3):173–7.
37. Frassoni C, Arcelli P, Selvaggio M, Spreafico R. Calretinin immunoreactivity in the developing thalamus of the rat: a marker of early generated thalamic cells. Neuroscience. 1998;83(4):1203–14.
38. Contestabile A, Villani L, Fasolo A, Franzoni MF, Gribaudo L, Oktedalen O, Fonnum F. Topography of cholinergic and substance P pathways in the habenulo-interpeduncular system of the rat. An immunocytochemical and microchemical approach. Neuroscience. 1987;21(1):253–70.
39. Bianco IH, Wilson SW. The habenular nuclei: a conserved asymmetric relay station in the vertebrate brain. Philos Trans R Soc Lond Ser B Biol Sci. 2009;364(1519):1005–20.
40. Contestabile A, Flumerfelt BA. Afferent connections of the interpeduncular nucleus and the topographic organization of the habenulo-interpeduncular pathway: an HRP study in the rat. J Comp Neurol. 1981;196(2):253–70.
41. Nishida A, Furukawa A, Koike C, Tano Y, Aizawa S, Matsuo I, Furukawa T. Otx2 homeobox gene controls retinal photoreceptor cell fate and pineal gland development. Nat Neurosci. 2003;6(12):1255–63.
42. Johansson PA, Irmler M, Acampora D, Beckers J, Simeone A, Gotz M. The transcription factor Otx2 regulates choroid plexus development and function. Development. 2013;140(5):1055–66.
43. Yang Y, Liu J, Mao H, Hu YA, Yan Y, Zhao C. The expression pattern of Follistatin-like 1 in mouse central nervous system development. Gene Expr Patterns. 2009;9(7):532–40.
44. Geng Y, Dong Y, Yu M, Zhang L, Yan X, Sun J, Qiao L, Geng H, Nakajima M, Furuichi T, et al. Follistatin-like 1 (Fstl1) is a bone morphogenetic protein (BMP) 4 signaling antagonist in controlling mouse lung development. Proc Natl Acad Sci U S A. 2011;108(17):7058–63.
45. Chatterjee M, Guo Q, Weber S, Scholpp S, Li JY. Pax6 regulates the formation of the habenular nuclei by controlling the temporospatial expression of Shh in the diencephalon in vertebrates. BMC Biol. 2014;12(1):13.
46. Vue TY, Aaker J, Taniguchi A, Kazemzadeh C, Skidmore JM, Martin DM, Martin JF, Treier M, Nakagawa Y. Characterization of progenitor domains in the developing mouse thalamus. J Comp Neurol. 2007;505(1):73–91.
47. Ferran JL, Sanchez-Arrones L, Bardet SM, Sandoval JE, Martinez-de-la-Torre M, Puelles L. Early pretectal gene expression pattern shows a conserved anteroposterior tripartition in mouse and chicken. Brain Res Bull. 2008;75(2–4):295–8.
48. Suda Y, Hossain ZM, Kobayashi C, Hatano O, Yoshida M, Matsuo I, Aizawa S. Emx2 directs the development of diencephalon in cooperation with Otx2. Development. 2001;128(13):2433–50.
49. Bramblett DE, Copeland NG, Jenkins NA, Tsai MJ. BHLHB4 is a bHLH transcriptional regulator in pancreas and brain that marks the dimesencephalic boundary. Genomics. 2002;79(3):402–12.
50. Martinez-Ferre A, Martinez S. Molecular regionalization of the diencephalon. Front Neurosci. 2012;6:73.
51. Jeong Y, Dolson DK, Waclaw RR, Matise MP, Sussel L, Campbell K, Kaestner KH, Epstein DJ. Spatial and temporal requirements for sonic hedgehog in the regulation of thalamic interneuron identity. Development. 2011;138(3):531–41.
52. Martinez-Ferre A, Lloret-Quesada C, Prakash N, Wurst W, Rubenstein JL, Martinez S. Fgf15 regulates thalamic development by controlling the expression of proneural genes. Brain Struct Funct. 2015;221(6):3095–109.
53. Danesin C, Peres JN, Johansson M, Snowden V, Cording A, Papalopulu N, Houart C. Integration of telencephalic Wnt and hedgehog signaling center activities by Foxg1. Dev Cell. 2009;16(4):576–87.
54. Hashimoto-Torii K, Motoyama J, Hui CC, Kuroiwa A, Nakafuku M, Shimamura K. Differential activities of sonic hedgehog mediated by Gli transcription factors define distinct neuronal subtypes in the dorsal thalamus. Mech Dev. 2003;120(10):1097–111.
55. Kiecker C, Lumsden A. Hedgehog signaling from the ZLI regulates diencephalic regional identity. Nat Neurosci. 2004;7(11):1242–9.
56. Scholpp S, Wolf O, Brand M, Lumsden A. Hedgehog signalling from the zona limitans intrathalamica orchestrates patterning of the zebrafish diencephalon. Development. 2006;133(5):855–64.
57. Vue TY, Bluske K, Alishahi A, Yang LL, Koyano-Nakagawa N, Novitch B, Nakagawa Y. Sonic hedgehog signaling controls thalamic progenitor identity and nuclei specification in mice. J Neurosci. 2009;29(14):4484–97.
58. Agren M, Kogerman P, Kleman MI, Wessling M, Toftgard R. Expression of the PTCH1 tumor suppressor gene is regulated by alternative promoters and a single functional Gli-binding site. Gene. 2004;330:101–14.
59. Persson M, Stamataki D, te Welscher P, Andersson E, Bose J, Ruther U, Ericson J, Briscoe J. Dorsal-ventral patterning of the spinal cord requires Gli3 transcriptional repressor activity. Genes Dev. 2002;16(22):2865–78.
60. Lim Y, Cho G, Minarcik J, Golden J. Altered BMP signaling disrupts chick diencephalic development. Mech Dev. 2005;122(4):603–20.
61. Louvi A, Yoshida M, Grove EA. The derivatives of the Wnt3a lineage in the central nervous system. J Comp Neurol. 2007;504(5):550–69.
62. Borello U, Cobos I, Long JE, McWhirter JR, Murre C, Rubenstein JL. FGF15 promotes neurogenesis and opposes FGF8 function during neocortical development. Neural Dev. 2008;3:17.

5

Targeting NMDA receptors in stroke: new hope in neuroprotection

Qiu Jing Wu[1,2] and Michael Tymianski[1,2,3*]

Abstract: NMDA (N-methyl-d-aspartate) receptors (NMDARs) play a central role in excitotoxic neuronal death caused by ischemic stroke, but NMDAR channel blockers have failed to be translated into clinical stroke treatments. However, recent research on NMDAR-associated signaling complexes has identified important death-signaling pathways linked to NMDARs. This led to the generation of inhibitors that inhibit these pathways downstream from the receptor without necessarily blocking NMDARs. This therapeutic approach may have fewer side effects and/or provide a wider therapeutic window for stroke as compared to the receptor antagonists. In this review, we highlight the key findings in the signaling cascades downstream of NMDARs and the novel promising therapeutics for ischemic stroke.

Keywords: Ischemic stroke, NMDA receptors, Excitotoxicity, Death signaling complexes, Neuroprotection

Introduction: stroke epidemiology and need for effective therapeutics

Stroke is the second most common cause of death and the third most common cause of disability worldwide. In 2010, about 10% of all deaths and 4% of DALYs lost (disability adjusted life years) were caused by stroke [1]. It consumes near 4% of total health care costs each year and creates a huge burden on the health care system [2]. With an aging global population, the mortality rate and burden due to stroke will keep increasing. By 2030, stroke is estimated to cause 12 million deaths, and more than 200 million DALYs lost globally [1].

The two main types of stroke are ischemic and hemorrhagic. Ischemic strokes comprise about 87% of all strokes [2]. Ischemic stroke arises from a thrombotic or embolic blockage of brain arteries resulting in limited blood flow to the affected brain tissue, followed by energy depletion. This triggers a series of complex pathophysiological events including the disruption of ionic homeostasis, accumulation of synaptic and extrasynaptic glutamate, ion channel dysfuntion, membrane and DNA damage, inflammation and so on, eventually lead to neuronal cell death and ischemic brain injury [3–6].

So far the only FDA-approved pharmacotherapy for acute stroke is with intravenous thrombolytic therapy using recombinant tissue plasminogen activator (rtPA) [7, 8]. However, this agent has a 3–4.5 h therapeutic window, and risks producing an intracerebral hemorrhage (6–7% cases). This has limited the use of rtPA to only about 5% of all stroke patients [2, 9–11]. Thus there remains a significant unmet medical need for identifying more effective and safer stroke drugs.

For the past decades, extensive research has advanced our understanding of the stroke pathology. Excitotoxicity mediated by N-methyl-D-aspartate (NMDA) type of glutamate receptors has been at the center stage of stroke research. In this review, we highlight recent key findings in ischemic cell death signaling pathways linked to or downstream of NMDARs and newly developed drug candidates that act as neuroprotectants, agents that reduce the vulnerability of ischemic brain to ischemia.

Understanding stroke: excitotoxicity and NMDA receptors

Excitotoxicity is among the first identified, and most intensively studied ischemic cell death mechanism. The term "excitotoxicity" describes the process in which excess quantities of the excitatory neurotransmitter glutamate over-activates NMDARs and induces neuronal toxicity [12–14]. This has been considered as one of the major pathogenic mechanisms underlying ischemic brain injury [4, 15, 16].

* Correspondence: mike.tymianski@uhn.ca
[1]Krembil Research Institute, University Health Network, 60 Leonard St, Toronto, ON M5T2S8, Canada
[2]Department of Physiology, University of Toronto, Toronto, ON, Canada
Full list of author information is available at the end of the article

During ischemia, restricted cerebral blood flow depletes the supply of oxygen and nutrients that are required by neurons to maintain ionic homeostasis [4]. Disrupted ionic gradients depolarize the cell and, among other things, trigger the release of excitatory neurotransmitters, namely glutamate, into the synaptic space. At the same time, energy depletion also impairs the function of re-uptake transporters so they are unable to clear excess glutamate. This results in the accumulation of excitatory glutamate in the extracellular space and the consequent over-activation of glutamate receptors of post-synaptic neurons.

Ionotropic glutamate receptors are ligand-gated ion channels that allow rapid ion influx in response to glutamate and comprise the gateway to excitotoxicity [17–20]. They contain both an extracellular glutamate binding site and a transmembrane ion channel. The two main subtypes of ionotropic glutamate receptors are NMDA (N-methyl-d-aspartate) receptors (NMDARs) and AMPA (α-amino-3-hydroxy-5-methylisoxazole-4-propionic acid) receptors (AMPARs). At the resting state, the channel pores of NMDARs are normally blocked by Mg^{2+}. When glutamate is released from pre-synaptic sites, activated AMPARs cause a partial depolarization in the post-synaptic membrane sufficient to remove the Mg^{2+} block from NMDARs. Once NMDARs are activated, they flux Na^+ and Ca^{2+} into the cell. The Ca^{2+} influx through NMDARs is not only critical for the normal physiological processes in neurons, but also plays a major role in initiating ischemic cell death [17–19, 21]. In excitotoxicity, excess glutamate release results in over-activation of NMDARs and leads to calcium overload inside the neurons. Calcium overload triggers a range of downstream pro-death signaling events such as calpain activation [22, 23], reactive oxygen species (ROS) generation [24–26], and mitochondrial damage [4, 24, 27], resulting in cell necrosis or apoptosis.

Given the pivotal role of NMDAR in excitotoxicity, the initial therapeutic approach was to block the receptors [4, 7, 28]. NMDAR antagonists were designed to target different sites: non-competitive antagonists that block the ion channels, competitive antagonists that prevent excitatory neurotransmitters from binding to the glutamate recognition site, and glutamate release inhibitors that blocked presynaptic voltage sensing Na^+ channels [29]. In pre-clinical studies in rats, NMDAR antagonists protected neurons from ischemic death in a model of middle cerebral artery occlusion (MCAO). The MCA can be occluded either transiently or permanently in these models, producing strokes of various severity [30–33]. However, despite initial promise in rodents such as rats, NMDAR antagonists have failed to be translated for clinical use in acute stroke [6, 34]. The explanation for these failures of translation is likely multi-factorial [7]. Two important drawbacks are the short therapeutic time window, and dose-limiting safety concerns [16, 29, 35]. The NMDAR antagonists have to be administered either before or immediately after stroke to be effective [7, 35, 36]. In addition, the NMDAR antagonists can cause severe side effects such as nausea, vomiting, cardiovascular and psychomimetic effects in treated patients [35, 37–39]. In retrospect it appears that NMDAR blockade will interfere with normal neuronal function and cause substantial side effects at potentially therapeutic doses.

Due to the lack of clinical success with NMDA receptor antagonists, the focus of stroke neuroprotection shifted towards the identification of downstream intracellular signaling pathways triggered by NMDARs.

NMDA receptors: dual roles in neuronal survival and death

Structurally, NMDARs are heterotetramers formed by two GluN1 subunits and two glutamate binding GluN2 subunits. The GluN2 subunits can be GluN2A-GluN2D, as well as GluN3A and GluN3B, all of which have distinguishing properties and expression patterns in the CNS [40]. The most widely expressed NMDARs contain GluN1 subunits in combination with either GluN2B or GluN2A. NMDARs play central roles in synaptic plasticity, brain development, learning and memory [41, 42]. However, when excessively activated in ischemic stroke, NMDARs initiate toxic cascades that kill the neurons. Recent studies suggest that the dual roles of NMDARs in neuronal survival and death may depend on the subcellular locations and subtypes of the receptors that are activated [16, 43–46] (Fig. 1).

In the receptor location hypothesis, stimulating synaptic NMDARs activates pro-survival signaling pathways, whereas the activation of extrasynaptic NMDARs is associated with pro-death pathways. Synaptic NMDAR stimulation activates the PI3K (Phosphoinositide-3-kinase)/AKt kinase pathway, CREB (cAMP-response element binding protein)-dependent gene expression and suppression of pro-death genes, all of which contribute to pro-survival effects [46]. Upon NMDAR opening, PI3K is activated by Ca^{2+} and calmodulin that phosphorylate membrane phospholipid PtdIns(4,5)*P*2) to PtdIns(3,4,5)*P*3 [47]. PtdIns(3,4,5)*P*3 interacting kinase PDK1 (phosphoinositide dependent protein kinase1) is then recruited to the membrane and activates Akt by phosphorylation [48]. Akt promotes cell survival by phosphorylating a number of downstream targets. It inactivates GSK3β (glycogen synthase kinase 3β), pro-apoptotic *Bcl-2* associated death promotor BAD [49], JNK (c-Jun N-terminal Kinase)/p38 activator ASK1 (apoptosis signal-regulating kinase 1) [50], and apoptotic p53 [51]. Synaptic NMDAR activation also induces the expression of pro-survival genes. Synaptic NMDAR activity and Ca^{2+} influx activates the Ras/ERK (extracellular signal regulated kinase) signaling and nuclear CAMKs (Ca^{2+}/calmodulin dependent protein

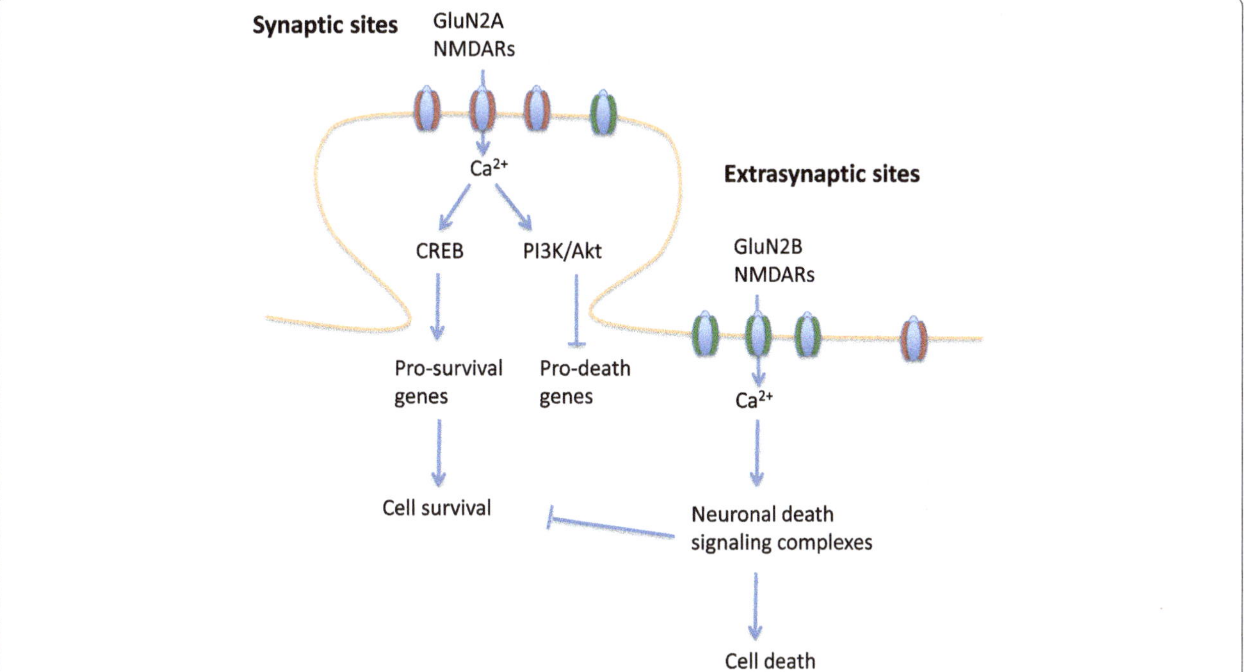

Fig. 1 Dual roles of NMDARs in cell survival and death. Activation of NMDARs can trigger pro-survival or pro-death signaling depending on the subcellular locations or subtypes of NMDARs. In mature neurons, GluN2A-containing NMDARs are abundant in the synapses, and GluN2B-containing NMDARs are enriched in the extrasynaptic sites. In general, synaptic/GluN2A-containing NMDARs are associated with pro-survival effects, whereas extrasynaptic/GluN2B-containing NMDARs are linked to pro-death signaling complexes

kinases), which then phosphorylates and activates CREB [52, 53]. Activation of CREB induces the expression of pro-survival genes that protect the neurons against apoptotic insults. CREB target genes include anti-apoptotic *BTG2*, apoptotic p53 suppressor *BCL6*, and survival promoting neurotrophin BDNF (brain derived neurotrophic factor) [44, 46].

In contrast with the pro-survival effect of synaptic NMDAR activities, extrasynaptic NMDARs are associated with pro-death signaling pathways. The activated extrasynaptic NMDARs attenuate the pro-survival signaling mediated by the synaptic NMDARs. For example, the activation of extrasynaptic NMDARs dephosphorylates and inactivates CREB [44]. They also dephosphorylate and inactivate ERK pathway, which prevents the activation of CREB and promote the expression of pro-death genes [46, 54]. Weak NMDAR antagonists such as memantine can selectively block extrasynaptic NMDARs, suggesting that there is a potential to modulate the balance between pro-survival and pro-death signaling in ischemic stroke [55, 56].

In addition, different NMDAR subunit combinations (receptor subtypes) may recruit different downstream signaling complexes resulting in distinct functional effects. GluN2A- and GluN2B-containing NMDARs are the two predominant types of NMDARs in the adult forebrain. During early development, GluN2B-containing NMDARs are abundant in the prenatal brain and then decreases postnatally, while the expression of GluN2A-containing NMDARs increases with development [40]. In the adult brain, GluN2B-containing NMDARs are enriched in the extrasynaptic sites, whereas GluN2A-containing NMDARs are highly expressed at the synapse. The GluN2A- and GluN2B- containing NMDARs also play different roles in response to ischemic insults: activation of either synaptic or extrasynaptic GluN2B-containing NMDARs results in excitotoxicity and neuronal apoptosis, whereas activation of synaptic or extrasynaptic GluN2A-containing NMDARs leads to neuronal survival and neuroprotection against ischemic insults [57, 58].

Given the dual roles of NMDARs, it would be ideal to selectively inhibit only the pro-death signaling from the receptors and not interfere with pro-survival pathways. One approach could be the targeting of extrasynaptic/GluN2B-containing NMDARs. However, the segregation of the different NMDAR subunits among synaptic vs. extrasynaptic sites is not absolute, hence blocking the extrasynaptic GluN2B-containing NMDARs may still antagonize synaptic GluN2A-containing NMDARs [5].

Targeting NMDAR pro-death pathways: potential therapeutics

An alternative to selectively targeting GluN2B- containing NMDARs may be to selectively target pro-death

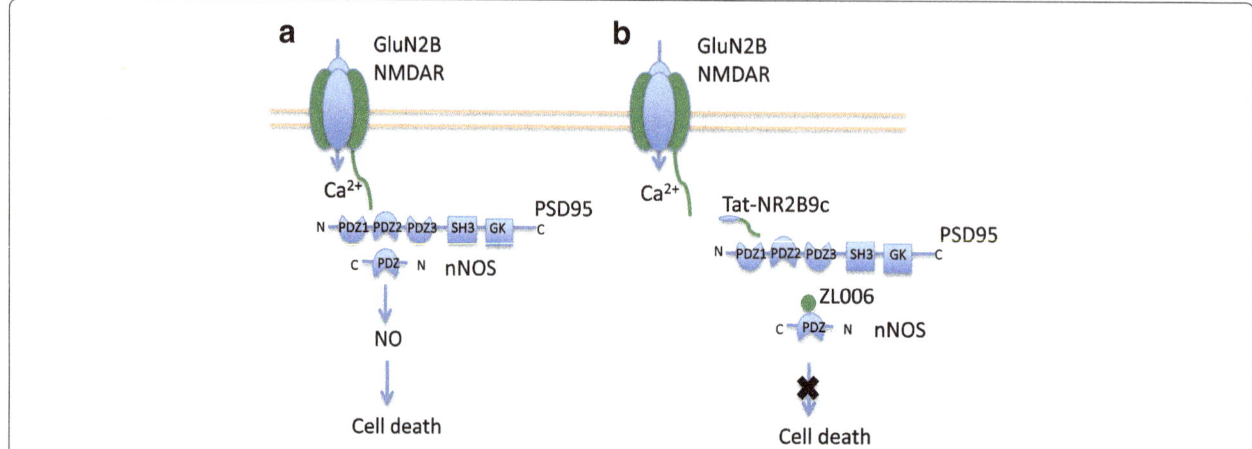

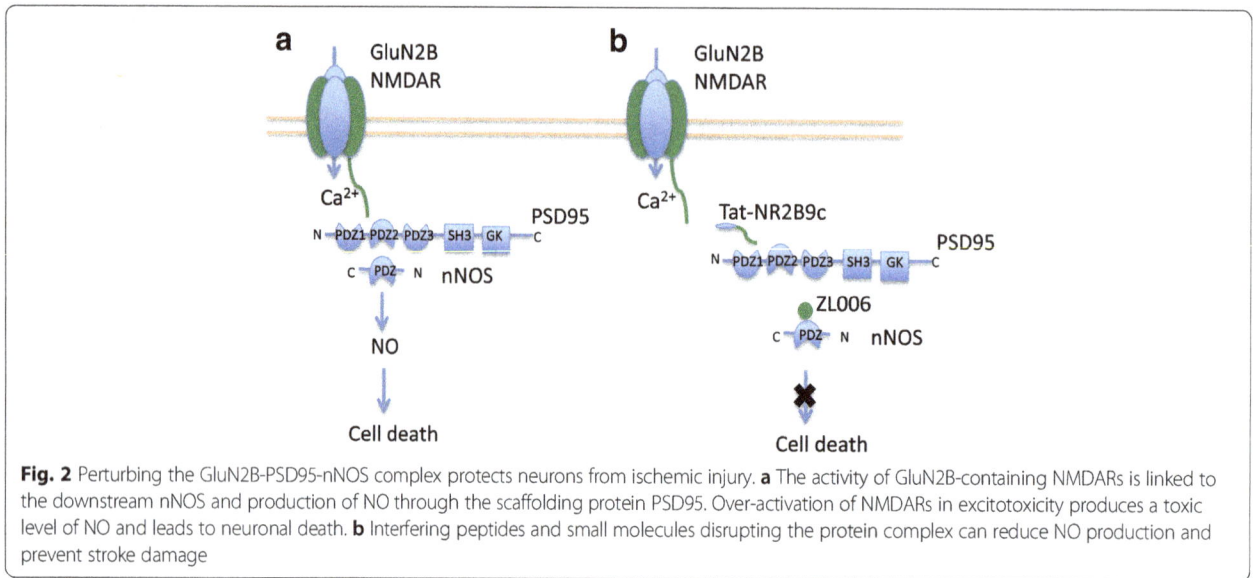

Fig. 2 Perturbing the GluN2B-PSD95-nNOS complex protects neurons from ischemic injury. **a** The activity of GluN2B-containing NMDARs is linked to the downstream nNOS and production of NO through the scaffolding protein PSD95. Over-activation of NMDARs in excitotoxicity produces a toxic level of NO and leads to neuronal death. **b** Interfering peptides and small molecules disrupting the protein complex can reduce NO production and prevent stroke damage

mechanisms downstream of NMDARs. This approach has shown significant promise in neuroprotection.

GluN2B-PSD95-nNOS complex

A well-characterized death-signaling pathway in ischemic stroke is found in the multi-protein complex associated with membrane-bound NMDARs. It is the GluN2B-PSD95-nNOS pathway, in which the scaffolding protein postsynaptic density-95 (PSD95) links NMDARs to downstream molecules including nitric oxide synthase (nNOS). PSD95 contains three PDZ domains (an acronym derived from post synaptic density protein-95, drosophila disc large tumor suppressor-1, and zonula occludens-1 protein-protein interaction domains). The PDZ1 and PDZ2 domains of PSD95 bind directly to the threonine/serine-X-valine-COOH (T/SXV) motif at the intracellular C-termini of GluN2 NMDAR subunits [59]. The PDZ2 domain of PSD95 also binds to the N-terminus of nNOS [60]. This molecular organization allows Ca^{2+} influx from over-activated NMDARs to cause overactivation of nNOS, which then produces nitric oxide (NO), a reactive nitrogen species and a known effector of excitotoxicity [61]. Disrupting the GluN2B-PSD95-nNOS complex suppresses NMDAR-mediated NO production and protects neurons from excitotoxicity [61–64] (Fig. 2).

Downstream of the complex: NO mediates neuronal death

NO reacts with superoxide free radicals to form the highly reactive oxidant peroxynitrite. That can cause protein oxidation, lipid peroxidation, and DNA damage [65–67]. Peroxynitrite mediated DNA damage can also activates poly (ADP)-ribose polymerase (PARP-1), a nuclear DNA repair enzyme, causing energy deprivation of ATP and NAD and triggering the mitochondrial release of apoptosis inducing factor (AIF) [26, 68, 69]. AIF then translocates into the nucleus and causes DNA fragmentation and cell death.

Clinical success of the PSD95 inhibitor Tat-NR2B9c (NA-1)

One approach to disrupting the production of NO in excitotoxicity is by using interfering peptides that bind either PSD95 or nNOS, thereby perturbing the ability of NMDAR activity to activate nNOS. One such interfering peptide had been termed "Tat-NR2B9c or NA-1", and is comprised of the 9 C-terminal residues of the GluN2B subunit fused with 11 residues of the cell membrane transduction facilitator Tat. Tat-NR2B9c was shown to uncouple NMDARs from PSD95 and attenuate downstream neurotoxic signaling [61, 70, 71] (Fig. 2). A number of in vivo studies in rats have demonstrated the neuroprotective effects of Tat-NR2B9c in reducing infarct volume and improving neurobehavioral outcomes when administered after ischemic stroke [61–63, 72].

To bridge the translational gap between rat animal models and human clinical trials, experiments were conducted to examine the effect of Tat-NR2B9c after MCAO in non-human primates with genetic, anatomic, and behavioral similarities to humans [64]. These experiments showed that stroke damage can be prevented in non-human primates in which a Tat-NR2B9c is administered after stroke onset in experimental paradigms that were designed to mimic clinically relevant situations. The treatment reduced infarct volumes as gauged by magnetic resonance imaging and histology, preserved the capacity of ischemic cells to maintain gene transcription in genome-wide screens of ischemic brain tissue, and significantly preserved neurological function in neuro- behavioral assays. These results show that the strategy of targeting PSD95 rather than NMDARs can reduce stroke damage in human-like brains, suggesting promise for future clinical use.

A clinical proof-of-concept study of NA-1 has been completed to assess whether NA-1 could reduce ischemic brain damage in human beings. This was a double-blind, randomized, controlled study conducted at 14 hospitals in Canada and the USA. The study enrolled patients who had a ruptured or unruptured intracranial aneurysm amenable to endovascular repair, as up to 90% of human beings undergoing endovascular intracranial aneurysm repair show small, embolic, procedurally induced ischemic strokes on diffusion-weighted (DWI) MRI. One hundred eighty-five patients were randomized to receive either NA-1 or saline control at the end of their endovascular procedure [71, 73]. Patient demographics, medical risks, adverse events and procedures were balanced between the groups. Patients who received NA-1 sustained fewer ischemic infarcts as gauged by MRI imaging. Among patients with ruptured, NA-1 treatment reduced the number and volume of strokes by all MRI criteria and improved neurological outcome. Thus, the strategy of treating a stroke with an agent that targets PSD95 after ischemia has begun has clinical promise.

Small molecules targeting the complex: ZL006, IC87201

Recent studies have discovered two small molecules ZL006 and IC87201 that are also reported to dissociate the GluN2B-PSD95-nNOS complex. A de novo small molecule ZL006 was synthesized to selectively inhibit the ischemia induced PSD95 and nNOS interaction (Fig. 2). This molecule showed neuroprotective effects in vitro and reduced cerebral ischemic injury in mouse and rat stroke models [74]. In addition, ZL006 is reported to cross the blood brain barrier and to not affect the normal function of NMDARs and nNOS. A similar compound IC87201 was discovered by *Florio* et al. using high throughput screening [75]. It was reported to disrupt the pathogenic PSD95-nNOS interaction without inhibiting the normal nNOS activity in neurons [75]. IC87201 has been tested for its anti-nociceptive effects, and was reported to reduce NMDA-induced hyperalgesia in mice, though its neuroprotective potential in stroke remains to be tested. Recent studies have challenged whether either of these molecules actually interact with the PDZ domains of nNOS or PSD-95, or inhibit the nNOS-PDZ/PSD-95-PDZ interface [76].

Peroxynitrite scavengers and antioxidants

The neuroprotective efficacy of peroxynitrite scavengers such as disufenton sodium (NXY-059) has been evaluated in rodent stroke models as well as in marmosets [77, 78]. However in a pivotal clinical trial, NXY-059 failed to show efficacy [79].

Uric acid is a powerful scavenger of free radicals in plasma [80]. Uric acid has been shown to attenuate peroxynitrite-mediated damage and alleviate ischemic injury in rodent stroke models [8, 81–83]. It also showed synergistic neuroprotection with thrombolytic agent rtPA (alteplase) in preclinical studies [82, 84]. The safety and efficacy of uric acid with thrombolytic therapy have been assessed in the phase 2b/3 URICOICTUS trial [85]. Although the combination of uric acid and rtPA did not prove efficacy in the primary outcome (modified Rankin score at 90 days follow-up), the treatment did not lead to safety concerns [8, 85]. In addition, the uric acid treatment was found to improve functional outcome in patient subgroups [8, 85–87]. More clinical trials studying the efficacy of uric acid are currently on going. In a recent study, the combined treatment of uric acid and rtPA prevented early ischemic stroke progression after acute ischemic stroke [84].

Edaravone is another anti-oxidant drug that scavenges hydroxyl, peroxyl, and superoxide radicals. It has been marketed in Japan since 2001 to treat acute ischemic patients within 24 h of stroke attack [88]. Edaravone was shown to reduce blood brain barrier dysfunction, reduce brain edema, decrease cortical infarct size, and decrease behavioral deficits in rodent and rabbit stroke models [88–92]. A recent review assessed clinical studies during years 1993–2008 has suggested that Edaravone may be a useful therapeutic treatment for ischemic stroke, but the efficacy of Edaravone should be further tested in randomized controlled clinical trials with standardized dosage, treatment time and duration [88].

GluN2B-DAPK1 interaction

DAPK1 (death-associated protein kinase 1) is a Ca^{2+}/calmodulin (CaM) dependent serine/threonine protein kinase whose activity is associated with apoptotic cell death [93]. DAPK1 is highly expressed in the brain. At basal condition, DAPK1 activity is suppressed by autophosphorylation at serine 308 in the CaM regulatory domain. Upon binding with Ca^{2+} activated CaM, the catalytic activity of DAPK1 is disinhibited and the pro-apoptotic activity is stimulated [94, 95]. In ischemic stroke, the over-activation of NMDAR leads to excessive Ca^{2+} influx into the cell and activates CaM and the calcinerin phosphatase (CaN), which in turn dephosphorylate and activate DAPK1 [96].

A recent study by Tu et al. demonstrated that activated DAPK1 is recruited to the GluN2B subunit of NMDARs after ischemic insults [97]. DAPK1 directly binds to amino acids 1292–1304 at the intracellular carboxyl tail region ($GluN2B^{CT}$) of the GluN2B subunit. DAPK1 activation increases phosphorylation at site Ser-1303 within the DAPK1 binding domain of GluN2B subunit, and enhances GluN2B-containing NMDAR channel conductance [97] (Fig. 3). Based on Tu et al.'s findings, GluN2B-DAPK1 may play an important role in mediating ischemic damage.

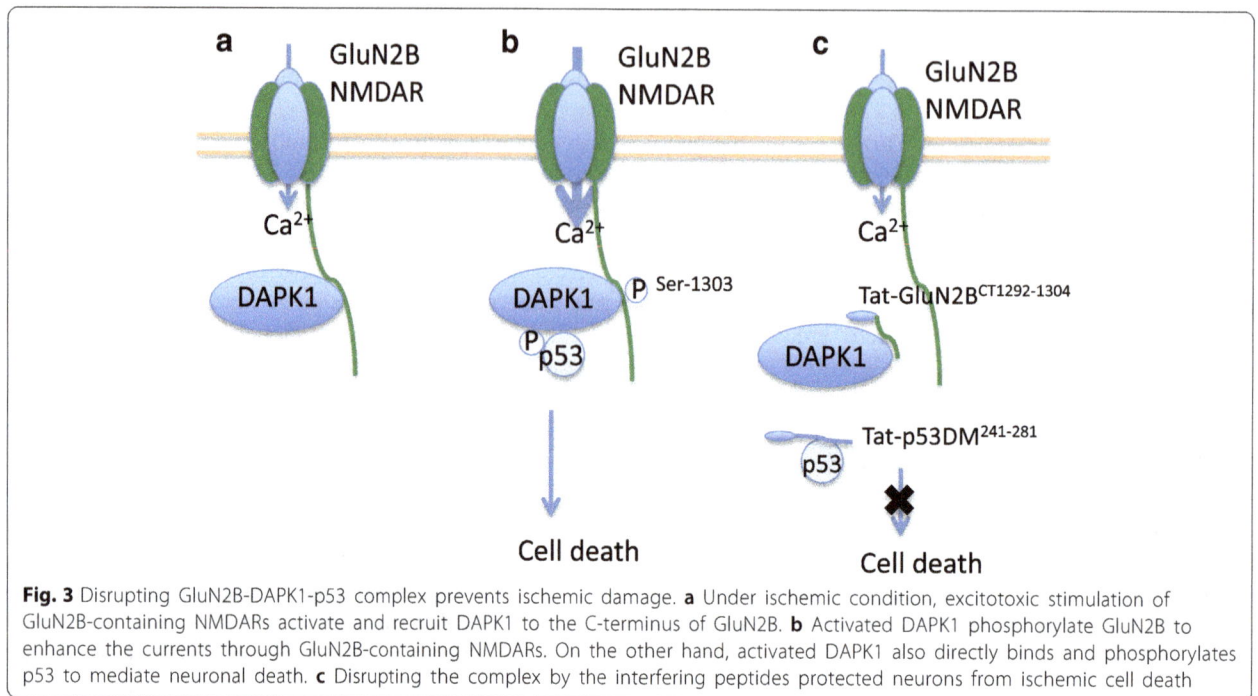

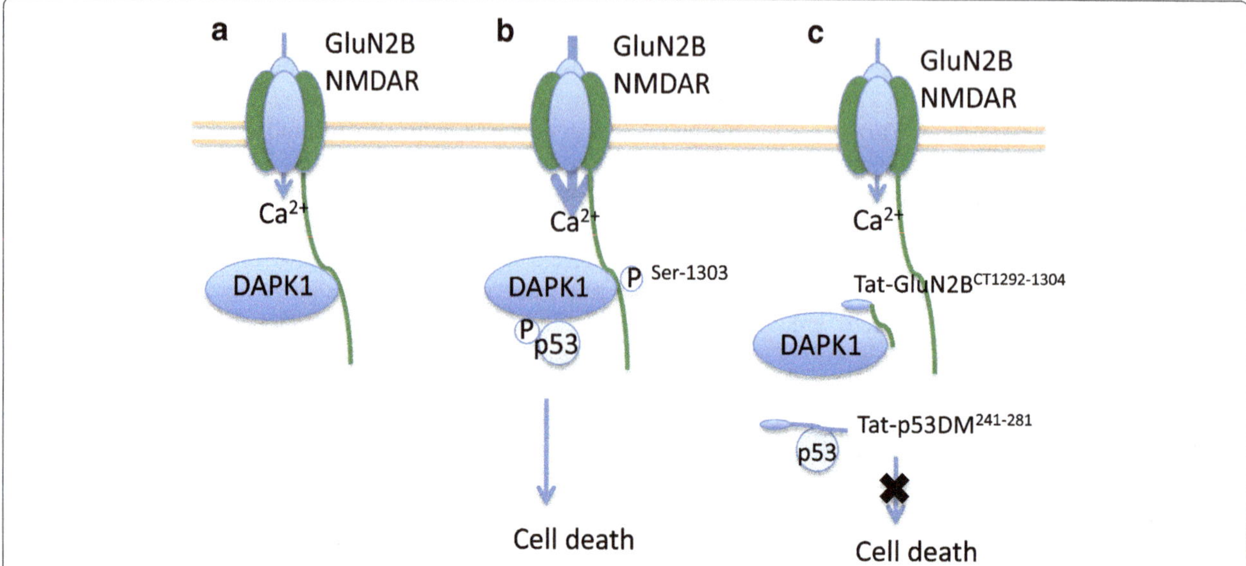

Fig. 3 Disrupting GluN2B-DAPK1-p53 complex prevents ischemic damage. **a** Under ischemic condition, excitotoxic stimulation of GluN2B-containing NMDARs activate and recruit DAPK1 to the C-terminus of GluN2B. **b** Activated DAPK1 phosphorylate GluN2B to enhance the currents through GluN2B-containing NMDARs. On the other hand, activated DAPK1 also directly binds and phosphorylates p53 to mediate neuronal death. **c** Disrupting the complex by the interfering peptides protected neurons from ischemic cell death

However, a more recent research by McQueen et al. has challenged previous report by Tu et al. [98] McQueen et al. observed that DAPK1 gene deletion did not protect neurons from excitotoxic and ischemic insults. The discrepancies between the two studies may need future investigation.

Development of Tat-GluN2B$^{CT1292-1304}$

Tu et al. has developed an interfering peptide Tat-GluN2B$^{CT1292-1304}$ to uncouple DAPK1 from the GluN2B subunit (Fig. 3). The administration of GluN2B$^{CT1292-1304}$ attenuates Ca^{2+} influx through extrasynaptic NMDARs and protects neurons from ischemic cell death in vivo, suggesting the therapeutic potential against ischemic injury. On the other hand, the recent study by McQueen et al. suggested that both Tat-GluN2B^{CT} and scrambled peptide Tat-GluN2B^{CT} are direct NMDAR antagonists [98]. The mechanism of action and the therapeutic potential of tat-GluN2B^{CT} may require future clarification.

Downstream of DAPK1: Tat-p53DM$^{241-281}$

One of the substrate for the DAPK1 kinase is the tumor suppressor p53, a transcriptional regulator that controls the cell death pathways in ischemic stroke and neurodegenerative diseases. Recently, Pei et al. found that activated DAPK1 phosphorylates p53 via direct protein-protein interaction [99]. The death domain of DAPK1 (DAPK1DD) directly binds to the p53 DNA binding motif consists of amino acids 241–281. The authors showed the significance of DAPK1-p53 interaction in mediating necrotic and apoptotic cell death [95, 99]. Based on this knowledge, an interfering peptide Tat-p53DM$^{241-281}$ was constructed to disrupt the interaction between DAPK1 and p53 (Fig. 3). Tat-p53DM$^{241-281}$ specifically inhibits the downstream signaling cascade of DAPK1, including p53-mediated expression of pro-apoptotic genes *Bax* and *Puma*, and apoptotic mediator caspase-3 [99]. In addition, Tat-p53DM$^{241-281}$ reduced infarct volume, and improved neurobehavioral outcomes even when administered 6 h after MCAO [100]. The long therapeutic time window of Tat-p53DM$^{241-281}$ makes it a potentially promising candidate for stroke treatment.

GluN2B NMDAR-PTEN

Phosphatase and tensin homolog deleted on chromosome ten (PTEN) is an important tumor suppressor with lipid and protein phosphatase activity. Previous research identified the involvement of PTEN in neuronal death after ischemia [101, 102]. PTEN can mediate apoptotic cell death by dephosphorylating phosphatidylinositol 3,4,5-trisphosphate (PIP3) and inhibiting the pro-survival Phosphatidylinositol-3-kinase (PI3K)/Akt signaling cascade [103, 104].

Once activated by the calcium influx through NMDARs, PTEN can be recruited to the neuronal death complex associated with the GluN2B-containing NMDARs. It directly interacts with the GluN1 subunit of GluN2B-containing NMDARs. This interaction augments the channel currents flow through GluN2B-containing NMDAR channel pores and further enhances the recruitment of PTEN to the GluN2B subunit mediated death-signaling complex. It is recently identified that excitotoxic stimulation of NMDARs can induce the PTEN nuclear translocation, which results in a marked reduction in pro-survival nuclear PIP3 and Akt phosphorylation [102, 105]. Increased nuclear PTEN accumulation and PTEN's cell death promoting activities contribute to the NMDAR mediated neuronal death in excitotoxicity.

Blocking PTEN nuclear translocation by Tat-K13

PTEN nuclear translocation is enabled by a single ubiquitination at residue K13 in neurons under excitotoxic stress [105]. In order to disrupt this cell death signaling, an interfering peptide Tat-K13 was developed. It consists of the transmembrane domain Tat protein and amino acids flanking the K13 ubiquitination site of PTEN [105]. Rats treated with Tat-K13 in an ischemic model had significantly reduced stroke lesion size even when administered 6 h after the stroke onset compared to the Tat-K289 control group [105]. The neuroprotective effect of Tat-K13 at 6 h supports the concept that disrupting the downstream pro-death signaling cascade can provide a wider therapeutic time window than blocking the upstream NMDAR channels.

NMDAR-SFK-Panx1

The pannexin (Panx) family of ion channels belongs to the gap junction superfamily. The intracellular gap junction channels form connexins that are permeable to a wide range of ions, second messengers and metabolites. Thompson et al. first discovered that pannexin channels were involved in anoxic depolarization and subsequent neuronal death under an ischemic condition OGD (oxygen glucose deprivation) [106–108]. Recently the same group showed NMDARs, Src kinases (SFK) and Pannexin-1 (Panx1) form a signaling complex in mediating ischemic injury [109, 110]. During ischemia, NMDAR activates SFKs, which in turn phosphorylates site Y308 in the C-terminal of Panx1 to activate Panx1 and induce secondary ischemic currents [108, 110].

Block Panx1 phosphorylation by Tat-Panx$_{308}$

Interfering peptide Tat-Panx$_{308}$ resembles the C-terminal epitope of Panx1 including the Y308 site. Tat-Panx$_{308}$ blocks the phosphorylation and activation of Panx1 by Src kinases during ischemia, and disrupts the NMDAR-Src-Panx1 complex [110]. Administration of Tat-Panx$_{308}$ before or 2 h after stroke onset reduced lesion size and sensorimotor deficits in rats, demonstrating the neuroprotective effect of dissociating the complex [110].

Further downstream death signaling proteins

Calpains: cleavage of NCX3, kidins220, STEP, mGluR1

Calpains are a family of calcium dependent cysteine proteases involved in NMDAR mediated excitotoxicity. Recent research suggests that stimulating the extrasynaptic subpopulation of NMDARs can activate calpains and induce cell death [22, 23, 111, 112] (Fig. 4). When activated, calpains can modulate substrate functions and regulate cellular mechanisms through substrate proteolysis. It's remarkable that a novel calpain inhibitor SNJ-

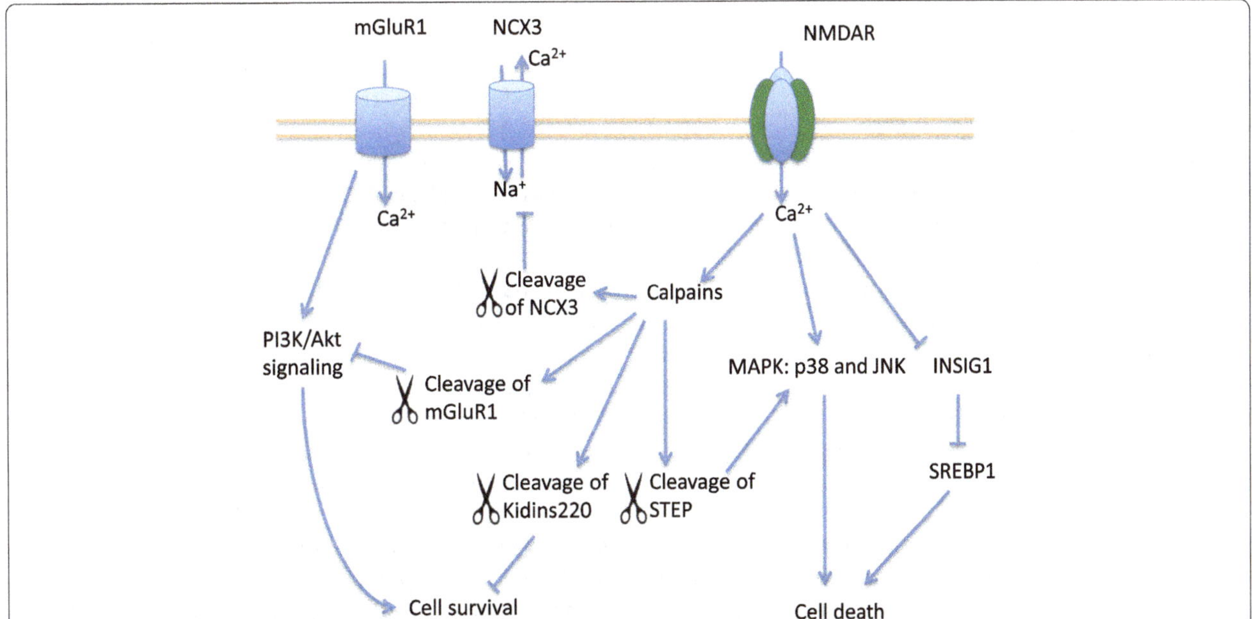

Fig. 4 Further downstream cell death signaling proteins activated by NMDARs. Stimulation of NMDARs in excitotoxicity activates calpain-mediated cleavage of proteins and contributes to cell death. Examples of the substrates for calpain-cleavage include NCX3, mGluR1, Kidins220, and STEP. In excitotoxicity, NMDARs also activate p38 and JNK to induce cell death. In addition, NMDAR stimulation triggers the degradation of INSIG1 and disinhibits SREBP1-mediated cell death

1945 demonstrated neuroprotection in cerebral ischemia in mice even when treatment was given 6 h post stroke [113].

Calpain cleavage of NCX-3

Excitotoxic calpain cleavage of plasma membrane sodium-calcium exchanger (NCX3) can induce calcium overload in the cytoplasm and mediate excitotoxic neuronal death. NCX is an important regulator of intracellular calcium level by removing Ca^{2+} from the cytoplasm. Following activation of NMDARs in excitotoxicity, NCX partially recovers the intracellular calcium concentration back to the physiological level [6, 114]. Inhibiting calpains or replacing NCX3 with another non-cleavable isoform NCX2 prevents calcium overload and neuronal death [115].

Calpain cleavage of Kidins220 and Tat-K

Kinase D-interacting substrate of 220 kDa (Kidins220) is involved in regulating and integrating signaling pathways that are essential for neuronal survival and function [116–118]. Kidins220 is involved in neurotrophin and ephrin receptors signaling [117, 118]. Excitotoxic stimulation of GluN2B-containing NMDARs activates calpains to truncate Kidins220, and impairs the neurotrophic signaling, evenally lead to ischemic neuronal damage [119].

To interfere with this process, a 25-amino acids peptide (Tat-K) was developed. It contains a short Kidins220 sequence enclosing the calpain cleavage site (AA1668–1681) linked to the Tat transmembrane protein [120]. Application of Tat-K in NMDA-treated neurons decreased calpain cleavage of Kidins220, preserved the activity of ERK and CREB that are critical for neuronal survival, and promoted cell viability [120].

Calpain cleavage of STEP and Tat-STEP

One of the substrates for calpain cleavage is the striatal enriched protein tyrosine phosphatase (STEP) [23]. STEP is an intracellular tyrosine phosphatase that antagonizes the activity dependent strengthening of synapses [121]. It dephosphorylates and inactivates a number of important synaptic signaling proteins including two of the mitogen activated protein kinases (MAPK): the extracellular signal-regulated kinase (ERK), and stress response protein kinase p38 [122, 123]. STEP was also shown to dephosphorylate GluN2B subunit at Tyr1472 and facilitates the internalization of GluN2B-containing NMDARs [124]. Activated synaptic NMDARs degrade STEP and promote pro-survival ERK signaling. In contrast, stimulating extrasynaptic NMDARs invokes calpain-mediated cleavage of STEP61 (full length protein) into STEP33 (cleavage product) [22, 23]. Truncated STEP loses its ability to bind and dephosphorylate the protein targets including p38 and GluN2B subunit of NMDARs that are enriched in the extrasynaptic region. The loss of function of STEP after calpain cleavage enhances p38 activity and prevents the endocytosis of GluN2B containing NMDARs, which contribute to ischemic damage and neuronal death.

As the activation of extrasynaptic NMDARs induces calpain mediated cleavage of STEP and causes cell death, an interfering peptide consisting of 16 amino acids spanning the cleavage site of STEP fused with TAT was developed [23]. Tat-STEP is reported to prevent the NMDAR mediated cleavage of STEP by calpains, reduces consequent p38 activation, and protects neurons from ischemic cell death in vitro [23, 125].

Calpain cleavage of mGluR1 and Tat-mGluR1

The activation of NMDARs in excitotoxicity and subsequent activated calpains have also been linked to the cleavage of metabotropic glutamate receptor 1 (mGluR1). Native mGluR1 interacts with the adaptor protein Homer and nuclear Phosphoinositide 3 kinase enhancer (PIKE) complex to activate the pro-survival PI3K/Akt signaling pathway and to protect neurons from apoptosis [126]. The calpain-mediated cleavage of mGluR1 converts the receptor from pro-survival into pro-death signaling in ischemia [6, 23]. Activation of NMDARs triggers calpains to truncate mGluR1 at Ser936 in the C-terminal domain [127]. The truncated mGluR1 is unable to activate the neuroprotective PI3K/Akt signaling pathway while its ability to increase cytosolic calcium remains intact [127].

To selectively block calpain-mediated cleavage of mGluR1, an interfering peptide was synthesized with an amino acid sequence spanning the calpain cleavage site and Tat protein transduction domain that renders the peptide permeable across cell membranes [127]. The interfering peptides compete with the endogenous mGluR1 for calpain truncation and protect the native mGluR1 receptors in neurons. Treatment with Tat-mGluR1 selectively reduced mGluR1 truncation at low concentrations (1-2uM), and prevented excitotoxic neuronal death in vitro and in vivo [127].

MAPKs: p38 inhibitors, D-JNKI-1

The mitogen-activated protein kinase (MAPK) consists of a family of serine/threonine kinases that mediate intracellular signaling associated with cellular functions such as proliferation, survival and death [128–131]. The three most extensively studied subfamilies of MAPKs are: extracellular signal-regulated kinase 1/2 (ERK1/2); p38 MAPK; and c-Jun amino terminal kinase (JNK). ERK1/2 signaling is involved in CREB activation and mainly pro-survival [128]. In contrast, p38 and JNK are stress response proteins that activate death-related transcription and mediate neuronal apoptosis [128–130, 132].

P38 and JNK MAPKs have been implicated in the NMDAR-dependent neuronal apoptosis after stroke [133–135] (Fig. 4). P38 is activated by Rho, a member of the Rho family GTPases, and induces neuronal death following excitotoxic NMDAR activation [135]. As mentioned above, calpain cleavage of STEP is also involved in p38 activation and excitotoxic cell death [23]. In addition, p38 activation may be downstream of the GluN2B-PSD95-nNOS complex, and partially contributes to the death-promoting activity of the complex in excitotoxicity [6, 136, 137]. p38 inhibitor SB239063 prevented excitotoxic neuronal death in vitro and in vivo rat focal ischemic stroke model [133, 138–140].

JNK, also known as stress-activated protein kinase (SAPK), is activated in excitotoxicity and mediates neuronal death. Mice lacking JNK3, an isoform of JNK highly expressed in the brain, are resistant to excitotoxic neuronal apoptosis [141]. A peptide inhibitor Tat-JBD_{20} (also known as JNK inhibitor-1) was designed to block JNK from binding with its downstream substrates including c-Jun, which is a major target of JNK involved in stress-induced apoptosis [142]. JNK inhibitor peptide Tat-JBD_{20} has a Tat transporter sequence plus 20 amino acid JNK binding motif of JNK interacting protein-1/islet-brain 1 (JIP-1/IB1) [143–145]. The interfering peptide is synthesized in D-retroinverso form (D-JNKI-1) to prevent protease-mediated degradation in neurons and expand its half-life in vivo [145, 146]. The JNK inhibitor D-JNKI-1 has been shown to protected neurons in vitro and reduce neuronal damage in animals subjected to focal ischemic stroke [145]. D-JNKI-1 shows neuroprotection even when administered as late as 6 or 12 h after the stroke onset [145]. Late administration in transient ischemic animal model also reduced behavioral impairment up to 14 days [145].

SREBP1: Indip

SREBP1 is a transcription factor and regulator for cholesterol, fatty acid, triglyceride, and phospholipid biosynthesis [147]. Recently SREBP1 has been identified as an NMDAR-dependent mediator of excitotoxic neuronal death

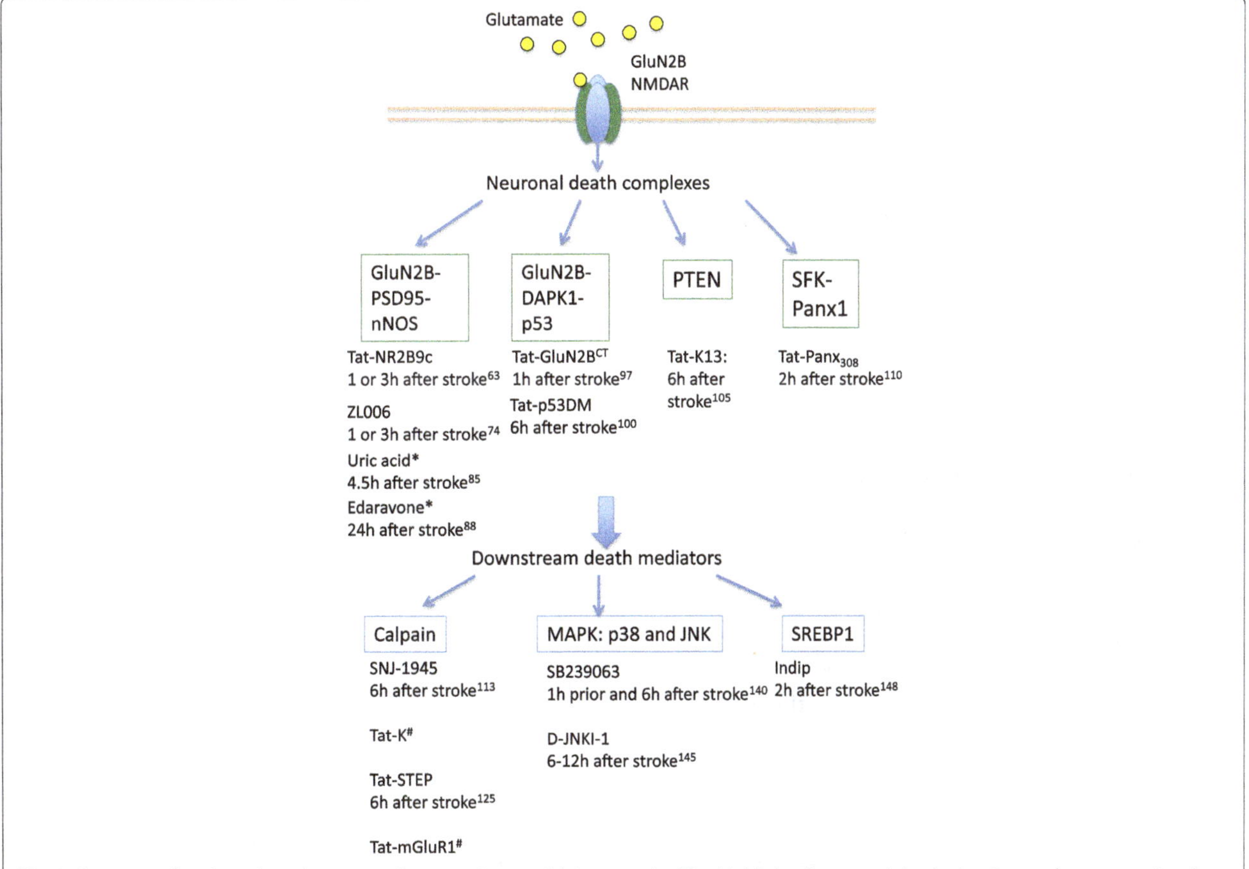

Fig. 5 Summary of excitotoxic pathways, mediators and potential therapeutics. The highlighted neuronal death signaling pathways associated with excitotoxicity are: GluN2B-PSD95-nNOS, GluN2B-DAPK1-p53, GluN2B NMDAR-PTEN, and NMDAR-SFK-Panx1. Further downstream death mediators of excitotoxicity are calpain, MAPK:p38 and JNK, and SREBP1. The interfering peptides and molecules targeting each neurotoxic pathway/mediator are listed in red, and their time windows of administration after stroke onset were previously tested in animal stroke models or clinical trials. *:Peroxynitrite scavengers and antioxidants that may act downstream of the GluN2B-PSD95-nNOS pathway to prevent neurotoxicity. #: Therapeutic time window of the peptides not yet examined in animal ischemic stroke model. Numbers in superscript indicates references in the manuscript

following ischemic stroke [6, 16, 148] (Fig. 4). Under ischemic conditions, the activation of NMDARs induces ubiquitination and proteasome-mediated degradation of insulin-induced gene 1 (INSIG1) at the endoplasmic reticulum (ER). Native INSIG1 inhibits and retains SREBP1 in the ER. The degradation of INSIG1 enables SREBP1 to travel to the Golgi apparatus where SREBP1 is cleaved and becomes activated. The active SREBP1 then translocates into the nucleus and modifies gene transcriptions to mediate neuronal death.

To block this pathway, an interfering peptide Indip (INSIG1 degradation inhibiting peptide) has been developed to inhibit INSIG1 degradation. Indip contains a Tat-linked peptide with amino acid sequence flanking the two lysine-156 and 158 ubiquitination sites of INSIG1 that are required for cleavage [149]. It inhibited INSIG1 degradation, prevented SREBP1 activation and protected neurons from neuronal death in vitro and in vivo stroke models. Indip was neuroprotective when administered 2 h after stroke, and improved neurobehavioral outcomes for up to 7 days [148].

Concluding remarks and future directions

NMDARs are essential in supporting neuronal functions under physiological functions, and also play a central role in excitotoxicity that causes neuronal death after ischemic stroke. Early treatments blocking NMDARs with antagonists failed to be translated into successful clinical neuroprotective therapies, mainly due to poor tolerance of the drugs and a short therapeutic time window. Because of the dual roles of NMDARs in pro-survival and pro-death signaling in neurons, NMDAR antagonism may eliminate survival signaling and impair neuronal function, resulting in severe adverse effects. Thus it would be better to selectively block only the pro-death effects of NMDARs while leaving pro-survival pathways intact. Moreover, once activated NMDARs trigger downstream pro-death signaling pathways, blocking the receptors may no longer be effective.

Now our understanding of ischemic mechanisms is evolving. Recent research has identified several key signaling complexes and downstream effectors in mediating neuronal death in excitotoxicity. Based on this knowledge, interfering peptides and pharmacological inhibitors have been developed to specifically uncouple the neuronal death signaling from NMDARs without affecting the functional and survival signaling of the receptors (Fig. 5). In addition, because these new potential therapeutics target the downstream pathways of NMDARs, they may provide a wider therapeutic time window.

Given the new advancements in stroke research as discussed above, the relative importance and interplay among these signaling pathways still remains to be determined. In addition, combining multiple therapies that target different pathways in stroke may have a synergistic effect in neuroprotection. Future experiments may be conducted to test the safety and efficacy of combined treatments in preventing ischemic injury.

Furthermore, ischemic stroke and neurodegenerative diseases are commonly concurrent in patients [150, 151], suggesting an overlap of pathologies in neurological diseases. Therefore, a knowledge of ischemic cell death signaling and the identified neuroprotective candidates may also benefit the development of therapies for other neurological disorders.

Abbreviations

AIF: Apoptosis inducing factor; AMPAR: α-amino-3-hydroxy-5-methylisoxazole-4-propionic acid receptors; ASK1: Apoptosis signal-regulating kinase 1; CAMKs: Ca^{2+}/calmodulin dependent protein kinases; CREB: cAMP-response element binding protein; DAPK1: Death-associated protein kinase 1; ERK: Extracellular signal-regulated kinase; INSIG1: Insulin-induced gene 1; JNK: c-Jun N-terminal Kinase; Kidins220: Kinase D-interacting substrate of 220 kDa; MAPK: Mitogen activated protein kinases; MCAO: Occlusion of the middle cerebral artery; NCX3: Sodium-calcium exchanger; NMDAR: N-methyl-d-aspartate receptors; nNOS: Nitric oxide synthase; OGD: Oxygen glucose deprivation; PI3K: Phosphoinositide-3-kinase; PSD95: Postsynaptic density protein95; PTEN: Phosphatase and tensin homolog deleted on chromosome ten; rtPA: Recombinant tissue plasminogen activator; STEP: Striatal enriched protein tyrosine phosphatase

Acknowledgements

Not applicable.

Funding

This work was supported by funds from the Canada Research Chairs program.

Authors' contributions

QJW prepared the manuscript and constructed the figures. MT edited the manuscript and figures. Both authors read and approved the final manuscript.

Competing interests

Dr. Michael Tymianski is M.T. is a Canada Research Chair (Tier 1) in Translational Stroke Research, and the CEO of NoNO Inc., a biotechnology company developing NA-1 for clinical use. QJW has no competing interests.

Author details

[1]Krembil Research Institute, University Health Network, 60 Leonard St, Toronto, ON M5T2S8, Canada. [2]Department of Physiology, University of Toronto, Toronto, ON, Canada. [3]Division of Neurosurgery, University of Toronto, Toronto, ON, Canada.

References

1. Feigin VL, Forouzanfar MH, Krishnamurthi R, Mensah GA, Connor M, Bennett DA, Moran AE, Sacco RL, Anderson L, Truelsen T, et al. Global and regional burden of stroke during 1990-2010: findings from the global burden of disease study 2010. Lancet. 2014;383(9913):245–54.
2. Donnan GA, Fisher M, Macleod M, Davis SM. Stroke. Lancet. 2008; 371(9624):1612–23.
3. Rothman SM, Olney JW. Excitotoxicity and the NMDA receptor–still lethal after eight years. Trends Neurosci. 1995;18(2):57–8.
4. Dirnagl U, Iadecola C, Moskowitz MA. Pathobiology of ischaemic stroke: an integrated view. Trends Neurosci. 1999;22(9):391–7.
5. Tymianski M. Emerging mechanisms of disrupted cellular signaling in brain ischemia. Nat Neurosci. 2011;14(11):1369–73.
6. Lai TW, Zhang S, Wang YT. Excitotoxicity and stroke: identifying novel targets for neuroprotection. Prog Neurobiol. 2014;115:157–88.
7. Gladstone DJ, Black SE, Hakim AM. Heart, Stroke Foundation of Ontario Centre of excellence in stroke R: toward wisdom from failure: lessons from neuroprotective stroke trials and new therapeutic directions. Stroke. 2002;33(8):2123–36.
8. Chamorro A, Dirnagl U, Urra X, Planas AM. Neuroprotection in acute stroke: targeting excitotoxicity, oxidative and nitrosative stress, and inflammation. Lancet Neurol. 2016;15(8):869–81.
9. California Acute Stroke Pilot Registry I. Prioritizing interventions to improve rates of thrombolysis for ischemic stroke. Neurology. 2005; 64(4):654–9.
10. Wahlgren N, Ahmed N, Davalos A, Ford GA, Grond M, Hacke W, Hennerici MG, Kaste M, Kuelkens S, Larrue V, et al. Thrombolysis with alteplase for acute ischaemic stroke in the safe implementation of thrombolysis in stroke-monitoring study (SITS-MOST): an observational study. Lancet. 2007;369(9558):275–82.
11. Larrue V, von Kummer R, del Zoppo G, Bluhmki E. Hemorrhagic transformation in acute ischemic stroke. Potential contributing factors in the European cooperative acute stroke study. Stroke. 1997;28(5): 957–60.
12. Olney JW. Brain lesions, obesity, and other disturbances in mice treated with monosodium glutamate. Science. 1969;164(3880):719–21.
13. Garthwaite G, Williams GD, Garthwaite J. Glutamate toxicity: an experimental and theoretical analysis. Eur J Neurosci. 1992;4(4):353–60.
14. Choi DW, Koh JY, Peters S. Pharmacology of glutamate neurotoxicity in cortical cell culture: attenuation by NMDA antagonists. J Neurosci. 1988;8(1):185–96.
15. Szydlowska K, Tymianski M. Calcium, ischemia and excitotoxicity. Cell Calcium. 2010;47(2):122–9.
16. Lai TW, Shyu WC, Wang YT. Stroke intervention pathways: NMDA receptors and beyond. Trends Mol Med. 2011;17(5):266–75.
17. Tymianski M, Charlton MP, Carlen PL, Tator CH. Source specificity of early calcium neurotoxicity in cultured embryonic spinal neurons. J Neurosci. 1993;13(5):2085–104.
18. Sattler R, Charlton MP, Hafner M, Tymianski M. Distinct influx pathways, not calcium load, determine neuronal vulnerability to calcium neurotoxicity. J Neurochem. 1998;71(6):2349–64.
19. Sattler R, Tymianski M. Molecular mechanisms of glutamate receptor-mediated excitotoxic neuronal cell death. Mol Neurobiol. 2001;24(1–3):107–29.
20. Aarts MM, Tymianski M. Novel treatment of excitotoxicity: targeted disruption of intracellular signalling from glutamate receptors. Biochem Pharmacol. 2003;66(6):877–86.
21. Choi DW. Glutamate neurotoxicity and diseases of the nervous system. Neuron. 1988;1(8):623–34.
22. Curcio M, Salazar IL, Mele M, Canzoniero LM, Duarte CB. Calpains and neuronal damage in the ischemic brain: the swiss knife in synaptic injury. Prog Neurobiol. 2016;143:1–35.
23. Xu J, Kurup P, Zhang Y, Goebel-Goody SM, Wu PH, Hawasli AH, Baum ML, Bibb JA, Lombroso PJ. Extrasynaptic NMDA receptors couple preferentially to excitotoxicity via calpain-mediated cleavage of STEP. J Neurosci. 2009; 29(29):9330–43.
24. Kristian T, Siesjo BK. Calcium in ischemic cell death. Stroke. 1998;29(3):705–18.
25. Eliasson MJ, Huang Z, Ferrante RJ, Sasamata M, Molliver ME, Snyder SH, Moskowitz MA. Neuronal nitric oxide synthase activation and peroxynitrite formation in ischemic stroke linked to neural damage. J Neurosci. 1999; 19(14):5910–8.
26. Lau A, Tymianski M. Glutamate receptors, neurotoxicity and neurodegeneration. Pflugers Arch. 2010;460(2):525–42.
27. Fujimura M, Morita-Fujimura Y, Murakami K, Kawase M, Chan PH. Cytosolic redistribution of cytochrome c after transient focal cerebral ischemia in rats. J Cereb Blood Flow Metab. 1998;18(11):1239–47.
28. Simon RP, Swan JH, Griffiths T, Meldrum BS. Blockade of N-methyl-D-aspartate receptors may protect against ischemic damage in the brain. Science. 1984;226(4676):850–2.
29. Muir KW, Lees KR. Clinical experience with excitatory amino acid antagonist drugs. Stroke. 1995;26(3):503–13.
30. Bordi F, Pietra C, Ziviani L, Reggiani A. The glycine antagonist GV150526 protects somatosensory evoked potentials and reduces the infarct area in the MCAo model of focal ischemia in the rat. Exp Neurol. 1997;145(2 Pt 1):425–33.
31. Takaoka S, Bart RD, Pearlstein R, Brinkhous A, Warner DS. Neuroprotective effect of NMDA receptor glycine recognition site antagonism persists when brain temperature is controlled. J Cereb Blood Flow Metab. 1997;17(2):161–7.
32. Warner DS, Martin H, Ludwig P, McAllister A, Keana JF, Weber E. In vivo models of cerebral ischemia: effects of parenterally administered NMDA receptor glycine site antagonists. J Cereb Blood Flow Metab. 1995;15(2): 188–96.
33. Pearlstein RD, Beirne JP, Massey GW, Warner DS. Neuroprotective effects of NMDA receptor glycine recognition site antagonism: dependence on glycine concentration. J Neurochem. 1998;70(5):2012–9.
34. Ginsberg MD. Neuroprotection for ischemic stroke: past, present and future. Neuropharmacology. 2008;55(3):363–89.
35. Wood PL, Hawkinson JE. N-methyl-D-aspartate antagonists for stroke and head trauma. Expert Opin Investig Drugs. 1997;6(4):389–97.
36. Dyker AG, Lees KR. Remacemide hydrochloride: a double-blind, placebo-controlled, safety and tolerability study in patients with acute ischemic stroke. Stroke. 1999;30(9):1796–801.
37. Albers GW, Atkinson RP, Kelley RE, Rosenbaum DM. Safety, tolerability, and pharmacokinetics of the N-methyl-D-aspartate antagonist dextrorphan in patients with acute stroke. Dextrorphan study group. Stroke. 1995;26(2):254–8.
38. Diener HC, AlKhedr A, Busse O, Hacke W, Zingmark PH, Jonsson N, Basun H. Study g: treatment of acute ischaemic stroke with the low-affinity, use-dependent NMDA antagonist AR-R15896AR. A safety and tolerability study. J Neurol. 2002;249(5):561–8.
39. Grotta J, Clark W, Coull B, Pettigrew LC, Mackay B, Goldstein LB, Meissner I, Murphy D, LaRue L. Safety and tolerability of the glutamate antagonist CGS 19755 (Selfotel) in patients with acute ischemic stroke. Results of a phase IIa randomized trial. Stroke. 1995;26(4):602–5.
40. Kohr G. NMDA receptor function: subunit composition versus spatial distribution. Cell Tissue Res. 2006;326(2):439–46.
41. Aamodt SM, Constantine-Paton M. The role of neural activity in synaptic development and its implications for adult brain function. Adv Neurol. 1999;79:133–44.
42. Bliss TV, Collingridge GL. A synaptic model of memory: long-term potentiation in the hippocampus. Nature. 1993;361(6407):31–9.
43. Sattler R, Xiong Z, Lu WY, JF MD, Tymianski M. Distinct roles of synaptic and extrasynaptic NMDA receptors in excitotoxicity. J Neurosci. 2000;20(1):22–33.
44. Hardingham GE, Fukunaga Y, Bading H. Extrasynaptic NMDARs oppose synaptic NMDARs by triggering CREB shut-off and cell death pathways. Nat Neurosci. 2002;5(5):405–14.
45. Leveille F, El Gaamouch F, Gouix E, Lecocq M, Lobner D, Nicole O, Buisson A. Neuronal viability is controlled by a functional relation between synaptic and extrasynaptic NMDA receptors. FASEB J. 2008;22(12):4258–71.
46. Hardingham GE. Coupling of the NMDA receptor to neuroprotective and neurodestructive events. Biochem Soc Trans. 2009;37(Pt 6):1147–60.
47. Joyal JL, Burks DJ, Pons S, Matter WF, Vlahos CJ, White MF, Sacks DB. Calmodulin activates phosphatidylinositol 3-kinase. J Biol Chem. 1997; 272(45):28183–6.
48. Alessi DR, James SR, Downes CP, Holmes AB, Gaffney PR, Reese CB, Cohen P. Characterization of a 3-phosphoinositide-dependent protein kinase which phosphorylates and activates protein kinase Balpha. Curr Biol. 1997;7(4):261–9.
49. Downward J. How BAD phosphorylation is good for survival. Nat Cell Biol. 1999;1(2):E33–5.

50. Kim AH, Khursigara G, Sun X, Franke TF, Chao MV. Akt phosphorylates and negatively regulates apoptosis signal-regulating kinase 1. Mol Cell Biol. 2001; 21(3):893–901.
51. Yamaguchi A, Tamatani M, Matsuzaki H, Namikawa K, Kiyama H, Vitek MP, Mitsuda N, Tohyama M. Akt activation protects hippocampal neurons from apoptosis by inhibiting transcriptional activity of p53. J Biol Chem. 2001; 276(7):5256–64.
52. Wu GY, Deisseroth K, Tsien RW. Activity-dependent CREB phosphorylation: convergence of a fast, sensitive calmodulin kinase pathway and a slow, less sensitive mitogen-activated protein kinase pathway. Proc Natl Acad Sci U S A. 2001;98(5):2808–13.
53. Impey S, Fong AL, Wang Y, Cardinaux JR, Fass DM, Obrietan K, Wayman GA, Storm DR, Soderling TR, Goodman RH. Phosphorylation of CBP mediates transcriptional activation by neural activity and CaM kinase IV. Neuron. 2002; 34(2):235–44.
54. Ivanov A, Pellegrino C, Rama S, Dumalska I, Salyha Y, Ben-Ari Y, Medina I. Opposing role of synaptic and extrasynaptic NMDA receptors in regulation of the extracellular signal-regulated kinases (ERK) activity in cultured rat hippocampal neurons. J Physiol. 2006;572(Pt 3):789–98.
55. Okamoto S, Pouladi MA, Talantova M, Yao D, Xia P, Ehrnhoefer DE, Zaidi R, Clemente A, Kaul M, Graham RK, et al. Balance between synaptic versus extrasynaptic NMDA receptor activity influences inclusions and neurotoxicity of mutant huntingtin. Nat Med. 2009;15(12):1407–13.
56. Xia P, Chen HS, Zhang D, Lipton SA. Memantine preferentially blocks extrasynaptic over synaptic NMDA receptor currents in hippocampal autapses. J Neurosci. 2010;30(33):11246–50.
57. Liu Y, Wong TP, Aarts M, Rooyakkers A, Liu L, Lai TW, Wu DC, Lu J, Tymianski M, Craig AM, et al. NMDA receptor subunits have differential roles in mediating excitotoxic neuronal death both in vitro and in vivo. J Neurosci. 2007;27(11):2846–57.
58. Chen M, Lu TJ, Chen XJ, Zhou Y, Chen Q, Feng XY, Xu L, Duan WH, Xiong ZQ. Differential roles of NMDA receptor subtypes in ischemic neuronal cell death and ischemic tolerance. Stroke. 2008;39(11):3042–8.
59. Kornau HC, Schenker LT, Kennedy MB, Seeburg PH. Domain interaction between NMDA receptor subunits and the postsynaptic density protein PSD-95. Science. 1995;269(5231):1737–40.
60. Tochio H, Mok YK, Zhang Q, Kan HM, Bredt DS, Zhang M. Formation of nNOS/PSD-95 PDZ dimer requires a preformed beta-finger structure from the nNOS PDZ domain. J Mol Biol. 2000;303(3):359–70.
61. Sattler R, Xiong Z, Lu WY, Hafner M, MacDonald JF, Tymianski M. Specific coupling of NMDA receptor activation to nitric oxide neurotoxicity by PSD-95 protein. Science. 1999;284(5421):1845–8.
62. Aarts M, Liu Y, Liu L, Besshoh S, Arundine M, Gurd JW, Wang YT, Salter MW, Tymianski M. Treatment of ischemic brain damage by perturbing NMDA receptor- PSD-95 protein interactions. Science. 2002;298(5594):846–50.
63. Sun HS, Doucette TA, Liu Y, Fang Y, Teves L, Aarts M, Ryan CL, Bernard PB, Lau A, Forder JP, et al. Effectiveness of PSD95 inhibitors in permanent and transient focal ischemia in the rat. Stroke. 2008;39(9):2544–53.
64. Cook DJ, Teves L, Tymianski M. Treatment of stroke with a PSD-95 inhibitor in the gyrencephalic primate brain. Nature. 2012;483(7388):213–7.
65. Lipton SA, Choi YB, Pan ZH, Lei SZ, Chen HS, Sucher NJ, Loscalzo J, Singel DJ, Stamler JS. A redox-based mechanism for the neuroprotective and neurodestructive effects of nitric oxide and related nitroso-compounds. Nature. 1993;364(6438):626–32.
66. Radi R, Beckman JS, Bush KM, Freeman BA. Peroxynitrite-induced membrane lipid peroxidation: the cytotoxic potential of superoxide and nitric oxide. Arch Biochem Biophys. 1991;288(2):481–7.
67. Salgo MG, Bermudez E, Squadrito GL, Pryor WA. Peroxynitrite causes DNA damage and oxidation of thiols in rat thymocytes [corrected]. Arch Biochem Biophys. 1995;322(2):500–5.
68. Zhang J, Dawson VL, Dawson TM, Snyder SH. Nitric oxide activation of poly(ADP-ribose) synthetase in neurotoxicity. Science. 1994;263(5147):687–9.
69. Yu SW, Wang H, Poitras MF, Coombs C, Bowers WJ, Federoff HJ, Poirier GG, Dawson TM, Dawson VL. Mediation of poly(ADP-ribose) polymerase-1-dependent cell death by apoptosis-inducing factor. Science. 2002;297(5579): 259–63.
70. Tymianski M. Can molecular and cellular neuroprotection be translated into therapies for patients?: yes, but not the way we tried it before. Stroke. 2010; 41(10 Suppl):S87–90.
71. Tymianski M. Novel approaches to neuroprotection trials in acute ischemic stroke. Stroke. 2013;44(10):2942–50.
72. Bratane BT, Cui H, Cook DJ, Bouley J, Tymianski M, Fisher M. Neuroprotection by freezing ischemic penumbra evolution without cerebral blood flow augmentation with a postsynaptic density-95 protein inhibitor. Stroke. 2011;42(11):3265–70.
73. Hill MD, Martin RH, Mikulis D, Wong JH, Silver FL, Terbrugge KG, Milot G, Clark WM, Macdonald RL, Kelly ME, et al. Safety and efficacy of NA-1 in patients with iatrogenic stroke after endovascular aneurysm repair (ENACT): a phase 2, randomised, double-blind, placebo-controlled trial. Lancet Neurol. 2012;11(11):942–50.
74. Zhou L, Li F, Xu HB, Luo CX, Wu HY, Zhu MM, Lu W, Ji X, Zhou QG, Zhu DY. Treatment of cerebral ischemia by disrupting ischemia-induced interaction of nNOS with PSD-95. Nat Med. 2010;16(12):1439–43.
75. Florio SK, Loh C, Huang SM, Iwamaye AE, Kitto KF, Fowler KW, Treiberg JA, Hayflick JS, Walker JM, Fairbanks CA, et al. Disruption of nNOS-PSD95 protein-protein interaction inhibits acute thermal hyperalgesia and chronic mechanical allodynia in rodents. Br J Pharmacol. 2009;158(2):494–506.
76. Bach A, Pedersen SW, Dorr LA, Vallon G, Ripoche I, Ducki S, Lian LY. Biochemical investigations of the mechanism of action of small molecules ZL006 and IC87201 as potential inhibitors of the nNOS-PDZ/PSD-95-PDZ interactions. Sci Rep. 2015;5:12157.
77. Marshall JW, Cummings RM, Bowes LJ, Ridley RM, Green AR. Functional and histological evidence for the protective effect of NXY-059 in a primate model of stroke when given 4 hours after occlusion. Stroke. 2003;34(9):2228–33.
78. Kuroda S, Tsuchidate R, Smith ML, Maples KR, Siesjo BK. Neuroprotective effects of a novel nitrone, NXY-059, after transient focal cerebral ischemia in the rat. J Cereb Blood Flow Metab. 1999;19(7):778–87.
79. Shuaib A, Lees KR, Lyden P, Grotta J, Davalos A, Davis SM, Diener HC, Ashwood T, Wasiewski WW, Emeribe U, et al. NXY-059 for the treatment of acute ischemic stroke. N Engl J Med. 2007;357(6):562–71.
80. Sautin YY, Johnson RJ. Uric acid: the oxidant-antioxidant paradox. Nucleosides Nucleotides Nucleic Acids. 2008;27(6):608–19.
81. Squadrito GL, Cueto R, Splenser AE, Valavanidis A, Zhang H, Uppu RM, Pryor WA. Reaction of uric acid with peroxynitrite and implications for the mechanism of neuroprotection by uric acid. Arch Biochem Biophys. 2000; 376(2):333–7.
82. Romanos E, Planas AM, Amaro S, Chamorro A. Uric acid reduces brain damage and improves the benefits of rt-PA in a rat model of thromboembolic stroke. J Cereb Blood Flow Metab. 2007;27(1):14–20.
83. Onetti Y, Dantas AP, Perez B, Cugota R, Chamorro A, Planas AM, Vila E, Jimenez-Altayo F. Middle cerebral artery remodeling following transient brain ischemia is linked to early postischemic hyperemia: a target of uric acid treatment. Am J Physiol Heart Circ Physiol. 2015;308(8):H862–74.
84. Amaro S, Laredo C, Renu A, Llull L, Rudilosso S, Obach V, Urra X, Planas AM, Chamorro A, Investigators U-I. Uric acid therapy prevents early ischemic stroke progression: a tertiary analysis of the URICO-ICTUS trial (efficacy study of combined treatment with uric acid and r-tPA in acute ischemic stroke). Stroke. 2016;47(11):2874–6.
85. Chamorro A, Amaro S, Castellanos M, Segura T, Arenillas J, Marti-Fabregas J, Gallego J, Krupinski J, Gomis M, Canovas D, et al. Safety and efficacy of uric acid in patients with acute stroke (URICO-ICTUS): a randomised, double-blind phase 2b/3 trial. Lancet Neurol. 2014; 13(5):453–60.
86. Llull L, Laredo C, Renu A, Perez B, Vila E, Obach V, Urra X, Planas A, Amaro S, Chamorro A. Uric acid therapy improves clinical outcome in women with acute ischemic stroke. Stroke. 2015;46(8):2162–7.
87. Amaro S, Llull L, Renu A, Laredo C, Perez B, Vila E, Torres F, Planas AM, Chamorro A. Uric acid improves glucose-driven oxidative stress in human ischemic stroke. Ann Neurol. 2015;77(5):775–83.
88. Lapchak PA. A critical assessment of edaravone acute ischemic stroke efficacy trials: is edaravone an effective neuroprotective therapy? Expert Opin Pharmacother. 2010;11(10):1753–63.
89. Nishi H, Watanabe T, Sakurai H, Yuki S, Ishibashi A. Effect of MCI-186 on brain edema in rats. Stroke. 1989;20(9):1236–40.
90. Watanabe T, Yuki S, Egawa M, Nishi H. Protective effects of MCI-186 on cerebral ischemia: possible involvement of free radical scavenging and antioxidant actions. J Pharmacol Exp Ther. 1994;268(3):1597–604.
91. Wu TW, Zeng LH, Wu J, Fung KP. MCI-186: further histochemical and biochemical evidence of neuroprotection. Life Sci. 2000;67(19):2387–92.
92. Lapchak PA, Zivin JA. The lipophilic multifunctional antioxidant edaravone (radicut) improves behavior following embolic strokes in rabbits: a

combination therapy study with tissue plasminogen activator. Exp Neurol. 2009;215(1):95–100.

93. Bialik S, Kimchi A. The death-associated protein kinases: structure, function, and beyond. Annu Rev Biochem. 2006;75:189–210.
94. Chen CH, Wang WJ, Kuo JC, Tsai HC, Lin JR, Chang ZF, Chen RH. Bidirectional signals transduced by DAPK-ERK interaction promote the apoptotic effect of DAPK. EMBO J. 2005;24(2):294–304.
95. Wang S, Shi X, Li H, Pang P, Pei L, Shen H, Lu Y. DAPK1 signaling pathways in stroke: from mechanisms to therapies. Mol Neurobiol. 2017;54(6):4716–22.
96. Marshall J, Dolan BM, Garcia EP, Sathe S, Tang X, Mao Z, Blair LA. Calcium channel and NMDA receptor activities differentially regulate nuclear C/EBPbeta levels to control neuronal survival. Neuron. 2003;39(4):625–39.
97. Tu W, Xu X, Peng L, Zhong X, Zhang W, Soundarapandian MM, Balel C, Wang M, Jia N, Zhang W, et al. DAPK1 interaction with NMDA receptor NR2B subunits mediates brain damage in stroke. Cell. 2010;140(2):222–34.
98. McQueen J, Ryan TJ, McKay S, Marwick K, Baxter P, Carpanini SM, Wishart TM, Gillingwater TH, Manson JC, Wyllie DJA, et al. Pro-death NMDA receptor signaling is promoted by the GluN2B C-terminus independently of Dapk1. Elife. 2017;6:e17161. https://doi.org/10.7554/eLife.17161.
99. Pei L, Shang Y, Jin H, Wang S, Wei N, Yan H, Wu Y, Yao C, Wang X, Zhu LQ, et al. DAPK1-p53 interaction converges necrotic and apoptotic pathways of ischemic neuronal death. J Neurosci. 2014;34(19):6546–56.
100. Wang X, Pei L, Yan H, Wang Z, Wei N, Wang S, Yang X, Tian Q, Lu Y. Intervention of death-associated protein kinase 1-p53 interaction exerts the therapeutic effects against stroke. Stroke. 2014;45(10):3089–91.
101. Gary DS, Mattson MP. PTEN regulates Akt kinase activity in hippocampal neurons and increases their sensitivity to glutamate and apoptosis. NeuroMolecular Med. 2002;2(3):261–9.
102. Ning K, Pei L, Liao M, Liu B, Zhang Y, Jiang W, Mielke JG, Li L, Chen Y, El-Hayek YH, et al. Dual neuroprotective signaling mediated by downregulating two distinct phosphatase activities of PTEN. J Neurosci. 2004;24(16):4052–60.
103. Stambolic V, Suzuki A, de la Pompa JL, Brothers GM, Mirtsos C, Sasaki T, Ruland J, Penninger JM, Siderovski DP, Mak TW. Negative regulation of PKB/Akt-dependent cell survival by the tumor suppressor PTEN. Cell. 1998;95(1):29–39.
104. Maehama T, Dixon JE. The tumor suppressor, PTEN/MMAC1, dephosphorylates the lipid second messenger, phosphatidylinositol 3,4,5-trisphosphate. J Biol Chem. 1998;273(22):13375–8.
105. Zhang S, Taghibiglou C, Girling K, Dong Z, Lin SZ, Lee W, Shyu WC, Wang YT. Critical role of increased PTEN nuclear translocation in excitotoxic and ischemic neuronal injuries. J Neurosci. 2013;33(18):7997–8008.
106. Thompson RJ, Zhou N, MacVicar BA. Ischemia opens neuronal gap junction hemichannels. Science. 2006;312(5775):924–7.
107. Thompson RJ, Jackson MF, Olah ME, Rungta RL, Hines DJ, Beazely MA, MacDonald JF, MacVicar BA. Activation of pannexin-1 hemichannels augments aberrant bursting in the hippocampus. Science. 2008; 322(5907):1555–9.
108. Thompson RJ. Pannexin channels and ischaemia. J Physiol. 2015; 593(16):3463–70.
109. Weilinger NL, Tang PL, Thompson RJ. Anoxia-induced NMDA receptor activation opens pannexin channels via Src family kinases. J Neurosci. 2012;32(36):12579–88.
110. Weilinger NL, Lohman AW, Rakai BD, Ma EM, Bialecki J, Maslieieva V, Rilea T, Bandet MV, Ikuta NT, Scott L, et al. Metabotropic NMDA receptor signaling couples Src family kinases to pannexin-1 during excitotoxicity. Nat Neurosci. 2016;19(3):432–42.
111. D'Orsi B, Bonner H, Tuffy LP, Dussmann H, Woods I, Courtney MJ, Ward MW, Prehn JH. Calpains are downstream effectors of bax-dependent excitotoxic apoptosis. J Neurosci. 2012;32(5):1847–58.
112. DeRidder MN, Simon MJ, Siman R, Auberson YP, Raghupathi R, Meaney DF. Traumatic mechanical injury to the hippocampus in vitro causes regional caspase-3 and calpain activation that is influenced by NMDA receptor subunit composition. Neurobiol Dis. 2006;22(1):165–76.
113. Koumura A, Nonaka Y, Hyakkoku K, Oka T, Shimazawa M, Hozumi I, Inuzuka T, Hara H. A novel calpain inhibitor, ((1S)-1((((1S)-1-benzyl-3-cyclopropylamino-2,3-di-oxopropyl)amino)carbonyl)-3-met hylbutyl) carbamic acid 5-methoxy-3-oxapentyl ester, protects neuronal cells from cerebral ischemia-induced damage in mice. Neuroscience. 2008;157(2):309–18.
114. White RJ, Reynolds IJ. Mitochondria and Na+/Ca2+ exchange buffer glutamate-induced calcium loads in cultured cortical neurons. J Neurosci. 1995;15(2):1318–28.
115. Bano D, Young KW, Guerin CJ, Lefeuvre R, Rothwell NJ, Naldini L, Rizzuto R, Carafoli E, Nicotera P. Cleavage of the plasma membrane Na+/Ca2+ exchanger in excitotoxicity. Cell. 2005;120(2):275–85.
116. Iglesias T, Cabrera-Poch N, Mitchell MP, Naven TJ, Rozengurt E, Schiavo G. Identification and cloning of Kidins220, a novel neuronal substrate of protein kinase D. J Biol Chem. 2000;275(51):40048–56.
117. Arevalo JC, Yano H, Teng KK, Chao MV. A unique pathway for sustained neurotrophin signaling through an ankyrin-rich membrane-spanning protein. EMBO J. 2004;23(12):2358–68.
118. Arevalo JC, Pereira DB, Yano H, Teng KK, Chao MV. Identification of a switch in neurotrophin signaling by selective tyrosine phosphorylation. J Biol Chem. 2006;281(2):1001–7.
119. Lopez-Menendez C, Gascon S, Sobrado M, Vidaurre OG, Higuero AM, Rodriguez-Pena A, Iglesias T, Diaz-Guerra M. Kidins220/ARMS downregulation by excitotoxic activation of NMDARs reveals its involvement in neuronal survival and death pathways. J Cell Sci. 2009;122(Pt 19):3554–65.
120. Gamir-Morralla A, Lopez-Menendez C, Ayuso-Dolado S, Tejeda GS, Montaner J, Rosell A, Iglesias T, Diaz-Guerra M. Development of a neuroprotective peptide that preserves survival pathways by preventing Kidins220/ARMS calpain processing induced by excitotoxicity. Cell Death Dis. 2015;6:e1939.
121. Braithwaite SP, Paul S, Nairn AC, Lombroso PJ. Synaptic plasticity: one STEP at a time. Trends Neurosci. 2006;29(8):452–8.
122. Munoz JJ, Tarrega C, Blanco-Aparicio C, Pulido R. Differential interaction of the tyrosine phosphatases PTP-SL, STEP and HePTP with the mitogen-activated protein kinases ERK1/2 and p38alpha is determined by a kinase specificity sequence and influenced by reducing agents. Biochem J. 2003; 372(Pt 1):193–201.
123. Paul S, Nairn AC, Wang P, Lombroso PJ. NMDA-mediated activation of the tyrosine phosphatase STEP regulates the duration of ERK signaling. Nat Neurosci. 2003;6(1):34–42.
124. Snyder EM, Nong Y, Almeida CG, Paul S, Moran T, Choi EY, Nairn AC, Salter MW, Lombroso PJ, Gouras GK, et al. Regulation of NMDA receptor trafficking by amyloid-beta. Nat Neurosci. 2005;8(8):1051–8.
125. Deb I, Manhas N, Poddar R, Rajagopal S, Allan AM, Lombroso PJ, Rosenberg GA, Candelario-Jalil E, Paul S. Neuroprotective role of a brain-enriched tyrosine phosphatase, STEP, in focal cerebral ischemia. J Neurosci. 2013;33(45):17814–26.
126. Rong R, Ahn JY, Huang H, Nagata E, Kalman D, Kapp JA, Tu J, Worley PF, Snyder SH, Ye K. PI3 kinase enhancer-Homer complex couples mGluRI to PI3 kinase, preventing neuronal apoptosis. Nat Neurosci. 2003;6(11):1153–61.
127. Xu W, Wong TP, Chery N, Gaertner T, Wang YT, Baudry M. Calpain-mediated mGluR1alpha truncation: a key step in excitotoxicity. Neuron. 2007;53(3):399–412.
128. Xia Z, Dickens M, Raingeaud J, Davis RJ, Greenberg ME. Opposing effects of ERK and JNK-p38 MAP kinases on apoptosis. Science. 1995;270(5240):1326–31.
129. Graves JD, Draves KE, Craxton A, Saklatvala J, Krebs EG, Clark EA. Involvement of stress-activated protein kinase and p38 mitogen-activated protein kinase in mIgM-induced apoptosis of human B lymphocytes. Proc Natl Acad Sci U S A. 1996;93(24):13814–8.
130. Verheij M, Bose R, Lin XH, Yao B, Jarvis WD, Grant S, Birrer MJ, Szabo E, Zon LI, Kyriakis JM, et al. Requirement for ceramide-initiated SAPK/JNK signalling in stress-induced apoptosis. Nature. 1996;380(6569):75–9.
131. Davis RJ. Signal transduction by the JNK group of MAP kinases. Cell. 2000; 103(2):239–52.
132. Gupta S, Barrett T, Whitmarsh AJ, Cavanagh J, Sluss HK, Derijard B, Davis RJ. Selective interaction of JNK protein kinase isoforms with transcription factors. EMBO J. 1996;15(11):2760–70.
133. Kawasaki H, Morooka T, Shimohama S, Kimura J, Hirano T, Gotoh Y, Nishida E. Activation and involvement of p38 mitogen-activated protein kinase in glutamate-induced apoptosis in rat cerebellar granule cells. J Biol Chem. 1997;272(30):18518–21.
134. Cao J, Semenova MM, Solovyan VT, Han J, Coffey ET, Courtney MJ. Distinct requirements for p38alpha and c-Jun N-terminal kinase stress-activated protein kinases in different forms of apoptotic neuronal death. J Biol Chem. 2004;279(34):35903–13.
135. Semenova MM, Maki-Hokkonen AM, Cao J, Komarovski V, Forsberg KM, Koistinaho M, Coffey ET, Courtney MJ. Rho mediates calcium-dependent activation of p38alpha and subsequent excitotoxic cell death. Nat Neurosci. 2007;10(4):436–43.
136. Cao J, Viholainen JI, Dart C, Warwick HK, Leyland ML, Courtney MJ. The PSD95-nNOS interface: a target for inhibition of excitotoxic p38 stress-

activated protein kinase activation and cell death. J Cell Biol. 2005; 168(1):117–26.
137. Li LL, Ginet V, Liu X, Vergun O, Tuittila M, Mathieu M, Bonny C, Puyal J, Truttmann AC, Courtney MJ. The nNOS-p38MAPK pathway is mediated by NOS1AP during neuronal death. J Neurosci. 2013;33(19):8185–201.
138. Legos JJ, McLaughlin B, Skaper SD, Strijbos PJ, Parsons AA, Aizenman E, Herin GA, Barone FC, Erhardt JA. The selective p38 inhibitor SB-239063 protects primary neurons from mild to moderate excitotoxic injury. Eur J Pharmacol. 2002;447(1):37–42.
139. Barone FC, Irving EA, Ray AM, Lee JC, Kassis S, Kumar S, Badger AM, White RF, McVey MJ, Legos JJ, et al. SB 239063, a second-generation p38 mitogen-activated protein kinase inhibitor, reduces brain injury and neurological deficits in cerebral focal ischemia. J Pharmacol Exp Ther. 2001;296(2):312–21.
140. Legos JJ, Erhardt JA, White RF, Lenhard SC, Chandra S, Parsons AA, Tuma RF, Barone FC. SB 239063, a novel p38 inhibitor, attenuates early neuronal injury following ischemia. Brain Res. 2001;892(1):70–7.
141. Yang DD, Kuan CY, Whitmarsh AJ, Rincon M, Zheng TS, Davis RJ, Rakic P, Flavell RA. Absence of excitotoxicity-induced apoptosis in the hippocampus of mice lacking the Jnk3 gene. Nature. 1997;389(6653):865–70.
142. Whitmarsh AJ, Kuan CY, Kennedy NJ, Kelkar N, Haydar TF, Mordes JP, Appel M, Rossini AA, Jones SN, Flavell RA, et al. Requirement of the JIP1 scaffold protein for stress-induced JNK activation. Genes Dev. 2001;15(18):2421–32.
143. Barr RK, Kendrick TS, Bogoyevitch MA. Identification of the critical features of a small peptide inhibitor of JNK activity. J Biol Chem. 2002;277(13):10987–97.
144. Bonny C, Oberson A, Negri S, Sauser C, Schorderet DF. Cell-permeable peptide inhibitors of JNK: novel blockers of beta-cell death. Diabetes. 2001;50(1):77–82.
145. Borsello T, Clarke PG, Hirt L, Vercelli A, Repici M, Schorderet DF, Bogousslavsky J, Bonny C. A peptide inhibitor of c-Jun N-terminal kinase protects against excitotoxicity and cerebral ischemia. Nat Med. 2003;9(9):1180–6.
146. Brugidou J, Legrand C, Mery J, Rabie A. The retro-inverso form of a homeobox-derived short peptide is rapidly internalised by cultured neurones: a new basis for an efficient intracellular delivery system. Biochem Biophys Res Commun. 1995;214(2):685–93.
147. Goldstein JL, DeBose-Boyd RA, Brown MS. Protein sensors for membrane sterols. Cell. 2006;124(1):35–46.
148. Taghibiglou C, Martin HG, Lai TW, Cho T, Prasad S, Kojic L, Lu J, Liu Y, Lo E, Zhang S, et al. Role of NMDA receptor-dependent activation of SREBP1 in excitotoxic and ischemic neuronal injuries. Nat Med. 2009;15(12):1399–406.
149. Gong Y, Lee JN, Lee PC, Goldstein JL, Brown MS, Ye J. Sterol-regulated ubiquitination and degradation of Insig-1 creates a convergent mechanism for feedback control of cholesterol synthesis and uptake. Cell Metab. 2006;3(1):15–24.
150. Leys D, Henon H, Mackowiak-Cordoliani MA, Pasquier F. Poststroke dementia. Lancet Neurol. 2005;4(11):752–9.
151. Cumming TB, Brodtmann A. Can stroke cause neurodegenerative dementia? Int J Stroke. 2011;6(5):416–24.

6

The DLGAP family: neuronal expression, function and role in brain disorders

Andreas H. Rasmussen[1], Hanne B. Rasmussen[2] and Asli Silahtaroglu[1*]

Abstract

The neurotransmitter glutamate facilitates neuronal signalling at excitatory synapses. Glutamate is released from the presynaptic membrane into the synaptic cleft. Across the synaptic cleft glutamate binds to both ion channels and metabotropic glutamate receptors at the postsynapse, which expedite downstream signalling in the neuron. The postsynaptic density, a highly specialized matrix, which is attached to the postsynaptic membrane, controls this downstream signalling. The postsynaptic density also resets the synapse after each synaptic firing. It is composed of numerous proteins including a family of Discs large associated protein 1, 2, 3 and 4 (DLGAP1-4) that act as scaffold proteins in the postsynaptic density. They link the glutamate receptors in the postsynaptic membrane to other glutamate receptors, to signalling proteins and to components of the cytoskeleton. With the central localisation in the postsynapse, the DLGAP family seems to play a vital role in synaptic scaling by regulating the turnover of both ionotropic and metabotropic glutamate receptors in response to synaptic activity. DLGAP family has been directly linked to a variety of psychological and neurological disorders. In this review we focus on the direct and indirect role of DLGAP family on schizophrenia as well as other brain diseases.

Keywords: DLGAP1, DLGAP2, DLGAP3, DLGAP4, SAPAP, PSD, GKAP, Schizophrenia, Scaffold proteins, Synaptic scaling

Introduction

The postsynaptic density (PSD) is a highly specialized matrix that is involved in transmission of neuronal signals across the synaptic junction. The PSD is found in the synaptic terminal of postsynaptic neurons. A variety of proteins is expressed in the PSD for transmitting neuronal signals from the PSD to the soma or other parts of the neuron. The PSD scaffolding proteins, Discs large scaffold proteins (DLGs) and the family of Src-homology (SH3) and multiple ankyrin repeat domain proteins (SHANK) are essential for proper function of both the ionotropic N-methyl-D-aspartate (NMDA) and α-amino-3-hydroxy-5-methyl-4-isoxazolepropionic acid (AMPA) receptors and the metabotropic glutamate receptors (mGluRs) [1–4]. The family of Discs large associated proteins (DLGAPs) are also important scaffold proteins in the PSD. There are five DLGAP proteins, DLGAP1 – DLGAP5 where DLGAP1 - DLGAP4 (DLGAP1–4) proteins interact directly with both DLG and SHANK through their multiple domains [2, 5, 6]. Via interaction partners, DLGAP1–4 proteins are likely to play a role in multiple processes of the PSD. For example, neuronal DLGAP proteins have key roles in synaptic scaling [7, 8]. DLGAP1–4 proteins have also been linked to a variety of neurological disorders including schizophrenia, autism spectrum disease (ASD), trichotillomania, obsessive compulsive disorder (OCD) and cerebellar ataxia [9–14] (see Table 1). Here we present the existing knowledge on the expression, function and the regulation of DLGAP1–4 in the brain. We also review the link of DLGAP1–4 to the various neurological disorders. DLGAP5 is not included in this review since it is mainly linked to various types of cancers and does not seem to play an important role in neuronal signalling [15–17].

Nomenclature

The DLGAP protein family is known under several different names. Initially DLGAP1 was named Guanylate kinase associated protein (GKAP) since it interacts with the guanylate kinase (GK) domain of SAP90/PSD-95 [5]. Shortly after, three other similar proteins were and the family of four proteins was subsequently named as SAP90/PSD95-associated

* Correspondence: asli@sund.ku.dk
[1]Department of Cellular and Molecular Medicine, Faculty of Medical and Health Sciences, University of Copenhagen, DK-2200 Copenhagen, Denmark
Full list of author information is available at the end of the article

Table 1 Table with the DLGAP subtypes expressed in the brain i.e. DLGAP1–4 and the corresponding CNS diseases and affected brain regions

DLGAP subtype	CNS disease	Brain region affected	References
DLGAP1	Schizophrenia	Nucleus accumbens	[9]
	Alzheimer's disease	Frontal cortex	[114]
	Major depressive disorder	Hippocampus	[115]
DLGAP2	Schizophrenia	na*	[99]
	Fragile x mental retardation	Hippocampus	[116]
	Post traumatic stress disorder	Hippocampus	[102]
	Autism spectrum disease	na*	[10, 100, 101]
DLGAP3	Trichotillomania	Striatum	[11, 12]
	Obsessive compulsive disorder	Striatum	[11, 13, 106]
	Parkinson's disease	na*	[117]
	Schizophrenia	na*	[98]
DLGAP4	Cerebellar ataxia	Cerebellum	[14]
	Bipolar disorder (indirectly linked)	na*	[118]

na* No proven affected brain region. DLGAP1 is thought to be involved in schizophrenia starting from nucleus accumbens, Alzheimer's disease in frontal cortex and major depressive disorder originating from hippocampus. DLGAP2 is linked to multiple diseases. First schizophrenia with no proven affected brain region, second autism spectrum disease also with no proven affected brain region and finally fragile x mental retardation and post-traumatic stress disorder both originating from the hippocampus. DLGAP3 is proven to be involved in both trichotillomania and OCD both starting in the striatum. DLGAP3 has also been linked to Parkinson's disease. Finally, DLGAP4 is proven to be involved in cerebellar ataxia coming from cerebellum and indirectly to bipolar disorder via the microRNA miR-1908-5p. The relevant references are linked in the fourth column, respectively

protein 1–4 (SAPAP1–4) [18]. DLGAP1 is, however, still referred to as GKAP in the literature. PSD-95 is also named Discs large scaffold protein 4 abbreviated DLG4. Therefore, the SAPAP family proteins were named discs large homolog associated protein (DLGAP) 1–4. PSD-95 will in this work be referred to as DLG4 and GKAP/SAPAP1–4 will be referred to as DLGAP1–4.

DLGAP chromosomal localisation, protein homology and conservation

Four DLGAP proteins are found in the human brain, which are all encoded from a different locus. This section contains an overview of the chromosomal locations and mRNA transcript variants of *DLGAP* genes in human. The DLGAP proteins have a high sequential homology that we will review in detail along with the conservation of the DLGAP family in mammals and vertebrates.

Chromosomal localisation and mRNA transcripts

The *DLGAP1–4* genes are located on 4 different chromosomes. *DLGAP1* is located on the short arm of chromosome 18 within the band 11.31 (18p11.31) and has 9 human transcript variants spanning from 2253 nucleotides to 6628 nucleotides (see Fig. 1a). *DLGAP2* is located on the short arm of chromosome 8, in the band 23.3 (8p23.3). Two transcript variants have been identified for *DLGAP2* having only one exon difference. Transcript variant 1 has 12 exons and transcript variant 2 has 11 exons (see Fig. 1a). *DLGAP3* is located on chromosome 1 in the band 34.3 on the short arm (1p34.3). Only one human *DLGAP3* transcript has been identified so far (see Fig. 1a). The *DLGAP4* gene is situated on the long arm of chromosome 20 within the band 11.23 (20q11.23). Three transcript variants with varying lengths from 3044 nucleotides to 5080 nucleotides have been found in human (see Fig. 1a).

DLGAP protein homology

The many mRNA transcripts of *DLGAP1–4* encode DLGAP proteins with various lengths and domains (see Fig. 2a). The pairwise homology between the DLGAP proteins differ by 26 to 48%. DLGAP1 compared to DLGAP2 show the highest homology and DLGAP3 compared to DLGAP4 show the lowest homology (see Fig. 1b). DLGAP1–4 have 3 domains, a 14 amino acids repeat domain, a dynein light chain (DLC) domain and a GKAP homology (GH1) domain (see section 4.1). Especially the GH1 domain by which the DLGAP proteins are characterized, shows a high degree of homology i.e. 61 to 75%. In addition, the last 40 residues next to the C-terminal also show a high degree of homology (see Fig. 1d).

Conservation

DLGAP1–4 are important proteins in the postsynaptic density. They act as scaffold proteins and are involved in signalling to and from glutamate receptors [19]. The

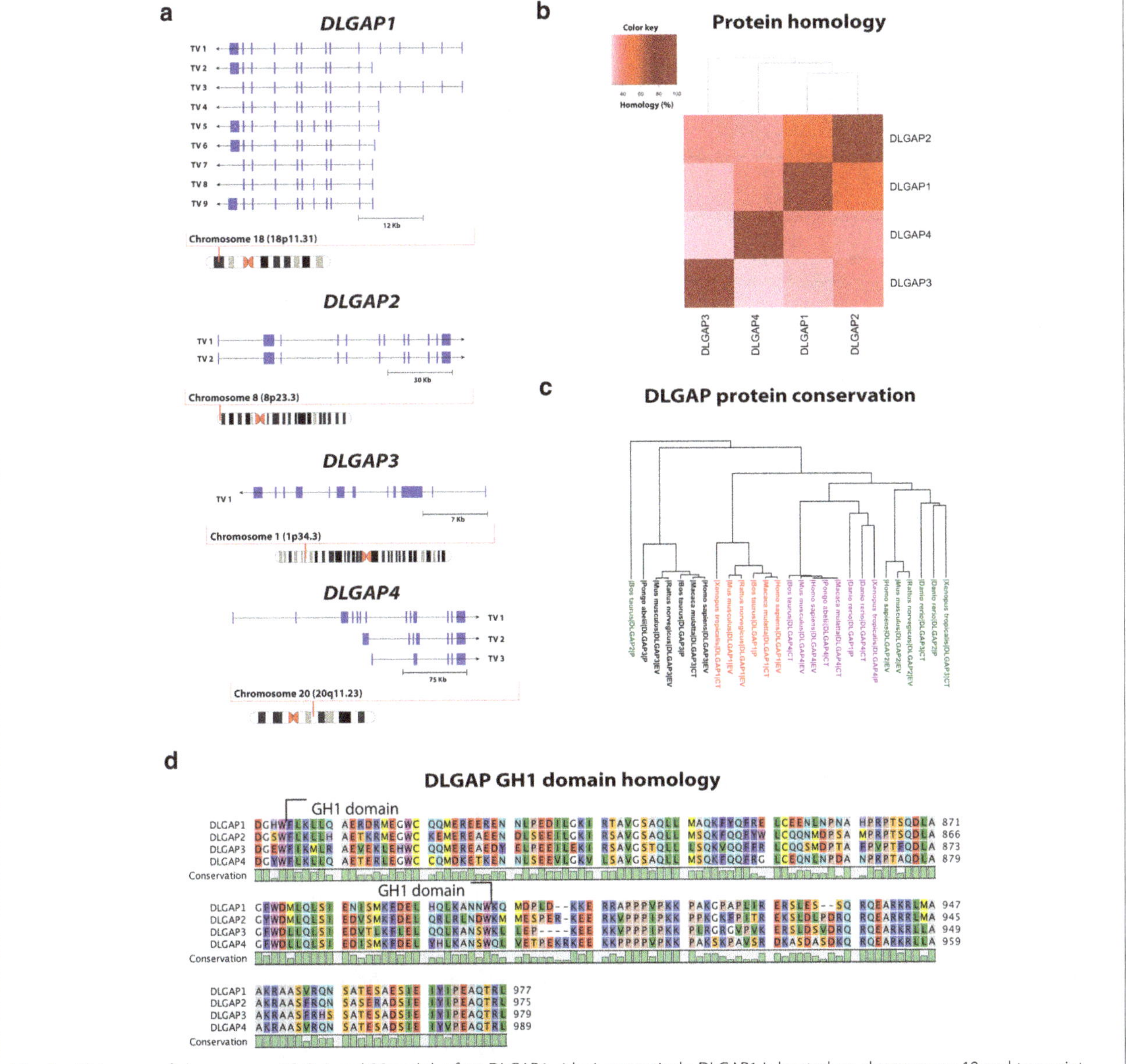

Fig. 1 **a** Pictogram of chromosome 18, 8, 1 and 20 and the four DLGAP1–4 loci, respectively. DLGAP1 is located on chromosome 18 and transcript variants 1 to 9 are illustrated. DLGAP2 is found on chromosome 8 and has two transcript variants. The DLGAP3 gene is located on chromosome 1 and has one transcript variant. DLGAP4 is located on chromosome 20 and has 3 transcript variants. **b** Heatmap showing the homology in percentage between the longest isoform, isoform a, of DLGAP1–4 proteins respectively. The color key indicates the respective percentage to each colour. The heatmap is created in RStudio v.0.99.484 with data from a multiple alignment made with clustal omega v.1.2.1. DLGAP1 isoform a: 977 amino acids (NP_004737.2), DLGAP2 isoform a: 975 amino acids (NP_004736.2), DLGAP3 isoform a: 979 amino acids (NP_001073887.1) and DLGAP4 isoform a: 989 amino acids (NP_055717.2). **c** Phylogenetic tree of DLGAP1–4 protein conservation in following species; *Homo sapiens* (NP_004737.2, NP_004736.2, NP_001073887.1, NP_001035951.1), *Macaca mulatta* (AFE64413.1, AFJ72104.1, AFE64177.1), *Bos taurus* (NP_001179558.1, DAA17363.1, NP_001179367.1, AAI26739.1), *Rattus norvegicus* (NP_075235.3, NP_446353.2, NP_775161.2), *Mus musculus* (NP_808307.2, NP_766498.2, AAH57615.1, NP_001035953.1), *Pongo abelii* (XP_009251088.1, NP_001127321.1), *Xenopus tropicalis* (NP_001123829.1, NP_001106458.1, XP_012827022.1) and *Danio rerio* (NP_001189384.1, XP_009291347.1, NP_001038179.1, AAI33919.1). EV: Experimentally validated, CT: Conceptual Translation, P: Predicted from genomic sequence. The phylogenetic tree is created in RStudio v.0.99.484 with data from a multiple alignment made with clustal omega v.1.2.1. **d** Figure of multiple alignment of DLGAP1–4 GH1 domain and C-terminal. The sequence homology of the GH1 domain is 61 to 75% between DLGAP1 – DLGAP4. The alignment and data is generated in clustal omega v.1.2.1 and visualized in CLC sequence viewer v.7.6

DLGAP proteins are conserved between species most likely because their function is highly essential. DLGAP proteins have been experimentally found or predicted from genomic sequences in *Homo sapiens, Macaca mulatta, Pongo abelii, Bos taurus, Rattus norvegicus, Mus musculus* and in the two vertebrates *Danio rerio* and *Xenopus tropicalis* (see Fig. 1c). DLGAP1–4 was originally found in rat [5, 18] but most research have

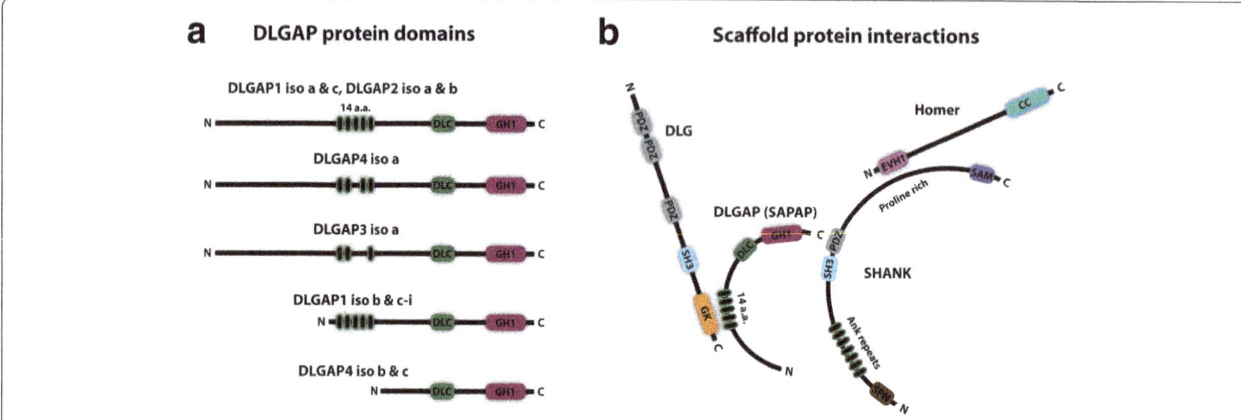

Fig. 2 **a** Pictogram of the DLGAP1–4 proteins with their respective domains. The DLGAP1–4 proteins have a 14 amino acid repeat domain (14-a.a. repeats) with 0 to 5 repeats depending on the DLGAP isoform, a Dynein light chain (DLC) domain and a GKAP homology domain 1 (GH1). **b** Illustration of how the four proteins interact. DLGAP binds via the C-terminal to the PDZ domain of SHANK. The 14-a.a. repeat domain of DLGAP binds the GK domain of DLG. Homer binds with the EVH1 domain to the proline rich domain of SHANK

since then been conducted in mouse and human where the genes and proteins also are described best.

Domain overview and protein interaction

The DLGAP1–4 proteins contain several characterized domains that enable them to interact with numerous proteins in the PSD either directly or indirectly via other scaffold proteins (see Fig. 2a-b). Some of these interacting proteins, namely the DLG4 protein, the SHANK family, the Homer family and the Stargazin protein will also be reviewed here. These proteins all have domains that have the capability to link DLGAP1–4 to the three major glutamate receptors in the PSD, namely the NMDA receptor, the AMPA receptor and the group I mGluRs [1–3, 5, 20, 21].

The DLGAP family

As mentioned, the DLGAP proteins have three known domains, a 14-a.a. repeat domain, a DLC domain and a GH1 domain (see Fig. 2a). With the 14-a.a. domain DLGAP proteins are capable of binding the GK domain of DLG1, DLG2 and DLG4 [5, 22–24]. Depending on the isoform, the 14-a.a. domain can be located in the middle of the protein or near the N-terminal. For example, in the long DLGAP1 isoforms (isoform a & c) the repeats are located in the middle whereas in the short isoforms (isoform b, d-i) the repeats are located near the N-terminal. DLGAP1 has five 14-a.a. repeats but some of the repeats are missing in the other DLGAP proteins. For example, the long DLGAP4 isoform a lacks the repeat number 3 and the short isoforms b and c do not contain any of the 5 repeats (see Fig. 2a) [18]. This diversity in repeats may contribute to their individual function and binding affinity to DLG4 at the synapse. The second domain, the DLC domain is located downstream of the repeats. This DLC domain interacts directly with DLC, a motor protein subunit found in the dendrites and PSD [25]. The last domain, the GH1 domain, is found at the C-terminal. GH1 is composed of 4 alpha helices and display a high sequence homology between the DLGAP proteins as previously mentioned (see Figs. 1d and 2a & b). However, the role of the GH1 domain is still unknown [5, 6, 26].

Proteins interacting with the DLGAP family

The DLG family The DLG family is a group of proteins also known as membrane-associated guanylate kinases (MAGUKs). Three of these proteins; DLG1, DLG2 and DLG4 also known as SAP97, PSD-93 and PSD-95, respectively, are known to interact directly with DLGAP [22–24]. The DLG proteins are important proteins in the PSD because they link other scaffold proteins and signalling molecules either directly or indirectly to the membrane bound ion channels. DLGs are known to stabilize the glutamate receptors upon binding and they may also trigger synaptic growth by modulation of growth-related proteins in the PSD [4]. DLGs, like DLGAP proteins, are also involved in synaptic scaling [4, 27–29], which is a process that is associated with schizophrenia [30]. The link of DLG1, DLG2 and DLG4 to schizophrenia has been well documented [31–36]. Additionally, DLG4 has been linked to ASD [37].

DLGs have three different types of domains where the first type is the Postsynaptic density protein; Drosophila disc large tumor suppressor; Zonula occludens-1 protein (PDZ) domain. In addition, DLGs have a Src Homology 3 (SH3) domain and a GK domain. DLGs have 3 PDZ domains (see Fig. 2b). The second PDZ domain binds the C-terminal of NMDA receptors [1]. Downstream of the PDZ domains, the SH3 domain is located, which has multiple binding partners including the A kinase anchor protein 150, AKAP150 [38]. Also, DLGs can create intramolecular interactions by binding the SH3 domain to the GK domain [39]. Most likely DLG proteins are also able to dimerize via SH3:GK interactions. With its GK domain DLGs interact directly with most DLGAP proteins through the 14-a.a. repeat domain [5] (see Fig. 2b). With the GK domain and the second PDZ domain DLGs acts as scaffolds between the DLGAP proteins and the NMDA receptors and AMPA receptors via Stargazin (see section 4.2.4) [3].

The SHANK family DLGAP proteins bind a second family of proteins, the SHANK proteins [2]. Most SHANK proteins are highly expressed in the PSD and they are important for the maturation of the PSD. Overexpression of SHANK leads to earlier maturation of the postsynapse by recruitment and interaction with other scaffold proteins. There are three *SHANK* genes in humans that encode 3 SHANK proteins (SHANK1–3). *SHANK3* has been linked to schizophrenia whereas *SHANK1–3* have all been linked to ASD [40].

SHANK proteins do not directly bind to glutamate receptors in the PSD but SHANK1–3 have the capability to link the ionotropic glutamate receptors to the metabotropic glutamate receptors by dimerization and molecular interaction with other scaffold proteins. Compared to DLGAP1–4 and DLG4, SHANK1–3 are longer proteins and have more domains (see Fig. 2b). Close to the N-terminal SHANK1–3 has a SHANK/ProSAP (SPN) domain followed by 7 Ankyrin (Ank) repeats. Like DLG4, SHANKs also have a SH3 domain and one PDZ domain. Downstream of PDZ, a proline rich domain is found, which is followed by a sterile alpha motif, SAM, domain close to the C-terminal. The SPN domain is largely uncharacterized. However, two binding partners have been reported for the Ank repeats, the protein alpha-Fodrin [41] and the Sharpin protein [42]. Both proteins bind to the cytoskeleton [43, 44]. Interestingly, the long isoform of SHANK2 with the Ank repeats, SHANK2E, seems not to be expressed in the PSD but mostly in epithelial cells [45]. SHANK1–3 has one SH3 domain like DLG4. In SHANK1–3, this domain mediates interaction with the PSD scaffold protein Densin-180. Densin-180 can promote dendritic branching. This feature is however negatively regulated when Densin-180 interacts with SHANK proteins [46]. Close to the SH3 domain, SHANK1–3 have a PDZ domain. The C-terminal of DLGAP1–4 interacts directly with SHANK1–3 via this domain [2] (see Fig. 2a & b). Hereby SHANK1–3 are linked to the postsynaptic plasma membrane via DLGAP1–4, PSD-95 and NMDA receptors. Downstream close to the N-terminal SHANK1–3 have a SAM domain, which bind other SAM domains for multimerization of SHANK1–3 proteins [47]. Multimerization of SHANK1–3 proteins can generate a network in the PSD that link numerous proteins to the postsynaptic receptors. This network also enables downstream signalling cascades from the postsynaptic glutamate receptors in which DLGAP proteins are an important element. Finally, SHANK1–3 also connects to the Homer family, via the proline rich domain [20].

The Homer family The Homer family consists of 3 proteins (Homer1–3) with various isoforms encoded by 3 *HOMER* genes. The Homer proteins have a function in neuronal development [48] and they play a central role in the PSD because these proteins bind to group I mGluRs and regulate the activity hereof [49, 50]. *Homer1* has been linked to mental retardation syndromes in Fragile X mental retardation patients and in *Fragile mental retardation 1 (FMR1)* knockout mice [51, 52]. Abnormal spine densities were found in the *FMR1* knockout mice, which support the importance for Homer proteins in neuronal development and proper PSD function.

Homer1–3 have two known domains. The first domain is the highly conserved Ena/VASP Homology 1 (EVH1) domain and the second domain is a coiled coil (CC) domain (see Fig. 2b). The EVH1 domain is located near the N-terminal and with this domain Homer1–3 interacts with the proline rich domain of SHANK1–3 [20]. In addition Homer1–3 have the ability to interact with group I mGluRs that also have a proline rich domain [21]. DLGAP1–4 is not directly associated with Homer1–3. However, Homer1–3 are interesting because they connect DLGAP1–4 to group I mGluR via SHANK1–3 (see Fig. 2b). Like DLG4 and SHANK1–3, Homer1–3 also have the capability to dimerize. The CC domain can bind other CC domains for homodimerization [53].

Stargazin DLGAP proteins indirectly interact with Stargazin via DLG4, which is interesting because it couples DLGAP proteins to the AMPA receptor. Stargazin is a tetraspanning transmembrane protein also known as calcium channel, voltage-dependent, gamma subunit 2. Stargazin shows structural resemblance to calcium channel, voltage-dependent, gamma subunit 1, which is a subunit in voltage gated calcium channels. Thus, it was first believed to be a calcium channel subunit [54], Stargazin is not a genuine subunit of calcium channels [55]. Stargazin is well known from the stargazer mouse, a model of ataxia and epilepsy where the *Stargazin* gene is deleted [56, 57]. Stargazin was found to interact with AMPA receptors and regulate their synaptic targeting, surface trafficking and trafficking to endosomes in ion channel scaling. This regulation require the C-terminal of Stargazin that interacts with the PDZ domain of DLG4 [3, 58–60]. Stargazin also plays an important role in the function of AMPA receptors. Stargazin can modulate the biophysical properties and channel gating of AMPA receptors [61–64]. Moreover, Stargazin can increase the efficacy of agonists on AMPA receptors and it can also act to slow down deactivation of AMPA receptors after glutamate binding [62, 65, 66].

DLGAP1–4 expression in the brain

DLGAP1–4 are expressed throughout the body but in general they are expressed in much higher levels in the brain [6]. DLGAP1–4 are mainly localized in the dendrites and the postsynapse of excitatory synapses (see Fig. 3) [18, 67, 68]. In the brain the expression of DLGAPs is widespread and the different isoforms show a somewhat different expression pattern. In situ hybridization experiments on rat and mouse brain tissue show that *Dlgap1* mRNA is expressed in cortex, hippocampus, olfactory bulb, striatum, thalamus as well as in both granule layer and Purkinje cells of cerebellum (see Table 2) [6, 68]. The expression of *Dlgap2* resembles that of *Dlgap1* with expression in cortex, hippocampus and olfactory bulb. However, *Dlgap2* is highly expressed in the striatum and interestingly *Dlgap2* is the only *Dlgap* that is not expressed in the cerebellum and in the thalamus [68]. Expression of *Dlgap3* mRNA is observed throughout the mouse brain including the cortex, thalamus, retina and olfactory bulb with high levels in the hippocampus, striatum and granule cells of cerebellum [68]. In cortex and cerebellum, the expression level of DLGAP3 varies in the postnatal rat brain. Around 3 weeks after birth the expression level peaks [69]. There are three transcript variants expressed from the *DLGAP4* locus, which are all present in the brain. Transcript variant 1 however, is totally brain specific whereas transcript variant 2 and 3 show tissue-wide expression [14]. In the brain *DLGAP4* shows high expression in the hippocampus, striatum, thalamus, amygdala, substantia nigra and in the Purkinje cells of cerebellum [14, 18, 68, 69].

Functional role of DLGAP proteins

DLGAP proteins are involved in ion channel scaling at the synapse

The DLGAP1 protein is enriched in the synapse where it acts as a scaffold protein and contributes to synaptic scaling [8]. Synaptic scaling, a form of homeostatic synaptic plasticity, is a function of the excitatory synapses to reset the neuronal firing rate to "normal" levels. The firing rate is normalized by a change in the postsynaptic response in every synapse of a neuron. The change in postsynaptic response results from alterations in the activity of neurotransmitter receptors like AMPA and NMDA receptors. For example, NMDA receptor scaling is regulated via the number of NMDA receptors at the synapse. The number of NMDA receptors functions as a bidirectional feedback mechanism. When the synapse is inactive, NMDA receptors are transported from the endoplasmic reticulum to the synapse. When the synapse is active, synaptic NMDA receptors undergo endocytosis and export of NMDA receptors from the endoplasmic reticulum slows down [70].

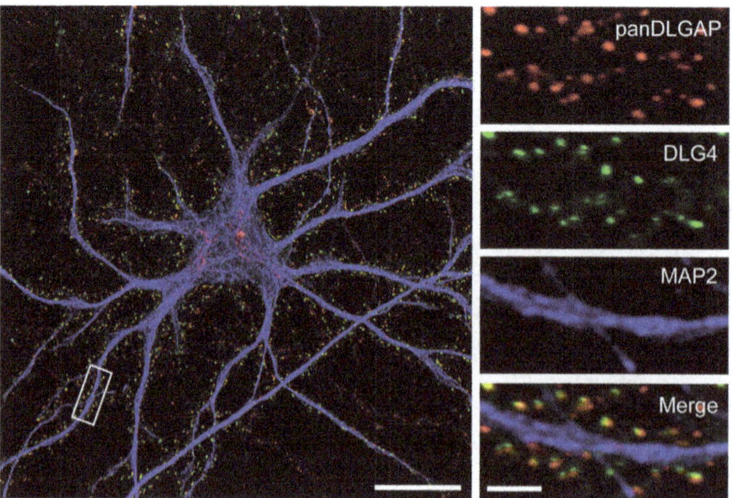

Fig. 3 DLGAPs are proteins of the postsynaptic density. The postsynaptic localization of DLGAPs in a cultured rat hippocampal neuron as revealed by a panDLGAP immunostaining. The excitatory postsynapses were visualized with an antibody directed against PSD-95 and MAP-2 used as a dendritic marker. Left scale bar, 20 μm; right scale bar, 3 μm

Table 2 The table shows where the DLGAP subtypes are expressed in the brain (Brain region, second column)

DLGAP subtype	Brain region	Brain region	References
DLGAP1	Cortex	↑	[6, 68]
	Hippocampus	↑	
	Cerebellum	↑	
	Olfactory bulbs	↑	
	Striatum	↓	
	Thalamus	M	
DLGAP2	Cortex	M	[68]
	Hippocampus	↑	
	Olfactory bulbs	M	
	Striatum	↑	
DLGAP3	Cortex	M	[68]
	Thalamus	M	
	Retina	M	
	Olfactory bulbs	M	
	Hippocampus	↑	
	Striatum	↑	
	Cerebellum	↑	
DLGAP4	Hippocampus	↑	[14, 18, 69]
	Striatum	↑	
	Cerebellum	↑	
	Thalamus	M	
	Amygdala	M	
	Substantia nigra	↓	

In the third column the expression level for the specific brain region is indicated. ↑; indicates high expression, M; indicates medium expression and ↓; indicates low expression levels. In the fourth column relevant references are linked

Synaptic scaling and the turnover of NMDA receptors are supplemented by a turnover of proteins in the PSD. The level of the scaffold protein DLG4, which interacts with the cytoplasmic tail of NMDA receptors (reviewed here: Sheng [71]) is reduced during NMDA receptor activity. Reduction of DLG4 at synaptic sites is a result of ubiquitination and proteasomal degradation [72, 73]. DLGAP proteins appear to control the DLG4 degradation indirectly. Upon dissociation of the DLGAP 14-a.a. domain from the DLG4 GK domain, both DLGAP1 and DLG4 are ubiquitinated and degraded [8, 74]. The DLG4-DLGAP1 interaction is disrupted by phosphorylation of DLGAP1, which is catalyzed by the Ca^{2+}/calmodulin-dependent protein kinase II alpha chain (αCaMKII). αCaMKII is activated by influx of Ca^{2+} ions through the NMDA receptors upon activation. The scaffold protein SHANK is also downregulated at the synapse as a result of DLGAP1 phosphorylation [8]. The phosphorylation most likely disrupts the interaction of the C-terminal of DLGAP1 with the PDZ domain of SHANK (see Fig. 4a) [75].

During synaptic inactivation DLGAP1, DLG4 and SHANK are, like the NMDA receptors, accumulating at the synapse again. DLGAP1 seems to be the linker in this accumulation. However, DLGAP1, DLG4 and SHANK are equally dependent on each other for accumulation (see Fig. 4a) [76]. It is believed that the scaffold proteins and NMDA receptors have a fast turnover with a short lifespan at the synapse [77].

DLGAP1 turnover seems to be important in synaptic scaling mediated by influx of Ca^{2+} ions through the NMDA receptors but it also plays a role in AMPA receptor scaling. It is known that DLG4 indirectly binds to AMPA receptors through Stargazin [3]. Further, DLGAP proteins interact with DLG4 as described above and phosphorylation of DLG4 by protein kinase A (PKA) leads to removal of AMPA receptors from the membrane by endocytosis [72]. Research has also shown, that loss of DLGAP3 causes silencing of AMPA receptors at the postsynapse [78]. In addition, overexpression of mutant DLGAP1 in hippocampal neurons eliminate homeostatic regulation of AMPA receptor surface expression [8].

DLGAP proteins clearly have a central role in ion channel synaptic scaling including both NMDARs and AMPARs. This function of DLGAPs appears to be achieved in concert with DLG4, SHANK, αCaMKII and possibly Stargazin.

DLGAP proteins control metabotropic glutamate receptor group I induced synaptic scaling

The group I metabotropic glutamate receptors (mGluRs) belong to a class of receptors in the mGluR family that is involved in synaptic scaling [79]. mGluRs are G-protein coupled receptors (GPCR) that bind glutamate. Upon glutamate binding of group I mGluRs, phospholipase C (PLC) hydrolyses phospholipids in the membrane. Subsequently inositol 1,4,5-triphosphate (IP3) and diacyl glycerol (DAG) are released, which can lead to activation of protein kinase C (PKC) and increased intracellular levels of Ca^{2+} (see Fig. 4b). The group I mGluR family includes two receptors, namely mGluR1 and mGluR5. Group I mGluRs can modulate NMDA and AMPA receptor activity and induce synaptic scaling upon activation. The scaffold protein Homer seems to be required for group I mGluR induced synaptic scaling [79] and for the crosstalk between group I mGluRs and the NMDA and AMPA receptors [80]. The crosstalk is likely mediated through a DLG4-DLGAP-SHANK-Homer complex [21]. Homer binds to the C-terminal of group I mGluR [81] and the coupling of Homer to the group

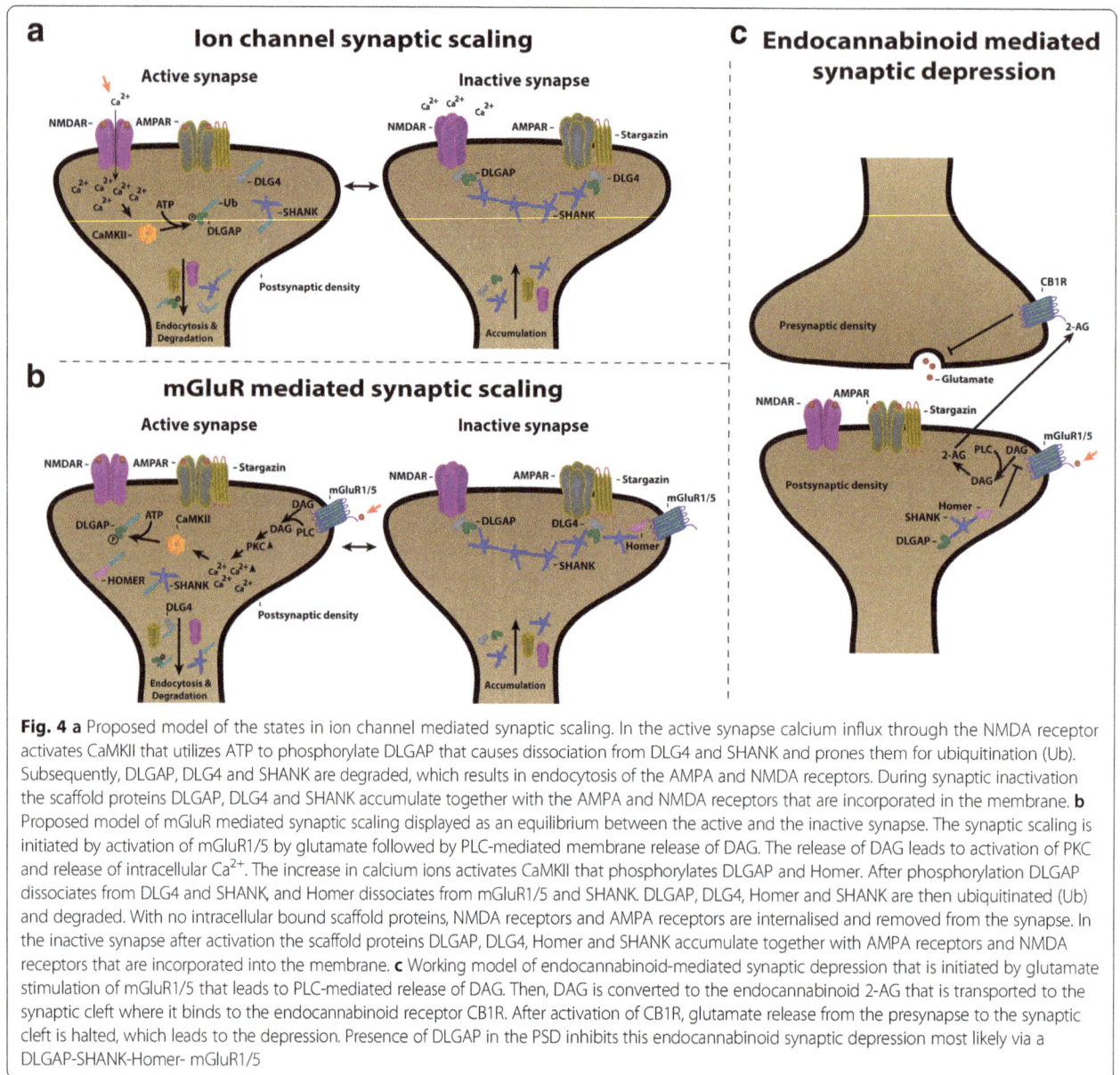

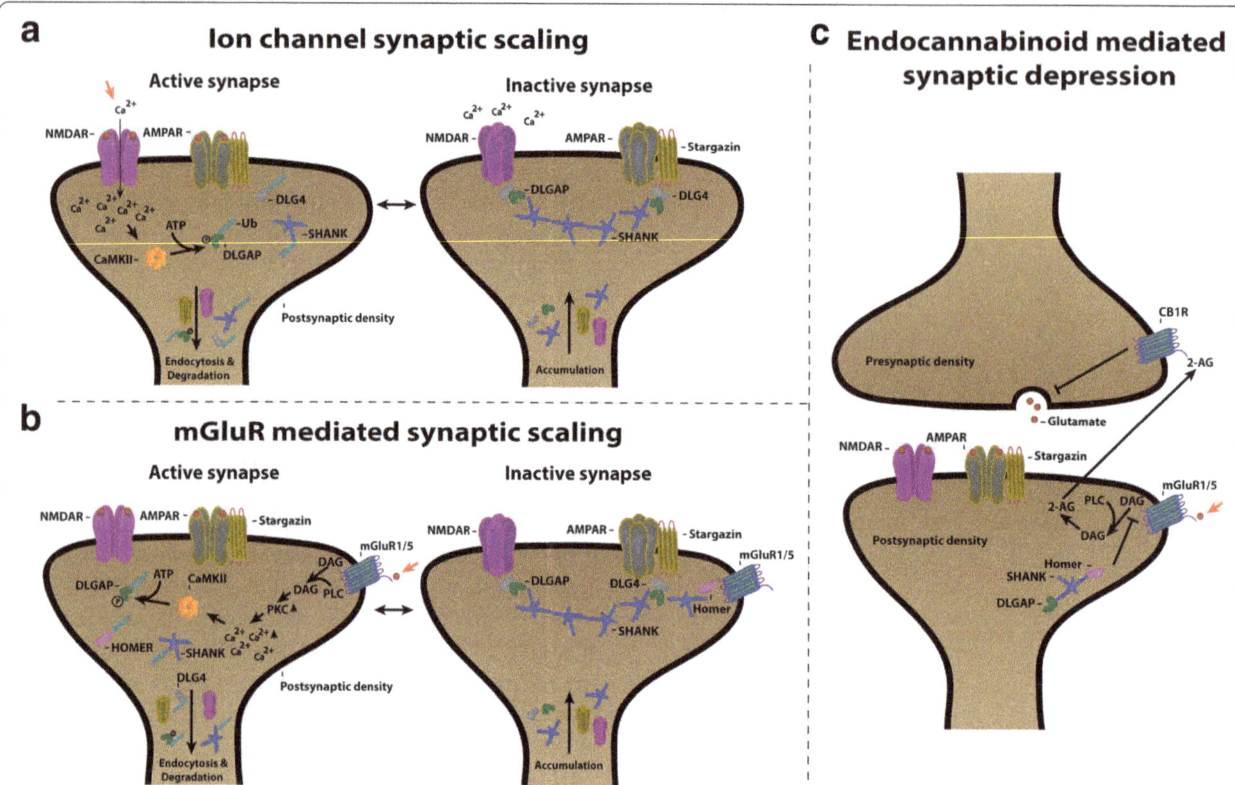

Fig. 4 a Proposed model of the states in ion channel mediated synaptic scaling. In the active synapse calcium influx through the NMDA receptor activates CaMKII that utilizes ATP to phosphorylate DLGAP that causes dissociation from DLG4 and SHANK and prones them for ubiquitination (Ub). Subsequently, DLGAP, DLG4 and SHANK are degraded, which results in endocytosis of the AMPA and NMDA receptors. During synaptic inactivation the scaffold proteins DLGAP, DLG4 and SHANK accumulate together with the AMPA and NMDA receptors that are incorporated in the membrane. **b** Proposed model of mGluR mediated synaptic scaling displayed as an equilibrium between the active and the inactive synapse. The synaptic scaling is initiated by activation of mGluR1/5 by glutamate followed by PLC-mediated membrane release of DAG. The release of DAG leads to activation of PKC and release of intracellular Ca^{2+}. The increase in calcium ions activates CaMKII that phosphorylates DLGAP and Homer. After phosphorylation DLGAP dissociates from DLG4 and SHANK, and Homer dissociates from mGluR1/5 and SHANK. DLGAP, DLG4, Homer and SHANK are then ubiquitinated (Ub) and degraded. With no intracellular bound scaffold proteins, NMDA receptors and AMPA receptors are internalised and removed from the synapse. In the inactive synapse after activation the scaffold proteins DLGAP, DLG4, Homer and SHANK accumulate together with AMPA receptors and NMDA receptors that are incorporated into the membrane. **c** Working model of endocannabinoid-mediated synaptic depression that is initiated by glutamate stimulation of mGluR1/5 that leads to PLC-mediated release of DAG. Then, DAG is converted to the endocannabinoid 2-AG that is transported to the synaptic cleft where it binds to the endocannabinoid receptor CB1R. After activation of CB1R, glutamate release from the presynapse to the synaptic cleft is halted, which leads to the depression. Presence of DLGAP in the PSD inhibits this endocannabinoid synaptic depression most likely via a DLGAP-SHANK-Homer- mGluR1/5

I mGluR and other interaction partners in the PSD is, like for DLGAP1, also controlled by phosphorylation catalysed by CaMKII [82]. In addition to Homer, DLGAPs are also believed to play an important role in group I mGluR induced synaptic scaling. This is due to the essential binding to both DLG4 and SHANK, and research show that loss of DLGAP2 causes significant downregulation of Homer and AMPA receptors [83]. DLGAP's role in group I mGluR synaptic scaling is probably not much different from its role in ion channel scaling. DLGAPs are likely phosphorylated by CaMKII upon group I mGluR activation. Phosphorylation of DLGAP and Homer leads to degradation or removal of DLGAP, Homer, DLG4 and SHANK from the PSD. Upon degradation or removal of scaffold proteins, the NMDA and AMPA receptors are unstable and subsequently removed from the membrane via endocytosis (see Fig. 4b).

The role of endocannabinoids in synaptic depression is guarded by DLGAP

The group I mGluRs can regulate synaptic plasticity via release of intracellular Ca^{2+} as described above. Another way group I mGluRs can regulate synaptic plasticity is through endocannabinoid mediated synaptic depression. Endocannabinoids are a class of lipids that are synthesized from membrane-bound phospholipids. The synthesis occurs after activation of group I mGluRs where the phospholipids are converted into endocannabinoids via different cleaving mechanisms. For example, DAG that is released from the membrane by PLC after group I mGluR activation is converted to the endocannabinoid 2-Arachidonoyl glycerol (2-AG). After synthesis the endocannabinoids are transported into the synaptic cleft and to the presynapse where the endocannabinoid receptor 1 (CB1R) is located. The CB1R is a GPCR and upon endocannabinoid binding, downstream signalling is initiated. One downstream signalling cascade results in inhibition of neurotransmitter release from the presynapse (see Fig. 4c) [84]. The scaffold protein Homer1 that binds group I mGluRs seems to play a role in the endocannabinoid signalling [85]. Homer1 expression regulates endocannabonoid production as a result of mGluR stimulation. Besides Homer1, DLGAP3 also regulates endocannabinoid mediated synaptic depression. In *Dlgap3* knockout mice, endocannabinoid-dependent synaptic depression is increased in the striatum in a mGluR dependent manner [7]. This indicates that the presence of DLGAP proteins in the PSD activates or promotes synaptic transmission by inhibiting mGluR-mediated endocannabinoid signalling. The scaffold protein SHANK binds both DLGAP and Homer why DLGAP3 most likely controls endocannabinoid signalling through a DLGAP3-SHANK-Homer-group I mGluR complex (see Fig. 4c).

DLGAP proteins in neurological and psychiatric disorders

The DLGAP proteins are expressed in the postsynapse and interact with several proteins involved in the function and maintenance of the NMDA, AMPA and group I mGluR glutamate receptors. DLGAPs play an important role in the PSD and even small changes in expression of DLGAPs could have severe consequences in the signalling within the PSD. It is therefore not surprising that all DLGAPs have been linked to various psychiatric and neurological disorders including schizophrenia, OCD and cerebellar ataxia (see Table 1) [9, 11, 14].

Schizophrenia and DLGAPs

Schizophrenia is a widespread, complex mental disorder that is characterized by symptoms like delusions, hallucinations and abnormal social behaviour. It affects approximately 1% of the population worldwide [86]. Schizophrenia has a high degree of heritability however, a large fraction of patients do not have a family history which can be explained by sporadic mutations [87, 88].

Schizophrenia is functionally associated with the NMDA receptors [89, 90]. One hypothesis behind the NMDA receptor influence in schizophrenia is explained by altered glutamate signalling as a result of reduced or increased incorporation of NMDA receptors in the postsynaptic membrane [91, 92]. As explained in section 6, DLGAPs influence NMDA receptor synaptic scaling via DLG4 and both DLG4 and DLGAP1 have been linked to schizophrenia. The DLG family members, DLG1 and DLG2, which also interact with DLGAPs and NMDA receptors [93–95] have been linked to schizophrenia as well [35–37].

Analysis of brain samples from post mortem schizophrenic patients revealed that the level of DLG4 was downregulated in anterior cingulate cortex [33]. Another study demonstrated increased expression of DLGAP1 in the nucleus accumbens [9]. Moreover, the expression level of DLG1 and DLG2 was also found to be significantly skewed in a schizophrenia rat model and in schizophrenic patients [32, 96–98]. The deregulation of DLGs and DLGAP1 in these patients could be an indication of malfunction of NMDA receptors. Especially the NMDA subunit, GluN2A shows altered expression in schizophrenic patients [91, 92]. The schizophrenia-related upregulation of DLGAP1 expression could be the result of a feedback mechanism where the neurons are trying to re-establish the normal function and signalling of the GluN2A containing NMDA receptor.

After the discovery of the potential role of DLGAP1 in schizophrenia, related gene family members have also been analysed extensively in genetic studies. Multiple single nucleotide variations (SNVs) have been reported in *DLGAP2* and *DLGAP3* genes in schizophrenia patient cohorts [99, 100]. In *DLGAP3* two SNVs were identified in the C-terminal, one of which was located in a domain which is believed to affect the post-translational modification of the DLGAP3 protein. It was speculated that all the *DLGAP3* SNVs would impact the interaction with protein kinases and thereby the function of DLGAP3 [99]. No functional studies have yet been conducted on *DLGAP2* and *DLGAP3* in relation to schizophrenia. *DLGAP2* and *DLGAP3* have only been linked to schizophrenia in genetic screens. Yet, genetic changes in *DLGAP2* and *DLGAP3* are considered as susceptibility factors for schizophrenia [99, 100].

Other brain disorders and DLGAPs

The DLGAPs have been linked to a number of brain disorders in addition to schizophrenia. *DLGAP2* was identified as a candidate gene for ASD where patients display impaired social interaction and communication skills in addition to having stereotyped interests and behaviours [10, 101, 102].

Animal studies have pinpointed a link between *DLGAP2* and post-traumatic stress disorder (PTSD), which is observed as a result of a traumatic experience. In a rat model of PTSD, a change in methylation and in expression of *Dlgap2* was shown in the hippocampus [103]. In individuals with PTSD the hippocampus is known to be smaller and less activated [104–106]. Moreover, *Dlgap2* knockout (*Dlgap2*$^{-/-}$) mice showed deficits in learning, abnormal social behaviour and intense aggressive behaviour, which is characteristic for both ASD and PTSD [83].

Biochemical studies revealed that specific subunits in the AMPA and NMDA receptors, the scaffold protein Homer1 and αCaMKII were significantly downregulated in the *Dlgap2*$^{-/-}$ mice resulting in disruption of both synaptic transmission and synaptic structure [83].

DLGAP3 has been associated with OCD, which arises from anomalous signalling in the striatum and develops into a phenotype where the patients need to check or perform certain things repeatedly. *Dlgap3* knockout (*Dlgap3*$^{-/-}$) mice showed increased self-grooming bouts compared to wild type mice, which resulted in lesions in their head and neck. In addition, the *Dlgap3*$^{-/-}$ mice exhibited increased anxiety-like behaviour, which is also characteristic for OCD [11].

Since *Dlgap3*$^{-/-}$ mice showed OCD-like symptoms, patients with the grooming disorder, trichotillomania (hair-pulling disorder) and OCD were genotyped for SNVs in the *DLGAP3* locus [12]. An association was found between variations in the *DLGAP3* gene and trichotillomania, which appeared to be familial. However, a coherence between variants in the *DLGAP3* gene and OCD was not obvious [12]. Other studies have nonetheless linked genetic variants in *DLGAP3* to OCD-like symptoms. In patients with OCD and trichotillomania, multiple and rare missense mutations were found in the *DLGAP3* gene [107].

The fourth *DLGAP* gene, *DLGAP4*, has been related to cerebellar ataxia. Our group had discovered a familial translocation between chromosome 8 and 20 t(8:20) segregating with early-onset cerebellar ataxia [108]. This translocation resulted in symptoms including ataxia, clumsiness, impaired hand coordination and tremors. The translocation disrupted the *DLGAP4* locus and separated the promoter and the first exon from the rest in transcript variant 1, which is brain-specific. In addition, the translocation disrupted the *DLGAP4* promoter associated CpG island which lead to epigenetic changes and increased expression of the *DLGAP4* transcript variant 2 [14].

The misregulation of *DLGAP4* could very likely lead to altered surface expression of both ionoptropic and metabotropic glutamate receptors in the PSD. Deregulation of glutamate receptor turnover, could potentially be followed by a faulted glutamate signalling from the presynapse to the postsynapse leading to the reported phenotype. In fact, both loss of AMPA receptors and loss of group I mGluR signalling have previously been associated with cerebellar ataxia [109–111].

Conclusions

In this review we have focused on members 1 to 4 of the DLGAP protein family with regard to their function in the brain and involvement in neurological diseases. The DLGAP proteins have multiple domains and act as scaffold proteins in the PSD where they enable crosstalk between metabotropic and ionotropic glutamate receptors via other scaffold proteins including DLG4, SHANK and Homer [1–5, 21, 47, 49, 50, 58–60]. DLGAPs are believed to control synaptic scaling as a result of NMDA receptor, AMPA receptor and group I mGluR activation [3, 5, 7, 8, 58–60]. Undoubtedly further research on this topic would be of great value to decipher the role of the individual DLGAP proteins and the interplay between the DLGAP proteins in neuronal synapses. To understand the implication of DLGAPs in neurological disorders will be of great importance. Multiple studies have been conducted on DLGAPs in relation to schizophrenia [37, 86, 112–114]. Specifically, there is heavy literature on involvement of DLGAP1 in schizophrenia and suggesting DLGAP2 as a candidate gene for ASD [10, 100, 101] and PTSD [83, 102]. It is likely that mutations in *DLGAP2* could lead to the symptoms seen in ASD and PTSD patients. The data convincingly depicts the *DLGAP3* gene as a disease gene for both OCD and trichotillomania [11–13, 106]. In contrast to DLGAP1–3, the general literature on DLGAP4 is very limited. *DLGAP4* is proposed as a candidate gene for cerebellar ataxia [14] but *DLGAP4* was never investigated in studies of the Stargazer mouse, a mouse model of cerebellar ataxia [3, 54, 56]. More research and data is expected in the coming years to clarify the role of DLGAP1, 2, 3 and 4 in synaptic plasticity and their involvement in schizophrenia and neurological diseases.

Abbreviations

AMPA: α-amino-3-hydroxy-5-methyl-4-isoxazolepropionic acid; Ank: Ankyrin; ASD: Autism spectrum disease; ASD: Autism spectrum disorder; CB1R: Endocannabinoid receptor 1; CC: Coiled coil; DAG: Diacyl glycerol; DLC: Dynein light chain; DLGAP1-4: Discs large associated protein 1, 2, 3 and 4; DLGAPs: Discs large associated proteins; DLGs: Discs large scaffold proteins; EVH1: Ena/VASP Homology 1; FMR1: Fragile mental retardation 1; GH1: GKAP homology; GK: Guanylate kinase; GKAP: Guanylate kinase associated protein; GPCR: G-protein coupled receptors; Homer1-3: Homer family consisting of 3 proteins; IP3: Inositol 1,4,5-triphosphate; MAGUKs: Membrane-associated guanylate kinases; mGluRs: Metabotropic glutamate receptors; NMDA: N-methyl-D-aspartate; OCD: Obsessive compulsive disorder; PDZ: Zonula occludens-1 protein; PKA: Protein kinase A; PKC: Protein kinase C; PLC: Phospholipase C; PSD: Postsynaptic density; PTSD: Post-traumatic stress disorder; SAPAP1-4: SAP90/PSD95-associated protein 1–4; SH3: Src Homology 3; SHANK: Src-homology (SH3) and multiple ankyrin repeat domain proteins; SHANK1-3: SHANK proteins; SNV: Single nucleotide variation; SPN: SHANK/ProSAP

Acknowledgements
We would like to thank and acknowledge Susanne Hoiberg for reading the manuscript.

Funding
This study is supported partially by a grant from the Lundbeck Foundation (AS) and a partial PhD fellowship for AHR from the ICMM, University of Copenhagen. The funding body had no influence in the design of the study, interpretation of data and writing the manuscript.

Authors' contributions
AHR has contributed significantly with ideas and reviewing the literature, putting figures together, and writing the preliminary version of the manuscript. HBR has contributed substantially with the design, making a new figure and revising the manuscript critically. AS has initiated the project and contributed significantly with ideas and by critically revising the manuscript as a whole. All authors have read and approved the final manuscript.

Authors' information
AHR is a PhD student in the Cellular and Genetic Medicine Program. HBR is Associate Professor in the Department of Biomedical Sciences interested in molecular and cellular neurobiology, AS is Associate Professor in the Medical Genetics Program, Department of Cellular and Molecular Medicine. AS is interested in genomic organization, gene expression and gene regulatory mechanisms in the brain, DLGAP4 gene, cytogenetics.

Competing interests
The authors declare that they have no competing interests.

Author details
[1]Department of Cellular and Molecular Medicine, Faculty of Medical and Health Sciences, University of Copenhagen, DK-2200 Copenhagen, Denmark. [2]Department of Biomedical Sciences, Faculty of Medical and Health Sciences, University of Copenhagen, DK-2200 Copenhagen, Denmark.

References
1. Kornau HC, Schenker LT, Kennedy MB, Seeburg PH. Domain interaction between NMDA receptor subunits and the postsynaptic density protein PSD-95. Science. 1995;269:1737–40.
2. Naisbitt S, Kim E, Tu JC, Xiao B, Sala C, Valtschanoff J, et al. Shank, a novel family of postsynaptic density proteins that binds to the NMDA receptor/PSD-95/GKAP complex and cortactin. Neuron. 1999;23:569–82.
3. Chen L, Chetkovich DM, Petralia RS, Sweeney NT, Kawasaki Y, Wenthold RJ, et al. Stargazin regulates synaptic targeting of AMPA receptors by two distinct mechanisms. Nature. Macmillian Magazines Ltd. 2000;408:936–43.
4. Steiner P, Higley MJ, Xu W, Czervionke BL, Malenka RC, Sabatini BL. Destabilization of the postsynaptic density by PSD-95 serine 73 Phosphorylation inhibits spine growth and synaptic plasticity. Neuron. 2008;60:788–802.
5. Kim E. GKAP, a novel synaptic protein that interacts with the Guanylate Kinase-like domain of the PSD-95/SAP90 family of channel clustering molecules. J Cell Biol. 1997;136:669–78.
6. Naisbitt S, Kim E, Weinberg RJ, Rao A, Yang F-C, Craig AM, et al. Characterization of Guanylate Kinase-associated protein, a postsynaptic density protein at excitatory synapses that interacts directly with postsynaptic density-95/synapse-associated protein 90. J Neurosci. 1997;17:5687–96.
7. Chen M, Wan Y, Ade K, Ting J, Feng G, Calakos N. Sapap3 deletion anomalously activates short-term endocannabinoid-mediated synaptic plasticity. J Neurosci. 2011;31:9563–73.
8. Shin SM, Zhang N, Hansen J, Gerges NZ, Pak DTS, Sheng M, et al. GKAP orchestrates activity-dependent postsynaptic protein remodeling and homeostatic scaling. Nat Neurosci. 2012;15:1655–66.
9. Kajimoto Y, Shirakawa O, Lin X-H, Hashimoto T, Kitamura N, Murakami N, et al. Synapse-associated protein 90/postsynaptic density-95-associated protein (SAPAP) is expressed differentially in phencyclidine-treated rats and is increased in the nucleus accumbens of patients with schizophrenia. Neuropsychopharmacology. 2003;28:1831–9.
10. Pinto D, Pagnamenta AT, Klei L, Anney R, Merico D, Regan R, et al. Functional impact of global rare copy number variation in autism spectrum disorders. Nature. 2010;466:368–72.
11. Welch JM, Lu J, Rodriguiz RM, Trotta NC, Peca J, Ding J-D, et al. Cortico-striatal synaptic defects and OCD-like behaviours in Sapap3-mutant mice. Nature. Nature Publishing Group. 2007;448:894–900.
12. Bienvenu OJ, Wang Y, Shugart YY, Welch JM, Grados MA, Fyer AJ, et al. Sapap3 and pathological grooming in humans: results from the OCD collaborative genetics study. Am J Med Genet B Neuropsychiatr Genet. 2009;150:710–20.
13. Ryu S, Oh S, Cho EY, Nam HJ, Yoo JH, Park T, et al. Interaction between genetic variants of DLGAP3 and SLC1A1 affecting the risk of atypical antipsychotics-induced obsessive-compulsive symptoms. Am J Med Genet B Neuropsychiatr Genet. 2011;156:949–59.
14. Minocherhomji S, Hansen C, Kim H-G, Mang Y, Bak M, Guldberg P, et al. Epigenetic remodelling and dysregulation of DLGAP4 is linked with early-onset cerebellar ataxia. Hum Mol Genet. 2014;23:6163–76.
15. Chiu AW, Huang Y-L, Huan SK, Wang Y-C, Ju J-P, Chen M-F, et al. Potential molecular marker for detecting transitional cell carcinoma. Urology. 2002;60:181–5.
16. Tang ZY, Ye SL, Liu YK, Qin LX, Sun HC, Ye QH, et al. A decade's studies on metastasis of hepatocellular carcinoma. J Cancer Res Clin Oncol. 2004;130:187–96.
17. Stangeland B, Mughal AA, Grieg Z, Sandberg CJ, Joel M, Nygård S, et al. Combined expressional analysis, bioinformatics and targeted proteomics identify new potential therapeutic targets in glioblastoma stem cells. Oncotarget. 2015;6:26192–215.
18. Takeuchi M. SAPAPs. A family of PSD-95/SAP90-associated proteins localized at postsynaptic density. J Biol Chem. 1997;272:11943–51.
19. O'Connor EC, Bariselli S, Bellone C. Synaptic basis of social dysfunction: a focus on postsynaptic proteins linking group-I mGluRs with AMPARs and NMDARs. Eur J Neurosci. 2014;39:1114–29.
20. Tu JC, Xiao B, Yuan JP, Lanahan AA, Leoffert K, Li M, et al. Homer binds a novel proline-rich motif and links group I metabotropic glutamate receptors with IP3 receptors. Neuron. 1998;21:717–26.
21. Tu JC, Xiao B, Naisbitt S, Yuan JP, Petralia RS, Brakeman P, et al. Coupling of mGluR/Homer and PSD-95 complexes by the shank family of postsynaptic density proteins. Neuron. 1999;23:583–92.
22. Wu H, Reissner C, Kuhlendahl S, Coblentz B, Reuver S, Kindler S, et al. Intramolecular interactions regulate SAP97 binding to GKAP. EMBO J. 2000;19:5740–51.
23. Sabio G, Arthur JSC, Kuma Y, Peggie M, Carr J, Murray-Tait V, et al. p38gamma regulates the localisation of SAP97 in the cytoskeleton by modulating its interaction with GKAP. EMBO J. 2005;24:1134–45.
24. Manneville JB, Jehanno M, Etienne-Manneville S. Dlg1 binds GKAP to control dynein association with microtubules, centrosome positioning, and cell polarity. J Cell Biol. 2010;191:585–98.
25. Naisbitt S, Valtschanoff J, Allison DW, Sala C, Kim E, Craig AM, et al. Interaction of the postsynaptic density-95/guanylate kinase domain-associated protein complex with a light chain of myosin-V and dynein. J Neurosci. 2000;20:4524–34.
26. Tong J, Yang H, Eom SH, Chun C, Im YJ. Structure of the GH1 domain of guanylate kinase-associated protein from Rattus Norvegicus. Biochem Biophys Res Commun. Elsevier Inc. 2014;452:130–5.
27. Waites CL, Specht CG, Härtel K, Leal-Ortiz S, Genoux D, Li D, et al. Synaptic SAP97 isoforms regulate AMPA receptor dynamics and access to presynaptic glutamate. J Neurosci. 2009;29:4332–45.
28. Li D, Specht CG, Waites CL, Butler-Munro C, Leal-Ortiz S, Foote JW, et al. SAP97 directs NMDA receptor spine targeting and synaptic plasticity. J Physiol. 2011;589:4491–510.

29. Sun Q, Turrigiano GG. PSD-95 and PSD-93 play critical but distinct roles in synaptic scaling up and down. J Neurosci. 2011;31:6800–8. http://www.jneurosci.org/content/31/18/6800.long.
30. Stephan KE, Friston KJ, Frith CD. Dysconnection in schizophrenia: from abnormal synaptic plasticity to failures of self-monitoring. Schizophr Bull. 2009;35:509–27.
31. Kristiansen LV, Meador-Woodruff JH. Abnormal striatal expression of transcripts encoding NMDA interacting PSD proteins in schizophrenia, bipolar disorder and major depression. Schizophr Res. 2005;78:87–93.
32. Kristiansen LV, Beneyto M, Haroutunian V, Meador-Woodruff JH. Changes in NMDA receptor subunits and interacting PSD proteins in dorsolateral prefrontal and anterior cingulate cortex indicate abnormal regional expression in schizophrenia. Mol. Psychiatry. 2006;11:737–47.
33. Funk AJ, Rumbaugh G, Harotunian V, McCullumsmith RE, Meador-Woodruff JH. Decreased expression of NMDA receptor-associated proteins in frontal cortex of elderly patients with schizophrenia. Neuroreport. 2009;20:1019–22.
34. Xing J, Kimura H, Wang C, Ishizuka K, Kushima I, Arioka Y, et al. Resequencing and association analysis of six PSD-95-related genes as possible susceptibility genes for schizophrenia and autism Spectrum disorders. Sci Rep. 2016;6:27491.
35. Uezato A, Kimura-Sato J, Yamamoto N, Iijima Y, Kunugi H, Nishikawa T. Further evidence for a male-selective genetic association of synapse-associated protein 97 (SAP97) gene with schizophrenia. Behav Brain Funct. 2012;8:2.
36. Sato J, Shimazu D, Yamamoto N, Nishikawa T. An association analysis of synapse-associated protein 97 (SAP97) gene in schizophrenia. J Neural Transm. 2008;115:1355–65.
37. Xing J, Kimura H, Wang C, Ishizuka K, Kushima I, Arioka Y, et al. Resequencing and association analysis of six PSD-95-related genes as possible susceptibility genes for schizophrenia and autism Spectrum disorders. Sci Rep. 2016;6:1–8.
38. Colledge M, Dean RA, Scott GK, Langeberg LK, Huganir RL, Scott JD. Targeting of PKA to glutamate receptors through a MAGUK-AKAP complex. Neuron. 2000;27:107–19.
39. Shin H, Hsueh YP, Yang FC, Kim E, Sheng M. An intramolecular interaction between Src homology 3 domain and guanylate kinase-like domain required for channel clustering by postsynaptic density-95/SAP90. J Neurosci. 2000;20:3580–7.
40. Guilmatre A, Huguet G, Delorme R, Bourgeron T. The emerging role of SHANK genes in neuropsychiatric disorders. Dev Neurobiol. 2014;74:113–22.
41. Böckers TM, Mameza MG, Kreutz MR, Bockmann J, Weise C, Buck F, et al. Synaptic scaffolding proteins in rat brain: Ankyrin repeats of the multidomain shank protein family interact with the cytoskeletal protein α-fodrin. J Biol Chem. 2001;276:40104–12.
42. Lim S, Sala C, Yoon J, Park S, Kuroda S, Sheng M, et al. Sharpin, a novel postsynaptic density protein that directly interacts with the shank family of proteins. Mol Cell Neurosci. 2001;17:385–97.
43. Levine J, Willard M. Fodrin: axonally transported polypeptides associated with the internal periphery of many cells. J Cell Biol. 1981;90:631–42.
44. Rantala JK, Pouwels J, Pellinen T, Veltel S, Laasola P, Mattila E, et al. SHARPIN is an endogenous inhibitor of β1-integrin activation. Nat Cell Biol. 2011;13:1315–24.
45. McWilliams RR, Gidey E, Fouassier L, Weed SA, Doctor RB. Characterization of an ankyrin repeat-containing Shank2 isoform (Shank2E) in liver epithelial cells. Biochem J. 2004;380:181–91.
46. Quitsch A, Berhörster K, Liew CW, Richter D, Kreienkamp H-J. Postsynaptic shank antagonizes dendrite branching induced by the leucine-rich repeat protein Densin-180. J Neurosci. 2005;25:479–87.
47. Sheng M, Kim E. The shank family of scaffold proteins. J Cell Sci. 2000;113:1851–6.
48. Shiraishi Y, Mizutani A, Bito H, Fujisawa K, Narumiya S, Mikoshiba K, et al. Cupidin, an isoform of Homer/Vesl, interacts with the actin cytoskeleton and activated rho family small GTPases and is expressed in developing mouse cerebellar granule cells. J Neurosci. 1999;19:8389–400.
49. Mao L, Yang L, Tang Q, Samdani S, Zhang G, Wang JQ. The scaffold protein Homer1b/c links metabotropic glutamate receptor 5 to extracellular signal-regulated protein kinase cascades in neurons. J Neurosci. 2005;25:2741–52.
50. Yamamoto K, Sakagami Y, Sugiura S, Inokuchi K, Shimohama S, Kato N. Homer 1a enhances spike-induced calcium influx via L-type calcium channels in neocortex pyramidal cells. Eur J Neurosci. 2005;22:1338–48.
51. Pieretti M, Zhang FP, Fu YH, Warren ST, Oostra BA, Caskey CT, et al. Absence of expression of the FMR-1 gene in fragile X syndrome. Cell. 1991;66:817–22.
52. Nimchinsky EA, Oberlander AM, Svoboda K. Abnormal development of dendritic spines in FMR1 knock-out mice. J Neurosci. 2001;21:5139–46.
53. Xiao B, Tu JC, Petralia RS, Yuan JP, Doan A, Breder CD, et al. Homer regulates the association of group 1 metabotropic glutamate receptors with multivalent complexes of Homer-related, synaptic proteins. Neuron. 1998;21:707–16.
54. Letts VA, Felix R, Biddlecome GH, Arikkath J, Mahaffey CL, Valenzuela A, et al. The mouse stargazer gene encodes a neuronal Ca2+–channel gamma subunit. Nat Genet. 1998;19:340–7.
55. Tselnicker I, Tsemakhovich VA, Dessauer CW, Dascal N. Stargazin modulates neuronal voltage-dependent ca(2+) channel ca(v)2.2 by a Gbetagamma-dependent mechanism. J Biol Chem. 2010;285:20462–71.
56. Noebels JL, Qiao X, Bronson RT, Spencer C, Davisson MT. Stargazer: a new neurological mutant on chromosome 15 in the mouse with prolonged cortical seizures. Epilepsy Res. 1990;7:129–35.
57. Menuz K, Nicoll RA. Loss of inhibitory neuron AMPA receptors contributes to ataxia and epilepsy in stargazer mice. J Neurosci. 2008;28:10599–603.
58. Chen L, El-Husseini A, Tomita S, Bredt DS, Nicoll RA. Stargazin differentially controls the trafficking of alpha-amino-3-hydroxyl-5-methyl-4-isoxazolepropionate and kainate receptors. Mol Pharmacol. 2003;64:703–6.
59. Bats C, Groc L, Choquet D. The interaction between Stargazin and PSD-95 regulates AMPA receptor surface trafficking. Neuron. 2007;53:719–34.
60. Matsuda S, Kakegawa W, Budisantoso T, Nomura T, Kohda K, Yuzaki M. Stargazin regulates AMPA receptor trafficking through adaptor protein complexes during long-term depression. Nat Commun Nat Res. 2013;4:1–12.
61. Priel A, Kolleker A, Ayalon G, Gillor M, Osten P, Stern-Bach Y. Stargazin reduces desensitization and slows deactivation of the AMPA-type glutamate receptors. J Neurosci. 2005;25:2682–6.
62. Tomita S, Adesnik H, Sekiguchi M, Zhang W, Wada K, Howe JR, et al. Stargazin modulates AMPA receptor gating and trafficking by distinct domains. Nature. 2005;435:1052–8.
63. Turetsky D, Garringer E, Patneau DK. Stargazin modulates native AMPA receptor functional properties by two distinct mechanisms. J Neurosci. 2005;25:7438–48.
64. Cho C-H, St-Gelais F, Zhang W, Tomita S, Howe JR. Two families of TARP Isoforms that have distinct effects on the kinetic properties of AMPA receptors and synaptic currents. Neuron. 2007;55:890–904.
65. MacLean DM, Ramaswamy SS, Du M, Howe JR, Jayaraman V. Stargazin promotes closure of the AMPA receptor ligand-binding domain. J Gen Physiol. 2014;144:503–12.
66. Carbone AL, Plested AJR. Superactivation of AMPA receptors by auxiliary proteins. Nat Commun. 2016;7:1–12.
67. Yao I, Iida J, Nishimura W, Hata Y. Synaptic localization of SAPAP1, a synaptic membrane-associated protein. Genes Cells. 2003;8:121–9.
68. Welch JM, Wang D, Feng G. Differential mRNA expression and protein localization of the SAP90/PSD-95-associated proteins (SAPAPs) in the nervous system of the mouse. J Comp Neurol. 2004;472:24–39.
69. Kindler S, Rehbein M, Classen B, Richter D, Böckers TM. Distinct spatiotemporal expression of SAPAP transcripts in the developing rat brain: a novel dendritically localized mRNA. Brain Res Mol Brain Res. 2004;126:14–21.
70. Pérez-Otaño I, Ehlers MD. Homeostatic plasticity and NMDA receptor trafficking. Trends Neurosci. 2005;28:229–38.
71. Sheng M. Molecular organization of the postsynaptic specialization. Proc Natl Acad Sci U S A. 2001;98:7058–61.
72. Colledge M, Snyder EM, Crozier RA, Soderling JA, Jin Y, Langeberg LK, et al. Ubiquitination regulates PSD-95 degradation and AMPA receptor surface expression. Neuron. 2003;40:595–607.
73. Na CH, Jones DR, Yang Y, Wang X, Xu Y, Peng J. Synaptic protein ubiquitination in rat brain revealed by antibody-based ubiquitome analysis. J Proteome Res. 2012;11:4722–32.
74. Hung AY, Sung CC, Brito IL, Sheng M. Degradation of postsynaptic scaffold GKAP and regulation of dendritic spine morphology by the TRIM3 ubiquitin ligase in rat hippocampal neurons. PLoS One. 2010;5:1–11.
75. Dosemeci A, Jaffe H. Regulation of phosphorylation at the postsynaptic density during different activity states of Ca2+/calmodulin-dependent protein kinase II. Biochem Biophys Res Commun. 2010;391:78–84.
76. Romorini S, Piccoli G, Jiang M, Grossano P, Tonna N, Passafaro M, et al. A functional role of postsynaptic density-95-guanylate kinase-associated protein complex in regulating shank assembly and stability to synapses. J Neurosci. 2004;24:9391–404.
77. Hanus C, Schuman EM. Proteostasis in complex dendrites. Nat Rev Neurosci. 2013;14:638–48.

78. Wan Y, Feng G, Calakos N. Sapap3 deletion causes mGluR5-dependent silencing of AMPAR synapses. J Neurosci. 2011;31:16685–91.
79. Hu JH, Park JM, Park S, Xiao B, Dehoff MH, Kim S, et al. Homeostatic scaling requires group I mGluR activation mediated by Homer1a. Neuron. 2010;68:1128–42.
80. Bertaso F, Roussignol G, Worley P, Bockaert J, Fagni L, Ango F. Homer1a-dependent crosstalk between NMDA and Metabotropic glutamate receptors in mouse neurons. PLoS One. 2010;5:1–6.
81. Brakeman PR, Lanahan AA, O'Brien R, Roche K, Barnes CA, Huganir RL, et al. Homer: a protein that selectively binds metabotropic glutamate receptors. Nature. 1997;386:284–8.
82. Mizutani A, Kuroda Y, Futatsugi A, Furuichi T, Mikoshiba K. Phosphorylation of Homer3 by calcium/calmodulin-dependent kinase II regulates a coupling state of its target molecules in Purkinje cells. J Neurosci. 2008;28:5369–82.
83. Jiang-Xie L-F, Liao H-M, Chen C-H, Chen Y-T, Ho S-Y, Lu D-H, et al. Autism-associated gene Dlgap2 mutant mice demonstrate exacerbated aggressive behaviors and orbitofrontal cortex deficits. Mol Autism. 2014;5:13.
84. Howlett AC, Barth F, Bonner TI, Cabral G, Casellas P, Devane WA, et al. International Union of Pharmacology. XXVII. Classification of cannabinoid receptors. Pharmacol Rev. 2002;54:161–202.
85. Roloff AM, Anderson GR, Martemyanov KA, Thayer SA. Homer 1a gates the induction mechanism for endocannabinoid-mediated synaptic plasticity. J Neurosci. 2010;30:3072–81.
86. Li JM, Lu CL, Cheng MC, Luu SU, Hsu SH, Chen CH. Genetic analysis of the DLGAP1 gene as a candidate gene for schizophrenia. Psychiatry Res. 2013;205:13–7.
87. Lichtenstein P, Yip BH, Björk C, Pawitan Y, Cannon TD, Sullivan PF, et al. Common genetic determinants of schizophrenia and bipolar disorder in Swedish families: a population-based study. Lancet. 2009;373:234–9.
88. Tang A-H, Alger BE. Homer protein-metabotropic glutamate receptor binding regulates endocannabinoid signaling and affects hyperexcitability in a mouse model of fragile X syndrome. J Neurosci. 2015;35:3938–45.
89. Malhotra AK, Pinals DA, Adler CM, Elman I, Clifton A, Pickar D, et al. Ketamine-induced exacerbation of psychotic symptoms and cognitive impairment in neuroleptic-free schizophrenics. Neuropsychopharmacology. 1997;17:141–50.
90. Kim JS, Kornhuber HH, Schmid-Burgk W, Holzmüller B. Low cerebrospinal fluid glutamate in schizophrenic patients and a new hypothesis on schizophrenia. Neurosci Lett. 1980;20:379–82.
91. Dracheva S, Marras SA, Elhakem SL, Kramer FR, Davis KL, Haroutunian V. N-methyl-D-aspartic acid receptor expression in the dorsolateral prefrontal cortex of elderly patients with schizophrenia. Am J Psychiatry. 2001;158:1400–10.
92. Woo T-UW, Walsh JP, Benes FM. Density of glutamic acid decarboxylase 67 messenger RNA-containing neurons that express the N-methyl-D-aspartate receptor subunit NR2A in the anterior cingulate cortex in schizophrenia and bipolar disorder. Arch Gen Psychiatry. 2004;61:649–57.
93. Gardoni F, Mauceri D, Fiorentini C, Bellone C, Missale C, Cattabeni F, et al. CaMKII-dependent phosphorylation regulates SAP97/NR2A interaction. J Biol Chem. 2003;278:44745–52.
94. Wang L, Piserchio A, Mierke DF. Structural characterization of the intermolecular interactions of synapse-associated protein-97 with the NR2B subunit of N-methyl-D-aspartate receptors. J Biol Chem. 2005;280:26992–6.
95. Sans N, Petralia RS, Wang YX, Blahos J, Hell JW, Wenthold RJ. A developmental change in NMDA receptor-associated proteins at hippocampal synapses. J Neurosci. 2000;20:1260–71.
96. Uezato A, Yamamoto N, Iwayama Y, Hiraoka S, Hiraaki E, Umino A, et al. Reduced cortical expression of a newly identified splicing variant of the DLG1 gene in patients with early-onset schizophrenia. Transl Psychiatry. 2015;5:e654.
97. Toyooka K, Iritani S, Makifuchi T, Shirakawa O, Kitamura N, Maeda K, et al. Selective reduction of a PDZ protein, SAP-97, in the prefrontal cortex of patients with chronic schizophrenia. J Neurochem. 2002;83:797–806.
98. Li JM, Lu CL, Cheng MC, Luu SU, Hsu SH, Chen CH. Exonic resequencing of the DLGAP3 gene as a candidate gene for schizophrenia. Psychiatry Res. 2013;208:84–7.
99. Li J-M, Lu C-L, Cheng M-C, Luu S-U, Hsu S-H, Hu T-M, et al. Role of the DLGAP2 gene encoding the SAP90/PSD-95-associated protein 2 in schizophrenia. PLoS One. 2014;9:1–8.
100. Marshall CR, Noor A, Vincent JB, Lionel AC, Feuk L, Skaug J, et al. Structural variation of chromosomes in autism Spectrum disorder. Am J Hum Genet. 2008;82:477–88.
101. Chien W-H, Gau SS-F, Liao H-M, Chiu Y-N, Wu Y-Y, Huang Y-S, et al. Deep exon resequencing of DLGAP2 as a candidate gene of autism spectrum disorders. Mol Autism. 2013;4:26.
102. Chertkow-Deutsher Y, Cohen H, Klein E, Ben-Shachar D. DNA methylation in vulnerability to post-traumatic stress in rats: evidence for the role of the post-synaptic density protein Dlgap2. Int J Neuropsychopharmacol. 2010;13:347–59.
103. Gilbertson MW, Shenton ME, Ciszewski A, Kasai K, Lasko NB, Orr SP, et al. Smaller hippocampal volume predicts pathologic vulnerability to psychological trauma. Nat Neurosci. 2002;5:1242–7.
104. Bremner JD, Vythilingam M, Vermetten E, Southwick SM, McGlashan T, Nazeer A, et al. MRI and PET study of deficits in Hippocampal structure and function in women with childhood sexual abuse and posttraumatic stress disorder. Am J Psychiatry. 2003;160:924–32.
105. Woon FL, Sood S, Hedges DW. Hippocampal volume deficits associated with exposure to psychological trauma and posttraumatic stress disorder in adults: a meta-analysis. Prog Neuro-Psychopharmacol Biol Psychiatry. 2010;34:1181–8.
106. Züchner S, Wendland JR, Ashley-Koch AE, Collins AL, Tran-Viet KN, Quinn K, et al. Multiple rare SAPAP3 missense variants in trichotillomania and OCD. Mol Psychiatry. Nature Publishing Group. 2009;14:6–9.
107. Hertz JM, Sivertsen B, Silahtaroglu A, Bugge M, Kalscheuer V, Weber A, et al. Early onset, non-progressive, mild cerebellar ataxia co-segregating with a familial balanced translocation t(8;20)(p22;q13). J Med Genet. 2004;41:1–3.
108. Hashimoto K, Fukaya M, Qiao X, Sakimura K, Watanabe M, Kano M. Impairment of AMPA receptor function in cerebellar granule cells of ataxic mutant mouse stargazer. J Neurosci. 1999;19:6027–36.
109. Coesmans M, Smitt PAS, Linden DJ, Shigemoto R, Hirano T, Yamakawa Y, et al. Mechanisms underlying cerebellar motor deficits due to mGluR1-autoantibodies. Ann Neurol. 2003;53:325–36.
110. Guergueltcheva V, Azmanov DN, Angelicheva D, Smith KR, Chamova T, Florez L, et al. Autosomal-recessive congenital cerebellar ataxia is caused by mutations in metabotropic glutamate receptor 1. Am J Hum Genet. 2012;91:553–64.
111. Aoyama S, Shirakawa O, Ono H, Hashimoto T, Kajimoto Y, Maeda K. Mutation and association analysis of the DAP-1 gene with schizophrenia. Psychiatry Clin Neurosci. 2003;57:545–7.
112. Pickard BS, Malloy MP, Clark L, Lehellard S, Ewald HL, Mors O, et al. Candidate psychiatric illness genes identified in patients with pericentric inversions of chromosome 18. Psychiatr Genet. 2005;15:37–44.
113. Kirov G, Pocklington AJ, Holmans P, Ivanov D, Ikeda M, Ruderfer D, et al. De novo CNV analysis implicates specific abnormalities of postsynaptic signalling complexes in the pathogenesis of schizophrenia. Mol Psychiatry. 2012;17:142–53.
114. Roselli F, Livrea P, Almeida OFX. CDK5 is essential for soluble amyloid β-induced degradation of GKAP and remodeling of the synaptic actin cytoskeleton. PLoS One. 2011;6:1–14.
115. Mathias SR, Knowles EEM, Kent JW, McKay DR, Curran JE, de Almeida MAA, et al. Recurrent major depression and right hippocampal volume: a bivariate linkage and association study. Hum Brain Mapp. 2016;37:191–202.
116. Schütt J, Falley K, Richter D, Kreienkamp H-J, Kindler S. Fragile X mental retardation protein regulates the levels of scaffold proteins and glutamate receptors in postsynaptic densities. J Biol Chem. 2009;284:25479–87.
117. Liu S, Zhang Y, Bian H, Li X. Gene expression profiling predicts pathways and genes associated with Parkinson's disease. Neurol Sci. 2016;37:73–9.
118. Kim Y, Zhang Y, Pang K, Kang H, Park H, Lee Y, et al. Bipolar disorder associated microRNA, miR-1908-5p, regulates the expression of genes functioning in neuronal Glutamatergic synapses. Exp Neurobiol. 2016;25:296–306.

RNAseq analysis of hippocampal microglia after kainic acid-induced seizures

Dale B. Bosco[1], Jiaying Zheng[1], Zhiyan Xu[2], Jiyun Peng[1], Ukpong B. Eyo[1], Ke Tang[3], Cheng Yan[3], Jun Huang[3], Lijie Feng[4], Gongxiong Wu[5], Jason R. Richardson[6], Hui Wang[2,7*] and Long-Jun Wu[1,8*]

Abstract

Microglia have been shown to be of critical importance to the progression of temporal lobe epilepsy. However, the broad transcriptional changes that these cells undergo following seizure induction is not well understood. As such, we utilized RNAseq analysis upon microglia isolated from the hippocampus to determine expression pattern alterations following kainic acid induced seizure. We determined that microglia undergo dramatic changes to their expression patterns, particularly with regard to mitochondrial activity and metabolism. We also observed that microglia initiate immunological activity, specifically increasing interferon beta responsiveness. Our results provide novel insights into microglia transcriptional regulation following acute seizures and suggest potential therapeutic targets specifically in microglia for the treatment of seizures and epilepsy.

Introduction

Temporal lobe epilepsy (TLE) represents the most common form of focal epileptic disorder. While several pharmaceutical treatments are currently available to mitigate and reduce seizure occurrence, as many as one third of patients display resistance to medication [1]. As such, an unmet need exists, requiring further investigation into the mechanisms underlying TLE. The rodent kainic acid (KA) epilepsy model can recapitulate many of the physical features of TLE including behavioral seizures and neuropathological lesions [2]. Therefore, many investigations have focused on how KA alters the activity and viability of neurons. However, comparatively little attention has been paid to glial cells, including astrocytes and microglia, in epileptogenesis [3, 4].

Comprising between 5 and 15% of total central nervous system (CNS) cells, microglia predominantly serve as the resident immune cell of the CNS. Recent evidence has also revealed that microglia have a diverse set of roles within the CNS, including directing neuronal maturation and supporting synaptic turnover [5, 6]. With regard to epilepsy, it was established relatively early that large numbers of reactive microglia can be found within the hippocampus of temporal lobe epilepsy patients [7, 8]. Our recent studies demonstrated that seizures can acutely induce microglia-neuron interaction as well as the changes in microglial landscape [9–12]. Microgliosis and inflammatory cytokine release has been observed within areas of neuronal damage implicating microglia in promotion of neuropathy [13]. However, microglia may also have neuroprotective roles such as modulating excitotoxicity.

Since microglia seem to be an important part of the epileptic response, we investigated how KA-induced seizures modulate microglial transcriptional activity and alters their phenotype. Specifically, we investigated hippocampal microglia since this brain region is one of the most affected by seizure [14]. To explore this, we performed RNAseq analysis, a powerful tool to determine wide scale phenotypic alterations, on isolated hippocampal microglia from mice that received KA. We report that KA-induced seizures resulted in significant transcriptional changes to microglia when compared to sham controls. Specifically, there are significant increases in the expression of metabolic and mitochondrial pathways. Coincidently, we observed that immune related factors were also being up-regulated, including several chemokine factors such as chemokine ligand 5 (CCL5) and C-X-C motif chemokine 10 (CXCL10). We also

* Correspondence: huiwangph@ntu.edu.cn; wu.longjun@mayo.edu
[2]Department of Pharmacology, School of Pharmacy, Nantong University, 19 Qixiu Road, Nantong 226001, Jiangsu, China
[1]Department of Neurology, Mayo Clinic, 200 First Street SW, Rochester, MN 55905, USA
Full list of author information is available at the end of the article

observed that microglia increased their responsiveness to interferon β, possibly through interferon regulatory factor 7 (Irf7). Thus, we show that KA-induced seizures significantly regulate the microglia transcriptome, providing novel directions for further investigation.

Results

Kainic acid induced seizures significantly alters microglial gene expression profile

To begin our investigation, heterozygote CX3CR1$^{GFP/+}$ mice were treated with kainic acid (KA) via ICV injection to induce an acute seizure response [12]. Microglia in the mouse hippocampus show dramatic reactivity following KA-induced seizure strating at as early as 1 day and peaks at 3 days after KA treatment [15]. We therefore focused on hippocampus microglia isolated via FACS 3 days after KA-induced seizures. RNAseq libraries were constructed using the isolated cells and loaded onto an Illumina Hiseq platform. DEseq was used to determine differential gene expression. From the results, over 2300 differentially expressed genes were identified (Fig. 1a, Additional file 1: Table S1). Of these, we observed many of the suggested microglia specific genes including P2Y12, Tmem119, and Olfml3 [16]. Additionally, we detected only slight increases to myelin (e.g., PLP), neuronal (e.g., Rbfox3, Map2), and astrocytes (e.g., Gfap, Aldh1l1) markers within samples isolated from KA treated mice, with only GFAP registering as significant. These factors were not detected within the control samples. Since it has been suggested that the phagocytic capacity of microglia is substantially reduced following KA-seizure [17] and that microglial could express GFAP [18] we believe that the genes alterations that were deemed significant reflect microglia specific alterations. These results demonstrated the purity of microglia sorting. The overwhelming majority of differentially expressed genes were up-regulated in the microglia samples from KA treated mice with few genes being down-regulated when compared to sham controls (Fig. 1b-c). Table 1 lists the top 25 up-regulated and Table 2 the identified down-regulated genes. Table 3 lists the top 25 genes found only in the KA-treated animals as determined by P_{adj} values.

We next determined whether KA-induced seizures affected microglial specific markers. Using the list determined by Hickman et al. [16], we found that seven of the listed microglial markers were differentially expressed (Fig. 2a, Additional file 2: Figure S1). These were adenosine A3 receptor (Adora 3), crystallin beta A4 (Cryba4), galactose-3-O-sulfotransferase 4 (Gal3st4), lipase member H (Liph), membrane-spanning 4-domains, subfamily A, member 6B (Ms4a6b), serine peptidase

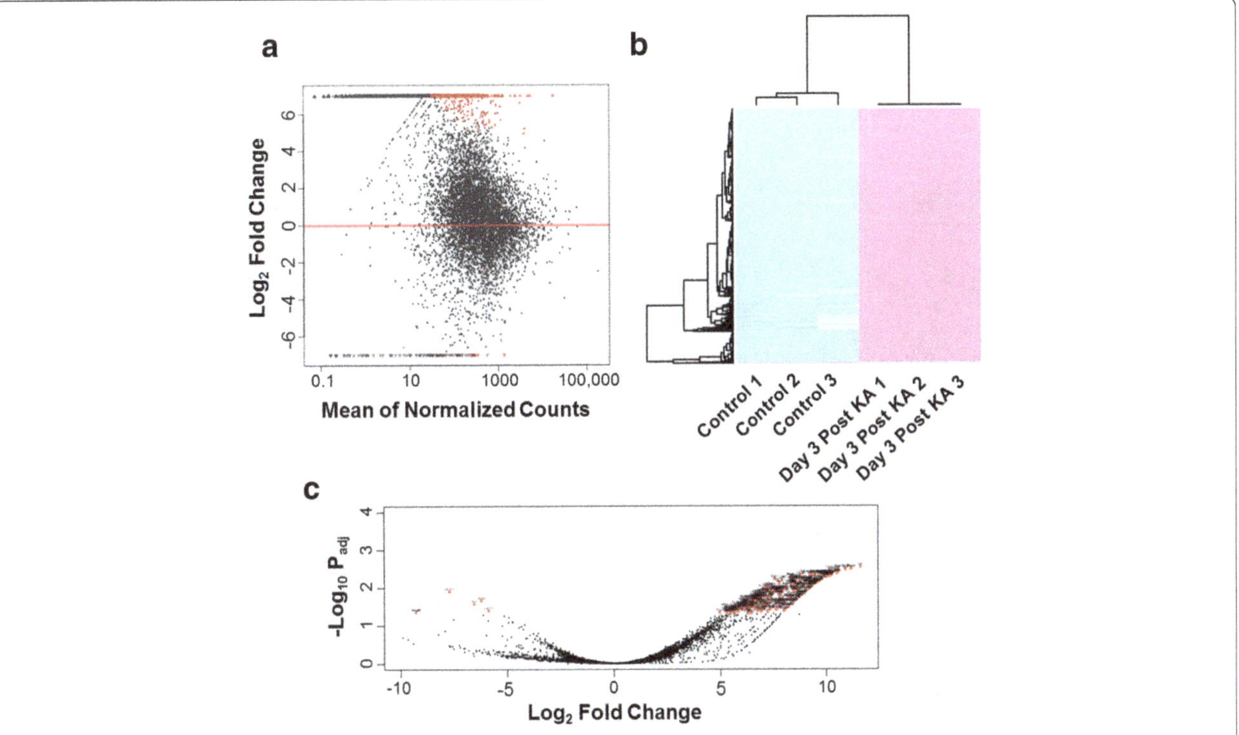

Fig. 1 Differentially expressed genes between the sham control and KA treated groups. **a** MA-plot of gene expression. All significant differentially expressed genes ($P_{adj} < 0.05$) and locally weighted smoothing (LOESS) line are colored in red. **b** Heat map and hierarchical clustering was performed based on all differentially expressed genes. Magenta indicates high relative expression, and cyan indicates low relative expression. **c** Volcano plot of gene expression. All significant differentially expressed genes are colored in red and labeled by gene symbols

Table 1 Top 25 most up-regulated genes

ENSEMBL	Gene ID	Gene Symbol	Gene Name	Log_2 Fold Change	P_{adj}
ENSMUSG00000019505	22187	Ubb	ubiquitin B(Ubb)	11.64	2.89E-03
ENSMUSG00000006418	81018	Rnf114	ring finger protein 114(Rnf114)	11.21	3.18E-03
ENSMUSG00000005881	66366	Ergic3	ERGIC and golgi 3(Ergic3)	11.17	3.27E-03
ENSMUSG00000090841	17904	Myl6	myosin, light polypeptide 6, alkali, smooth muscle and non- muscle(Myl6)	10.91	3.39E-03
ENSMUSG00000040952	20085	Rps19	ribosomal protein S19(Rps19)	10.90	3.07E-03
ENSMUSG00000042650	268420	Alkbh5	alkB homolog 5, RNA demethylase(Alkbh5)	10.58	3.27E-03
ENSMUSG00000047215	20005	Rpl9	ribosomal protein L9(Rpl9)	10.54	3.27E-03
ENSMUSG00000020664	13382	Dld	dihydrolipoamide dehydrogenase(Dld)	10.54	4.14E-03
ENSMUSG00000025959	93691	Klf7	Kruppel-like factor 7 (ubiquitous)(Klf7)	10.52	4.28E-03
ENSMUSG00000022982	20655	Sod1	superoxide dismutase 1, soluble(Sod1)	10.51	4.21E-03
ENSMUSG00000026213	71728	Stk11ip	serine/threonine kinase 11 interacting protein(Stk11ip)	10.49	4.28E-03
ENSMUSG00000031483	244373	Erlin2	ER lipid raft associated 2(Erlin2)	10.45	3.66E-03
ENSMUSG00000029298	236573	Gbp9	guanylate-binding protein 9(Gbp9)	10.27	4.58E-03
ENSMUSG00000034855	15945	Cxcl 10	chemokine (C-X-C motif) ligand 10(Cxcl10)	10.27	3.78E-03
ENSMUSG00000070031	434484	Sp140	Sp140 nuclear body protein(Sp140)	10.24	4.59E-03
ENSMUSG00000054920	71778	Klhl5	kelch-like 5(Klhl5)	10.22	4.74E-03
ENSMUSG00000040447	216892	Spns2	spinster homolog 2(Spns2)	10.17	4.91E-03
ENSMUSG00000022884	13682	Eif4a2	eukaryotic translation initiation factor 4A2(Eif4a2)	10.16	3.39E-03
ENSMUSG00000028962	20535	Slc4a2	solute carrier family 4 (anion exchanger), member 2(Slc4a2)	10.15	4.93E-03
ENSMUSG00000047153	219094	Khnyn	KH and NYN domain containing(Khnyn)	10.15	5.07E-03
ENSMUSG00000030298	110379	Sec13	SEC13 homolog, nuclear pore and COPII coat complex component(Sec13)	10.12	4.98E-03
ENSMUSG00000031378	11666	Abcd1	ATP-binding cassette, sub-family D (ALD), member 1(Abcd1)	10.11	4.28E-03
ENSMUSG00000004568	102098	Arhgef18	rho/rac guanine nucleotide exchange factor (GEF) 18(Arhgef18)	10.02	5.27E-03
ENSMUSG00000030577	12483	Cd22	CD22 antigen(Cd22)	10.02	5.22E-03
ENSMUSG00000031858	74549	Mau2	MAU2 sister chromatid cohesion factor(Mau2)	10.01	4.58E-03

Table 2 Down-regulated genes

ENSEMBL	Gene ID	Gene Symbol	Gene Name	Log_2 Fold Change	P_{adj}
ENSMUSG00000000562	11542	Ccdc171	adenosine A3 receptor(Adora3)	−5.87	3.98E-02
ENSMUSG00000090137	22186	Uba52	ubiquitin A-52 residue ribosomal protein fusion product 1(Uba52)	−6.22	2.17E-02
ENSMUSG00000052407	320226	Atn1	coiled-coil domain containing 171(Ccdc171)	−6.55	2.65E-02
ENSMUSG00000092995	387134	Mir16–1	microRNA 16–1(Mir16–1)	−7.71	1.23E-02
ENSMUSG00000004263	13498	Adora3	atrophin 1(Atn1)	−9.29	4.39E-02
ENSMUSG00000074344	69296	Tmigd3	transmembrane and immunoglobulin domain containing 3(Tmigd3)	−9.29	4.39E-02

Table 3 Top 25 differentially expressed genes only observed in KA treated group

ENSEMBL	Gene ID	Gene Symbol	Gene Name	P_{adj}
ENSMUSG00000069516	17105	Lyz2	lysozyme 2	6.62E-04
ENSMUSG00000060938	19941	Rpl26	ribosomal protein L26	1.15E-03
ENSMUSG00000002602	26362	Axl	AXL receptor tyrosine kinase	2.25E-03
ENSMUSG00000031320	20102	Rps4x	ribosomal protein S4, X-linked	2.25E-03
ENSMUSG00000049313	20660	Sorl 1	sortilin-related receptor, LDLR class A repeats-containing	2.25E-03
ENSMUSG00000062006	68436	Rpl34	ribosomal protein L34	2.25E-03
ENSMUSG00000063524	619547	Rpl34-ps1	ribosomal protein L34, pseudogene 1	2.25E-03
ENSMUSG00000069516	100043876	Gm4705	predicted gene 4705	2.25E-03
ENSMUSG00000063524	13806	Eno1	enolase 1, alpha non-neuron	2.25E-03
ENSMUSG00000069892	245240	9,930,111 J21 Rik2	RIKEN cDNA 9,930,111 J21 gene 2	2.25E-03
ENSMUSG00000089809	319818	A930011G23Rik	RIKEN cDNA A930011G23 gene	2.25E-03
ENSMUSG00000090733	57294	Rps27	ribosomal protein S27	2.25E-03
ENSMUSG00000073418	12268	C4b	complement component 4B	2.83E-03
ENSMUSG00000001794	12336	Capns1	calpain, small subunit 1	2.94E-03
ENSMUSG00000003518	72349	Dusp3	dual specificity phosphatase 3	2.94E-03
ENSMUSG00000005566	21849	Trim28	tripartite motif-containing 28	2.94E-03
ENSMUSG00000009687	18301	Fxyd5	FXYD domain-containing ion transport regulator 5	2.94E-03
ENSMUSG00000022415	20972	Syngr1	synaptogyrin 1	2.94E-03
ENSMUSG00000022477	11429	Aco2	aconitase 2, mitochondrial	2.94E-03
ENSMUSG00000022565	18810	Plec	plectin	2.94E-03
ENSMUSG00000024679	68774	Ms4a6d	membrane-spanning 4-domains, subfamily A, member 6D	2.94E-03
ENSMUSG00000025498	54123	Irf7	interferon regulatory factor 7	2.94E-03
ENSMUSG00000026222	20684	Sp100	nuclear antigen Sp100	2.94E-03
ENSMUSG00000026430	54354	Rassf5	Ras association (RalGDS/AF-6) domain family member 5	2.94E-03
ENSMUSG00000034854	73822	Mfsd12	major facilitator superfamily domain containing 12	2.94E-03

inhibitor Kunitz type 1 (Spint1), and toll-like receptor 12 (Tlr12). Since KA treatment has also been shown to induce inflammatory responses [15], we also investigated our list of differentially expressed genes for potential inflammatory markers. Indeed, we found a number of inflammatory factors are increased within microglia isolated from KA treated mice, including C-C motif chemokine ligand 5 (Ccl5), Ccl7, and C-X-C motif chemokine ligand 10 (Cxcl10) (Fig. 2b, Additional file 2: Figure S2). We determined that expression of several inflammatory and immunological response receptors are also increased (Fig. 2c). These receptors included C-C motif chemokine receptor 2 (Ccr2), C-X-C motif chemokine receptor 4 (Cxcr4), and Tlr1. Finally, a significant number cluster of differentiation (CD) markers were significantly increased (Fig. 2d). The majority of identified CD markers are related to immunological responses including CD40, CD69, and CD80 [19, 20]. These results suggest that microglia are undergoing immunological activation in response to KA-induced seizures.

Gene ontology analysis indicates significant increases to metabolic processes

Our next step was to identify if any unifying features existed within our differential expression data set. As such, we utilized clusterProfiler to perform gene ontology (GO) analysis [21]. We investigated our data set using the three major classifications, cellular component, biological process, and molecular function (Additional file 3: Table S2, Additional file 4: Table S3 and Additional file 5: Table S4). To further visualize our results, identified GO terms were input into REViGO [22]. This web-based application allows for long lists of GO terms to be summarized and grouped based on semantic similarities. REViGO analysis was run using the associated P_{adj} for each identified GO term, with medium allowed similarity (0.7), and SimRel similarity measurement. TreeMaps were then generated for each ontology classification. Each box represents GO terms that are then grouped and colored based on keyword similarities. Box size indicates each terms level of significance as determined by input P_{adj} values. Added labels highlight overarching grouping terms. As Fig. 3a illustrates there are significant alterations

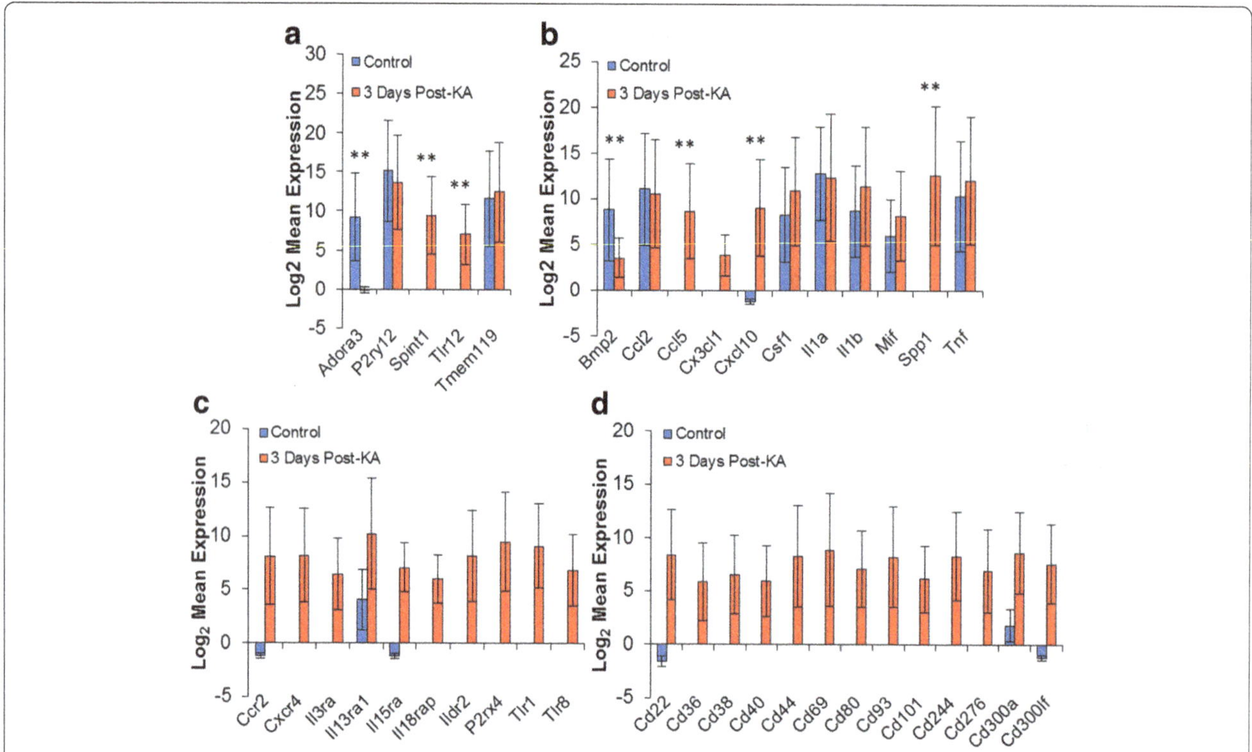

Fig. 2 Selected differential expressed genes. Expression results were investigated for genes relating to microglial specificity and inflammatory and immunological regulation. **a** Microglial markers. **b** Secreted factors. **c** Related receptors. **d** CD markers. Values are expressed and mean ± standard error. $^{**}P_{adj} < 0.05$. All gene listed in panel (**c** and **d**) had a $P_{adj} < 0.05$

to intracellular factor expression, especially within the mitochondria. Moreover, Biological process GO analysis showed that there seems to be significant alterations to microglial metabolism, with catabolism being at the forefront (Fig. 3b). It also identified that microglia were activating viral defense mechanisms following seizure. Finally, we observed that a number of transferase activities were being undertaken following seizure (Fig. 3c).

Kainic acid treatment may sensitize microglia to interferon beta

Delving deeper into the identified GO terms it was observed that a number of related terms were pertinent to type I interferons, specifically interferon β (IFN-β). Table 4 summarizes these identified GO terms. IFN-β is a type-I interferon that binds interferon-α/β receptor (IFNAR) to regulate a multitude of signaling cascades particularly the JAK/STAT pathway [23]. IFN-β has also been suggested to modulate microglial activity in multiple sclerosis and pathological neovascularization [24, 25]. Since IFN-β signaling was well represented within our GO analysis, we believe that IFN-β is important to the microglial modulation that occurs following KA-induced seizures.

Pathway analysis reveals both metabolic and immune response processes are altered

Finally, we performed pathway analysis on the differential expression data set using the clusterProfiler enrichKEGG function (Fig. 4). Unsurprisingly, this analysis corroborated our GO analysis results in that metabolism was significantly enriched in our data set. We also identified several pathways relating to neurological diseases (i.e., Parkinson's, Alzheimer's, and Huntington's disease) (Fig. 4). Using KEGGmapper we were able to further investigate which specific metabolic pathway were being affected. We found that Glycan, fatty acid and lipid, and nucleotide metabolism are all up-regulated within the KA treated samples. Moreover, we observed several pathways involving glutamate utilization and isoprenoid biosynthesis were also affected (Fig. 5a).

While metabolism was by far the most significantly altered pathway term identified, several other pathways of note were identified, specifically those relating to neurodegenerative diseases (i.e., Parkinson's, Huntington's, Alzheimer's) and viral response (i.e., Herpes simplex, Epstein-Barr, viral carcinogenesis). While it was consistent with our exploration avenue to observe pathways relating to neurodegenerative diseases, we observed viral responses in both GO and pathway analysis. As such, we further explored the gene relationships underlying these

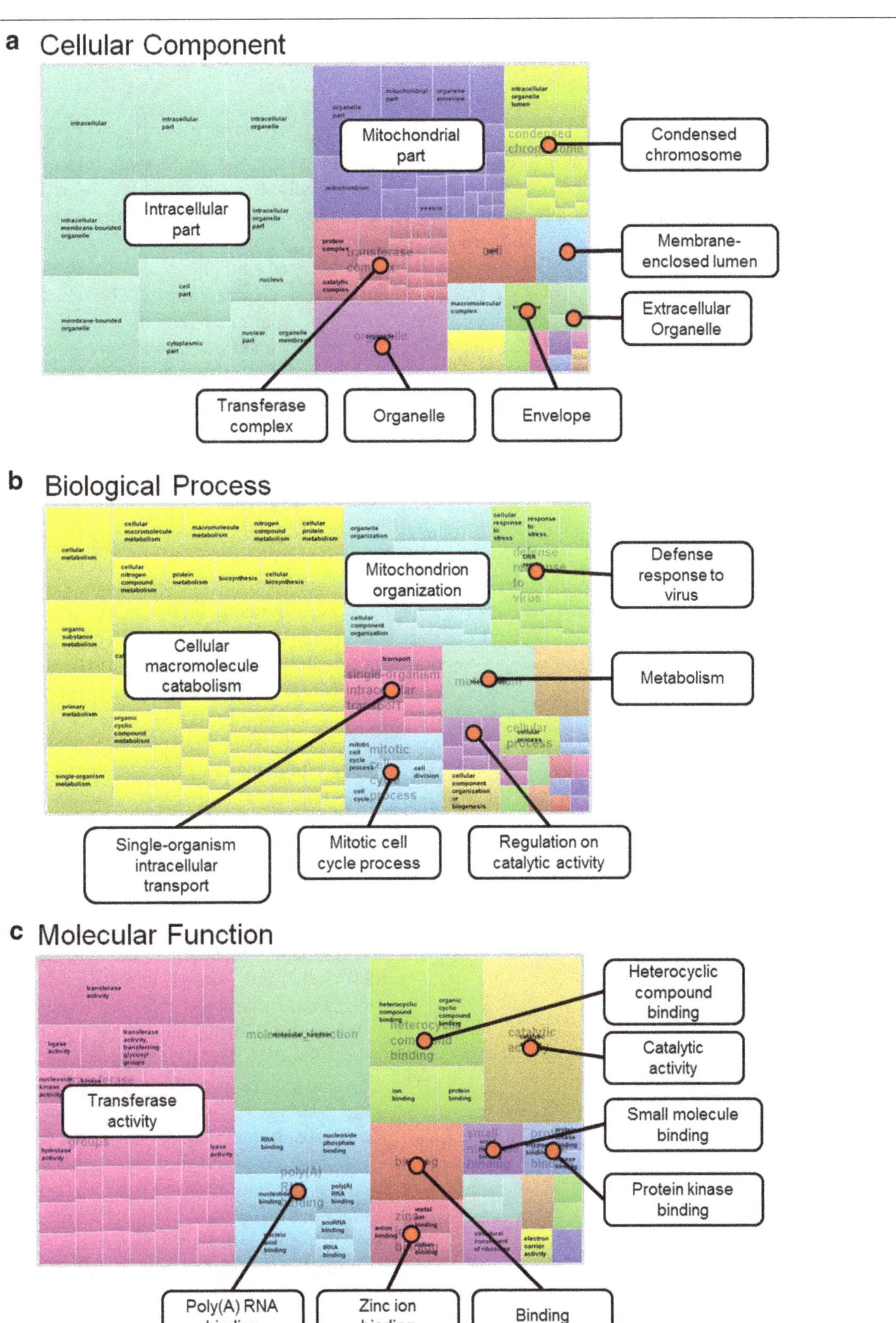

Fig. 3 (See legend on next page.)

(See figure on previous page.)
Fig. 3 Functional classification of the differentially expressed genes. **a** Cellular component. **b** Biological process. **c** Molecular function. Visualization of identified Gene Ontology terms was completed using REViGO [22]. Analysis was run using the P_{adj} for each identified term, medium allowed similarity (0.7), and SimRel similarity measurement. Individual term size weight within each TreeMap was determined by associated P_{adj}.

identified pathway terms. Differential expressed genes identified to be part of the indicated KEGG pathway terms were analyzed with the GeneMANIA application for Cytoscape V3.5.1 [26]. GeneMANIA utilizes both published information and computational predictions to identify relationships between input genes. It will also suggest possible interaction partners not initially input into the query. Indeed, we demonstrate that the overwhelming majority of genes associated with the identified neurodegenerative pathways were related to mitochondrial function, specifically the electron transport chain (Fig. 5b). This is consistent with our GO analysis. Investigation of viral pathway term genes however revealed a more diverse set of groupings (Fig. 5c). These include genes related to RNA polymerase complexes and histones. Both of which are consistent with the high levels of transcriptional modulation observed. Additionally, several genes were associated with immunological regulation, such as complement C3, signal transducer and activator of transcription 2 (Stat2), and antigen peptide transporter 1 (Tap1).

Discussion

The majority of research into epilepsy has focused on neuronal hyperactivities and cell death. However, the role of glia, particularly microglia, in the pathogenesis of epilepsy is an important emerging area of study. Specifically, the transcriptomic alterations of microglia following KA-induced seizure have not been well studied. In this regard, we utilized RNAseq analysis on isolated hippocampal microglia to investigate microglial response during the acute phase after seizure. In total, our results clearly demonstrate that microglia undergo significant alterations following KA-induced seizures, including up-regulation of several inflammatory factors and modulation of mitochondrial activity.

Table 4 Type I interferon related GO terms

GO Term ID	Term Name	P_{adj}
GO:0032480	negative regulation of type I interferon production	0.0012
GO:0032479	regulation of type I interferon production	0.0019
GO:0034340	response to type I interferon	0.0046
GO:0032606	type I interferon production	0.0055
GO:0032648	regulation of interferon-beta production	0.0109
GO:0032608	interferon-beta production	0.0166
GO:0035456	response to interferon-beta	0.0173
GO:0060337	type I interferon signaling pathway	0.0204
GO:0071357	cellular response to type I interferon	0.0204
GO:0032688	negative regulation of interferon-beta production	0.0375
GO:0060340	positive regulation of type I interferon-mediated signaling pathway	0.0375
GO:0035458	cellular response to interferon-beta	0.0429
GO:0060338	regulation of type I interferon-mediated signaling pathway	0.0497

Microglia may undergo oxidative stress response following KA-induced seizure

The most obvious phenotypic alteration was mitochondrial activity in microglia after seizures. While it is possible that up-regulation of mitochondrial genes is merely indicative of microglia transitioning from a resting to active state, it is also possible that microglia are increasing production of mitochondria-derived reactive oxygen species (ROS). While NADPH oxidase has often been described as the primary source of ROS, it has been well established that NADH dehydrogenase (electron transport chain complex I) can also contribute to ROS formation [27]. Indeed, several complex I subunits (e.g., Ndufs8, Ndufa5, Ndufb8) were differentially expressed in our dataset but no NADPH oxidase subunits were up-regulated. This idea is also supported by the observed up-regulation of superoxide dismutase (Sod) 1 and 2, both of which can convert the superoxide generated by the electron transport chain into hydrogen peroxide [28]. Sod 1 and 2 are critically important for the mitigation of oxidative stress and are altered during epilepsy.

When considering our other results, specifically the observed utilization of glutamate, there is further indication that microglia are responding to oxidative stressors. Our results identified two possible means by which glutamate could be utilized, conversion to either 1) proline or 2) glutathione. Of these, the generation of glutathione may be of significance. From our results we observed differential expression of glutathione peroxidase 3 (Gpx3), glutathione S-transferase omega 1 (Gsto1), glutathione transferase zeta 1 (Gstz1), and glutathione reductase (Gsr) expression, all of which are important to the mitigation of oxidative stress [29, 30]. Understanding the consequence of this response could open new avenues into attenuating oxidative damage following seizures. Moreover, it is interesting that of the four main glutathione peroxidase variants, we only observed

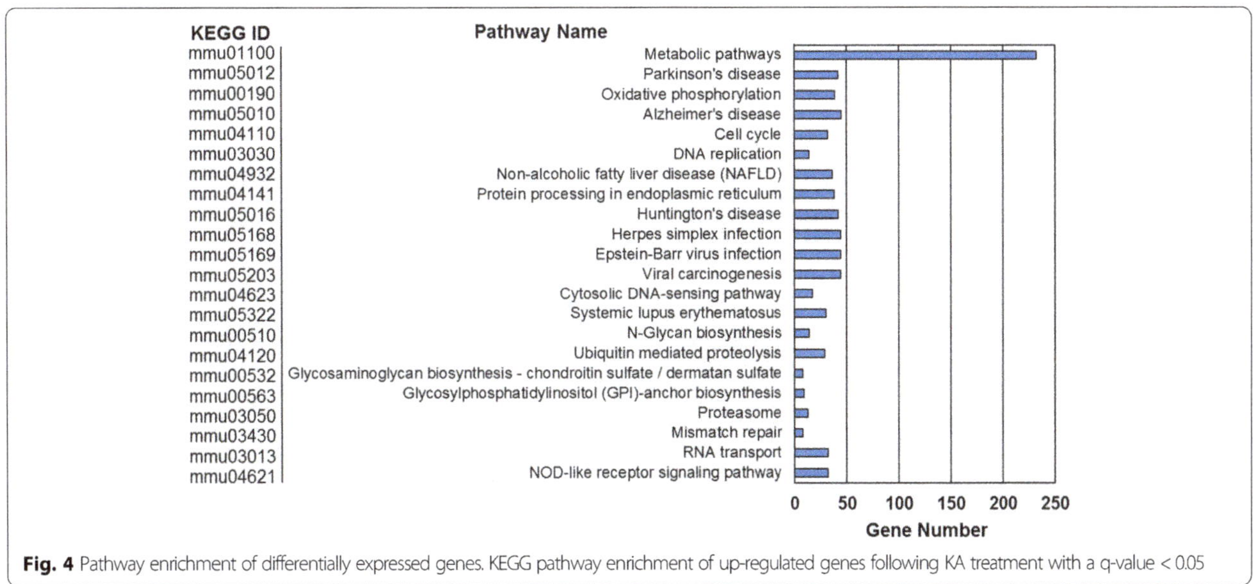

Fig. 4 Pathway enrichment of differentially expressed genes. KEGG pathway enrichment of up-regulated genes following KA treatment with a q-value < 0.05

increases in Gpx3, which is found within the extracellular space [31]. It is possible that microglia are attempting to mitigate not only their own endogenous oxidative stress but also that within the environment.

Microglia increase metabolic activity in response to KA-induced seizure

Our results also showed that many genes relating to metabolic activity are significantly up-regulated. Specifically, GO and pathway analysis determined that microglia up-regulated lipid, nucleotide, and glycan metabolism. These metabolic activities have also been observed during transcriptional analysis of total rat cortex following sarin-induced seizure [32]. We also identified that geranylgeranyl diphosphate synthase 1 (Ggps1) was up-regulated. Ggps1 is responsible for synthesis of the isoprenoid intermediate geranylgeranyl diphosphate (GGPP), which can be attached to a wide assortment of proteins via geranylgeranyltransferases (GGT) like Rab GGT, whose alpha subunit was differentially expressed in our data set [33, 34]. Within Alzheimer's disease it was shown that GGPP may influence microglial inflammatory response via modulation of Rho GTPase [35]. Moreover, many of the positive effects of statin drugs (e.g., reducing excitotoxicity and inflammation) within Alzheimer's disease, Parkinson's disease, and multiple sclerosis could be attributed to mitigation of isoprenoid intermediates, like GGPP [36–39]. The observed mitigation of KA induced seizure symptoms by statins may also involve similar mechanisms [40]. Given our results, it would be of interest to determine if statins improve seizure recovery by attenuating microglial inflammatory response.

Microglia undergo immunological activation in response to KA-induced seizure

Microglia as a principal immune cell in the brain are activated in human epileptic brain and rodent seizure models [4]. Not surprisingly, we also observed that microglia underwent immunological activation, as seen by enrichment of viral response pathways, at 3 days post KA-induced seizures in mice. However, underlying each of these pathways was a shared set of up-regulated genes, including a number of histocompatibility genes, many of which seem to correlate with non-classical major histocompatibility complexes. More specifically, we observed that H2-T23, which encodes Qa-1, and several genes that make up Qa-2 (i.e., H2-Q6, H2-Q7, and H2-Q8) were differentially expressed within our data set [41, 42]. These histocompatibility complexes have been shown to modulate the activity of natural killer (NK) cells [43, 44]. In regards to neuroinflammation, it was reported that the soluble forms of MHC-E and MHC-G might be related to inflammation protection within multiple sclerosis [45]. However, very little has been done to investigate the roles of these histocompatibility complexes within epilepsy. Given the indications that NK cells are increased following temporal lobe epilepsy, it is worth investigating whether microglia are modulating NK cell activity within the hippocampal region following seizure induction, and whether this modulation is inhibitory of stimulatory.

Interferon beta may modulate microglial activity following KA-induced seizure

Another sign of microglial immunomodulation was the identification of a number of IFN-β responsive terms during GO analysis. IFN-β is typically seen as being

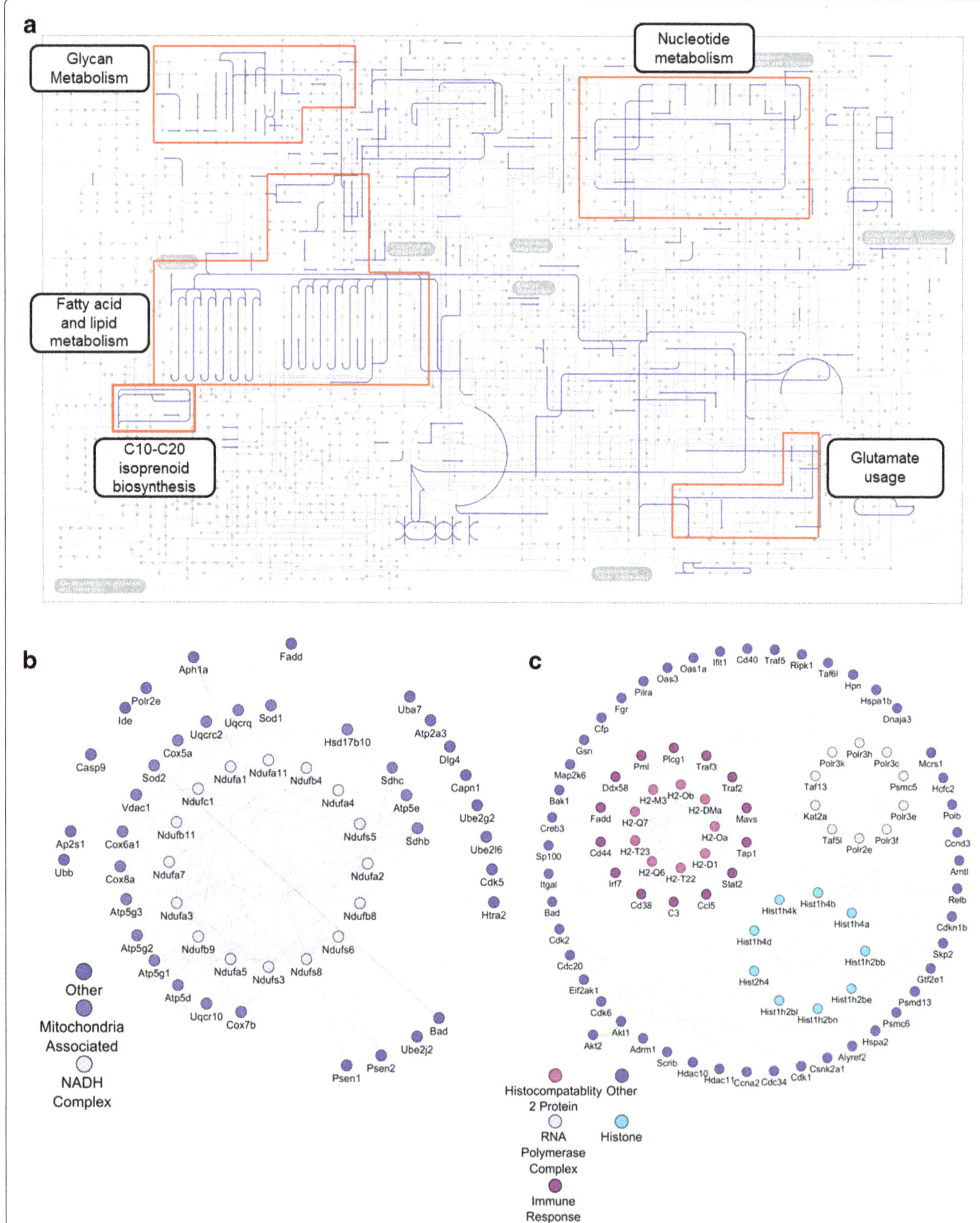

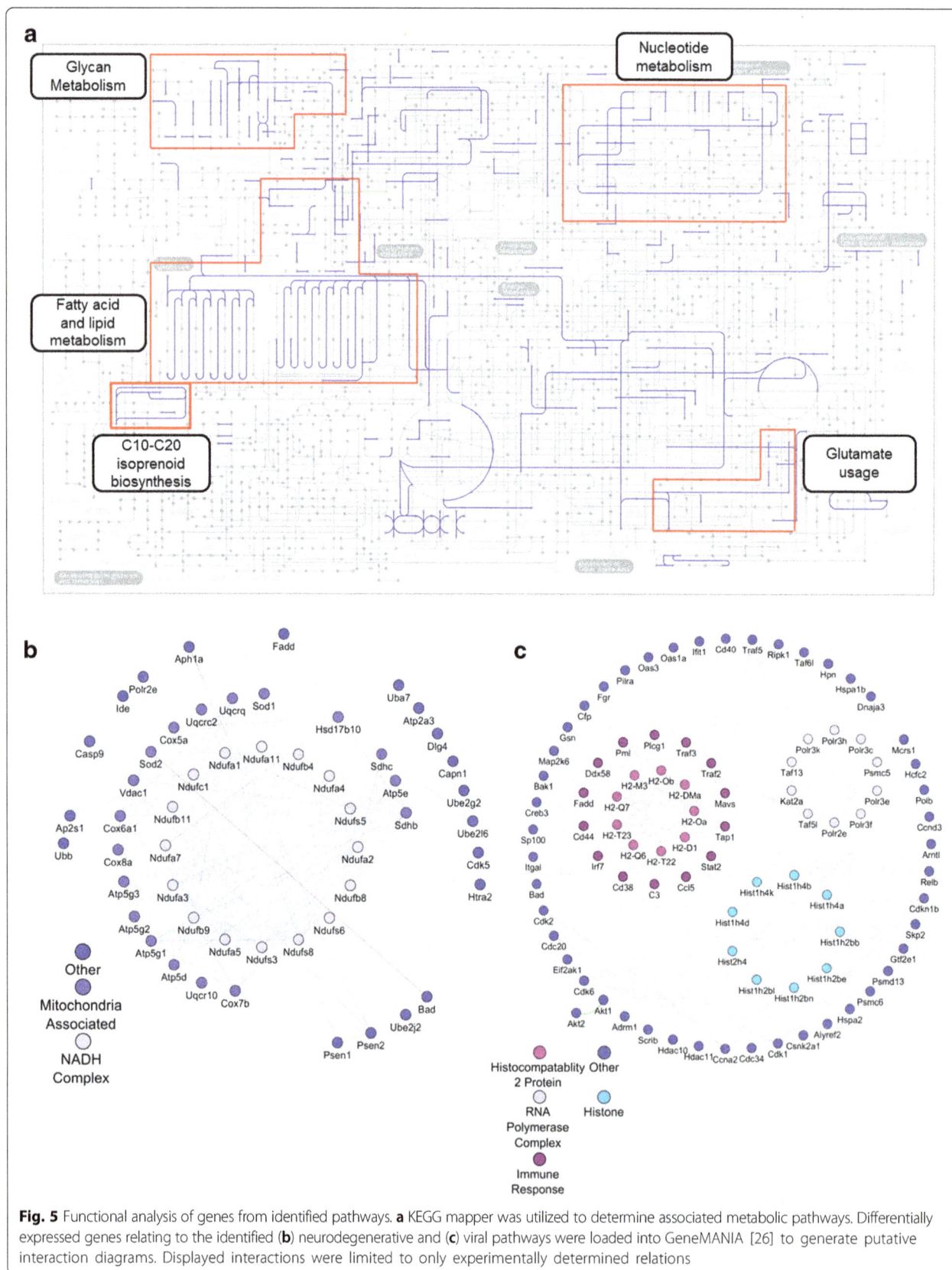

Fig. 5 Functional analysis of genes from identified pathways. **a** KEGG mapper was utilized to determine associated metabolic pathways. Differentially expressed genes relating to the identified (**b**) neurodegenerative and (**c**) viral pathways were loaded into GeneMANIA [26] to generate putative interaction diagrams. Displayed interactions were limited to only experimentally determined relations

anti-inflammatory and has become a common treatment option for relapsing-remitting multiple sclerosis patients [46]. However, there are also indications that type-I interferons may negatively regulate brain activity during aging [47]. Thus, IFN-β may have differential roles depending on disease context. In relation to microglia it has been shown that IFN-β can induce chemokine CCL5 expression, which was highly up-regulated in our data set and in our recent cytokine array [15] after KA-induced seizures. It has also been shown that interferon regulatory factor 7 (Irf7), which is suggested to be the master regulator of type-I interferon-dependent immune response, can modulate CCL5 expression [48]. We observed that Irf7 was differently expressed following KA treatment, indicating a possible means by which IFN-β could modulate microglia inflammatory responses following seizures. As a final note, it has been shown that some Irf7 activity may be tightly regulated by non-degenerative ubiquitination [49, 50]. One of the most up-regulated genes in our data set following seizure was ubiquitin (Ubb). Consequently, our data set indicates that several facets of gene regulation are at play within microglia following KA treatment.

Identified differentially expressed genes warranting further investigation

Finally, while over 2300 differentially expressed genes were identified, we believe that the following selection may be of interest for further investigation. First is osteopontin (secreted phosphoprotein 1; Spp1), which has been observed within neuronal injuries, particularly ischemic stroke [51, 52]. However, little is known about how Spp1 is involved in epileptic seizures even though other less targeted profiling analyses have also noted its up-regulation following seizures [53, 54]. What is known is that its expression seems to be localized to certain areas of the brain, including the CA1 and CA3 regions of the hippocampus [55, 56]. Moreover, it has been suggested that only a sub-set of microglia actively express Spp1, with a possible role in phagocytosis [55]. However, the exact role of Spp1 following epilepsy requires further evaluation.

Next is the adenosine A_3 receptor (Adora3/A3ar). This gene is of interest as it was the only receptor to be down-regulated within our data set. Adenosine has long been viewed as an endogenous anticonvulsive and will increase dramatically during epileptic seizures [57]. As for Adora3, it was reported that its specific agonist, IB-MECA, could protect against seizures [58]. It was found that Adora3 is highly expressed in microglia and that LPS treatment down-regulates its expression [59]. Moreover, externally induced activation of Adora3 could reduce LPS-induced tumor necrosis factor alpha (TNFα) in both RAW 264.7 macrophages and BV2 microglia [60, 61]. Yet, little else is known about how Adora3 can modulate microglial activity, let alone why we observed a significant down-regulation in expression following KA-induced seizure.

Lastly, while several purinergic receptors have been shown to modulate microglial function during epilepsy, including P2ry12 and P2rx7, we only observed significantly increased expression of P2rx4 [12]. This receptor has been observed to be important to the pathogenesis of several neurological conditions including neuropathic pain and epilepsy [62, 63]. In regards to microglia, P2rx4 expression can be up-regulated via fibronectin, which was differentially expressed in our data set [64]. Within models of neuropathic pain, it has been suggested that activation of P2rx4 induced microglia to release brain-derived neurotropic factors (BDNF), which then affected neuronal activity by modulating GABAergic activity [65, 66]. Since the hippocampus has a significant population of GABAergic interneurons, particularly in the CA1 and CA3 regions, it may be of interest to determine to what extent this crosstalk exists and whether or not blockage of this communication could alleviate seizure symptoms [67].

In conclusion, our results demonstrate that KA-induced seizure acutely affects the phenotypic character of microglia within the hippocampus. Specifically, microglia seem to be undergoing a variety of activations, which could potentially regulate neuronal hyperactivities and seizure behaviors. We have identified a number of mechanisms and gene targets that could provide future directions for therapeutic intervention.

Methods

Mice

The described In vivo procedures were approved by Institutional Animal Care and Use Committee (IACUC) in both Rutgers University and Mayo Clinic. We followed the guidelines set forth by the Guide of the Care and Use of Laboratory Animals 8th Edition. Both male and female adult heterozygous microglia GFP reporter mice at two months of age were used. The mice express GFP under control of the fractalkine receptor promoter($CX3CR1^{GFP/+}$) that selectively label microglia in the CNS [68].

KA administration

An injection of kainic acid (KA) (Tocris Biosciences, Bristol, UK) via direct intracerebroventricular (ICV) injection to induce seizure was performed as previously described [12, 15]. Briefly, a guide tube (24 gauge) was implanted into $CX3CR1^{+/GFP}$ mice prior to KA injection. After a 24 h recovery period, a 30 gauge needle was inserted through the cannula to deliver the KA solution

(0.2 μg in 5 μl). Mice were then observed for induction of seizure response using the method described previously [12]. Briefly, seizure behavior was monitored under a modified Racine scale as follows [12, 15, 69]: (1) freezing behavior; (2) rigid posture with raised tail; (3) continuous head bobbing and forepaws shaking; (4) rearing, falling, and jumping; (5) continuous level 4; and (6) loss of posture and generalized convulsion activity. Mice progressed at least to stage 3 and were sacrificed 3d after seizure. Sham controls did not receive KA administration.

Microglia isolation

All mice were perfused with ice cold PBS (pH 7.4) 3 days post KA treatment. Hippocampi were excised, minced on ice, and suspended in a trypsin/EDTA solution for 20 mins, in a 37 °C shaker. After incubation, 3 ml DMEM and 50ul DNase was added to the cell suspension. Cell pellets where then suspended in 5 ml HEPES (4-(2-hydroxyethyl)-1- piperazineethanesulfonic acid) buffer, then centrifuged again. Pellets were finally re-suspended in 800 ml HEPES buffer and transferred into a sorting tube on ice. GFP-labeled microglia were isolated via FACS on a MoFlo XDP Cell Sorter (Beckman Coulter, CA, USA). Microglia from sham controls were isolated in the same manner after a corresponding length of time.

RNAseq analysis

RNA was isolated with the RNeasy Plus Micro Kit (Qiagen, Hilden, Germany). RNA quality was evaluated by Tapestation RNA HS Assay (Agilent Technologies, CA, USA) and Bioanalyzer 2100 Eukaryote Total RNA Nano Kit (Agilent Technologies). Libraries were constructed with the SMART-Seq v4 Ultra Low Input RNA Kit (Takara-Clontech, CA, USA) using manufacturer's instructions. Final library quantity was determined by KAPA SYBR® FAST qPCR and library quality evaluated by Tapestation RNA HS Assay (Agilent Technologies, CA, USA). Equimolar pooling of libraries were performed based on qPCR values and loaded onto an Illumina Hiseq platform (Illumina, CA, USA).

Differential gene expression analysis

RNA-seq data were aligned to the mouse reference genome using STAR mapping tool [70]. Read counts were then quantified using HTSeq-count [71]. DESeq, an R Bioconductor package, was used for differential gene expression analysis [72]. It estimates variance-mean dependence in RNA-seq count data and tests for differential expression using a negative binomial distribution model. Heat map and hierarchical clustering of differentially expressed genes was performed using the heatmap function in stats package in R.

Functional classification of differentially expressed genes

Gene Ontology (GO) analysis is a commonly used approach for functional studies of RNA-seq data. To functional classify the differentially expressed genes between the control and KA treated groups, GO enrichment analysis using clusterProfiler was performed. Additionally, significant KEGG pathways were identified using the enrichKEGG function in clusterProfiler package with FDR < 0.05.

Statistics

Both KA-treated and control were collected with n = 3 mice. The R package DESeq was used on our RNA-seq counts to estimate the variance-mean dependence and to test for differential expression. Differentially expressed proteins with adjusted p-values < 0.05 using the Benjamini-Hochberg procedure. These proteins were then subjected to pathway enrichment/gene ontology analysis. A Benjamini-Hochberg adjusted p-value of < 0.05 was used to identify significantly enriched pathways.

Additional files

Additional file 1: Table S1. List of all identified differentially expressed genes. (XLSX 336 kb)

Additional file 2: Figure S1. Expression profiles of microglia specific markers. The expression of microglia specific markers, as determined by Hickman et al. [16] was investigated. The Log_2 base mean expression of each condition is presented for each gene. Presented error bars are standard error using the Log_2 standard deviation of each mean. $^{**}P_{adj} < 0.05$. **Figure S2.** Expression profiles of cytokine markers. The expression of a variety of cytokines was investigated. The Log_2 base mean expression of each condition is presented for each gene. Presented error bars are standard error using the Log_2standard deviation of each mean. $^{**}P_{adj} < 0.05$. (PDF 114 kb)

Additional file 3: Table S2. List of all identified biological process GO terms. (XLSX 44 kb)

Additional file 4: Table S3. List of all identifed molecular function GO terms. (XLSX 23 kb)

Additional file 5: Table S4. List of all identifed cellular compartment GO terms. (XLSX 24 kb)

Acknowledgements

The authors would like to thank all members of Wu lab at Mayo for the insightful discussions and Dr. Paul A. Stewart (The Moffitt Cancer Center, Tampa, FL) for the technical assistance.

Funding

This work was supported by National Institute of Health (R01NS088627, R21DE025689, K22NS104392), and National Natural Science Foundation of China (No. 31500845).

Authors' contributions

DB, JRR, WH and WLJ designed the study and wrote the manuscript; DB, JZ, JP, and LF generated mouse seizure model; JZ, ZX, JP, UBE, LF, GW performed the cell sorting experiments; KT, CY and JH performed RNAseq and data analysis; DB and WLJ analyzed the data and revised the manuscript. All authors read and approved the final manuscript.

Competing interests

The authors declare that they have no competing interests.

Author details

[1]Department of Neurology, Mayo Clinic, 200 First Street SW, Rochester, MN 55905, USA. [2]Department of Pharmacology, School of Pharmacy, Nantong University, 19 Qixiu Road, Nantong 226001, Jiangsu, China. [3]Admera Health LLC, South Plainfield, NJ 07080, USA. [4]Department of Histology and Embryology, School of Basic Medical Sciences, Anhui Medical University, Hefei 230032, Anhui, China. [5]One Harvard Street Institute of Health, Brookline, MA 02446, USA. [6]Department of Pharmaceutical Sciences and Center for Neurodegenerative Disease and Aging, Northeast Ohio Medical University, Rootstown, OH 44272, USA. [7]Department of Neuroscience and Cell Biology, Rutgers-Robert Wood Johnson Medical School, Piscataway, NJ 08854, USA. [8]Department of Neuroscience, Mayo Clinic, Jacksonville, FL 32224, USA.

References

1. Kwan P, Brodie MJ. Clinical trials of antiepileptic medications in newly diagnosed patients with epilepsy. Neurology. 2003;60(11 Suppl 4):S2–12.
2. Levesque M, Avoli M. The kainic acid model of temporal lobe epilepsy. Neurosci Biobehav Rev. 2013;37(10 Pt 2):2887–99.
3. Wilcox KS, Gee JM, Gibbons MB, Tvrdik P, White JA. Altered structure and function of astrocytes following status epilepticus. Epilepsy Behav. 2015;49:17–9.
4. Eyo UB, Murugan M, Wu LJ. Microglia-neuron communication in epilepsy. Glia. 2017;65(1):5–18.
5. Eyo UB, Wu LJ. Bi-directional microglia-neuron communication in the healthy brain. Neural Plast. 2013;2013:456857.
6. Parkhurst CN, Yang G, Ninan I, Savas JN, Yates JR 3rd, Lafaille JJ, Hempstead BL, Littman DR, Gan WB. Microglia promote learning-dependent synapse formation through brain-derived neurotrophic factor. Cell. 2013;155(7):1596–609.
7. Beach TG, Woodhurst WB, MacDonald DB, Jones MW. Reactive microglia in hippocampal sclerosis associated with human temporal lobe epilepsy. Neurosci Lett. 1995;191(1–2):27–30.
8. Wyatt-Johnson SK, Herr SA, Brewster AL. Status epilepticus triggers time-dependent alterations in microglia abundance and morphological phenotypes in the Hippocampus. Front Neurol. 2017;8:700.
9. Eyo UB, Gu N, De S, Dong H, Richardson JR, Wu LJ. Modulation of microglial process convergence toward neuronal dendrites by extracellular calcium. J Neurosci. 2015;35(6):2417–22.
10. Eyo UB, Mo M, Yi MH, Murugan M, Liu J, Yarlagadda R, Margolis DJ, Xu P, Wu LJ. P2Y12R-dependent translocation mechanisms gate the changing microglial landscape. Cell Rep. 2018;23(4):959–66.
11. Eyo UB, Peng J, Murugan M, Mo M, Lalani A, Xie P, Xu P, Margolis DJ, Wu LJ. Regulation of physical microglia-neuron interactions by Fractalkine signaling after status epilepticus. eNeuro. 2017;3(6)
12. Eyo UB, Peng J, Swiatkowski P, Mukherjee A, Bispo A, Wu LJ. Neuronal hyperactivity recruits microglial processes via neuronal NMDA receptors and microglial P2Y12 receptors after status epilepticus. J Neurosci. 2014; 34(32):10528–40.
13. Mika J. Modulation of microglia can attenuate neuropathic pain symptoms and enhance morphine effectiveness. Pharmacol Rep. 2008;60(3):297–307.
14. Bronen RA. The status of status: seizures are bad for your brain's health. AJNR Am J Neuroradiol. 2000;21(10):1782–3.
15. Tian DS, Peng J, Murugan M, Feng LJ, Liu JL, Eyo UB, Zhou LJ, Mogilevsky R, Wang W, Wu LJ. Chemokine CCL2-CCR2 signaling induces neuronal cell death via STAT3 activation and IL-1beta production after status epilepticus. J Neurosci. 2017;37(33):7878–92.
16. Hickman SE, Kingery ND, Ohsumi TK, Borowsky ML, Wang LC, Means TK, El Khoury J. The microglial sensome revealed by direct RNA sequencing. Nat Neurosci. 2013;16(12):1896–905.
17. Abiega O, Beccari S, Diaz-Aparicio I, Nadjar A, Laye S, Leyrolle Q, Gomez-Nicola D, Domercq M, Perez-Samartin A, Sanchez-Zafra V, et al. Neuronal hyperactivity disturbs ATP microgradients, impairs microglial motility, and reduces phagocytic receptor expression triggering apoptosis/microglial phagocytosis uncoupling. PLoS Biol. 2016;14(5):e1002466.
18. Trias E, Díaz-Amarilla P, Olivera-Bravo S, Isasi E, Drechsel DA, Lopez N, Bradford CS, Ireton KE, Beckman JS, Barbeito L. Phenotypic transition of microglia into astrocyte-like cells associated with disease onset in a model of inherited ALS. Front Cell Neurosci. 2013;7:274.
19. Brown A. Understanding the MIND phenotype: macrophage/microglia inflammation in neurocognitive disorders related to human immunodeficiency virus infection. Clin Translat Med. 2015;4:7.
20. Louveau A, Nerriere-Daguin V, Vanhove B, Naveilhan P, Neunlist M, Nicot A, Boudin H. Targeting the CD80/CD86 costimulatory pathway with CTLA4-Ig directs microglia toward a repair phenotype and promotes axonal outgrowth. Glia. 2015;63(12):2298–312.
21. Yu G, Wang LG, Han Y, He QY. clusterProfiler: an R package for comparing biological themes among gene clusters. Omics. 2012;16(5):284–7.
22. Supek F, Bosnjak M, Skunca N, Smuc T. REVIGO summarizes and visualizes long lists of gene ontology terms. PLoS One. 2011;6(7):e21800.
23. Schreiber G, Piehler J. The molecular basis for functional plasticity in type I interferon signaling. Trends Immunol. 2015;36(3):139–49.
24. Kawanokuchi J, Mizuno T, Kato H, Mitsuma N, Suzumura A. Effects of interferon-beta on microglial functions as inflammatory and antigen presenting cells in the central nervous system. Neuropharmacology. 2004;46(5):734–42.
25. Luckoff A, Caramoy A, Scholz R, Prinz M, Kalinke U, Langmann T. Interferon-beta signaling in retinal mononuclear phagocytes attenuates pathological neovascularization. EMBO Mol Med. 2016;8(6):670–8.
26. Montojo J, Zuberi K, Rodriguez H, Kazi F, Wright G, Donaldson SL, Morris Q, Bader GD. GeneMANIA Cytoscape plugin: fast gene function predictions on the desktop. Bioinformatics (Oxford, England). 2010;26(22):2927–8.
27. Murphy MP. How mitochondria produce reactive oxygen species. Biochem J. 2009;417(1):1–13.
28. Dan Dunn J, Alvarez LA, Zhang X, Soldati T. Reactive oxygen species and mitochondria: a nexus of cellular homeostasis. Redox Biol. 2015;6:472–85.
29. Allen M, Zou F, Chai HS, Younkin CS, Miles R, Nair AA, Crook JE, Pankratz VS, Carrasquillo MM, Rowley CN, et al. Glutathione S-transferase omega genes in Alzheimer and Parkinson disease risk, age-at-diagnosis and brain gene expression: an association study with mechanistic implications. Mol Neurodegener. 2012;7:13.
30. Couto N, Wood J, Barber J. The role of glutathione reductase and related enzymes on cellular redox homoeostasis network. Free Radic Biol Med. 2016;95:27–42.
31. Olson GE, Whitin JC, Hill KE, Winfrey VP, Motley AK, Austin LM, Deal J, Cohen HJ, Burk RF. Extracellular glutathione peroxidase (Gpx3) binds specifically to basement membranes of mouse renal cortex tubule cells. Am J Physiol Renal Physiol. 2010;298(5):F1244–53.
32. Spradling KD, Lumley LA, Robison CL, Meyerhoff JL, Dillman JF 3rd. Transcriptional analysis of rat piriform cortex following exposure to the organophosphonate anticholinesterase sarin and induction of seizures. J Neuroinflammation. 2011;8:83.
33. Maurer-Stroh S, Washietl S, Eisenhaber F. Protein prenyltransferases. Genome Biol. 2003;4(4):212.
34. Wiemer AJ, Hohl RJ, Wiemer DF. The intermediate enzymes of isoprenoid metabolism as anticancer targets. Anti Cancer Agents Med Chem. 2009;9(5): 526–42.
35. Cordle A, Landreth G. 3-Hydroxy-3-methylglutaryl-coenzyme a reductase inhibitors attenuate beta-amyloid-induced microglial inflammatory responses. J Neurosci. 2005;25(2):299–307.
36. Kuipers HF, van den Elsen PJ. Immunomodulation by statins: inhibition of cholesterol vs. isoprenoid biosynthesis. Biomed Pharmacother. 2007;61(7): 400–7.
37. Li L, Zhang W, Cheng S, Cao D, Parent M. Isoprenoids and related pharmacological interventions: potential application in Alzheimer's disease. Mol Neurobiol. 2012;46(1):64–77.
38. Wahner AD, Bronstein JM, Bordelon YM, Ritz B. Statin use and the risk of Parkinson disease. Neurology. 2008;70(16 Pt 2):1418–22.

39. Roy A, Pahan K. Prospects of statins in Parkinson disease. Neuroscientist. 2011;17(3):244–55.
40. Lee JK, Won JS, Singh AK, Singh I. Statin inhibits kainic acid-induced seizure and associated inflammation and hippocampal cell death. Neurosci Lett. 2008;440(3):260–4.
41. Lo WF, Woods AS, DeCloux A, Cotter RJ, Metcalf ES, Soloski MJ. Molecular mimicry mediated by MHC class Ib molecules after infection with gram-negative pathogens. Nat Med. 2000;6(2):215–8.
42. Cai W, Cao W, Wu L, Exley GE, Waneck GL, Karger BL, Warner CM. Sequence and transcription of Qa-2-encoding genes in mouse lymphocytes and blastocysts. Immunogenetics. 1996;45(2):97–107.
43. Chiang EY, Henson M, Stroynowski I. The nonclassical major histocompatibility complex molecule Qa-2 protects tumor cells from NK cell- and lymphokine-activated killer cell-mediated cytolysis. J Immunol. 2002;168(5):2200–11.
44. Gays F, Fraser KP, Toomey JA, Diamond AG, Millrain MM, Dyson PJ, Brooks CG. Functional analysis of the molecular factors controlling Qa1-mediated protection of target cells from NK lysis. J Immunol. 2001;166(3):1601–10.
45. Morandi F, Venturi C, Rizzo R, Castellazzi M, Baldi E, Caniatti ML, Tola MR, Granieri E, Fainardi E, Uccelli A, et al. Intrathecal soluble HLA-E correlates with disease activity in patients with multiple sclerosis and may cooperate with soluble HLA-G in the resolution of neuroinflammation. J Neuroimmune Pharmacol. 2013;8(4):944–55.
46. Limmroth V, Putzki N, Kachuck NJ. The interferon beta therapies for treatment of relapsing-remitting multiple sclerosis: are they equally efficacious? A comparative review of open-label studies evaluating the efficacy, safety, or dosing of different interferon beta formulations alone or in combination. Ther Adv Neurol Disord. 2011;4(5):281–96.
47. Baruch K, Deczkowska A, David E, Castellano JM, Miller O, Kertser A, Berkutzki T, Barnett-Itzhaki Z, Bezalel D, Wyss-Coray T, et al. Aging. Aging-induced type I interferon response at the choroid plexus negatively affects brain function. Science (New York, NY). 2014;346(6205):89–93.
48. Honda K, Yanai H, Negishi H, Asagiri M, Sato M, Mizutani T, Shimada N, Ohba Y, Takaoka A, Yoshida N, et al. IRF-7 is the master regulator of type-I interferon-dependent immune responses. Nature. 2005;434(7034):772–7.
49. Huye LE, Ning S, Kelliher M, Pagano JS. Interferon regulatory factor 7 is activated by a viral oncoprotein through RIP-dependent ubiquitination. Mol Cell Biol. 2007;27(8):2910–8.
50. Ning S, Campos AD, Darnay BG, Bentz GL, Pagano JS. TRAF6 and the three C-terminal lysine sites on IRF7 are required for its ubiquitination-mediated activation by the tumor necrosis factor receptor family member latent membrane protein 1. Mol Cell Biol. 2008;28(20):6536–46.
51. Gliem M, Krammes K, Liaw L, van Rooijen N, Hartung HP, Jander S. Macrophage-derived osteopontin induces reactive astrocyte polarization and promotes re-establishment of the blood brain barrier after ischemic stroke. Glia. 2015;63(12):2198–207.
52. Chiu IM, Morimoto ETA, Goodarzi H, Liao JT, O'Keeffe S, Phatnani HP, Muratet M, Carroll MC, Levy S, Tavazoie S, et al. A neurodegeneration-specific gene expression signature and immune profile of acutely isolated microglia from an ALS mouse model. Cell Rep. 2013;4(2):385–401.
53. Hunsberger JG, Bennett AH, Selvanayagam E, Duman RS, Newton SS. Gene profiling the response to kainic acid induced seizures. Brain Res Mol Brain Res. 2005;141(1):95–112.
54. Gorter JA, van Vliet EA, Aronica E, Breit T, Rauwerda H, Lopes da Silva FH, Wadman WJ. Potential new antiepileptogenic targets indicated by microarray analysis in a rat model for temporal lobe epilepsy. J Neurosci. 2006; 26(43):11083–110.
55. Kim SY, Choi YS, Choi JS, Cha JH, Kim ON, Lee SB, Chung JW, Chun MH, Lee MY. Osteopontin in kainic acid-induced microglial reactions in the rat brain. Mol Cells. 2002;13(3):429–35.
56. Borges K, Gearing M, Rittling S, Sorensen ES, Kotloski R, Denhardt DT, Dingledine R. Characterization of osteopontin expression and function after status epilepticus. Epilepsia. 2008;49(10):1675–85.
57. Pedata F, Pugliese A, Sebastião A, Ribeiro J: Adenosine A3 receptor signaling in the central nervous system; 2010.
58. Von Lubitz DK, Carter MF, Deutsch SI, Lin RC, Mastropaolo J, Meshulam Y, Jacobson KA. The effects of adenosine A3 receptor stimulation on seizures in mice. Eur J Pharmacol. 1995;275(1):23–9.
59. Bennett ML, Bennett FC, Liddelow SA, Ajami B, Zamanian JL, Fernhoff NB, Mulinyawe SB, Bohlen CJ, Adil A, Tucker A, et al. New tools for studying microglia in the mouse and human CNS. Proc Natl Acad Sci U S A. 2016; 113(12):E1738–46.
60. Martin L, Pingle SC, Hallam DM, Rybak LP, Ramkumar V. Activation of the adenosine A3 receptor in RAW 264.7 cells inhibits lipopolysaccharide-stimulated tumor necrosis factor-alpha release by reducing calcium-dependent activation of nuclear factor-kappaB and extracellular signal-regulated kinase 1/2. J Pharmacol Exp Ther. 2006;316(1):71–8.
61. Lee JY, Jhun BS, Oh YT, Lee JH, Choe W, Baik HH, Ha J, Yoon KS, Kim SS, Kang I. Activation of adenosine A3 receptor suppresses lipopolysaccharide-induced TNF-alpha production through inhibition of PI 3-kinase/Akt and NF-kappaB activation in murine BV2 microglial cells. Neurosci Lett. 2006; 396(1):1–6.
62. Ulmann L, Levavasseur F, Avignone E, Peyroutou R, Hirbec H, Audinat E, Rassendren F. Involvement of P2X4 receptors in hippocampal microglial activation after status epilepticus. Glia. 2013;61(8):1306–19.
63. Ulmann L, Hatcher JP, Hughes JP, Chaumont S, Green PJ, Conquet F, Buell GN, Reeve AJ, Chessell IP, Rassendren F. Up-regulation of P2X4 receptors in spinal microglia after peripheral nerve injury mediates BDNF release and neuropathic pain. J Neurosci. 2008;28(44):11263–8.
64. Tsuda M, Toyomitsu E, Komatsu T, Masuda T, Kunifusa E, Nasu-Tada K, Koizumi S, Yamamoto K, Ando J, Inoue K. Fibronectin/integrin system is involved in P2X(4) receptor upregulation in the spinal cord and neuropathic pain after nerve injury. Glia. 2008;56(5):579–85.
65. Trang T, Beggs S, Wan X, Salter MW. P2X4-receptor-mediated synthesis and release of brain-derived neurotrophic factor in microglia is dependent on calcium and p38-mitogen-activated protein kinase activation. J Neurosci. 2009;29(11):3518–28.
66. Malcangio M. GABAB receptors and pain. Neuropharmacology. 2017. https://www.sciencedirect.com/science/article/pii/S0028390817302186?via%3Dihub.
67. Pelkey KA, Chittajallu R, Craig MT, Tricoire L, Wester JC, McBain CJ. Hippocampal GABAergic inhibitory interneurons. Physiol Rev. 2017;97(4):1619–747.
68. Jung S, Aliberti J, Graemmel P, Sunshine MJ, Kreutzberg GW, Sher A, Littman DR. Analysis of fractalkine receptor CX(3)CR1 function by targeted deletion and green fluorescent protein reporter gene insertion. Mol Cell Biol. 2000; 20(11):4106–14.
69. Racine RJ. Modification of seizure activity by electrical stimulation. II. Motor seizure. Electroencephalogr Clin Neurophysiol. 1972;32(3):281–94.
70. Dobin A, Davis CA, Schlesinger F, Drenkow J, Zaleski C, Jha S, Batut P, Chaisson M, Gingeras TR. STAR: ultrafast universal RNA-seq aligner. B ioinformatics (Oxford England). 2013;29(1):15–21.
71. Anders S, Pyl PT, Huber W. HTSeq–a Python framework to work with high-throughput sequencing data. Bioinformatics (Oxford England). 2015;31(2): 166–9.
72. Anders S, Huber W. Differential expression analysis for sequence count data. Genome Biol. 2010;11(10):R106.

8

TLR4-mediated autophagic impairment contributes to neuropathic pain in chronic constriction injury mice

Yibo Piao[1†], Do Hyeong Gwon[2†], Dong-Wook Kang[2†], Tae Woong Hwang[2], Nara Shin[1,2], Hyeok Hee Kwon[1,2], Hyo Jung Shin[2], Yuhua Yin[1,2], Jwa-Jin Kim[2,3], Jinpyo Hong[2], Hyun-Woo Kim[2], Yonghyun Kim[4], Sang Ryong Kim[5], Sang-Ha Oh[1,2*] and Dong Woon Kim[2*]

Abstract

Neuropathic pain is a complex, chronic pain state characterized by hyperalgesia, allodynia, and spontaneous pain. Accumulating evidence has indicated that the microglial Toll-like receptor 4 (TLR4) and autophagy are implicated in neurodegenerative diseases, but their relationship and role in neuropathic pain remain unclear. In this study, we examined TLR4 and its association with autophagic activity using a chronic constriction injury (CCI)-induced neuropathic pain model in wild-type (WT) and TLR4-knockout (KO) mice. The mice were assigned into four groups: WT-Contralateral (Contra), WT-Ipsilateral (Ipsi), TLR4 KO-Contra, and TLR4 KO-Ipsi. Behavioral and mechanical allodynia tests and biochemical analysis of spinal cord tissue were conducted following CCI to the sciatic nerve. Compared with the Contra group, mechanical allodynia in both the WT- and TLR4 KO-Ipsi groups was significantly increased, and a marked decrease of allodynia was observed in the TLR4 KO-Ipsi group. Although glial cells were upregulated in the WT-Ipsi group, no significant change was observed in the TLR4 KO groups. Moreover, protein expression and immunoreactive cell regulation of autophagy (Beclin 1, p62) were significantly increased in the neurons, but not microglia, of WT-Ipsi group compared with the WT-Contra group. The level of PINK1, a marker for mitophagy was increased in the neurons of WT, but not in TLR4 KO mice. Together, these results show that TLR4-mediated p62 autophagic impairment plays an important role in the occurrence and development of neuropathic pain. And what is more, microglial TLR4-mediated microglial activation might be indirectly coupled to neuronal autophage.

Keywords: TLR4, Autophagy, Glia, Neuropathic pain, CCI

Introduction

Neuropathic pain is a complex, chronic pain state characterized by hyperalgesia, allodynia, and spontaneous pain [1]. It is caused by a lesion or dysfunction of the peripheral or central nervous system (PNS and CNS, respectively) [2]. Although it is undisputed that neurons play a fundamental role in neuropathic pain, the management of the suppression of aberrant neuronal activity has limited effectiveness and/or undesirable side effects [3]. Thus, despite progress in the development of pharmacological agents, various therapeutic agents capable of blocking abnormal pain sensation without impairing normal abilities need to be proposed.

Recently, investigations that focus on the role of the PNS immune responses after nerve injuries have highlighted the active participation of glial cells in the maintenance of chronic pain in different pathological conditions. In particular, it has been confirmed that peripheral nerve injury can induce microglia and astrocyte activation in several chronic neuropathic pain models [4, 5]. Activated microglia release various algesic substances that enhance pain transmission by neurons; particularly, proinflammatory cytokines were shown to be common mediators of allodynia and hyperalgesia [6].

* Correspondence: djplastic@cnu.ac.kr; visnu528@cnu.ac.kr
†Equal contributors
[1]Department of Plastic and Reconstructive Surgery, Department of Pediatrics, Department of Anesthesiology and Pain Medicine, Chungnam National University Hospital, Daejeon 35015, Republic of Korea
[2]Department of Medical Science, Department of Physiology, Department of Anatomy, Brain Research Institute, Chungnam National University School of Medicine, Daejeon 35015, Republic of Korea
Full list of author information is available at the end of the article

Among these glial activation signals, Toll-like receptors (TLRs), particularly Toll-like receptor 4 (TLR4), have been demonstrated as initiators and mediators of neuropathic pain, [7].

TLR4 is an important pattern recognition receptor that has recently been implicated in chronic neuropathic pain [8, 9]. It recognizes pathogen-associated molecular patterns (PAMPs) and damage-associated molecular patterns (DAMPs) and regulates the innate or adaptive immune response. TLR4 has been shown to be highly expressed by microglia in the CNS of rodents [10]. Genetically altered mice with TLR4 deficiency have demonstrated significantly reduced microglia activation and pain hypersensitivity following nerve injury [7].

Autophagy is a highly regulated process involved in the turnover of long-lived proteins and damaged organelles. It involves the sequestration of regions of the cytosol within double-membrane-bound compartments and delivery of the contents to the lysosome for degradation [11]. Pain is a common feature of various neurodegenerative diseases, in which autophagy plays a critical role in the progression of the pathology and is being studied as a possible therapeutic target [12, 13]. A recent study demonstrated that autophagy is modulated differently in the spinal cord of mice in several neuropathic pain models [14]. As the most thoroughly characterized type of pattern recognition receptor, TLR4 enhances the elimination of phagocytosed mycobacteria to activate autophagy and serves as an environmental sensor for autophagy. The stimulation of TLR4 with lipopolysaccharide (LPS) induces autophagosome formation in macrophages by the TIR-domain-containing adapter-inducing interferon β (TRIF)-p38 axis and its downstream signaling pathways [15]. These results indicate that TLR4 and autophagy play a pivotal role in chronic neuropathic pain, but the mechanism remains poorly understood. Thus, in the present study, we investigated the spinal modulation of the main autophagic markers in chronic constriction injury (CCI)-induced neuropathic pain models established with wild-type and TLR4-knockout (KO) mice.

Results

Spinal nerve injury following CCI surgery induces mechanical allodynia in mice

Mechanical allodynia is a typical representation of neuropathic pain. CCI of different intensities causes an increase in mechanical allodynia [16]. To determine mechanical allodynia following CCI, we measured the hind paw PWF of mice after CCI of the sciatic nerve. In the WT group, CCI-induced mechanical allodynia caused a significant increase in PWF on the ipsilateral side compared with the contralateral side from day 1 post-surgery and was maintained for up to 7 days. A similar development of PWF on the ipsilateral side was also found in the TLR4 KO group but was significantly decreased compared with the WT group (but not on the contralateral side) in the days after surgery (Fig. 1).

Different nociceptive effects between WT and TLR4 KO mice on CCI-induced CatWalk analysis

CatWalk gait analysis has been used to assess gait variation and is recommended as an objective method to evaluate sensory neuropathy induced by CCI surgery [16, 17]. In the present study, we measured two parameters that were altered significantly in the ipsilateral hind paw of CCI mice: the print area was measured by calculating the surface area of the complete print of the hind paw, and the single stance was measured using the duration of the single hind paw touching the glass plate. The percentage of the print area and single stance (% ipsilateral/contralateral) was almost 100% before CCI

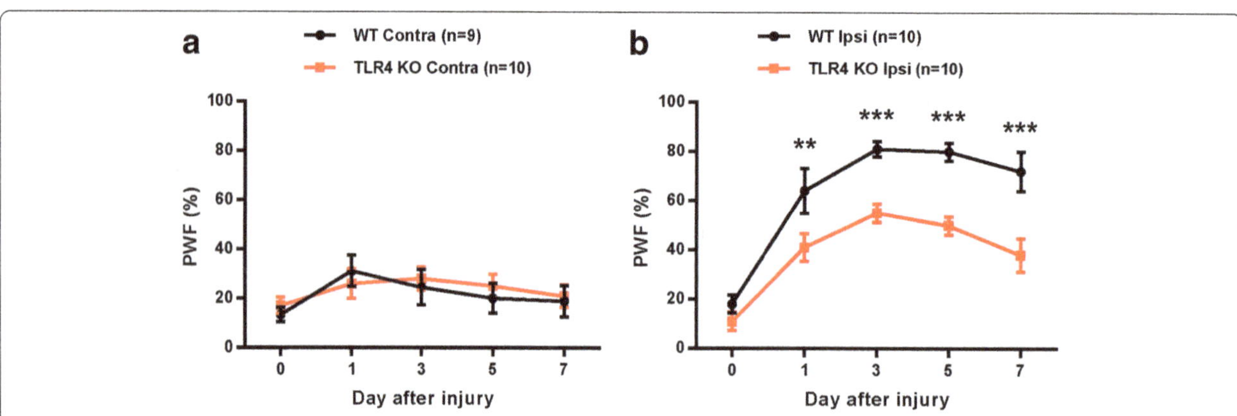

Fig. 1 Chronic constriction injury (CCI) induces mechanical allodynia in wild-type (WT) and Toll-like receptor 4 (TLR4) knockout (KO) mice. (**a**, **b**) The paw withdrawal frequency (% PWF) was measured on days 0 (baseline), 1, 3, 5, and 7 after surgery. Mechanical allodynia was separately compared in each group of contralateral (Contra) and ipsilateral (Ipsi) in CCI mice. Two-way analysis of variance (ANOVA); all the data are shown as mean ± standard error of the mean (SEM), where $*P < 0.05$, $**P < 0.01$, $***P < 0.001$, and $n = 10$ compared with the WT Ipsi group

surgery in either WT or TLR4 KO mice. However, in the WT group, the percentage was decreased almost to 0% on day 3 after CCI surgery and increased to 20% on subsequent days (Fig. 2a and c). The decreased percentage in the TLR4 KO mouse groups was observed, but reduced 50% on day 3 after surgery (Fig. 2a and c). The typical graph demonstrated that the print area and single stance disappeared in CCI mice because the mice did not step on the glass plate (Fig. 2b and d).

Activation of microglia in the spinal dorsal horn following CCI

Recent studies have indicated a critical role of spinal cord microglia in the genesis of neuropathic pain [16, 18, 19]. To demonstrate the induction of neuropathic pain in our CCI model, microglia activation in the spinal cord was examined by immunohistochemical analysis with the microglia marker Iba1. CCI induced the upregulation of Iba1 in the ipsilateral spinal cord of WT mice, especially in the lamina 1–2 of the dorsal horn; however, in the contralateral spinal cord, few Iba1-immunoreactive (IR) cells could be detected (Fig. 3a). Compared with the WT mice, there was no significant increase in IR cells in the ipsilateral spinal cord compared with the contralateral spinal cord in TLR4 KO mice (Fig. 3b).

Activation of astrocytes in the spinal dorsal horn following CCI

Astrocyte and microglia have different effects on neuronal activity; however, they share some common functions and are both activated in neuropathic pain [20, 21]. Therefore, we measured astrocyte activation in the same way as microglia. Similar to microglia, the upregulation of astrocytes was significantly increased in the superficial lumbar dorsal horn of the ipsilateral spinal cord compared with the contralateral spinal cord in WT mice, while no significant difference was found in TLR4 KO mice (Fig. 4).

LC3 levels in the spinal dorsal horn following CCI

Microtubule-associated protein 1 light chain 3 (LC3) was the first mammalian protein demonstrated to be specifically associated with autophagosomal membranes [22]. It has two forms—non-lipidated and lipidated—known as LC3-I and LC3-II, respectively. LC3-II plays an essential role during the expansion step of autophagosome formation and is regarded as the most representative marker of macroautophagy [23]. The expression of LC3 was examined by immunohistochemical analysis in the spinal dorsal horn 7 days after CCI. CCI induced no significant upregulation of LC3 between the ipsilateral and contralateral

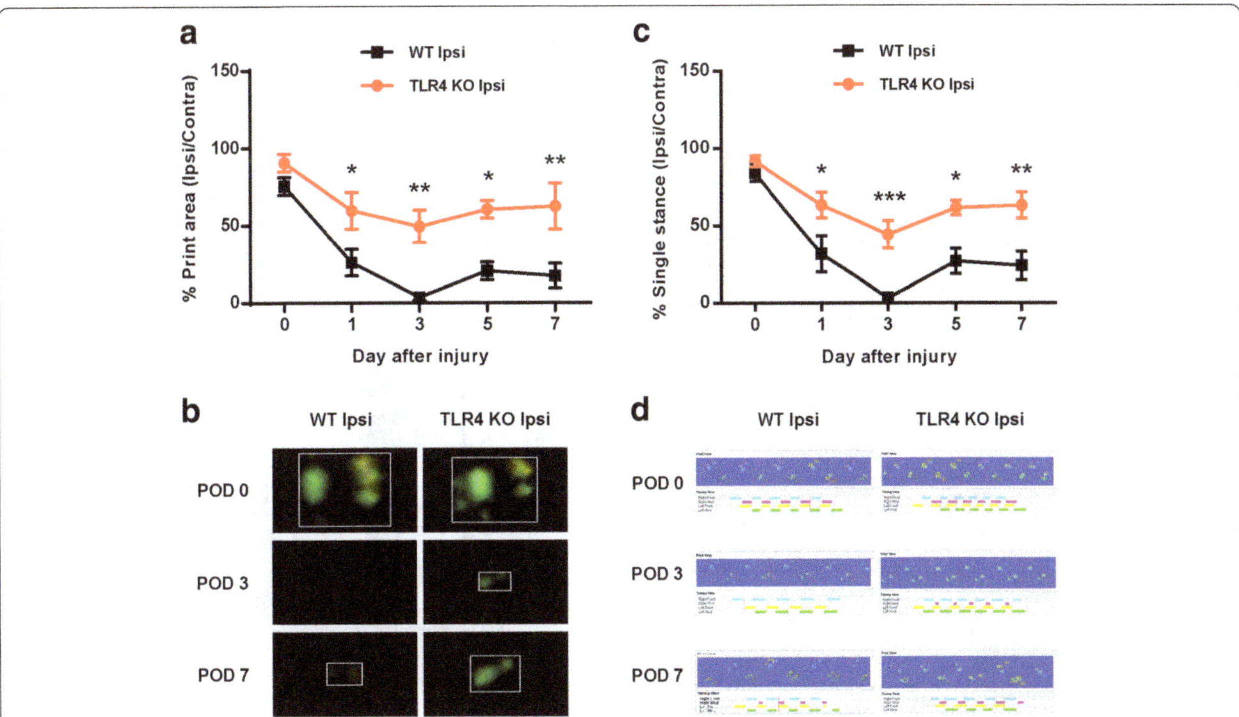

Fig. 2 Walking track analysis in CCI mice. **a** Percentage of the Ipsi paw print area (% ipsilateral/total area) assessed in the CatWalk analysis. The paw print area (%) was increased in TLR4 KO mice. **b** Combined paw print image. **c** Percentage of the Ipsi paw single stance (% Ipsi/Contra single stance). **d** Representative digitized paw prints and associated step cycles. Two-way ANOVA; all the data are shown as mean ± SEM, where $*P < 0.05$, $**P < 0.01$, and n = 10 compared with the WT Ipsi group

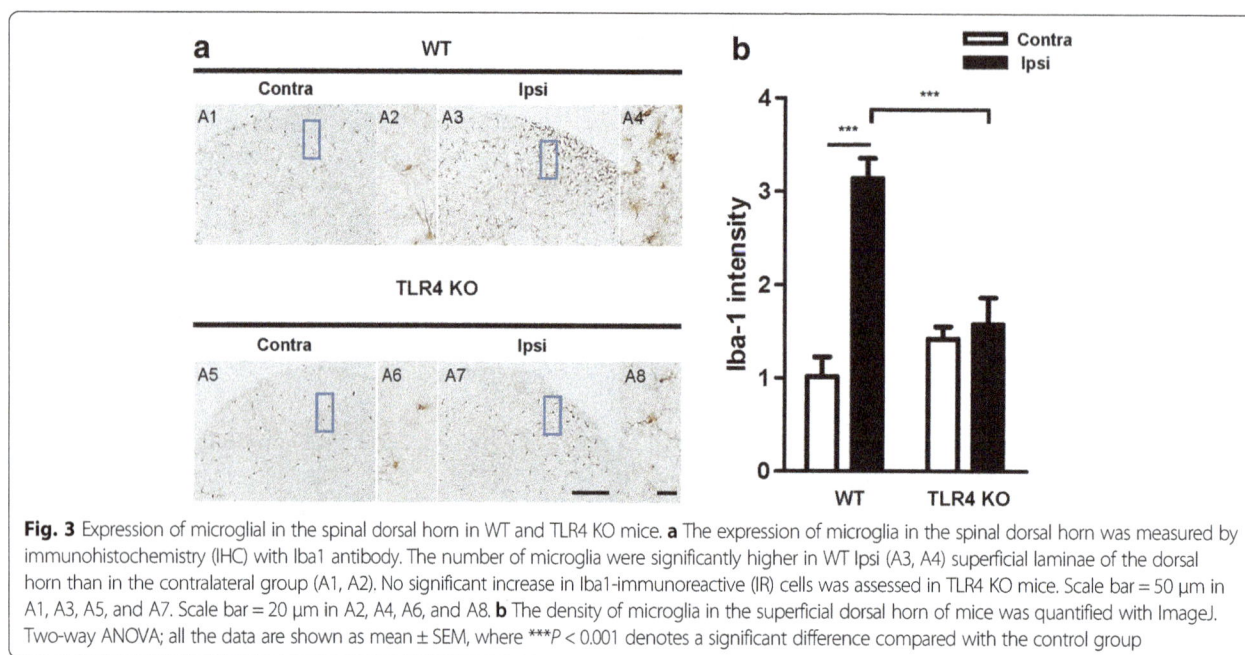

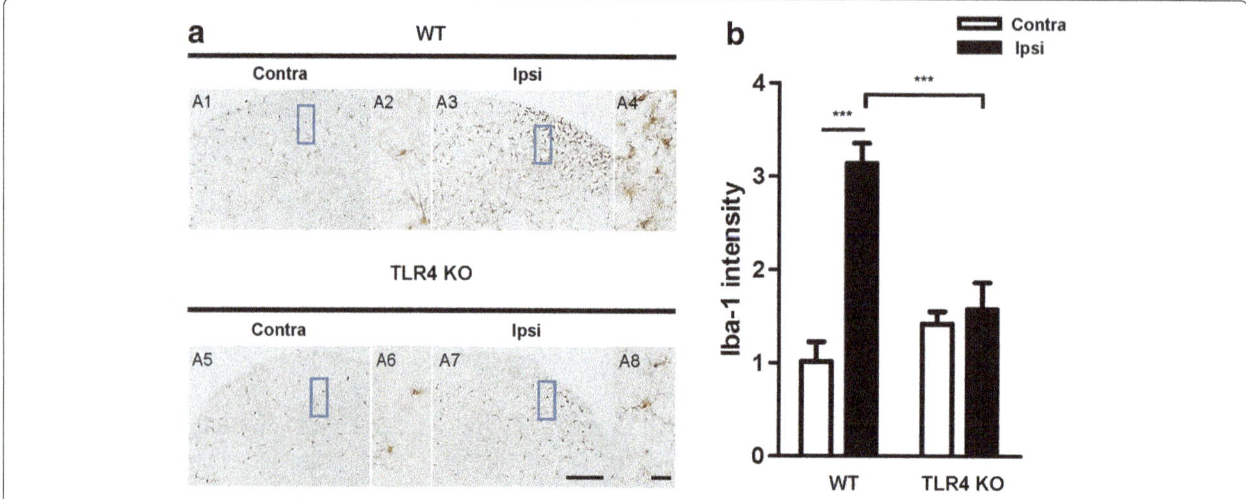

Fig. 3 Expression of microglial in the spinal dorsal horn in WT and TLR4 KO mice. **a** The expression of microglia in the spinal dorsal horn was measured by immunohistochemistry (IHC) with Iba1 antibody. The number of microglia were significantly higher in WT Ipsi (A3, A4) superficial laminae of the dorsal horn than in the contralateral group (A1, A2). No significant increase in Iba1-immunoreactive (IR) cells was assessed in TLR4 KO mice. Scale bar = 50 μm in A1, A3, A5, and A7. Scale bar = 20 μm in A2, A4, A6, and A8. **b** The density of microglia in the superficial dorsal horn of mice was quantified with ImageJ. Two-way ANOVA; all the data are shown as mean ± SEM, where $^{***}P < 0.001$ denotes a significant difference compared with the control group

spinal dorsal horn in either WT or TLR4 KO mice (Fig. 5a and b). Similarly, Western blot analysis exhibited no statistically significant variation in LC3-II expression between the ipsilateral and contralateral sides of the dorsal horn in both WT and TLR4 KO mice (Fig. 5c). Double immunofluorescence staining to detect the cellular localization of LC3 showed LC3 was expression in neuronal cells, not astrocyte and microglia in spinal dorsal horn (Fig. 5d).

Beclin 1 levels in the spinal dorsal horn following CCI

Activation of autophagy does not only depend on LC3 but also on a series of related proteins coordinated in various steps from initiation to degradation. Beclin 1 is one of the protein markers of autophagy that plays an essential role in the induction and formation of autophagosomes [24]. Thus, we measured the expression of Beclin 1 in the spinal cord of mice by immunohistochemical and Western blot analyses. CCI induced the

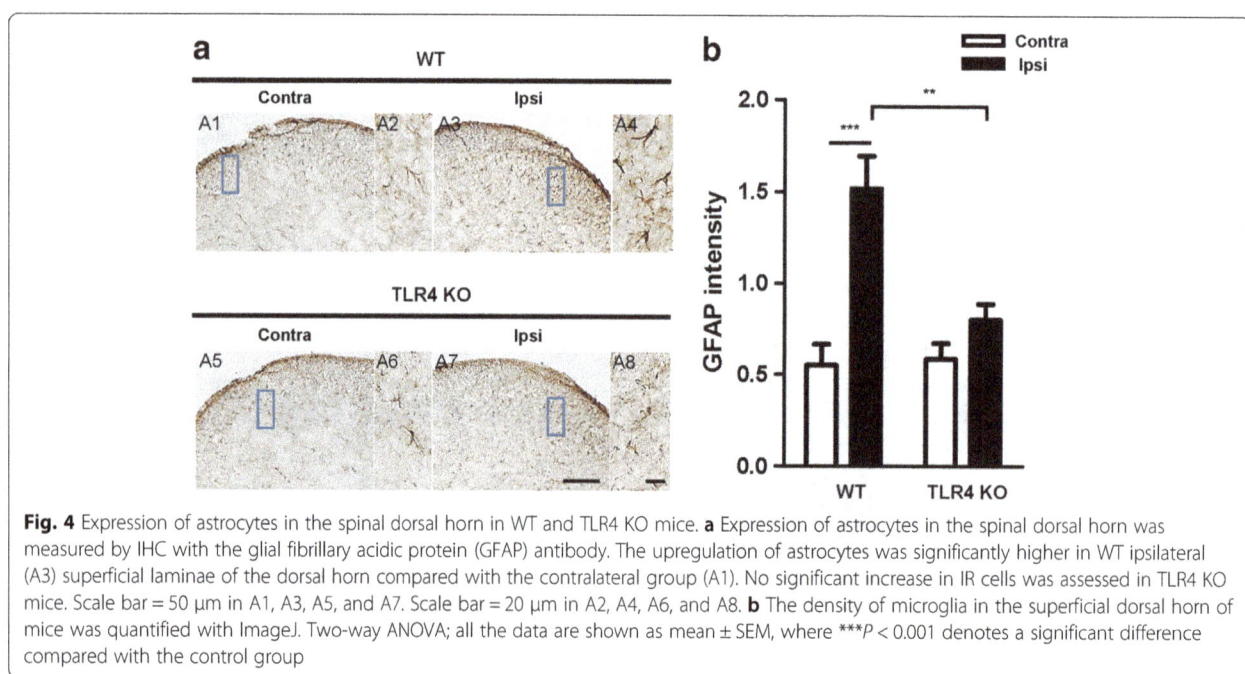

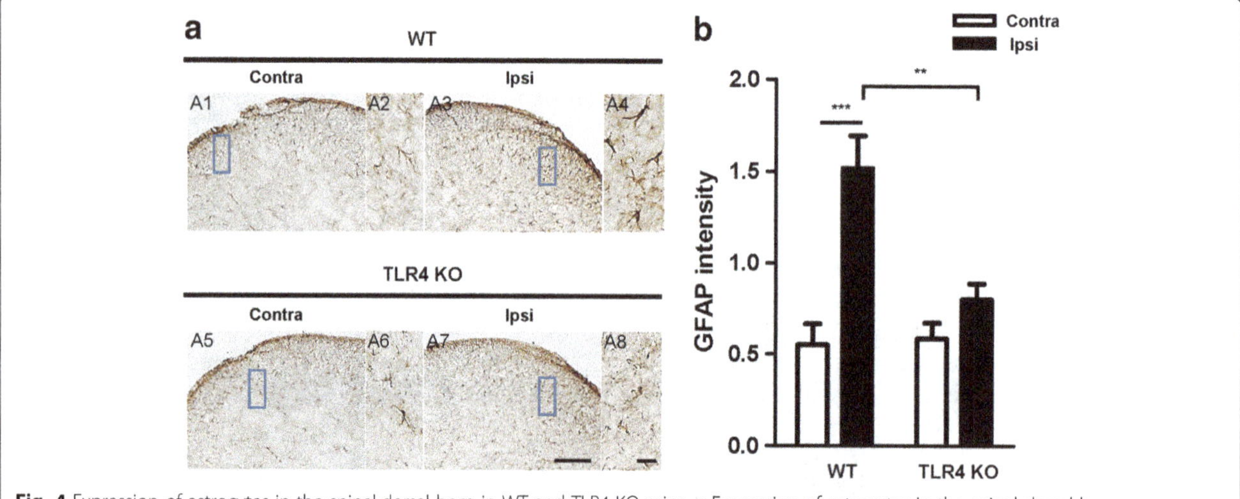

Fig. 4 Expression of astrocytes in the spinal dorsal horn in WT and TLR4 KO mice. **a** Expression of astrocytes in the spinal dorsal horn was measured by IHC with the glial fibrillary acidic protein (GFAP) antibody. The upregulation of astrocytes was significantly higher in WT ipsilateral (A3) superficial laminae of the dorsal horn compared with the contralateral group (A1). No significant increase in IR cells was assessed in TLR4 KO mice. Scale bar = 50 μm in A1, A3, A5, and A7. Scale bar = 20 μm in A2, A4, A6, and A8. **b** The density of microglia in the superficial dorsal horn of mice was quantified with ImageJ. Two-way ANOVA; all the data are shown as mean ± SEM, where $^{***}P < 0.001$ denotes a significant difference compared with the control group

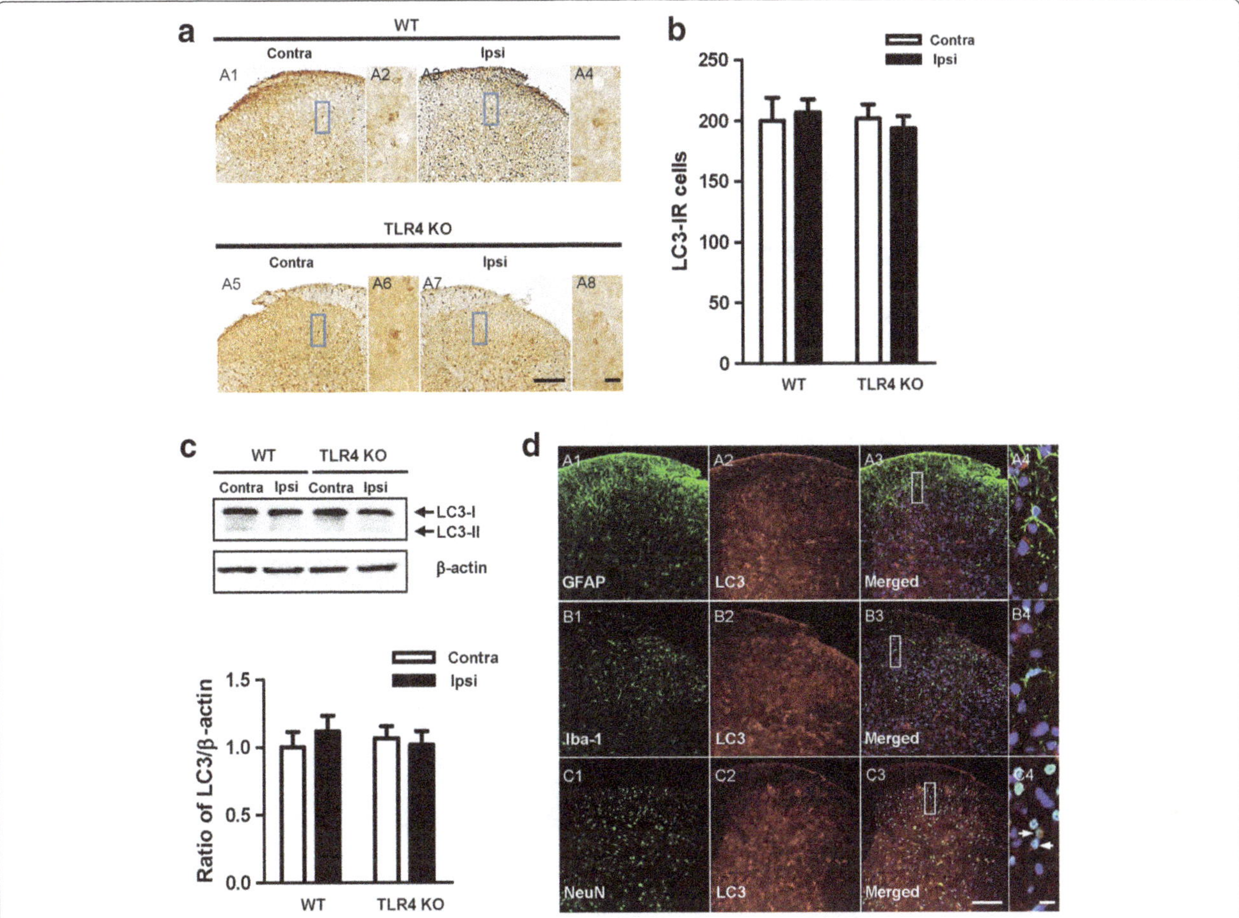

Fig. 5 Regulation of the autophagic marker microtubule-associated protein 1 light chain 3 (LC3) in WT and TLR4 KO mice. **a** LC3 immunoreactivity can be observed in the spinal dorsal horn of CCI mice. Compared with the contralateral side, no significant increase was shown in the ipsilateral side. Scale bar = 50 μm in A1, A3, A5, and A7. Scale bar = 20 μm in A2, A4, A6, and A8. **b** The number of LC3 IR cells showed no difference in WT and TLR4 KO mice in the superficial dorsal horn. **c** The protein levels of LC3-I and LC3-II were detected with immunoblotting. Levels of β-actin were used as the loading control. Western blot analysis revealed that the levels of LC3 showed no difference in CCI mice. The band densities were analyzed with ImageJ and are expressed as a percentage of the control. The bars indicate mean ± SEM. **d** Frozen sections (WT-CCI, POD7) were stained with LC3 and co-stained with anti-GFAP (A1–4), anti-iba-1 (B1–4), and anti-NeuN antibodies (C1–4). A4, B4 and C4 is rectangular magnification of merged A3, B3 and C3, respectively. Scale bar = 50 μm in A, B, C1–3. Scale bar = 20 μm in A, B, C4

upregulation of Beclin 1 in the ipsilateral spinal dorsal horn in WT mice, particularly in the lamina 1–2 of the dorsal horn. Beclin 1-immunoreactive cells were increased significantly in the ipsilateral compared with the contralateral spinal dorsal horn. There was no upregulation of Beclin 1 in the spinal dorsal horn of TLR4 KO mice, and there were no significant differences between the ipsilateral and contralateral dorsal horn (Fig. 6a and b). Western blot analysis indicated a significant increase in Beclin 1 expression in the ipsilateral compared with the contralateral spinal cord in WT mice. In contrast, no significant difference in Beclin 1 expression was observed in TLR4 KO mice (Fig. 6c). Double immunofluorescence staining to detect the cellular localization of Beclin 1 showed that Beclin 1 was expressed in neuronal cells, not astrocyte in spinal dorsal horn (Fig. 6d).

p62 levels in the spinal dorsal horn following CCI

As one of the well-known autophagy substrates, p62/SQSTM1 is widely used to monitor autophagic flux [25]. p62 binds to LC3 directly in autophagosomes and is degraded in functional autolysosomes [26, 27]. Therefore, p62 serves as a target marker to analyze autophagic degradation. Here, we evaluated p62 expression by immunohistochemical and Western blot analyses in the spinal dorsal horn of mice. In WT mice, p62 was upregulated significantly in the ipsilateral side of the spinal dorsal horn compared with the contralateral side, but no significant change was observed in TLR4 KO mice (Fig. 7a and b). Western blot analysis exhibited the same pattern as the immunohistochemical analysis (Fig. 7c). Double immunofluorescence staining also showed that p62 was expression in neuronal cells, not astrocyte in spinal dorsal horn (Fig. 7d).

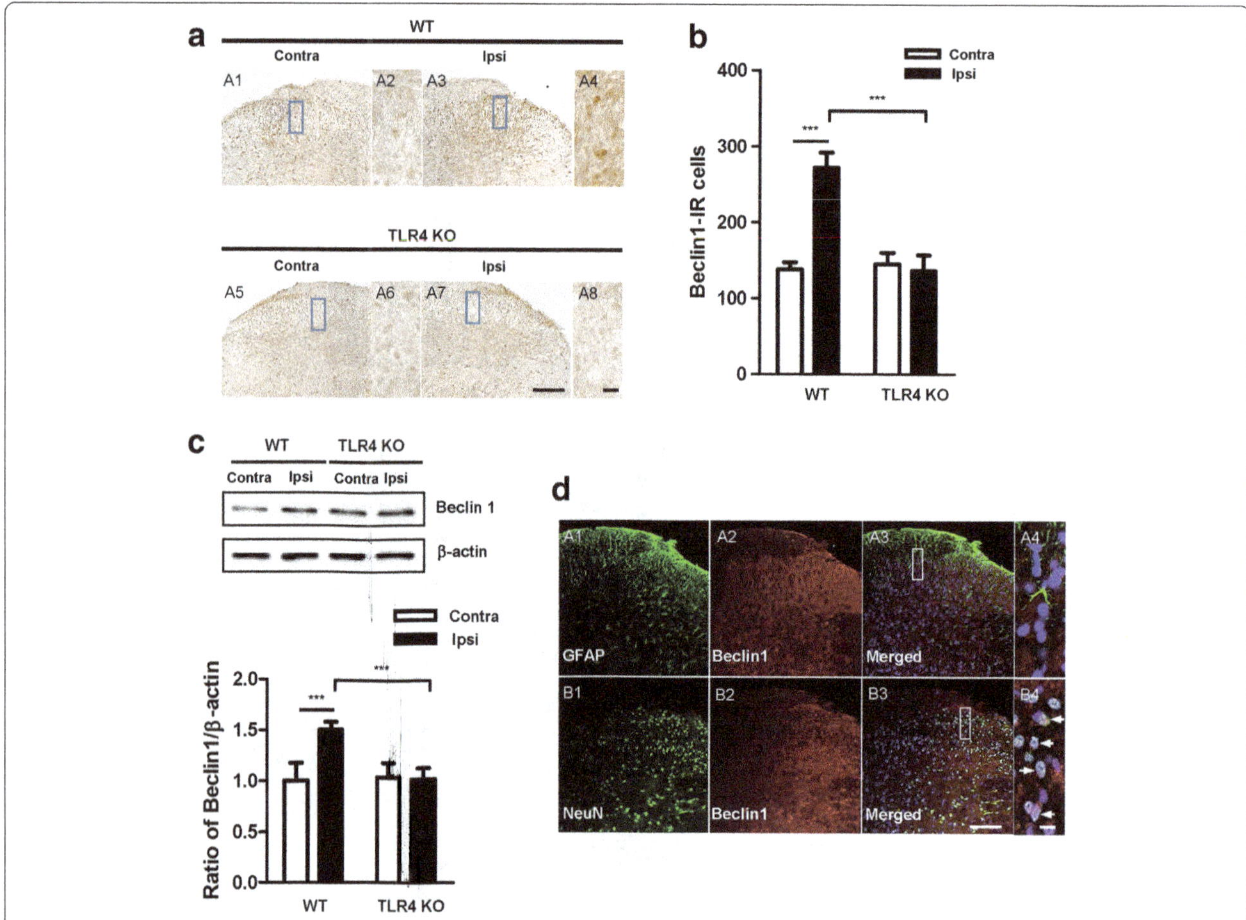

Fig. 6 CCI induces a change in Beclin1 modulation in WT and TLR4 mice. **a** Beclin1 immunoreactivity was observed in the spinal dorsal horn of CCI mice. Compared with the contralateral side, a significant increase was shown in the ipsilateral side of WT mice, and no significant difference was found in TLR4 KO mice. Scale bar = 50 μm in A1, A3, A5, and A7. Scale bar = 20 μm in A2, A4, A6, and A8. **b** The number of Beclin 1 IR cells was significantly increased in the ipsilateral side compared with the contralateral side of WT mice. **c** The protein levels of Beclin1 were detected with immunoblotting. Western blot analysis indicated an increase in the levels of Beclin1 in the ipsilateral side compared with the contralateral side of WT mice. The band densities were analyzed with Image J and expressed as a percentage of the control. Two-way ANOVA; all the data are shown as mean ± SEM, where $*P < 0.05$ denotes a significant difference compared with the control group. **d** Frozen sections (WT-CCI, POD7) were stained with Beclin1 and co-stained with anti-GFAP (A1–4) anti-NeuN antibodies (B1–4). A4 and B4 is rectangular magnification of merged A3 and B3, respectively. Scale bar = 50 μm in A, B1–3. Scale bar = 20 μm in A, B4

Expression of PINK1 in the spinal dorsal horn following CCI

Mitophagy, the selective degradation of mitochondria by autophagy, often occurs in defective mitochondria following damage or stress [28]. PINK1 is a neuroprotective protein that has been implicated in the activation of mitophagy by selectively accumulating in depolarized mitochondria and promoting PARK2/Parkin translocation [29]. The expression of PINK1 was examined in the spinal cord by immunohistochemical and Western blot analyses. The immunoreactive cells and protein expression of PINK1 were both significantly increased in the ipsilateral side of the spinal dorsal horn and contralateral side in the WT mice, but no significant differences were observed in either side of the spinal dorsal horn of TLR4 KO mice (Fig. 8a, b). Western blot analysis exhibited the same pattern as the immunohistochemical analysis (Fig. 8c). Double immunofluorescence staining to detect the cellular localization of PINK1 showed that PINK1 was expressed in neuronal cells, not astrocyte or microglia in spinal dorsal horn (Fig. 8d).

Inhibition of autophagy reduced pain behavior

To investigate the role of autophagic flux impairment in the development of neuropathic pain, the autophagic inhibitor, Chlorquine was injected subcutaneously (15 mg/kg/day). After 30 min, the paw withdrawal frequency was measured on days 0 (baseline), 1, 3, 5, and 7 after surgery. Compared with WT ipsi group, Chlorquine treatment significantly reduced the mechanical allodynia at 5 and 7 days in TLR4 KO CQ ipsi group similar with TLR4 KO ipsi group (Fig. 9).

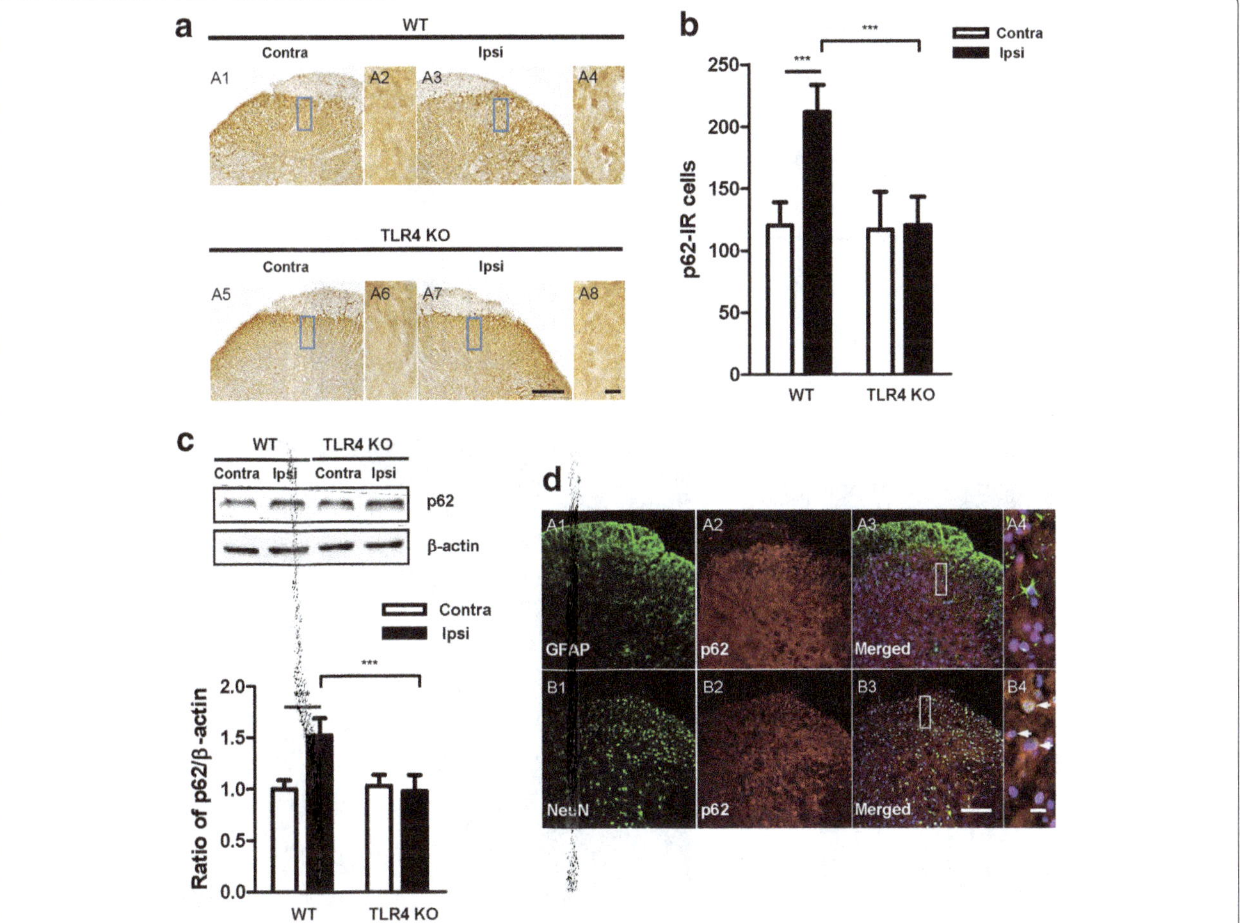

Fig. 7 Activation of p62 in WT and TLR4 mice. **a** p62 immunoreactivity was observed in the spinal dorsal horn of CCI mice. Compared with the contralateral side, a significant increase in p62 IR cells was shown in the ipsilateral side of WT mice, and no significant difference was found in TLR4 KO mice. Scale bar = 50 μm in A1, A3, A5, and A7. Scale bar = 20 μm in A2, A4, A6, and A8. **b** The number of p62 IR cells was significantly increased in the ipsilateral side compared with the contralateral of WT mice. **c** Western blotting was performed to measure the protein expression of p62. Western blot analysis indicated an increase in the levels of p62 in the ipsilateral compared with the contralateral side of WT mice. The corresponding densitometric analysis is shown as bar graphs using Image J. Two-way ANOVA; all the data are shown as mean ± SEM, where $*P < 0.05$ denotes a significant difference compared with the control group. **d** Frozen sections (WT-CCI, POD7) were stained with p62 and co-stained with anti-GFAP (A1–4) and anti-NeuN antibodies (B1–4). A4 and B4 is rectangular magnification of merged A3 and B3, respectively. Scale bar = 50 μm in A, B1–3. Scale bar = 20 μm in A, B4

Discussion

Damage or disease to the somatosensory nervous system that results in disorders of the PNS often leads to chronic neuropathic pain, a debilitating condition resulting from sensitization of the nociceptive pathway. A recent report suggested that the activation of glial cells, especially microglia located in the sensory laminae of the spinal dorsal horn, is the main cause of this process [30]. Activated microglia following peripheral nerve injury changes the morphology and releases neuroactive factors and cytokines that contribute to neuropathic pain [31]. Although the mechanism underlying microglial proliferation following nerve damage remains unclear, it has recently been reported that TLRs play a critical role in neuropathic pain after peripheral nerve injury [7, 32], particularly in microglia activation and driving pain hypersensitivity after nerve injury. TLR4 is an important PAMP and DAMP that regulates the innate or adaptive immune response. TLR4 has been shown to be highly expressed in the CNS of rodents by microglia [10], and genetically altered mice lacking TLR4 showed significantly reduced microglia activation and pain hypersensitivity following nerve injury [7]. Our results showed that the TLR4 KO in mice reduced pain hypersensitivity and proliferation of microglia following CCI-induced nerve injury, verifying the relationship between TLR4 and microglia in neuropathic pain (Fig. 1). CatWalk analysis also showed the correlation between TLR4 and pain hypersensitivity in neuropathic pain. Nerve injury following CCI decreased the percentages of the print

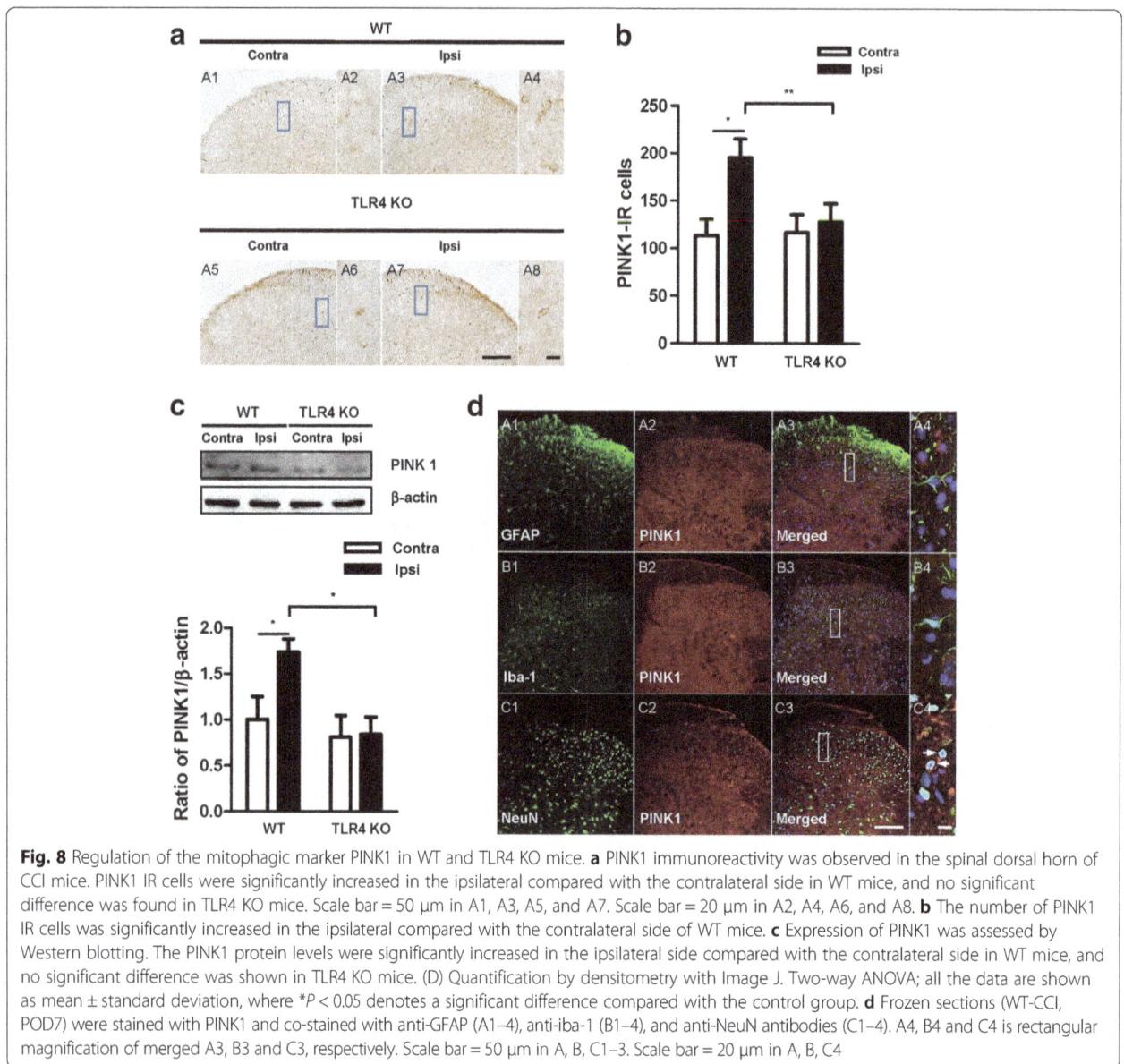

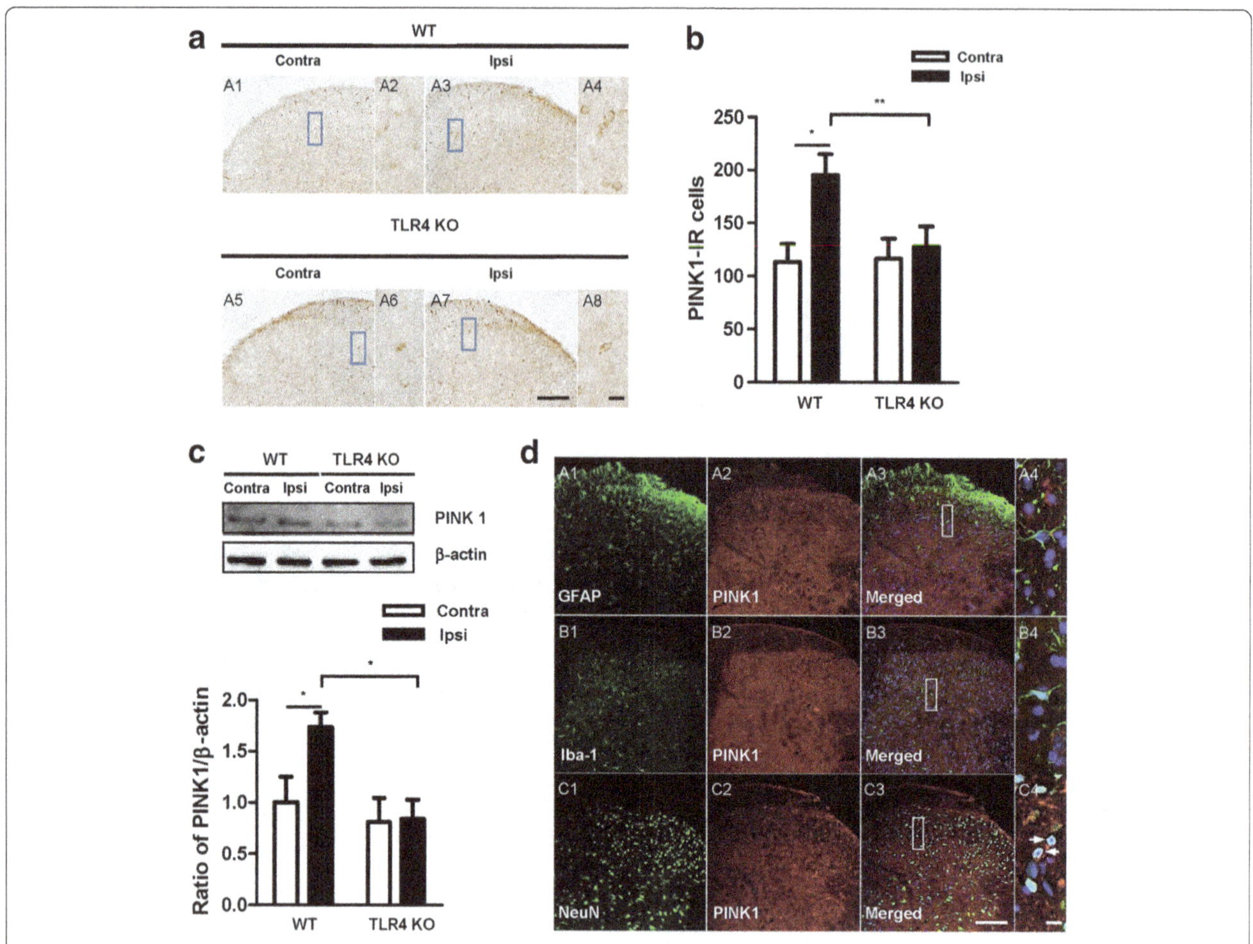

Fig. 8 Regulation of the mitophagic marker PINK1 in WT and TLR4 KO mice. **a** PINK1 immunoreactivity was observed in the spinal dorsal horn of CCI mice. PINK1 IR cells were significantly increased in the ipsilateral compared with the contralateral side in WT mice, and no significant difference was found in TLR4 KO mice. Scale bar = 50 μm in A1, A3, A5, and A7. Scale bar = 20 μm in A2, A4, A6, and A8. **b** The number of PINK1 IR cells was significantly increased in the ipsilateral compared with the contralateral side of WT mice. **c** Expression of PINK1 was assessed by Western blotting. The PINK1 protein levels were significantly increased in the ipsilateral side compared with the contralateral side in WT mice, and no significant difference was shown in TLR4 KO mice. (D) Quantification by densitometry with Image J. Two-way ANOVA; all the data are shown as mean ± standard deviation, where $^{*}P < 0.05$ denotes a significant difference compared with the control group. **d** Frozen sections (WT-CCI, POD7) were stained with PINK1 and co-stained with anti-GFAP (A1–4), anti-iba-1 (B1–4), and anti-NeuN antibodies (C1–4). A4, B4 and C4 is rectangular magnification of merged A3, B3 and C3, respectively. Scale bar = 50 μm in A, B, C1–3. Scale bar = 20 μm in A, B, C4

area and single stance on the ipsilateral side of mice, and the percentages were significantly increased in TLR4 KO compared with WT mice (Fig. 2).

Autophagy has recently been shown to be a mechanism by which host cells capture and eliminate intracellular pathogens. Pain is a common feature of various neurodegenerative diseases in which autophagy plays a critical role in the progression of the pathology and is being studied as a possible therapeutic target [12, 13]. A recent study demonstrated that autophagy was differently modulated in the spinal cord of mice in several neuropathic pain models [14]. As the most thoroughly characterized type of pattern recognition receptor, TLR4 enhances the elimination of phagocytosed mycobacteria to activate autophagy and serves as an environmental sensor for autophagy. The stimulation of TLR4 with LPS induces autophagosome formation in macrophages by the TRIF-p38 axis and its downstream signaling pathways [15]. Therefore, we hypothesized that the TLR4-mediated autophagy pathway may play a critical role in neuropathic pain. We investigated the spinal modulation of some autophagy markers (e.g., LC3, Beclin 1, and p62) in mice after CCI (Figs. 5–7). In WT mice, increased Beclin 1 levels were paralleled by strong p62 accumulation in the ipsilateral compared with the contralateral side but without a significant increase in LC3-I and LC3-II in both sides of the spinal dorsal horn, suggesting a block in the late phase of autophagic flux rather than an induction of the process. In TLR4 KO mice, however, no significant changes in the three

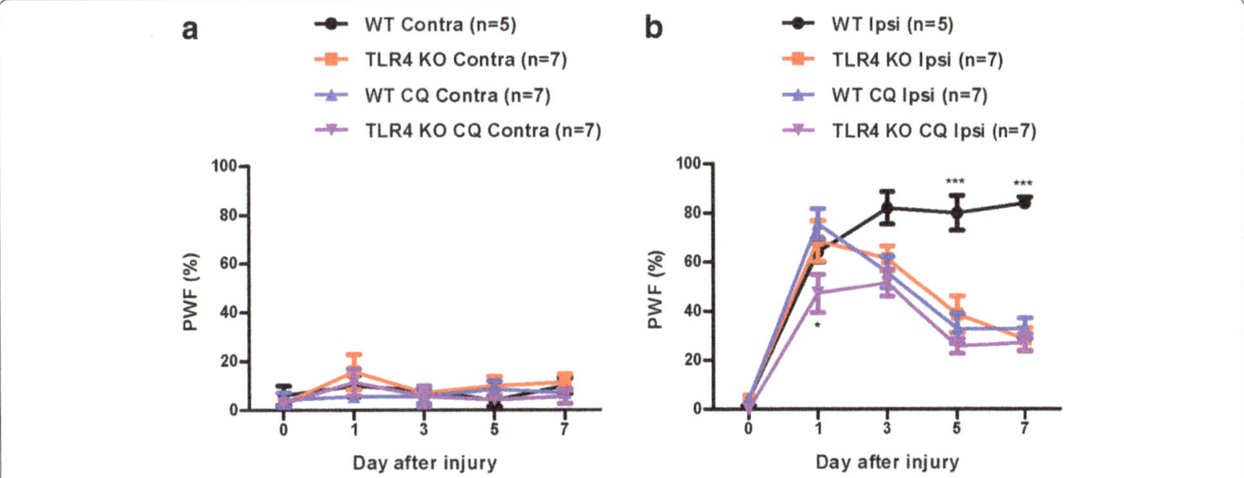

Fig. 9 Chloroquine attenuates dramatically mechanical allodynia induced by CCI in WT mice. **a, b** Chloroquine was administrated subcutaneously at 15 mg/kg/day. After 30 min, the paw withdrawal frequency (%PWF) was measured on days 0 (baseline), 1, 3, 5, and 7 after surgery. Mechanical allodynia was separately compared in each group of contralateral (Contra) and ipsilateral (Ipsi) in CCI mice. Two-way analysis of variance (ANOVA); all the data are shown as mean ± SEM, where $*P < 0.05$ denotes a significant different between TLR4 KO Ipsilateral with TLR4 KO CQ Ipsilateral, $***P < 0.001$ WT-CCI ipsilateral vs. the TLR4 KO-CCI ipsilateral

markers were observed in either the ipsilateral or contralateral sides of the spinal dorsal horn, suggesting that the modulation of autophagy was almost blocked due to the lack of TLR4 signaling.

Indeed, Beclin 1 upregulation in WT mice may indicate an increased autophagic flux but also defective autophagosome clearance. In the latter case, Beclin 1 upregulation will be associated with p62 accumulation because this autophagy substrate will not be efficiently degraded by the autophagosomes [23, 33]. Studies on the regulatory role of Beclin 1 in autophagy have suggested that the Beclin 1 complex is involved in autophagosome formation at an early stage [24], and this complex is essential for the recruitment of other autophagy-related proteins to the pre-autophagosomal structure [34].

No significant changes were observed in the expression of LC3-I and LC3-II in both WT and TLR4 KO mice (Fig. 5), and the lipidated form is known to be associated with autophagosomes [22]. Monitoring LC3-II conversion is considered one of the most reliable methods for monitoring autophagy. However, a concomitant increase in both the rate of autophagosome formation and LC3 downstream degradation can show normal steady-state levels in LC3-II despite enhanced autophagy activity [35]. Moreover, LC3 accumulation can result from autophagy induction, but also from impairment at one of the last steps such as fusion with the lysosomes or cargo degradation [33]. Therefore, it is preferable to integrate LC3 studies with the analysis of other components of the autophagic machinery such as members of the initiation complex (e.g., Beclin 1) or autolysosome substrates (i.e., SQSTM1/p62) [23].

One of the best-known autophagic substrates is p62/SQSTM1, a key LC3-binding protein, which serves as a link between LC3 and ubiquitinated proteins [27]. p62 and p62-bound polyubiquitinated proteins become incorporated into the completed autophagosome and are degraded in autolysosomes. Because of the correlation between autophagy modulation and p62 levels [27, 36, 37], this substrate is considered a useful readout of autophagic degradation [23, 38]. Indeed, p62 levels increase when autophagy is impaired [37]. In WT mice, ipsilateral p62 accumulation was observed to significantly increase compared with the contralateral side, suggesting a block in the final degradative steps of autophagy. However, in the TLR4 KO mice, no significant change in the p62 level was observed between the two sides of the spinal dorsal horn (Fig. 7). Altogether, the analysis of LC3, Beclin 1, and p62 in this study indicated that autophagy impairment in CCI-induced neuropathic pain may be due to the occurrence of a block in the late phase of autophagic flux rather than in the induction of the process, and this autophagy seems to be mediated by TLR4 signaling. Moreover, mitophagy was assessed by monitoring the expression of the protein marker PINK1 (Fig. 8). Expression of PINK1 was increased in WT mice after CCI but showed no significant change in TLR4 KO mice, indirectly supporting our hypothesis regarding TLR4-mediated autophagy.

Although it was early reported that TLR4 is expressed primarily in microglia, but not astrocytes or neurons [39], it was also found that neurons do express TLR4 and that TLR signaling in neurons regulates neural precursor cell proliferation axonal growth, adult neurogenesis, and neuronal plasticity [40]. In this study, we found that the expression of LC3, Beclin 1, and p62 associated with autophagy impairment in CCI-induced neuropathic pain was localized with neuronal cell, not astrocyte or microglia, in spinal dorsal horn. Previously, Tanga et al., reported that the genetically altered mice displayed significantly attenuated behavioral hypersensitivity and decreased expression of spinal microglial markers and proinflammatory cytokine [7]. Therefore, it is reasonable that TLR4-mediated pro-inflammatory cytokine release in microglia and TLR4-mediated autophagic impairment in neurons contribute pain sensory hypersensitivity synergically.

Our immunohistochemical studies were supported with autophagic inhibitor, Chlorquine treatment. Chloroquine (Sigma-Aldrich, St. Louis, MO) is one of many compounds which have shown to reverse autophagy by accumulating in lysosomes, disturbing the vacuolar H^+ ATPase, which is responsible for lysosomal acidification and blocking autophagy [41]. When injected intrathecally in WT, Chloroquine induced a significant reduction in threshold of mechanical sensitivity (Fig. 9b). This data is in perfect agreement with previous paper [14]. In that paper, the authors showed chloroquine was able to modulate the spinal autophagic machinery by the increase in p62, indicative of autophagosome accumulation. However, they did not show data on comparison with TLR4 KO mice. Our data showed that CCI-induced mechanical allodynia in TLR4 KO with Chloroquine treatment attenuated pain threshold compared to TLR4 KO. This data strongly supported TLR4-mediated autophagic impairment in neurons contribute pain sensory hypersensitivity with microglia activation, whereas, microglial TLR4-mediated microglial activation might be indirectly coupled to autophage.

In conclusion, the present study demonstrated that the deficiency of glial TLR4 could decrease mechanical allodynia with synergic TLR4 mediated blockade of impaired spinal autophagy induction in CCI-induced neuropathic pain mice (Fig. 10). Additionally, our study improves our understanding of TLR4 autophagy-related neuropathic pain and provides the scientific basis for the use of TLR4 and autophagy as potential therapeutic targets in the clinical management of neuropathic pain.

Methods

Experimental animals

Eight-week-old male C57BL/6j mice (Narabiotech, Seoul, Korea) were used in this study. C57BL/10ScNJ TLR4-KO (TLR4$^{-/-}$) mice were purchased from the Jackson Laboratories (Bar Harbor, ME, USA). All the mice were individually housed in cages on a standard 12 h/12 h light/dark cycle, and water and food were available ad libitum.

Mechanical allodynia assay

To assess the sensitization to innocuous mechanical stimulation (mechanical allodynia), we measured the paw withdrawal response frequency (PWF) using a von Frey filament (North Coast Medical, Morgan Hill, CA, USA) as described in a previous study [42]. Based on that study, a von Frey filament with a force of 2.0 g was selected for testing. Mice were placed on a metal mesh flooring, and the von Frey filament was applied from

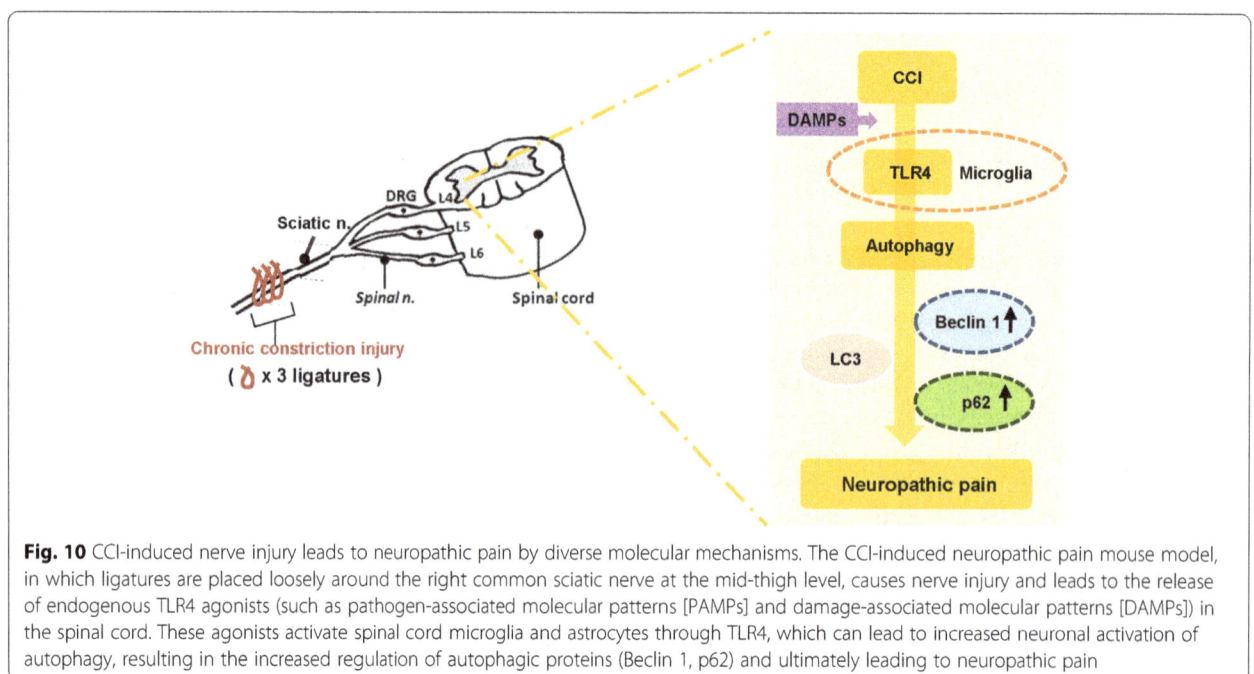

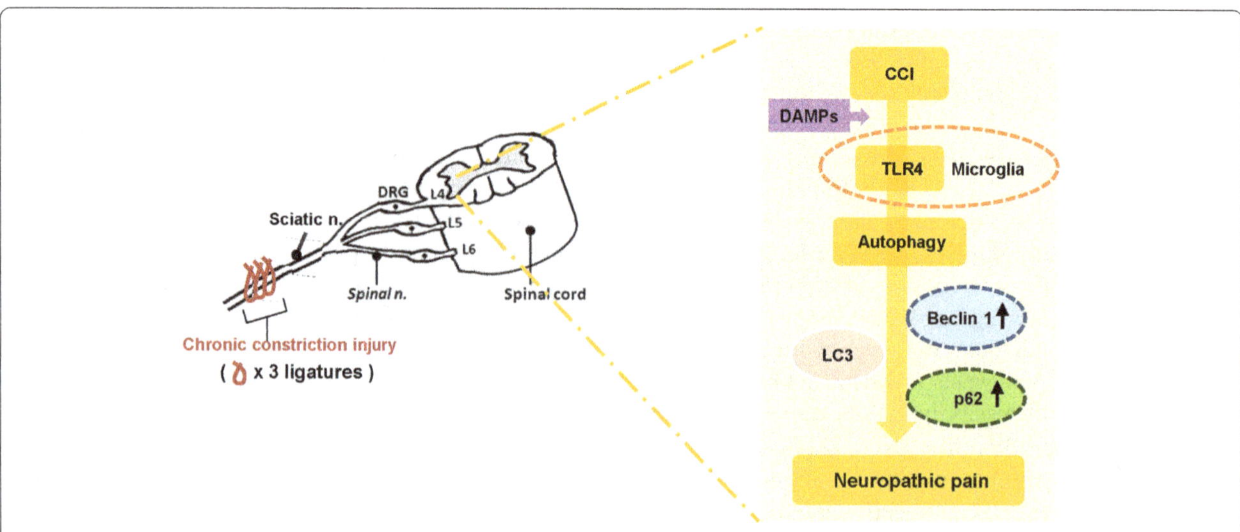

Fig. 10 CCI-induced nerve injury leads to neuropathic pain by diverse molecular mechanisms. The CCI-induced neuropathic pain mouse model, in which ligatures are placed loosely around the right common sciatic nerve at the mid-thigh level, causes nerve injury and leads to the release of endogenous TLR4 agonists (such as pathogen-associated molecular patterns [PAMPs] and damage-associated molecular patterns [DAMPs]) in the spinal cord. These agonists activate spinal cord microglia and astrocytes through TLR4, which can lead to increased neuronal activation of autophagy, resulting in the increased regulation of autophagic proteins (Beclin 1, p62) and ultimately leading to neuropathic pain

underneath the metal mesh flooring to each plantar of the hind paw. The filament was applied 10 times to each paw at intervals of 10 s, and the number of paw withdrawal responses following each filament stimulus was counted. The result of each experimental animal was expressed as a percentage of the paw withdrawal response frequency (% PWF). Paw withdrawal responses were measured day 0 (baseline), 1, 3, 5, and 7 after CCI surgery in each set.

CCI-induced neuropathic pain

CCI of the common sciatic nerve was performed based on the method described by Bennett and Xie [18]. Mice were anesthetized with an intraperitoneal injection (i.p.) of Avertin (2,2,2-tribromoethanol, 50% *w*/*v* in tertiary amyl alcohol, diluted 1:40 in H_2O; 20 ml/kg, i.p.; Sigma-Aldrich, St. Louis, MO, USA). The right common sciatic nerve was exposed at the mid-thigh level and was dissected from the connective tissue. Three loose ligatures of the 4–0 chromic gut were tied around the nerve with an interval of 1.0 to 1.5 mm between each ligature. After surgery, mice recovered on the heating pad at 27 °C.

CatWalk-automated gait analysis

The CatWalk XT system (Noldus Information Technology, Wageningen, The Netherlands) was used for the quantitative assessment of the gait parameter and footfalls in rodents. CatWalk is a verified system in the research of several pain models such as spinal cord injury, traumatic brain injury, and neuropathic pain. During the test, the mice traversed a dark tunnel with a glass plate from one side to the other. Their footprints were illuminated by fluorescent light from the glass plate and were captured by a high-speed camera positioned underneath the plate. The captured images were immediately processed by CatWalk XT software, and numerous parameters were analyzed, such as the print area, swing speed, and single stance. In this study, we measured the print area and single stance to assess differences in nociceptive responses between WT and TLR4-KO CCI mice. The print area is the contacting area between the hind paw and glass, and a single stance is the duration of the contralateral or ipsilateral hind paw touching the glass plate in the step cycle. CatWalk gait analysis was measured before and 1, 3, 5, and 7 days after CCI surgery in each set.

Immunostaining analysis

Immunohistochemistry was performed 7 days after surgery. The mice were anesthetized with sodium pentobarbital (50 mg/kg, i.p.) and perfused transcardially with heparinized phosphate-buffered saline (PBS, pH 7.4), followed by perfusion with 4% paraformaldehyde for 15 min. The lumbar enlargement (L4–L6) regions of the spinal cords were removed immediately, immersed in the same fixative overnight, and embedded in paraffin. The paraffin-embedded tissue arrays were performed in 4-μm sections and deparaffinized and rehydrated in a graded alcohol solution. The sections were soaked in 0.01 M citrate buffer (pH 6.0) and heated in a microwave vacuum histoprocessor (RHS-1, Milestone, Bergamo, Italy) at a controlled final temperature of 121 °C for 15 min for antigen retrieval. For immunohistochemical analyses as previously [43], endogenous peroxidase activity was blocked using 0.3% hydrogen peroxide. After primary antibody reaction (4 °C, overnight) as follows; Becline1(1:400; #AP1818a, ABGENT), p62 (1:400; #p0067, Sigma-Aldrich), PINK1 (1:400; #NBP2–36488, Novus Biologicals, Littleton, CO, USA), LC3 (1:200; #sc376404, Santa Cruz Biotechnology, Santa Cruz, CA, USA), NeuN (1:200; #24307S, Bioncompare), NeuN (1:200; #MAB377, Millpore), GFAP (1:2000, #Z0334, Dako), GFAP (1:2000; #MAB360, Millpore), Iba-1 (1:400; #019–19,741, Wako), Iba-1 (1:400; #016–26,721, Wako), the tissues were exposed to biotinylated anti-rabbit IgG and streptavidin peroxidase complex (Vector Laboratories, Inc., Burlingame, CA, USA). Immunostaining was visualized with diaminobenzidine (DAB), and the specimens were mounted using Polymount (Polysciences, Inc., Warrington, PA, USA).

Western blot analysis

The lumbar enlargement (L4-L6) regions of the spinal cord from WT and TLR4 KO mice were dissected and homogenized in lysis buffer. The lysates of the spinal cord (20 μg) were separated by 12 or 15% sodium dodecyl sulfate-polyacrylamide gel electrophoresis (SDS-PAGE) and transferred to nitrocellulose membranes. The blots were probed with the following primary antibodies: Becline 1 (1:1000; #sc-11,427, Santa Cruz Biotechnology, Santa Cruz, CA, USA), LC3 (1:1000; #L8918, Sigma-Aldrich), p62 (1:1000; #P0067, Sigma-Aldrich), PINK1 (1:1000; #NBP1–39667, Novus Biologicals, Littleton, CO, USA), and β-actin (1:500; #2965, Cell Signaling Technology, Danvers, MA, USA). The immune complexes were identified using an enhanced chemiluminescence (ECL) detection system (Habersham, Little Chalfont, United Kingdom).

Statistical analysis

All the data are presented as mean ± standard error of the mean. Quantitative analysis of immunostaining was performed using ImageJ (National Institutes of Health, Bethesda, MD, USA) as previously [43]. Statistical analyses were performed using the statistical software Prism 6.0 program (Graph Pad Software, San Diego, CA, USA), and repeated measurements from behavioral studies were analyzed by two-way analysis of variance. The results were considered significant at $^{*}P < 0.05$, $^{**}P < 0.01$, and $^{***}P < 0.001$.

Acknowledgments
We gratefully acknowledge Juhee Shin and Hyewon Park for expert technical assistance.

Funding
This research was supported by the Brain Research Program through the National Research Foundation of Korea (NRF) funded by the Ministry of Science, ICT & Future Planning (NRF-2016M3C7A1905074), and by the Korea government (MSIP) (2016R1A2B4009409, 2013R1A1A1057928, 2017R1D1A1B03028839).

Authors' contributions
YP, SO and DWK designed and performed experiments, analyzed the data and wrote the manuscript; GDH and DK performed Chloroquine experiments; TWH, NS, DHG, HHK and HJS performed histological and behavioral analysis; DK, YY and JK generated mouse model and performed genotype analysis; JH and HK analyzed the data and revised the manuscript; YK and SRK designed experiments and wrote the manuscript. All authors read and approved the final manuscript.

Competing interests
The author(s) declared no potential conflicts of interest with respect to the research, authorship, and/or publication of this article.

Author details
[1]Department of Plastic and Reconstructive Surgery, Department of Pediatrics, Department of Anesthesiology and Pain Medicine, Chungnam National University Hospital, Daejeon 35015, Republic of Korea. [2]Department of Medical Science, Department of Physiology, Department of Anatomy, Brain Research Institute, Chungnam National University School of Medicine, Daejeon 35015, Republic of Korea. [3]LES Corporation Inc., Gung-Dong 465-16, Yuseong-Gu, Daejeon 305-335, Republic of Korea. [4]Department of Chemical and Biological Engineering, The University of Alabama, Tuscaloosa, AL 35487, USA. [5]School of Life Sciences, BK21 plus KNU Creative BioResearch Group, Institute of Life Science & Biotechnology, Kyungpook National University, Daegu 41566, South Korea.

References
1. Basbaum AI, Bautista DM, Scherrer G, Julius D. Cellular and molecular mechanisms of pain. Cell. 2009;139:267–84.
2. Veldhuijzen DS, Lenz FA, LaGraize SC, Greenspan JD. What can neuroimaging tell us about central pain? In: Kruger L, Boca Raton LAR, editors. Translational pain research: from mouse to man. FL: Frontiers in Neuroscience; 2010.
3. Varrassi G, Muller-Schwefe G, Pergolizzi J, Oronska A, Morlion B, Mavrocordatos P, Margarit C, Mangas C, Jaksch W, Huygen F, et al. Pharmacological treatment of chronic pain - the need for CHANGE. Curr Med Res Opin. 2010;26:1231–45.
4. Tsuda M, Inoue K, Salter MW. Neuropathic pain and spinal microglia: a big problem from molecules in "small" glia. Trends Neurosci. 2005;28:101–7.
5. Watkins LR, Milligan ED, Maier SF. Glial activation: a driving force for pathological pain. Trends Neurosci. 2001;24:450–5.
6. Sommer C. Painful neuropathies. Curr Opin Neurol. 2003;16:623–8.
7. Tanga FY, Nutile-McMenemy N, DeLeo JA. The CNS role of toll-like receptor 4 in innate neuroimmunity and painful neuropathy. Proc Natl Acad Sci U S A. 2005;102:5856–61.
8. Tanga FY, Raghavendra V, DeLeo JA. Quantitative real-time RT-PCR assessment of spinal microglial and astrocytic activation markers in a rat model of neuropathic pain. Neurochem Int. 2004;45:397–407.
9. Cao L, Tanga FY, Deleo JA. The contributing role of CD14 in toll-like receptor 4 dependent neuropathic pain. Neuroscience. 2009;158:896–903.
10. Lehnardt S, Massillon L, Follett P, Jensen FE, Ratan R, Rosenberg PA, Volpe JJ, Vartanian T. Activation of innate immunity in the CNS triggers neurodegeneration through a toll-like receptor 4-dependent pathway. Proc Natl Acad Sci U S A. 2003;100:8514–9.
11. Yorimitsu T, Klionsky DJ. Autophagy: molecular machinery for self-eating. Cell Death Differ. 2005;12(Suppl 2):1542–52.
12. Rubinsztein DC, Gestwicki JE, Murphy LO, Klionsky DJ. Potential therapeutic applications of autophagy. Nat Rev Drug Discov. 2007;6:304–12.
13. Raudino F. Non-cognitive symptoms and related conditions in the Alzheimer's disease: a literature review. Neurol Sci. 2013;34:1275–82.
14. Berliocchi L, Maiaru M, Varano GP, Russo R, Corasaniti MT, Bagetta G, Tassorelli C. Spinal autophagy is differently modulated in distinct mouse models of neuropathic pain. Mol Pain. 2015;11:3.
15. Xu Y, Jagannath C, Liu XD, Sharafkhaneh A, Kolodziejska KE, Eissa NT. Toll-like receptor 4 is a sensor for autophagy associated with innate immunity. Immunity. 2007;27:135–44.
16. Chiang CY, Sheu ML, Cheng FC, Chen CJ, Su HL, Sheehan J, Pan HC. Comprehensive analysis of neurobehavior associated with histomorphological alterations in a chronic constrictive nerve injury model through use of the CatWalk XT system. J Neurosurg. 2014;120:250–62.
17. Vrinten DH, Hamers FF. CatWalk' automated quantitative gait analysis as a novel method to assess mechanical allodynia in the rat; a comparison with von Frey testing. Pain. 2003;102:203–9.
18. Bennett GJ, Xie YK. A peripheral mononeuropathy in rat that produces disorders of pain sensation like those seen in man. Pain. 1988;33:87–107.
19. Tsuda M, Inoue K. Role of molecules expressed in spiral microglia in neuropathic pain. Nihon Shinkei Seishin Yakurigaku Zasshi. 2006;26:57–61.
20. Milligan ED, Watkins LR. Pathological and protective roles of glia in chronic pain. Nat Rev Neurosci. 2009;10:23–36.
21. Hald A. Spinal astrogliosis in pain models: cause and effects. Cell Mol Neurobiol. 2009;29:609–19.
22. Kabeya Y, Mizushima N, Ueno T, Yamamoto A, Kirisako T, Noda T, Kominami E, Ohsumi Y, Yoshimori T. LC3, a mammalian homologue of yeast Apg8p, is localized in autophagosome membranes after processing. EMBO J. 2000;19:5720–8.
23. Klionsky DJ, Abdelmohsen K, Abe A, Abedin MJ, Abeliovich H, Acevedo Arozena A, Adachi H, Adams CM, Adams PD, Adeli K, et al. Guidelines for the use and interpretation of assays for monitoring autophagy (3rd edition). Autophagy. 2016;12:1–222.
24. Pattingre S, Espert L, Biard-Piechaczyk M, Codogno P. Regulation of macroautophagy by mTOR and Beclin 1 complexes. Biochimie. 2008; 90:313–23.
25. Mizushima N, Komatsu M. Autophagy: renovation of cells and tissues. Cell. 2011;147:728–41.
26. Johansen T, Lamark T. Selective autophagy mediated by autophagic adapter proteins. Autophagy. 2011;7:279–96.
27. Bjorkoy G, Lamark T, Brech A, Outzen H, Perander M, Overvatn A, Stenmark H, Johansen T. p62/SQSTM1 forms protein aggregates degraded by autophagy and has a protective effect on huntingtin-induced cell death. J Cell Biol. 2005;171:603–14.
28. Lemasters JJ. Selective mitochondrial autophagy, or mitophagy, as a targeted defense against oxidative stress, mitochondrial dysfunction, and aging. Rejuvenation Res. 2005;8:3–5.
29. Gelmetti V, De Rosa P, Torosantucci L, Marini ES, Romagnoli A, Di Rienzo M, Arena G, Vignone D, Fimia GM, Valente EM. PINK1 and BECN1 relocalize at mitochondria-associated membranes during mitophagy and promote ER-mitochondria tethering and autophagosome formation. Autophagy. 2017; 13:654–69.
30. Inoue K, Tsuda M. Purinergic systems, neuropathic pain and the role of microglia. Exp Neurol. 2012;234:293–301.

31. Inoue K, Tsuda M, Tozaki-Saitoh H. Modification of neuropathic pain sensation through microglial ATP receptors. Purinergic Signal. 2007;3:311–6.
32. Buchanan MM, Hutchinson M, Watkins LR, Yin H. Toll-like receptor 4 in CNS pathologies. J Neurochem. 2010;114:13–27.
33. Mizushima N, Yoshimori T, Levine B. Methods in mammalian autophagy research. Cell. 2010;140:313–26.
34. Suzuki K, Ohsumi Y. Molecular machinery of autophagosome formation in yeast, Saccharomyces Cerevisiae. FEBS Lett. 2007;581:2156–61.
35. Castillo K, Valenzuela V, Matus S, Nassif M, Onate M, Fuentealba Y, Encina G, Irrazabal T, Parsons G, Court FA, et al. Measurement of autophagy flux in the nervous system in vivo. Cell Death Dis. 2013;4:e917.
36. Pankiv S, Clausen TH, Lamark T, Brech A, Bruun JA, Outzen H, Overvatn A, Bjorkoy G, Johansen T. p62/SQSTM1 binds directly to Atg8/LC3 to facilitate degradation of ubiquitinated protein aggregates by autophagy. J Biol Chem. 2007;282:24131–45.
37. Komatsu M, Waguri S, Koike M, Sou YS, Ueno T, Hara T, Mizushima N, Iwata J, Ezaki J, Murata S, et al. Homeostatic levels of p62 control cytoplasmic inclusion body formation in autophagy-deficient mice. Cell. 2007;131:1149–63.
38. Sahani MH, Itakura E, Mizushima N. Expression of the autophagy substrate SQSTM1/p62 is restored during prolonged starvation depending on transcriptional upregulation and autophagy-derived amino acids. Autophagy. 2014;10:431–41.
39. Lehnardt S, Lachance C, Patrizi S, Lefebvre S, Follett PL, Jensen FE, Rosenberg PA, Volpe JJ, Vartanian T. The toll-like receptor TLR4 is necessary for lipopolysaccharide-induced oligodendrocyte injury in the CNS. J Neurosci. 2002;22:2478–86.
40. Okun E, Griffioen KJ, Mattson MP. Toll-like receptor signaling in neural plasticity and disease. Trends Neurosci. 2011;34:269–81.
41. Nalbandian A, Llewellyn KJ, Nguyen C, Yazdi PG, Kimonis VE. Rapamycin and chloroquine: the in vitro and in vivo effects of autophagy-modifying drugs show promising results in Valosin containing protein multisystem Proteinopathy. PLoS One. 2015;10(4):e0122888.
42. Roh DH, Kim HW, Yoon SY, Seo HS, Kwon YB, Kim KW, Han HJ, Beitz AJ, Na HS, Lee JH. Intrathecal injection of the sigma(1) receptor antagonist BD1047 blocks both mechanical allodynia and increases in spinal NR1 expression during the induction phase of rodent neuropathic pain. Anesthesiology. 2008;109:879–89.
43. Zhang EJ, Yi MH, Shin N, Baek H, Kim S, Kim E, Kwon K, Lee S, Kim HW, Bae YC, et al. Endoplasmic reticulum stress impairment in the spinal dorsal horn of a neuropathic pain model. Sci Rep. 2015;5:11555.

9

Stimulation-induced structural changes at the nucleus, endoplasmic reticulum and mitochondria of hippocampal neurons

Jung-Hwa Tao-Cheng

Abstract

Neurons exhibit stimulation-induced ultrastructural changes such as increase of thickness and curvature of the postsynaptic density, decrease in contact area between subsurface cistern and plasma membrane, and formation of CaMKII clusters and synaptic spinules. These structural characteristics help in identifying the activity state of the neuron and should be taken into consideration when interpreting ultrastructural features of the neurons. Here in organotypic hippocampal slice cultures where experimental conditions can be easily manipulated, two additional features are documented in forebrain neurons as reliable benchmarks for stimulation-induced structural changes: (1) The neuronal nucleus showed conspicuous clustering of dark chromatin, and (2) the endoplasmic reticulum formed stacks with a uniform gap of ~ 13 nm filled with dark materials. Both structural changes progressed with time and were reversible upon returning the slice cultures to control medium. These stimulation-induced structural changes were also verified in dissociated hippocampal neuronal cultures and perfusion-fixed brains. In hippocampal slice cultures, the neuronal chromatin clustering was detectable within 30 s of depolarization with high K^+ (90 mM) or treatment with NMDA (50 μM). In contrast, the formation of ER cisternal stacks did not become apparent for another 30 s. Importantly, in dissociated neuronal cultures, when the extracellular calcium was chelated by EGTA, treatment with high K^+ no longer induced these changes. These results indicate that the stimulation-induced chromatin clustering and formation of ER stacks in neurons are calcium-dependent. Additionally, mitochondria in neuronal somas of tissue culture samples consistently became swollen upon stimulation. However, swollen mitochondria were also present in some neurons of control samples, but could be eliminated by blocking basal activity or calcium influx. This calcium-dependent structural change of mitochondria is specific to neurons. These structural changes may bring insights to the neuron's response to intracellular calcium rise upon stimulation.

Keywords: Electron microscopy, ER, Calcium regulation, Chromatin, Nucleus

Introduction

Excitable cells like neurons and muscles show morphological changes under excitatory conditions. Prominent examples include electron microscopy (EM) studies that shed lights on synaptic vesicle recycling in frog neuromuscular junctions [1], and mouse hippocampal neurons in cell cultures [2]. Other EM studies on mouse and rat neurons have shown stimulation-induced increases in the thickness and curvature of the postsynaptic density (PSD) [3, 4], decrease in number and contact areas of subsurface cisterns with the plasma membrane [5], and formation of calcium calmodulin-dependent kinase II (CaMKII) clusters [4, 6] and synaptic spinules [7]. While some of the features require precise quantification to document, the presence of CaMKII clusters and synaptic spinules, in themselves, provides strong evidence that the samples are under stimulated conditions. Although the stimulation protocols employed in these studies are beyond normal physiological conditions and thus may render neurons under excitatory stress, all of these stimulation-induced structural changes are nevertheless reversible. These structural benchmarks are useful in interpreting whether structural characteristics are caused by heightened neuronal activity or other factors such as genetic manipulations. The present study set out to

Correspondence: chengs@ninds.nih.gov
NINDS Electron Microscopy Facility, National Institute of Neurological Disorders and Stroke, National Institutes of Health, Bethesda, MD 20892, USA

document additional stimulation-induced structural changes that may serve as helpful benchmarks to detect acute excitation in neurons, and to determine whether these effects are calcium-dependent.

One striking feature is manifested as clustering of dark chromatin in neuronal nucleus from rat hippocampal slice cultures within 30 s upon stimulation. Whether this feature is consistently induced by stimulation or hypoxic excitatory stress is examined in rat dissociated hippocampal cultures and in perfusion-fixed rat and mouse brains.

A second stimulation-induced benchmark structure is the stacking of endoplasmic reticulum (ER) with a uniform gap of ~ 13 nm between stacks. In Purkinje neurons of the cerebellum, formation of ER cisternal stacks is induced by hypoxic and hypoglycemic conditions that were caused by a few minutes of delay in perfusion fixation [4, 8]. Here, hippocampal neurons from all three experimental systems were examined to verify whether similar ER stacks form in forebrain neurons upon stimulation. Furthermore, the time course and reversibility of the formation of ER stacks were examined in hippocampal slice cultures.

A third structural change is that mitochondria in neuronal soma became swollen upon stimulation. Similar ultrastructural changes in mitochondria has been reported in rat dissociated hippocampal cultures upon excitotoxic injury [9] and in mice after hypoxic-ischemic brain injury [10]. The present study tested whether the swollen mitochondria are induced by activity and calcium influx.

Methods

Preparation, treatment and fixation of rat dissociated hippocampal neuronal cultures

Most samples were from a previously published report [5] and reexamined here for additional structural changes. Briefly, cell cultures were prepared from embryonic 20-day-old rat fetuses by papain dissociation, and then plated on glial feeder cultures, and experiments were carried out with three-week-old cultures. Culture dishes were placed on a floating platform in a water bath maintained at 37 °C. Control incubation medium was HEPES-based Kreb's Ringer at pH 7.4. High K^+ medium was at 90 mM KCl. N-methyl-D-aspartic acid (NMDA) medium contained 30–250 μM NMDA in the control medium. APV (50 μM), an NMDA antagonist, was included in the NMDA medium (50 μM) for some experiments. Cell cultures were washed with control medium and treated for 2–3 min with either control or high K^+ media, or with 2–15 min with NMDA, or 2 min of NMDA+APV. In order to test whether extracellular calcium is involved in stimulation-induced structural changes, a calcium chelator, EGTA (1 mM), was included in a calcium-free control or high K^+ medium where osmolarity was compensated with sucrose. In some experiments, basal activity of cultures was blocked by 1 h incubation in culture media containing tetrodotoxin (TTX at 0.5 μM) to block action potential, D(–)-amino-7-phosphonovaleric acid (APV at 50 μM) to block NMDA receptor activation, and 6-cyano-7-nito-quinoxaline-2,3-dione (CNQX at 20 μM) to block AMPA receptor activation. Treated samples were then fixed immediately with 4% glutaraldehyde in 0.1 N cacodylate buffer at pH 7.4 for 30 min at room temperature and then stored in fixative at 4 °C.

Preparation, treatment and fixation of rat organotypic hippocampal slice cultures

Most samples were from a previously published report [7] and reexamined here for additional structural changes. Briefly, the hippocampus was removed from postnatal 6–8-day old rats and cut at 250 μm thickness with a tissue chopper. Slices were placed on a cell culture inserts in six-well culture dishes and used 10-14 days in vitro with the dishes on a floating platform in a water bath at 37 °C. Normal, high K^+ and

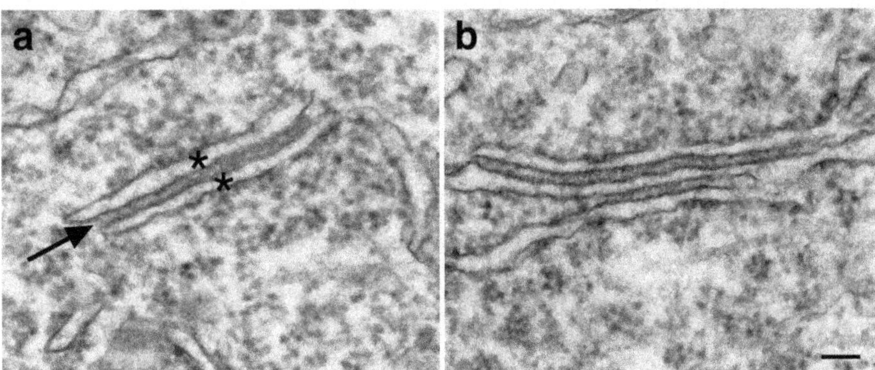

Fig. 1 ER cisternal stacks, defined by at least two ER cisterns (asterisks in a) apposed with a uniform ~ 13 nm gap (arrow in a). Images taken from hippocampal slice cultures treated with 3 min of 90 mM high K^+ (**a**) or 5 min of 50 μM NMDA (**b**). Scale bar = 0.1 μm

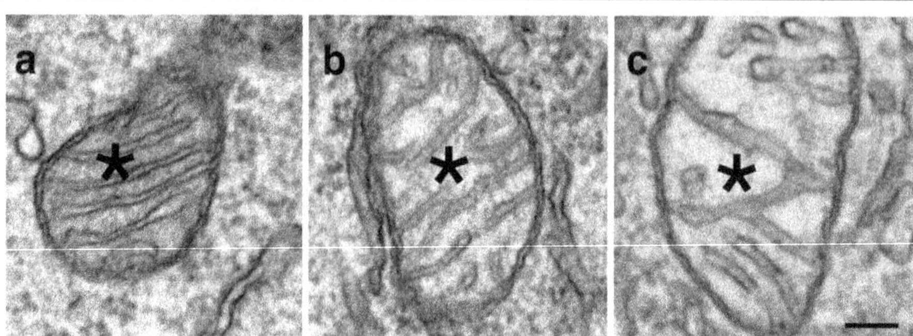

Fig. 2 Neuronal mitochondria are classified as "not swollen" if the matrix (marked by *) is dark (**a**), or "swollen" if the matrix is light (* in **b**, **c**). Images taken from dissociated hippocampal cultures treated for 2 min with calcium-free medium containing EGTA (1 mM; **a**), control medium (**b**), and high K^+ medium (90 mM; **c**). Scale bar = 0.1 μm

NMDA medium were the same as used for dissociated cells. Both high K^+ and NMDA treatments were for 0.5, 1, 2, 3, or 5 min. To examine recovery after depolarization, high K^+ medium was removed and the samples were washed three to four times in normal incubation medium for a total of 1, 2, 5, 10, 30 and 60 min. Experimental controls were processed in parallel, including all the medium changes and washing steps. Slice cultures were fixed with 2% glutaraldehyde and 2% paraformaldehyde, or 4% glutaraldehyde in 0.1 N cacodylate buffer at pH 7.4 for 1–3 h at room temperature and then stored at 4 °C.

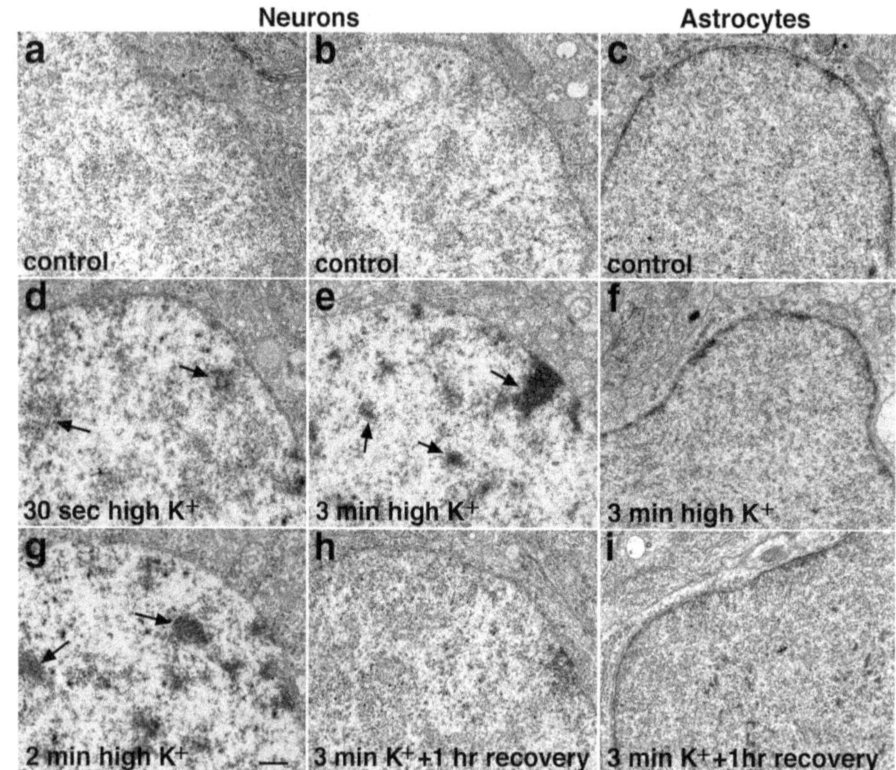

Fig. 3 Chromatin in neurons aggregates into dark clusters upon depolarization. Electron micrographs of neuronal nuclei from CA1 region of the hippocampus in slice cultures under different experimental conditions. (left column) – Chromatin appeared non-clustered under control conditions (**a**), but became aggregated into dark clusters (arrows) at 30 s after depolarization with high K^+ (90 mM, **d**), and progressed into even more pronounced clustering after 2 min of treatment (**g**). (middle column) – In a second series of experiments, the chromatin was again non-clustered under control conditions (**b**), became extensively clustered upon 3 min of depolarization with high K^+ (**e**), and reverted to the non-clustered appearance upon washout of the high K^+ medium and returning the samples to control medium for 1 h (**h**). (right column) – In contrast, nucleoplasm of fibrous astrocytes had a thin but dense rim of dark material of irregular thickness around the edge of the nucleus, and this configuration was not affected by high K^+ (**c**, **f**, **i**). Scale bar = 0.5 μm

Perfusion fixation of rat and mouse brains

Most samples were from previously published reports [4, 6] and reexamined here for additional structural changes. Briefly, adult rats were deeply anesthetized with Nembutal, and mice from 17-day to 3-month-old were deeply anesthetized with isoflurane. Animals were perfusion fixed through the heart with 2% glutaraldehyde + 2% paraformaldehyde in 0.1 M sodium cacodylate buffer at pH 7.4, or first perfused with 3.75% acrolein+ 2% paraformaldehyde, then followed by 2% paraformaldehyde. The time interval starting from the moment the diaphragm was cut to the moment when the outflow from the atrium turned from blood to clear fixative was recorded. Those animals that were successfully perfused within 100 s were classified as "fast" perfusion. For the "delayed" perfusion experiments, phosphate buffered saline containing calcium and magnesium was first perfused through the heart for 5 min before the start of the fixative. Neurons were under basal state after fast perfusion, and under ischemic excitatory conditions after delayed perfusion fixation [4, 6]. The perfusion-fixed brains were dissected and vibratomed into 100 μm thick coronal slices and stored in 2% glutaraldehyde in buffer at 4 °C.

Electron microscopy

Most fixed samples were washed in buffer and treated with 1% osmium tetroxide in 0.1 N cacodylate buffer at pH 7.4 for 1 h on ice. Some dissociated cells samples were treated with "reduced osmium" (1% osmium tetroxide + 1% potassium ferrocyanide in 0.1 N cacodylate buffer at pH 7.4 for 1 h on ice). Samples were then washed and en bloc stained with 0.25–1% uranyl acetate in 0.1 N acetate buffer at pH 5.0 overnight at 4 °C, dehydrated with a series of graded ethanol, and finally embedded in epoxy resins. Thin sections (70–90 nm thick) were counterstained with uranyl acetate and lead citrate, examined under a JEOL1200EX transmission electron microscope, and photographed with a bottom-mounted digital CCD camera (AMT XR-100, Danvers, MA, USA) at 4–10,000× for nucleus and at 10–40,000× for ER cisternal stacks and mitochondria.

Morphometry

Sampling of neuronal vs. astroglial nucleus

In perfusion-fixed brains and in hippocampal slice cultures, sampling of neuronal nuclei was restricted to the pyramidal cells in the CA1 region of the hippocampus. In

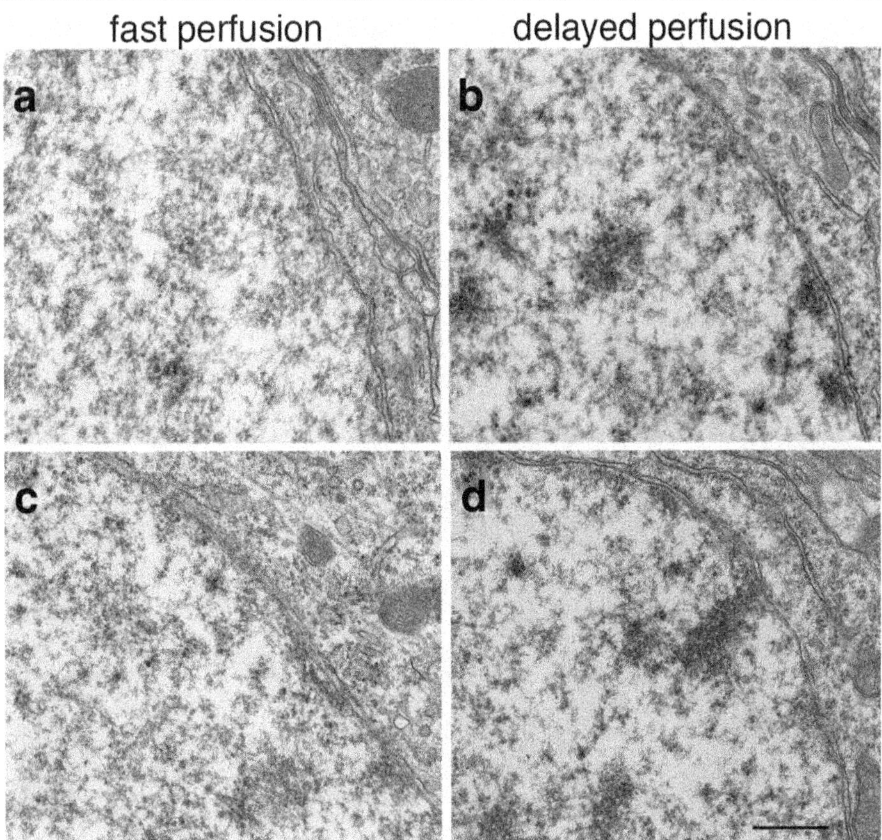

Fig. 4 Chromatin appeared non-clustered in fast perfusion-fixed mouse brains where neurons are under a basal state (**a**, **c**), but aggregated into dark clusters in delayed perfusion-fixed brains where neurons are under excitatory stress (b, d). Samples were from the CA1 region of the hippocampus (**a**, **b**) and layer III of cerebral cortex (**c**, **d**). Scale bar = 0.5 μm

dissociated cultures, neurons were mixed with astrocytes; the nuclei of the two cell types can be identified by their distinct ultrastructure [11]. For all three experimental systems, every neuronal soma encountered was photographed at 4–10,000× to document chromatin clustering.

The predominant type of astrocytes in slice cultures is "fibrous" (see [11] for classification of types of astrocytes), and every fibrous astroglial nucleus encountered was photographed until at least 10 astroglial nuclei were imaged per slice culture. More than 132 astroglial nuclei were imaged from 11 samples.

Scoring of ER cisternal stacks in neuronal somas

In both slice and dissociated cultures, every soma encountered was scored for presence of ER stacks. An ER cisternal stack is defined as two ER cisterns (marked by asterisks in Fig. 1a) closely apposed with a uniform gap of ~ 13 nm (arrows in Fig. 1a), filled with dense material, and the membranes facing the gap are free of ribosomes. Multiple cisterns closely apposed were sometimes present upon more intense stimuli (Fig. 1b). Every ER cisternal stack encountered, whether it consisted of 2 or more cisterns was counted as one entity in the present study. The frequency of ER stacks for each sample was expressed as total number of ER stacks per 100 neuronal somas.

At least 10 somal profiles were scored for each sample, with ~ 600 somas scored from 30 samples of slice cultures and more then 500 somas scored form 25 samples of dissociated cultures. Neurons that were partially under the grid bar were still included in the sampling as long as at least half of the nucleus was visible. Due to the fact that many neurons were scored with partial profiles, the total number of ER stacks from each sample was pooled from all somas that were scored, and then divided by the number of neurons and normalized as number of SSCs per 100 neuronal somas. This practice ensures that each sample is treated the same, resulting in one data point per sample.

Scoring of mitochondria morphology in neuronal somas

Mitochondria morphology was scored in every neuronal soma encountered. Based on the appearance of the matrix (asterisks in Fig. 2a-c), mitochondria were classified as "not swollen" (Fig. 2a) with a dark matrix, or "swollen" with a light matrix, including slightly swollen (Fig. 2b) and extensively swollen (Fig. 2c) ones. A neuron is classified as containing swollen mitochondria if any of

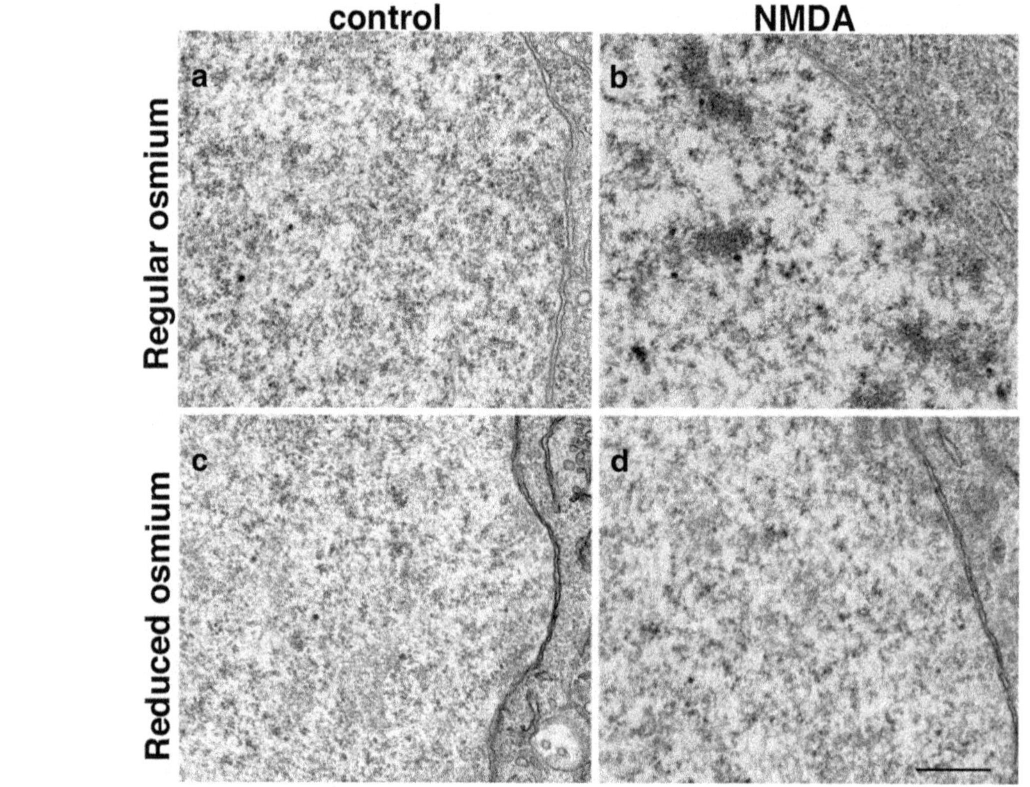

Fig. 5 While neuronal chromatin appear non clustered under control conditions (**a**, **c**), NMDA-induced clustering of dark chromatin was prominent in neuronal nucleus from dissociated hippocampal cultures post-fixed with regular osmium tetroxide (**b**) but far less obvious in samples post-fixed with "reduced osmium" (1% ferrocyanide mixed with 1% osmium tetroxide, (**d**). Samples were sister cultures with the same NMDA treatment and processed in parallel. Scale bar = 0.5 μm

its mitochondria appeared swollen. A percentage of neurons containing swollen mitochondria was calculated for each sample.

Statistical analysis

Comparisons between two groups were tested by Student's t test or paired t test. Comparisons among three groups or more were tested by one-way ANOVA with Tukey's post-test.

Results

Stimulation-induced changes in chromatin configuration in neuronal nucleus

One striking feature of acutely stimulated neurons was the appearance of clusters of dark chromatin in the nuclei. Figure 3 shows the nuclei of neurons and astrocytes in the CA1 region of the hippocampus in organotypic slice cultures. Under control conditions, the nucleoplasm of the pyramidal neurons had a non-clustered appearance at low magnification (Fig. 3a) in all 15 samples examined. Upon depolarization with high K^+ (90 mM), chromatin became clustered as dark aggregates (arrows in Fig. 3) in all 13 samples examined. This clustering of chromatin progressed with treatment time, from a less dense appearance at 30 s (Fig. 3d) to a more condensed form at 2 min (Fig. 3g) of treatment, and with lighter areas interspersed among the dark chromatin clusters. NMDA treatment (50 μM) induced a similar clustering of dark chromatin, which also progressed with treatment time in all 14 samples examined (Additional file 1).

This chromatin reorganization was reversible, as the appearance of the clustered chromatin upon depolarization (Fig. 3e) reverted back to that similar to the control conditions (Fig. 3b) upon cessation of stimulation and recovery in control medium (Fig. 3h). At least 10 min recovery in control medium was needed for the nucleus to revert back to its non-clustered appearance after a 3 min high K^+ treatment. In another experiment, at 5 min recovery after a 1 min high K+ treatment, the chromatin was still somewhat clustered. This

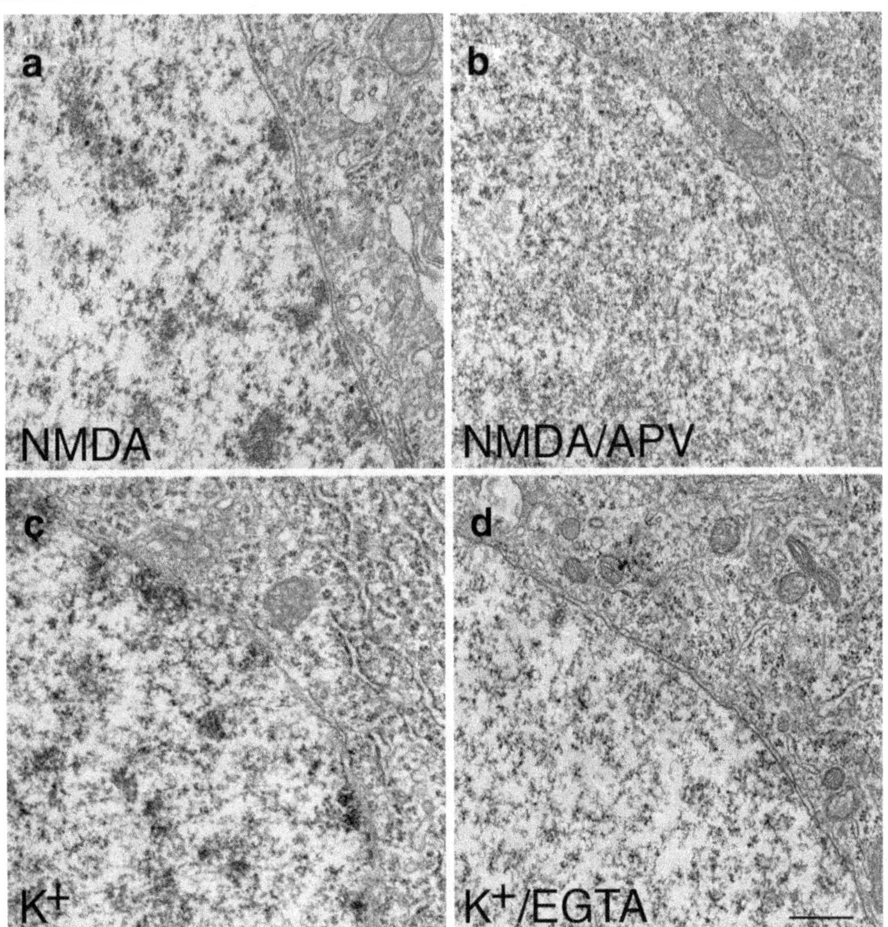

Fig. 6 Stimulation-induced clustering of chromatin is calcium-dependent. In dissociated hippocampal cultures, the NMDA-induced clustering of chromatin (**a**) was blocked by APV (**b**). The depolarization-induced clustering of chromatin (**c**) was blocked by chelation of extracellular calcium with EGTA (**d**). Scale bar = 0.5 μm

stimulation-induced clustering of chromatin is specific to neurons, as astroglial nuclei (Fig. 3c, f, j) from the same slice cultures did not show similar chromatin clustering upon depolarization (consistent in 4 experiments; Additional file 2).

This stimulation-induced chromatin clustering was also observed in other experimental systems. In fast perfusion-fixed mouse or rat brains, where neurons are presumed to be under basal conditions [4], the nuclei of neurons in 13 animals had a non-clustered appearance (Fig. 4a, c), consistent with images shown in a classic neurocytology atlas [11] where brains were optimally perfusion-fixed. In contrast, in 7 delayed perfusion-fixed brains, where neurons were under hypoxic excitatory stress [4], chromatin became aggregated as dark clusters (Fig. 4b, d) in different regions of the brain, including pyramidal neurons in the CA1 region and granules cells of the dentate gyrus of the hippocampus, pyramidal neurons in layer III of the cerebral cortex, and Purkinje cells of the cerebellum.

Likewise, in dissociated hippocampal neuronal cultures, neuronal nuclei had a non-clustered appearance under control conditions (Fig. 5a) in all 18 samples examined, but the chromatin consistently became clustered upon treatment with high K^+ (11 samples; Additional file 1) or with NMDA (8 samples; Fig. 5b). Thus, in all three experimental systems studied here, this clustering of dark chromatin in neuronal nucleus is a reliable indicator that neurons are under heightened excitatory conditions.

Interestingly, this stimulation-induced clustering of the chromatin was readily detectible only when samples were stained with regular osmium tetroxide treatment (Fig. 5b), but much less noticeable with "reduced osmium" treatment (Fig. 5d; [12]) where osmium tetroxide was mixed with potassium ferrocyanide, indicating that the clustered chromatin or its associated histones was selectively stained upon regular osmium treatment but not upon "reduced osmium" treatment. Thus, absence of chromatin clustering in samples stained with "reduced osmium" is not an indication that neurons are at a basal state.

The nuclear chromatin clustering induced by NMDA (Fig. 6a) in these dissociated hippocampal neurons was blocked by APV (Fig. 6b), an NMDA antagonist (3 exp). Since activation of NMDA receptors triggers calcium influx, the calcium-dependency of chromatin clustering was further tested. When the extracellular calcium was chelated by EGTA, the high K^+-induced nuclear chromatin clustering (Fig. 6c) was indeed blocked (Fig. 6d; 3 exp).

Stimulation-dependent formation of endoplasmic reticulum (ER) cisternal stacks in neuronal cytoplasm

ER cisternal stacks form in cerebellar Purkinje neurons under hypoxia-induced excitatory stress [4, 8]. Here, hippocampal slice cultures were used to determine if similar ER stacks form in forebrain neurons, and to examine the time course and reversibility of the formation of these ER stacks. As seen in Fig. 7a, ER stacks were absent in neurons under control conditions in all 15 samples, but were consistently prevalent in slice cultures treated for at least 2 min with high K^+ (Fig. 7b) in 8 samples, or NMDA (Fig. 7c) in 10 samples. Thus, ER stacks indeed form in hippocampal neurons during heightened stimulation.

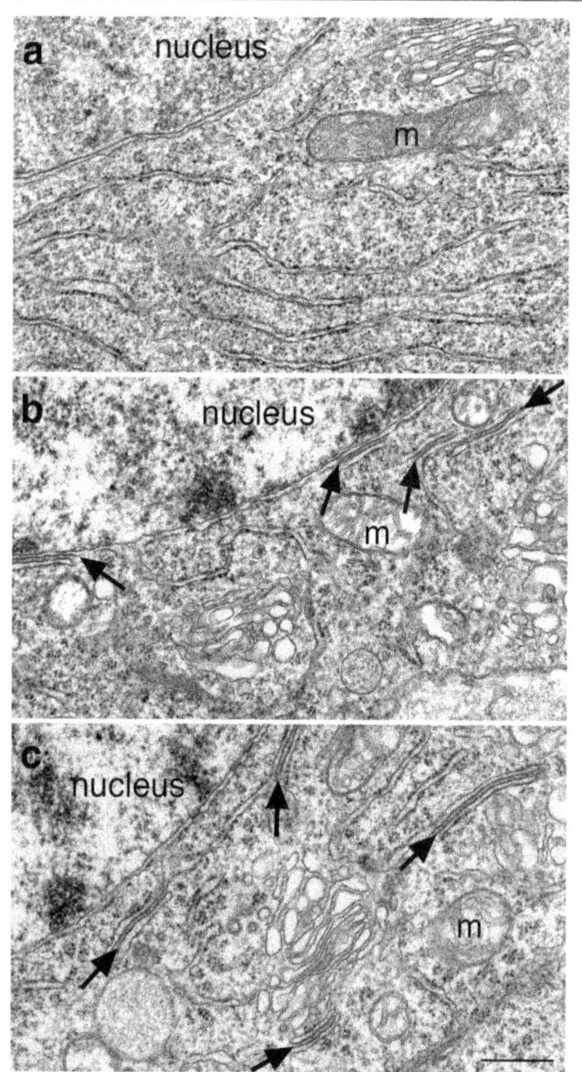

Fig. 7 ER cisternal stacks (arrows in **b**, **c**) were absent in neuronal somas under control conditions (**a**), but appeared upon stimulation, such as depolarization with high K^+ (90 mM, 3 min, **b**) or treatment with NMDA (50 μM, 2 min, **c**). Samples were from the CA1 region of the hippocampal slice cultures. Consistent with Fig. 3, the nuclei of these pyramidal neurons appeared non-clustered under control conditions (**a**), but the chromatin aggregated into dark clusters upon stimulation (**b**, **c**). Additionally, mitochondria (m) appeared swollen upon stimulation (**b**, **c**). Scale bar = 0.5 μm

Table 1 Effect of depolarization with high K^+ on number of ER cisternal stacks in neuronal somas in slice cultures, expressed as number per 100 neuronal somas

Exp	Cont	30″ K^+	1′ K^+	2′ K^+	3′ K^+	5′ K^+	K^+ + 1′ rec	K^+ + 2′ rec	K^+ + 5′ rec	K^+ + 10′ rec	K^+ + 1 h rec
1	0 (23)	14 (21)		241 (22)		659 (17)					
2	0 (21)				376 (21)						
3	0 (14)				167 (21)		305 (21)		20 (15)		
4	0 (22)				327 (22)					0 (27)	0 (24)
5	0 (19)		10 (21)					85 (13)			
6	0 (21)		57 (23)				55 (20)		0 (17)		
Mean ± SEM	0	27 ± 15		278 ± 46					7 ± 7		

Statistical analysis by ANOVA with Tukey's post-test: data points from 30″ and 1′ K^+, 2–3′ K^+, and 5–10′ recovery were pooled, respectively (mean values of each listed in the last row). 2–3′K^+ is highly significant over other conditions ($P < 0.0001$ vs. cont, 30′-1′K^+, 5–10′ rec). Not significant among all other multiple comparisons including cont, 30′-1′K^+ and 5–10′ rec

(n) number of somas examined

rec recovery in control medium

The stimulation-induced formation of ER cisternal stacks in hippocampal slice cultures progressed with treatment time as indicated by exp. 1 in Table 1 and exp. 1 and 2 in Table 3. There were only a few ER stacks at 30 s (0–14 per 100 neurons) to 1 min (6–57 per 100 neurons) of treatment, and ER stacks were more prevalent at 2–3 min (167–688 per 100 neurons). The formation of ER stacks was reversible as indicated by experiments 4 and 6 in Table 1, where ER stacks were no longer observed after the high K^+ medium was washed out and samples were allowed to recover in control medium for the indicated periods of time. As expected, a longer treatment time (3 min in exp. 4 vs. 1 min in exp. 6) required a longer recovery time (10 min in exp. 4 vs. 5 min in exp. 6). Interestingly, as indicated in exp. 3 and 5, ER stack formation did not stop with the cessation of treatment, and ER stacks still continued to form 1–2 min after the washout of high K^+ medium.

The formation of neuronal ER cisternal stacks was stimulation-dependent in all three experimental systems examined here, with identical configuration and gap width (~ 13 nm), in brain (Fig. 8a), in organotypic slice cultures (Fig. 8b), and in dissociated cultures (Fig. 8c). The gap is typically filled with dense materials that sometimes appear with a periodicity [13].

In fast perfusion-fixed brains, no ER cisternal stacks were detected in any brain areas examined including cerebral cortex, hippocampus and cerebellum from one adult rat and twelve mice at ages ranging from 17 days to 3 months. In seven delayed perfusion-fixed rat and mouse brains, ER stacks were especially abundant in cerebellar Purkinje cells from soma to spines, and multiple stacks were common (Fig. 8a inset; [4]). These ER stacks of Purkinje neurons contain high concentrations of inositol 1, 4, 5-triphosphate receptors (IP_3R) [13–15], a protein involved in calcium release from the ER lumen. Here in the present study, structurally identical ER stacks were present in hippocampus and cerebral cortex, but at much lower frequencies than those in Purkinje cells. Additionally, unlike in Purkinje somas, multiple stacks were rarely seen in the forebrain neurons. These observations are consistent with the overwhelmingly high levels of IP_3R in Purkinje cells over other neuronal cell types [15, 16].

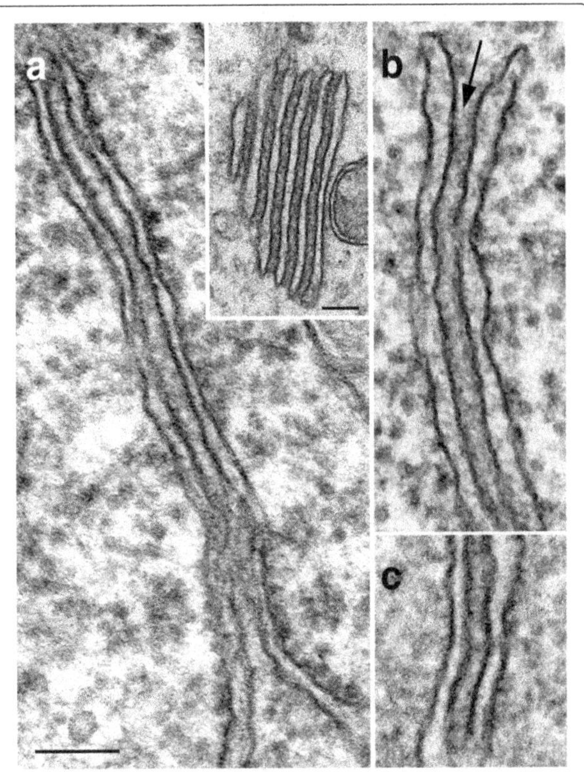

Fig. 8 ER cisternal stacks from different experimental systems display the same configuration and gap width of ~ 13 nm (arrow in **b**). **a** Images from delayed perfusion-fixed brains: pyramidal neuronal soma of the CA1 region of the mouse hippocampus, and Purkinje dendrites of the rat cerebellum (inset in a). **b** Hippocampal slice cultures depolarized with high K^+. **c** Dissociated hippocampal neurons treated with NMDA. Scale bar = 0.1 μm

In dissociated hippocampal neuronal cultures, as in slice cultures, ER cisternal stacks were absent under control conditions, and only present when cells were treated with high K^+ media (Table 2) or with NMDA (exp 3–5 in Table 3). However, upon identical treatment of 2 min of high K^+ or NMDA, neurons in dissociated cultures typically formed fewer ER stacks (12 and 3% for high K^+ or NMDA, respectively) than those in slice cultures. This stimulation-induced formation of ER stacks is calcium-dependent. No ER stacks were present when EGTA was included in the high K^+ medium (exp 5–7 in Table 2).

Notably, whenever ER cisternal stacks were observed in neuronal somas, the nuclei of these neurons always contained clustered chromatin (cf. Fig. 7). Furthermore, ER cisternal stacks were consistently present along with other benchmarks for stimulation-induced structural changes (Fig. 9), including the formation of CaMKII clusters [4, 6, 17] and synaptic spinules [7], as well as an increase in thickness and curvature of PSD [3, 4]. These observations further verified that presence of ER cisternal stacks is a reliable indicator that neurons are under heightened excitatory conditions.

Structural changes of neuronal mitochondria under different conditions

A third stimulation-induced structural change is that mitochondria in neuronal somas became swollen. In hippocampal slice cultures, virtually all mitochondria in neuronal somas appeared swollen upon high K^+ (Figs. 7b, 10c and 11e) or NMDA (Figs. 7c and 11c) treatment. This structural change is specific to neurons as the ultrastructure of mitochondria in astrocytes did not change upon depolarization (Fig. 10b, d).

However, neuronal mitochondria in control samples often also appeared swollen in slice cultures (Fig. 11a) as well as in dissociated cell cultures (Fig. 11d, g). The

Table 2 Effect of depolarization with high K^+ on number of ER cisternal stacks in neuronal somas in dissociated cultures, expressed as number per 100 neuronal somas

Exp	Cont	2′ K^+	3′ K^+	2′K^+/EGTA	3′K^+/EGTA
1	0 (20)	20 (20)			
2	0 (31)	0 (16)			
3	0 (22)	83 (18)			
4	0 (20)	32 (28)	110 (20)		
5	0 (20)	15 (20)		0 (20)	
6	0 (20)	31 (16)	65 (17)		0 (20)
7	0 (20)		74 (23)		0 (20)
Mean ± SEM	0	30 ± 12	83 ± 14		0

Statistical analysis by ANOVA with Tukey's post-test: 3′ K^+ is significant over other conditions ($P < 0.0005$ vs. cont; $P < 0.05$ vs. 2′K^+; $P < 0.005$ vs. 3′ K/EGTA). 2′ K^+ is barely significant over control ($P < 0.1$). Other multiple comparisons are all non-significant

(n) number of somas examined

Table 3 Effect of NMDA treatment on number of ER cisternal stacks in neuronal somas in slice cultures (exp 1–2) as well as in dissociated cultures (exp 3–5), expressed as number per 100 neuronal somas

Slice exp	Cont	30″ NMDA	1′ NMDA	2′ NMDA	3′ NMDA
1	0 (17)	0 (20)	6 (16)	461 (18)	
2	0 (20)	5 (20)	55 (20)	289 (18)	688 (17)
Mean ± SEM	0	2.5 ± 2.5	31 ± 25	375 ± 86	
Cells exp	Cont			2′ NMDA	
3	0 (20)			25 (20)	
4	0 (20)			0 (20)	
5	0 (16)			10 (20)	
Mean ± SEM	0			12 ± 7	

Statistical analysis by ANOVA with Tukey's post-test:

For slice culture experiments, 3′ NMDA is highly significant over other conditions ($P < 0.0001$ vs. cont, 30″NMDA, 1′NMDA; $P < 0.005$ vs. 2′ NMDA). 2′ NMDA is highly significant over other conditions ($P < 0.0001$ vs. cont; $P < 0.0005$ vs. 30′ NMDA, 1′ NMDA). Not significant among all other multiple comparisons including cont, 30″ NMDA and 1′ NMDA

For dissociated cell culture experiments, not significant between control and 2′NMDA

(n) number of somas examined

swollen mitochondria in control samples were only seen in some neurons, and not all mitochondria in the same neuron were swollen to the same degree. For example, mitochondria at different degrees of swelling from control samples were shown in Fig. 11 a and b for slice cultures, and Fig. 11 d and g for dissociated neurons. To test the possibility that these control neurons containing the swollen mitochondria had higher basal level activity, TTX (plus APV and CNQX) was applied to dissociated cell cultures to suppress neuronal activity. Indeed, the great majority of mitochondria in TTX-treated samples were not swollen (Fig. 11h). In two experiments, the percent of cells displaying swollen mitochondria was 50 and 67% for control samples, and 0 and 8% for TTX-treated samples.

Interestingly, while examining the high K^+-treated samples of dissociated cell cultures with or without EGTA, it became apparent that most mitochondria in neuronal somas in the presence of calcium were swollen (Fig. 11e) while those in the presence of EGTA were not (Fig. 11f). In 3 experiments, the average percentages of cells displaying swollen mitochondria in control, high K^+ and high K^+/EGTA samples were 67 ± 11, 92 ± 4 and 0%, respectively. The high K^+/EGTA samples were significantly different from control and high K^+ samples ($P < 0.005$ vs. control; $P < 0.0005$ vs. high K^+; ANOVA with Tukey's post-test). Thus, calcium influx during activity may be crucial in producing swollen mitochondria. In order to test whether the swelling in mitochondria in control samples can also be suppressed by blocking calcium influx, extracellular calcium was eliminated by treating the samples with calcium-free control media containing EGTA for 2 min. Indeed, mitochondria were not swollen (Fig. 11i). Altogether, these observations

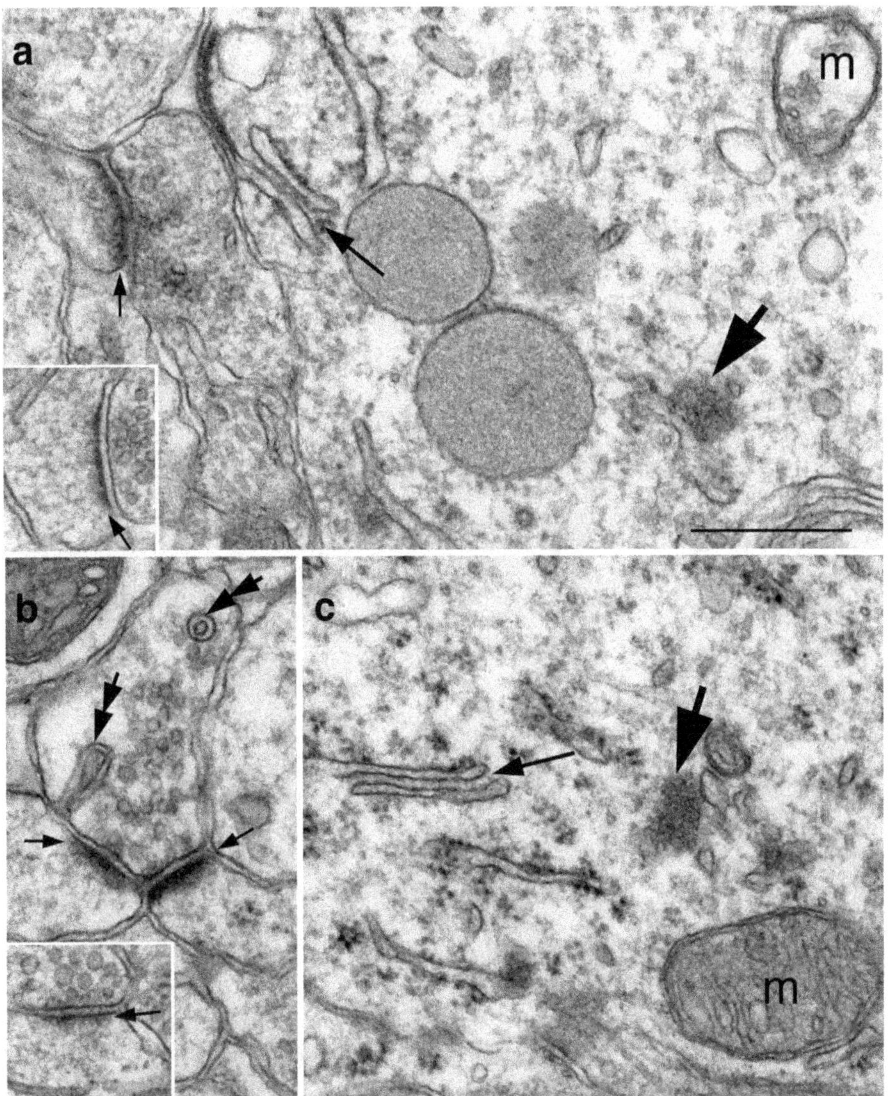

Fig. 9 Images of the CA1 region of the hippocampus from a slice culture treated with 50 μM NMDA for 5 min (**a**), and from a delayed perfusion-fixed mouse brain (**b**, **c**). In addition to ER cisternal stacks (long small arrows), presence of CaMKII clusters (large arrows) and spinules (double arrows in **b**) indicates that these neurons are under heightened excitatory conditions. Furthermore, the thickness of PSD (short small arrows in **a**, **b**) is conspicuously greater than those of the control samples (inset of a is from a sister slice culture under control conditions; inset of b is from an age-matched mouse with fast perfusion-fixation). Mitochondria (m) appeared swollen in (**a**) but not in (**b**). Scale bar = 0.5 μm

suggest that neuronal mitochondria appear to be an extremely sensitive indicator for the activity state of neurons in slice as well as in dissociated cultures, and that the swelling of mitochondria is dependent on calcium influx.

When perfusion-fixed brains from two sets of matched animals were scored for mitochondria morphology, relatively few mitochondria were swollen compared to those of in vitro samples. The great majority of mitochondria were not swollen in fast perfusion-fixed brains (Fig. 11j), and percentages of neurons containing swollen mitochondria were 0 and 7%. In two delayed perfusion-fixed brains, 22 and 33% of neurons contained swollen mitochondria (Fig. 11k) while the majority of mitochondria were not swollen (Fig. 11l). However, swollen mitochondria were consistently seen in poorly perfusion-fixed brains where fixative was not effectively delivered via blood vessels to surrounding tissues, evidenced by presence of blood cells in collapsed vessels.

Discussion

The present study describes three stimulation-induced structural changes in neurons that are easily detectible: clustering of nuclear chromatin, formation of ER cisternal stacks in the cytoplasm, and swelling of mitochondrial matrix. The first two structural benchmarks are unequivocal and useful indicators that neurons are

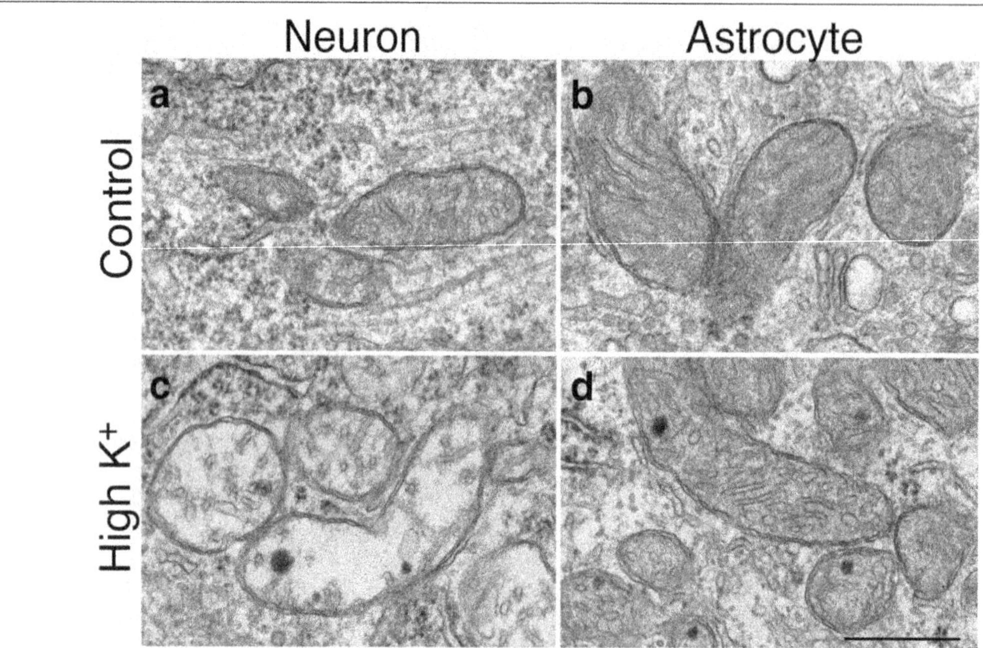

Fig. 10 Mitochondria in neuronal somas became swollen upon depolarization (**c** vs. **a**; **c** was treated with 90 mM K^+ for 3 min), while mitochondria in astrocytes displayed similar features under control conditions (**b**) or upon depolarization (**d**). Images of neurons and astrocytes were collected from the same samples of hippocampal slice cultures. Scale bar = 0.5 μm

under heightened excitatory conditions, while the swollen mitochondria could be induced by basal levels of activity. Excitatory conditions can be produced inadvertently during experimental manipulations such as transfer and mechanical handling of cell cultures. This consideration is especially important when interpreting results from perfusion-fixed brains, where the procedure of perfusion itself, if not performed well, may introduce ischemic stress, and possibly induce excitotoxicity [4].

Physiological consequences of the described stimulation-induced structural changes are at present largely undefined. Structural changes in chromatin have been linked to development and activity [18, 19], including long-term potentiation [20]. Additionally, upon 20 min of transient global ischemia, neuronal nuclei displayed chromatin clustering, which is reversed 3 h after reperfusion [21]. Of particular interest is the resemblance of the nuclear structural change induced by ischemia to the acute stimulation-induced chromatin clustering presented here. Although the earliest time point was set at 20 min after ischemia [21], chromatin clustering may have started sooner. Indeed, it is shown here that a delay of a few minutes in perfusion fixation that mimics ischemia [4] induced chromatin clustering in neuronal nuclei. Furthermore, in hippocampal slice cultures, 30 s of stimulation already induced chromatin clustering. Activity-dependent movement of postsynaptic proteins into the nucleus may trigger changes in gene expression [22, 23]. However, signaling via transport of synaptic proteins seems too slow to explain the current results. A more likely candidate to mediate such a rapid, activity-dependent nuclear response is calcium signaling. One consequence of depolarization and NMDA receptor activation is a rapid rise in intracellular calcium concentration, which is easily equilibrated across the nuclear membrane, and can trigger calcium-dependent transcriptional regulation in the nucleus [22, 24]. Indeed, the present study demonstrated that the stimulation-induced chromatin clustering in the neuronal nucleus is calcium-dependent. It is generally assumed that dark chromatin is transcriptionally inactive while loosely arranged chromatin in the lighter space of the nucleus may be transcriptionally active [18]. Accordingly, the stimulation-induced clustering of dark chromatin presented here may cause certain genes to become less accessible for transcription.

A second stimulation-induced structural benchmark presented here is the ER cisternal stacks. In Purkinje cells, ER stacks contain high concentrations of IP_3R on the side of the ER membranes that face the narrow gap, while the side of the ER membranes that face the cytoplasm have low levels of IP_3R [13, 15]. Interestingly, the uniform gap of the ER stack is filled with dark material, suggesting that protein interactions may tether the two membranes, potentially restricting the diffusion of molecules between the gap and the cytoplasm. Since IP_3R are involved in IP_3-induced calcium release from the ER to the cytoplasm,

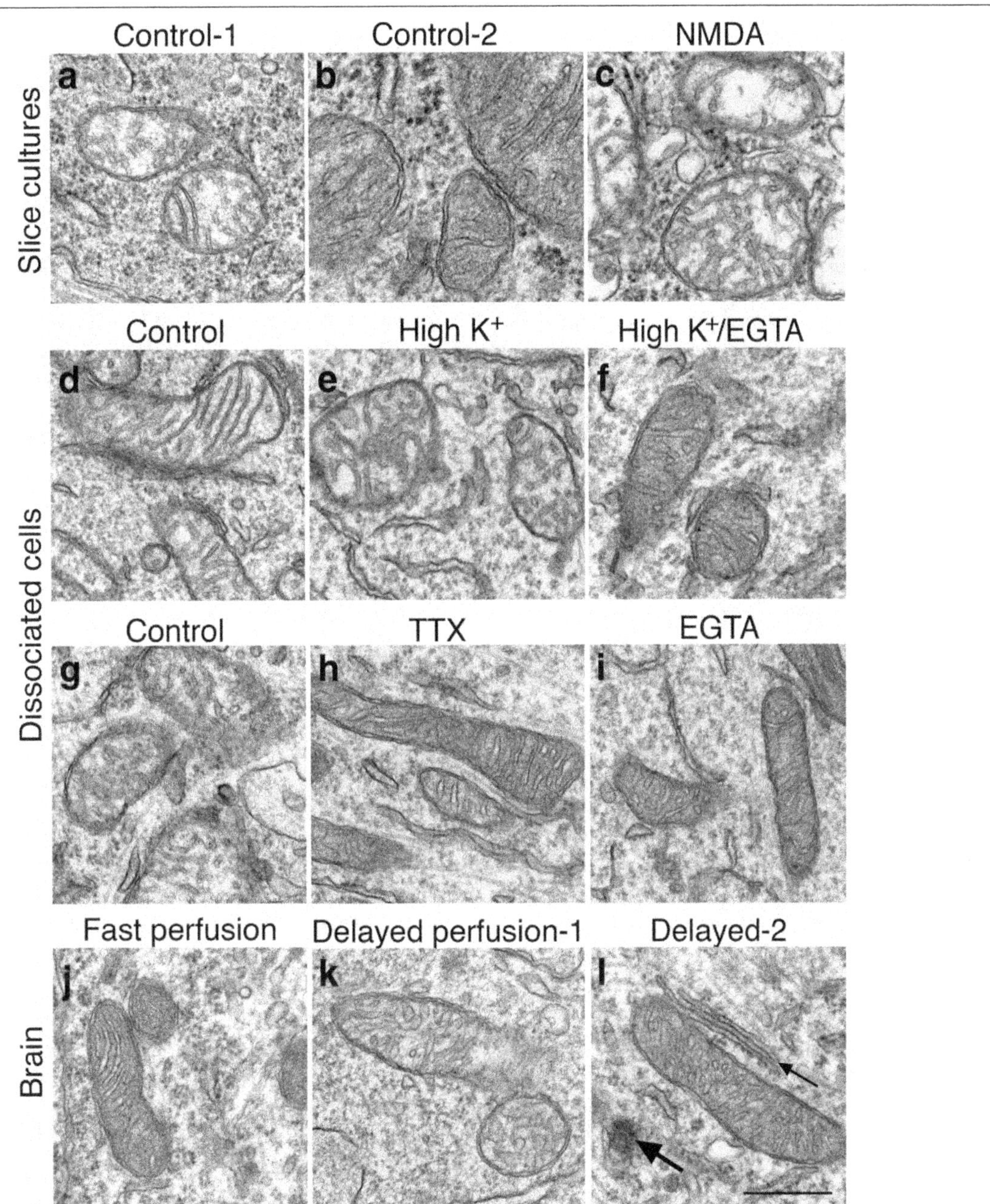

Fig. 11 Structural change of mitochondria in three experimental systems under different conditions. In hippocampal slice cultures, mitochondria in control samples could appear swollen (**a**) or not (**b**) while those in NMDA-treated samples were consistently swollen (**c**). In dissociated hippocampal cell cultures, 55–90% of neurons contained swollen mitochondria in control samples (**d**). Upon 2–3 min depolarization with high K^+, 87–100% neurons contain swollen mitochondria (**e**). When EGTA, a calcium chelator, is included in the high K^+ medium, mitochondria were not swollen (**f**). When dissociated cell cultures were incubated for 1 h with or without TTX, 50–67% of neurons contained swollen mitochondria in control samples (**g**) while the great majority (more than 90%) of mitochondria in TTX-treated samples were not swollen (**h**). Washing control samples with EGTA for 2 min also prevented mitochondria from swelling (**i**). In perfusion-fixed mouse brains, the great majority of mitochondria in fast perfusion-fixed brains were not swollen (**j**), while some swollen mitochondria were seen in delayed perfusion-fixed brains (**k**). However, many mitochondria in delayed-fixed brains were not swollen (**l**), and co-existed with CaMKII clusters (large arrow in l) and ER cisternal stacks (small arrows in l), two structural benchmarks indicating that this neuron was under hypoxic excitatory stress. Scale bar = 0.5 μm

formation of ER stacks that localizes IP_3R in this pattern may restrict the receptor's accessibility to cytosolic IP_3, thereby reducing calcium release into the cytoplasm. Importantly, the stimulation-induced formation of ER stacks is calcium-dependent and progresses with treatment time, correlating with a rise in intracellular calcium concentration. Thus, formation of ER stacks could prevent further calcium overload during heightened stimulation by restricting calcium release from ER to the cytoplasm.

These stimulation-induced ER stacks resemble another ER structural specialization, termed lamellar bodies [25, 26]. Both structures are composed of stacks of ER with a uniform gap between stacks, and lack ribosomes in the membranes facing the gaps. However, the two structures display different spacing: the gap width is ~ 13 nm for the ER stacks, and 30 nm for the lamellar bodies in adult animals [25, 26] (Additional file 3). This difference in gap width suggests that different proteins may be present in the gaps tethering the membranes of these two structural specializations of the ER. Additionally, the ER cisterns in lamellar bodies can become flattened while those in ER stacks never do. Furthermore, lamellar bodies are present in control samples (Additional file 3) while ER stacks are not.

The time course of formation and recovery of the two stimulation-induced structural change reported here are different in slice cultures. Chromatin clustering was consistently apparent at 30 s of stimulation while the formation of ER stacks typically needed a minute or more to become readily detectible. On the other hand, the recovery of ER stacks was faster than the chromatin clustering. For example, upon 5 min of recovery following 1 min of high K^+ treatment, ER stacks were no longer present while nuclear chromatin clustering still partially remained. Thus, these two calcium-dependent structural changes respond differently to the rise and fall of calcium, and the formation of ER stacks probably requires a higher threshold of calcium concentration.

A third finding here is that neuronal mitochondria from in vitro samples became swollen upon stimulation, consistent with a report on calcium-dependent mitochondria changes upon excitotoxic NMDA treatment [9]. However, neurons in control samples also contained a noticeable number of swollen mitochondria which could be blocked by suppressing basal activity or by eliminating calcium influx. Thus, neuronal mitochondria in tissue culture systems are very sensitive to basal activity and calcium entry. Very few swollen mitochondria were seen in fast perfusion-fixed brains. It is possible that the neurons in deeply anesthetized animals had lower activity than control neurons in tissue culture. Surprisingly, even in delayed perfusion-fixed brains where neurons were under hypoxic excitatory stress, only ~ 30% of neurons contained swollen mitochondria, in contrast to the > 90% of neurons with swollen mitochondria in the stimulated in vitro samples. Considering that the delay in perfusion was 5–8 min, a time that is longer than the 2–3 min treatment time for the in vitro samples, it is possible that the calcium regulation and its effects on mitochondria are different at these different time points. Alternatively, an ischemia-like stress in brain could produce different effects on mitochondria than the heightened stimulations applied to neurons in culture. It is also possible that mitochondria in neurons maintained in vitro are more vulnerable to activity-induced swelling. Notably, in poorly perfusion-fixed brains where fixative was not effectively delivered to surrounding tissues, all neuronal mitochondria were swollen. Neurons in these samples likely underwent a longer period of hypoxic stress before they were fixed. This finding is consistent with the report that mitochondria were swollen after 30 min of ischemia [27].

The stimulation-induced structural changes presented here consistently co-existed with other structural benchmarks including CAMKII clusters, synaptic spinules, and increase in thickness and curvature of the PSD, that are induced by neuronal activity [3, 4, 7]. Interestingly, the formation of many of these stimulation-induced structural changes is calcium-dependent [6, 28] and may also offer protection against calcium overload during heightened activity. For example, stimulation-induced formation of CaMKII clusters with tightly bound molecules may limit the access of this enzyme to substrate [17], and a decrease in ER and plasma membrane contact area may limit calcium influx during intense activity [5]. The present study added two more reliable structural benchmarks, chromatin clustering and ER cisternal stacks, that are induced by stimulation in forebrain neurons. The present study also demonstrated that the morphology of mitochondria from neurons in tissue culture is affected by basal level of activity and calcium influx. These stimulation-induced structural changes may provide new insights into the neuron's response to intracellular calcium rise.

Additional files

Additional file 1: Neural chromatin clustering upon stimulation. (PDF 2492 kb)

Additional file 2: Chromatin clustered upon depolarization in neurons but not in astrocytes. (PDF 5705 kb)

Additional file 3: Structural differences between ER lamellar bodies and ER cisternal stacks. (PDF 3994 kb)

Acknowledgements

I thank Rita Azzam, Virginia Crocker and Sandra Lara for expert EM technical support, Christine A Winters for hippocampal dissociated and organotypic cultures, Drs. Paul Gallant and Milton Brightman for perfusion fixation, Drs. Ayse Dosemeci and Paul Gallant for helpful discussions and critical reading of the manuscript, and the reviewers for in depth comments to improve this manuscript.

Funding

Supported by National Institute of Neurological Disorders and Stroke (NINDS) intramural funds.

Author's contributions

This is a solo author manuscript. The author read and approved the final manuscript.

Competing interests

The author declares that she has no competing interests.

References

1. Heuser JE, Reese TS. Evidence for recycling of synaptic vesicle membrane during transmitter release at the frog neuromuscular junction. J Cell Biol. 1973;57:315–44.
2. Watanabe S, Rost BR, Camacho-Pérez M, Davis MW, Söhl-Kielczynski B, Rosenmund C, Jorgensen EM. Ultrafast endocytosis at mouse hippocampal synapses. Nature. 2013;504:242–7.
3. Dosemeci A, Tao-Cheng J-H, Vinade L, Winters CA, Pozzo-Miller L, Reese TS. Glutamate-induced transient modification of the postsynaptic density. PNAS. 2001;98:10428–32.
4. Tao-Cheng J-H, Gallant PE, Brightman MW, Dosemeci A, Reese TS. Effects of delayed perfusion fixation on postsynaptic density and CaMKII clustering in different regions of the mouse brain. J Comp Neurol. 2007;501:731–40.
5. Tao-Cheng J-H. Activity-dependently structural decrease of contact area between subsurface cisterns and plasma membrane in hippocampal neurons. Mol Brain. 2018;11:23.
6. Tao-Cheng J-H, Vinade L, Smith C, Winters CA, Ward R, Brightman MW, Reese TS, Dosemeci A. Sustained elevation of calcium induces ca^{2+}/calmodulin-dependent protein kinase II clusters in neurons. Neuroscience. 2001;106:69–78.
7. Tao-Cheng J-H, Dosemeci A, Gallant PE, Miller S, Galbraith JA, Winters CA, Azzam R, Reese TS. Rapid turnover of spinules at synaptic terminals. Neuroscience. 2009;160:42–50.
8. Takei K, Mignery GA, Mugnaini E, Sudhof TC, De Camilli P. Inositol 1,4,5-trisphosphate receptor causes formation of ER cisternal stacks in transfected fibroblasts and in cerebellar Purkinje cells. Neuron. 1994;12:327–42.
9. Pivovarova NB, Nguyen HV, Winters CA, Brantner CA, Smith CL, Andrews SB. Excitotoxic calcium overload in a subpopulation of mitochondria triggers delayed death in hippocampal neurons. J Neurosci. 2004;24:5611–22.
10. Nichols M, Elustondo PA, Warford J, Thirumaran A, Pavlov EV, Robertson GS. Global ablation of the mitochondrial calcium uniporter increases glycolysis in cortical neurons subjected to energetic stressors. J Cereb Blood Flow Metab. 2017;37:3027–41.
11. Peters A, Palay SL, Webster HD. The fine structure of the nervous system. New York: Oxford University Press; 1991.
12. Wittmann M, Queisser G, Eder A, Wiegert JS, Bengtson CP, Hellwig A, Wittum G, Bading H. Synaptic activity induces dramatic changes in the geometry of the cell nucleus: interplay between nuclear structure, histone H3 phosphorylation, and nuclear calcium signaling. J Neurosci. 2009;29:14687–700.
13. Takei K, Stukenbrok H, Metcalf A, Mignery GA, Südhof TC, Volpe P, De Camilli P. Ca2+ stores in Purkinje neurons: endoplasmic reticulum subcompartments demonstrated by the heterogeneous distribution of the InsP3 receptor, ca(2+)-ATPase, and calsequestrin. J Neurosci. 1992;12:489–505.
14. Mignery GA, Südhof TC, Takei K, De Camilli P. Putative receptor for inositol 1,4,5-trisphosphate similar to ryanodine receptor. Nature. 1989;342:192–5.
15. Satoh T, Ross CA, Villa A, Supattapone S, Pozzan T, Snyder SH, Meldolesi J. The inositol 1,4,5,-trisphosphate receptor in cerebellar Purkinje cells: quantitative immunogold labeling reveals concentration in an ER subcompartment. J Cell Biol. 1990;111:615–24.
16. Sharp AH, McPherson PS, Dawson TM, Aoki C, Campbell KP, Snyder SH. Differential immunohistochemical localization of inositol 1,4,5-trisphosphate- and ryanodine-sensitive Ca2+ release channels in rat brain. J Neurosci. 1993;13:3051–63.
17. Dosemeci A, Reese TS, Petersen J, Tao-Cheng JH. A novel particulate form of ca(2+)/calmodulin-dependent protein kinase II in neurons. J Neurosci. 2000;20:3076–84.
18. Wilczynski GM. Significance of higher-order chromatin architecture for neuronal function and dysfunction. Neuropharmacology. 2014;80:28–33.
19. Medrano-Fernández A, Barco A. Nuclear organization and 3D chromatin architecture in cognition and neuropsychiatric disorders. Mol Brain. 2016;9:83.
20. Billia F, Baskys A, Carlen PL, De Boni U. Rearrangement of centromeric satellite DNA in hippocampal neurons exhibiting long-term potentiation. Brain Res Mol Brain Res. 1992;14:101–8.
21. Zhu L, Wang L, Ju F, Khan A, Cheng X, Zhang S. Reversible recovery of neuronal structures depends on the degree of neuronal damage after global cerebral ischemia in mice. Exp Neurol. 2017;289:1–8.
22. Lim AF, Lim WL, Ch'ng TH. Activity-dependent synapse to nucleus signaling. Neurobiol Learn Mem. 2017;138:78–84.
23. Herbst WA, Martin KC. Regulated transport of signaling proteins from synapse to nucleus. Curr Opin Neurobiol. 2017;45:78–84.
24. Hagenston AM, Bading H. Calcium signaling in synapse-to-nucleus communication. Cold Spring Harb Perspect Biol. 2011;3:a004564.
25. Le Beux YJ. Subsurface cisterns and lamellar bodies: particular forms of the endoplasmic reticulum in the neurons. Z Zellforsch Mikrosk Anat. 1972;133:327–52.
26. Synapseweb. https://synapseweb.clm.utexas.edu/112-endoplasmic-reticulum-6.
27. Ganesana M, Venton BJ. Early changes in transient adenosine during cerebral ischemia and reperfusion injury. PLoS One. 2018;13:e0196932.
28. Tao-Cheng JH, Dosemeci A, Gallant PE, Smith C, Reese T. Activity induced changes in the distribution of shanks at hippocampal synapses. Neuroscience. 2010;168:11–7.

10

Hippocampal calpain is required for the consolidation and reconsolidation but not extinction of contextual fear memory

Taikai Nagayoshi[1†], Kiichiro Isoda[1†], Nori Mamiya[1] and Satoshi Kida[1,2*]

Abstract

Memory consolidation, reconsolidation, and extinction have been shown to share similar molecular signatures, including new gene expression. Calpain is a Ca^{2+}-dependent protease that exerts its effects through the proteolytic cleavage of target proteins. Neuron-specific conditional deletions of calpain 1 and 2 impair long-term potentiation in the hippocampus and spatial learning. Moreover, recent studies have suggested distinct roles of calpain 1 and 2 in synaptic plasticity. However, the role of hippocampal calpain in memory processes, especially memory consolidation, reconsolidation, and extinction, is still unclear. In the current study, we demonstrated the critical roles of hippocampal calpain in the consolidation, reconsolidation, and extinction of contextual fear memory in mice. We examined the effects of pharmacological inhibition of calpain in the hippocampus on these memory processes, using the N-Acetyl-Leu-Leu-norleucinal (ALLN; calpain 1 and 2 inhibitor). Microinfusion of ALLN into the dorsal hippocampus impaired long-term memory (24 h memory) without affecting short-term memory (2 h memory). Similarly, this pharmacological blockade of calpain in the dorsal hippocampus also disrupted reactivated memory but did not affect memory extinction. Importantly, the systemic administration of ALLN inhibited the induction of c-fos in the hippocampus, which is observed when memory is consolidated. Our observations showed that hippocampal calpain is required for the consolidation and reconsolidation of contextual fear memory. Further, the results suggested that calpain contributes to the regulation of new gene expression that is necessary for these memory processes as a regulator of Ca^{2+}-signal transduction pathway.

Keywords: Calpain, Hippocampus, Fear conditioning, ALLN, c-fos

Introduction

Short-term memory (STM) is labile. The generation of stable long-term memory (LTM) requires the stabilization of a memory via a process known as memory consolidation [1–3]. The consolidated memory returns to the labile state following the retrieval and is re-stabilized through reconsolidation, which is a similar process to consolidation [4–7]. Conversely, the continuous or repeated retrieval of a conditioned fear memory initiates memory extinction, inhibiting fear responses [8–11]. The most common and critical biochemical signature of consolidation, reconsolidation, and extinction is the requirement for new gene expression [2, 7, 12–15].

* Correspondence: kida@nodai.ac.jp
†Equal contributors
[1]Department of Bioscience, Faculty of Applied Bioscience, Tokyo University of Agriculture, Tokyo, Japan
[2]Core Research for Evolutional Science and Technology, Japan Science and Technology Agency, Saitama, Japan

Previous studies showed that protein degradation is involved in the molecular processes necessary for synaptic plasticity and learning and memory [16–20]. Calpain is a Ca^{2+}-dependent cysteine protease involved in Ca^{2+} signaling pathway [21, 22]. It specifically cleaves substrates in neurons, including synaptic proteins such as membrane receptors, cytoskeletal proteins, postsynaptic density proproteins, and intracellular mediators, which are critical for synaptic function, and learning and memory [23–31]. Therefore, calpains have been known to contribute to neuronal processes, such as excitability, neurotransmitter release, synaptic plasticity, signal transduction, vesicular trafficking, structural stabilization, and gene transcription [32–34]. For instance, calpain specifically cleaves NMDA receptor 2B subunits (GluN2B), and p35, the neuronal-specific activator of cyclin-dependent kinase 5 (Cdk5) [25, 32, 35, 36], both of which play critical roles in learning and memory [37–40]. Calpain proteolysis targets the C-terminal of GluN2B, potentially changing the level of NMDA receptors and its activity at synapses [26]. Activated calpain cleaves the Cdk5 activator p35 in the N-terminal domains [41], generating a C-terminal-truncated product, i.e., p25, which plays critical roles in hippocampus-dependent memory [42, 43]. Importantly, neuron-specific conditional deletions of calpain 1 and 2 reduces dendritic branching complexity and spine density of hippocampal CA1 pyramidal neurons, which in turn impairs long-term potentiation (LTP) in the hippocampus and spatial learning [44]. Moreover, recent studies suggested that calpain 1 and 2 play distinct roles in synaptic plasticity [45]. However, the role of hippocampal calpain in memory processes, such as memory encoding, consolidation, reconsolidation, and extinction, remains unclear.

A contextual fear memory is an associative memory of a context with conditioned fear arising from a stimulus or event, such as an electric footshock. Memory consolidation and reconsolidation, but not extinction, of contextual fear requires the activation of gene expression in the hippocampus [13, 46–49]. In the present study, we clarified the role of hippocampal calpain in memory processes of contextual fear in mice. We analyzed the effects of the pharmacological inhibition of hippocampal calpain on memory consolidation, reconsolidation, and extinction of contextual fear. Further, since previous studies have suggested sex differences in molecular processes of learning and memory [50, 51], we also separately compared the role of calpains in female and male mice.

Results

Hippocampal calpain is required for the consolidation of contextual fear memory

The hippocampus plays a crucial role in contextual fear conditioning and consolidation of this memory [46, 52–54]. To understand the role of calpain in memory formation, we investigated whether hippocampal calpain was required for the LTM of contextual fear. Importantly, the effects of a calpain inhibitor was separately examined in male and female mice, since recent studies suggested that sex differences are critical modulators of memory performance [50, 51]. The female mice were trained with a single footshock and tested 24 h later. They received a microinfusion of the calpain 1 and 2 inhibitor N-Acetyl-Leu-Leu-norleucinal (ALLN; low-dose, 0.2 μg/side; middle-dose, 1 μg/side; high-dose, 2 μg/side), or vehicle (VEH) into the dorsal hippocampus immediately after the training. A one-way analysis of variance (ANOVA) revealed a significant effect of drug ($F(3,73) = 5.931$, $p < 0.05$; Fig. 1a). Post hoc Newman-Keuls analysis revealed that mice treated with ALLN froze significantly less than VEH-treated mice in a dose-dependent manner (low-dose, $p > 0.05$; middle-dose, $p > 0.05$; high-dose, $p < 0.05$; Fig. 1a). Similarly, male mice treated with ALLN showed significantly less freezing compared to VEH-treated mice (one-way ANOVA, $F(1,23) = 5.731$, $p < 0.05$; Post hoc Newman-Keuls, $p < 0.05$; Fig. 1b). These observations indicated that the microinfusion of ALLN into the dorsal hippocampus impaired LTM of contextual fear.

Next, we examined the effect of an ALLN microinfusion on STM (2 h memory). The experiment was similar to that outlined in Fig. 1a and b, except that the mice were tested at 2 h after the training. A one-way ANOVA revealed no significant effect of drug (female, $F(1,19) = 0.019$, $p > 0.05$; male, $F(1,18) = 0.287$, $p > 0.05$; Fig. 1c and d). This observation indicated that female and male mice treated with ALLN showed normal STM. Taken together, these results demonstrated that the inhibition of hippocampal calpain by ALLN infusion impaired LTM formation of contextual fear, without affecting STM. In addition, the effects of sex differences of memory performance were not observed. Our observations suggested that hippocampal calpain is required for the consolidation of contextual fear memory.

Hippocampal calpain is required for the reconsolidation of contextual fear memory

Reconsolidation involves similar molecular processes to consolidation [4–7, 13, 48]. Importantly, similarly to consolidation, reconsolidation of contextual fear memory depends on new gene expression in the hippocampus [13, 48, 55, 56]. Therefore, it is possible that hippocampal calpain is required for the reconsolidation of contextual fear memory. Next, we examined whether inhibition of hippocampal calpain affected the reconsolidation of contextual fear. Mice were trained, and re-exposed to the training context for 3 min (re-exposure) 24 h later. Reactivated fear memory was tested at 24 h after re-exposure (test). As illustrated in Fig. 1, the mice received a microinfusion of ALLN (2 μg/side) or VEH into the dorsal hippocampus immediately after the re-exposure. A two-way ANOVA revealed significant effects of drug (VEH vs. ALLN; female, $F(1,46) = 7.201$, $p < 0.05$; male, $F(1,40) = 8.179$, $p < 0.05$) and time (re-exposure vs. test; female, $F(1,46) = 4.796$, $p < 0.05$; male, $F(1,40) = 7.139$, $p < 0.05$), and a drug × time interaction (female, $F(1,46) = 6.064$, $p < 0.05$; male, $F(1,40) = 4.39$, $p < 0.05$; Fig. 2a and b). Post hoc Newman-Keuls analysis revealed that, during the test, ALLN-treated female and male mice froze significantly less than VEH-treated female and male mice, respectively (female, $p < 0.05$; male, $p < 0.05$; Fig. 2a and b). These results indicated that the inhibition of hippocampal calpain disrupted the reactivated contextual fear memory, which suggested that

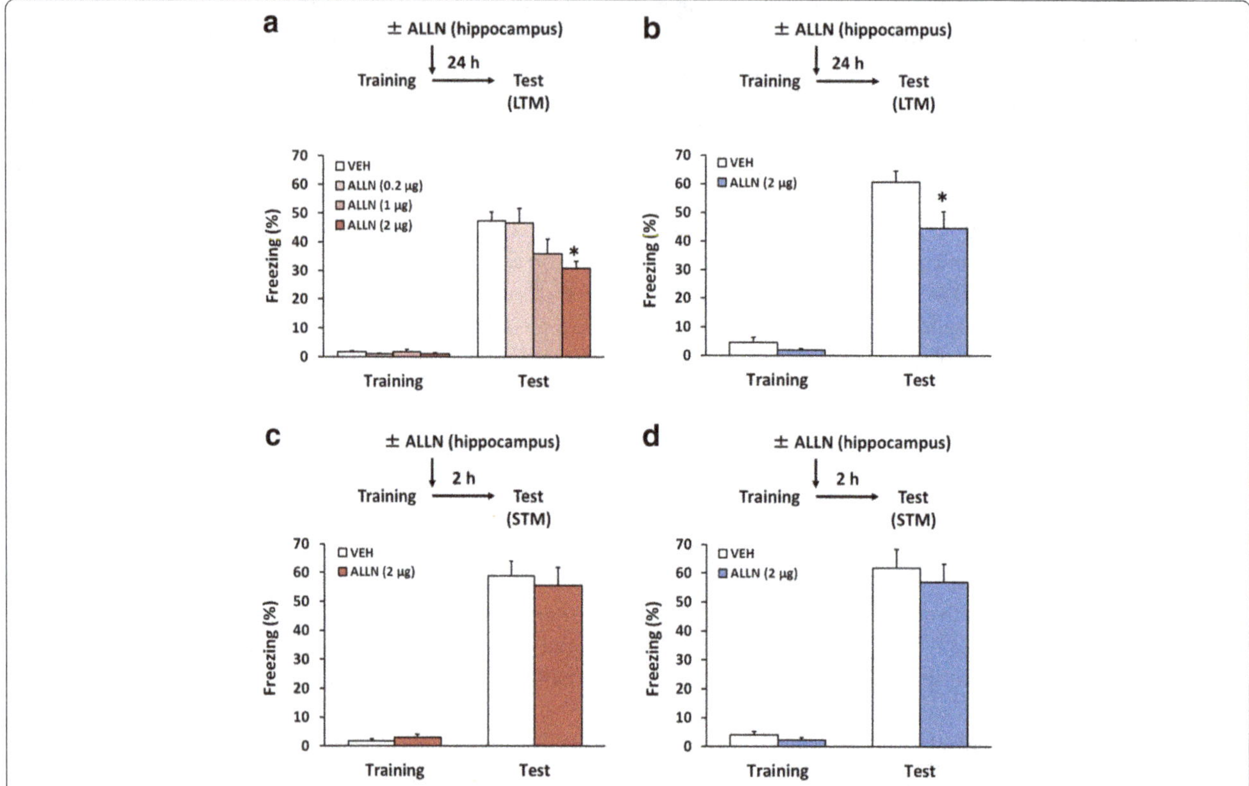

Fig. 1 Inhibition of hippocampal calpain blocks the consolidation of contextual fear memory. **a** and **b** Effects of a microinfusion of a low-, middle-, or high-dose of N-Acetyl-Leu-Leu-norleucinal (ALLN) into the dorsal hippocampus immediately after the training on LTM in female (**a**) or male (**b**) mice (**a**: VEH, $n = 28$; ALLN 0.2 μg, $n = 14$; ALLN 1 μg, $n = 10$; ALLN 2 μg, $n = 25$; **b**: VEH, $n = 14$; ALLN, $n = 11$). **c** and **d** Effects of a microinfusion of ALLN into the dorsal hippocampus immediately after the training on STM in female (**c**) or male (**d**) mice (c: VEH, $n = 11$; ALLN, $n = 10$; d: VEH, $n = 10$; ALLN, $n = 10$). *$p < 0.05$, compared with the VEH group at the test. Error bars indicate standerd error of mean (SEM)

hippocampal calpain is required for the reconsolidation of contextual fear memory.

Hippocampal calpain is not required for the extinction of contextual fear memory

Since the long-term extinction of contextual fear memory requires new gene expression, it shows similar molecular signatures as consolidation and reconsolidation [15, 48, 57]. However, a previous study showed that the extinction of contextual fear memory requires gene expression in the amygdala and mPFC, but not the hippocampus [48], suggesting that the hippocampus shows distinct impacts on consolidation/reconsolidation and extinction. Therefore, we attempted to further clarify the role of hippocampal calpain in the extinction of contextual fear memory. The mice were trained, and 24 h later were re-exposed to the training context for 30 min. Long-term extinction was tested at 24 h after the re-exposure. The mice received a microinfusion of ALLN (2 μg/side) or VEH into the dorsal hippocampus at 10 min before (Fig. 3a and b) or immediately after (Fig. 3c and d) the re-exposure. Mice in the VEH and ALLN groups showed decreased freezing levels, over time with re-exposure (pre-re-exposure infusion: female, $F(5,120) = 23.272$, $p < 0.05$; male, $F(5,95) = 27.700$, $p < 0.05$; post-re-exposure infusion: female, $F(5,130) = 60.161$, $p < 0.05$; male, $F(5,95) = 49.793$, $p < 0.05$; Fig. 3a–d). Further, overall freezing levels did not significantly differ during re-exposure (pre-re-exposure infusion: female, $F(1,24) = 0.391$, $p > 0.05$; male, $F(1,19) = 1.467$, $p > 0.05$; post-re-exposure infusion: female, $F(1,26) = 0.001$, $p > 0.05$; male, $F(1,19) = 0.514$, $p > 0.05$; Fig. 3a–d). These results indicated that the VEH and ALLN groups displayed comparable within-session extinction. Importantly, observations from the pre-re-exposure group suggested that the inhibition of hippocampal calpain did not affect within-session extinction. A two-way ANOVA comparing the freezing scores during the last 5 min in the re-exposure session and test revealed no significant effect of drug and the drug × time (re-exposure vs. test) interaction (pre-re-exposure infusion: female, drug, $F(1,48) = 0.684$, $p > 0.05$; time, $F(1,48) = 1.542$, $p > 0.05$; interaction, $F(1,48) = 0.039$, $p > 0.05$; male, drug, $F(1,38) = 0.711$, $p > 0.05$; time, $F(1,38) = 2.024$, $p > 0.05$; interaction, $F(1,38) = 0.008$, $p > 0.05$; post-

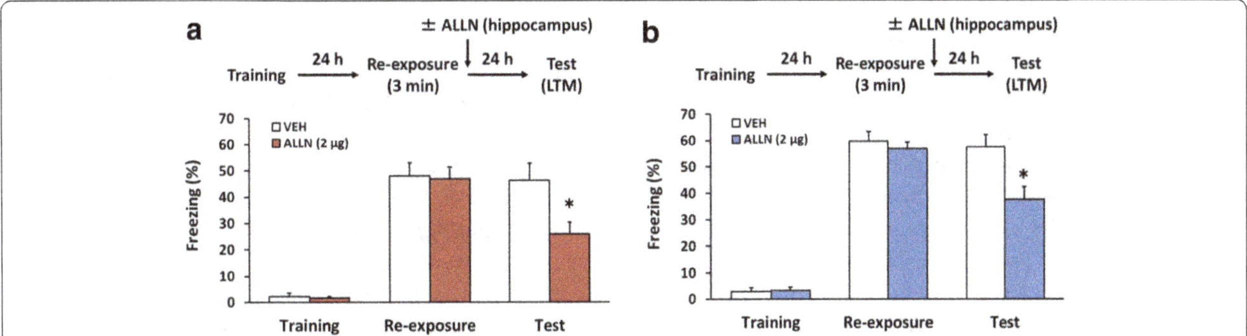

Fig. 2 Inhibition of hippocampal calpain impairs the reconsolidation of contextual fear memory. Effects of a microinfusion of ALLN into the dorsal hippocampus immediately after the 3-min re-exposure on reactivated memory in female (**a**) or male (**b**) mice (**a**: VEH, $n = 10$; ALLN, $n = 15$; **b**: VEH, $n = 10$; ALLN, $n = 12$). *$p < 0.05$, compared with the VEH group at the test. Error bars indicate SEM

re-exposure infusion: female, drug, $F(1,52) = 0.816$, $p > 0.05$; time, $F(1,52) = 5.344$, $p < 0.05$; interaction, $F(1,52) = 0.228$, $p > 0.05$; male, drug, $F(1,38) = 0.005$, $p > 0.05$; time, $F(1,38) = 6.364$, $p < 0.05$; interaction, $F(1,38) = 0.296$, $p > 0.05$; Fig. 3a – d). Thus, the inhibition of hippocampal calpain had no effect on long-term extinction. Taken together, our results suggest that hippocampal calpain is not required for within-session and long-term extinction in both sexes.

Calpain is required for c-fos induction when contextual fear memory is generated

It is possible that calpain contributes to the activation of gene expression that is required for the consolidation of contextual fear memory, since calpain activity is required for the modification of GluN2B, which occurs an upstream of activity-dependent gene expression in excitatory neurons [25, 30, 46, 47, 49, 58]. To assess this, we examined how inhibiting calpain in the hippocampus

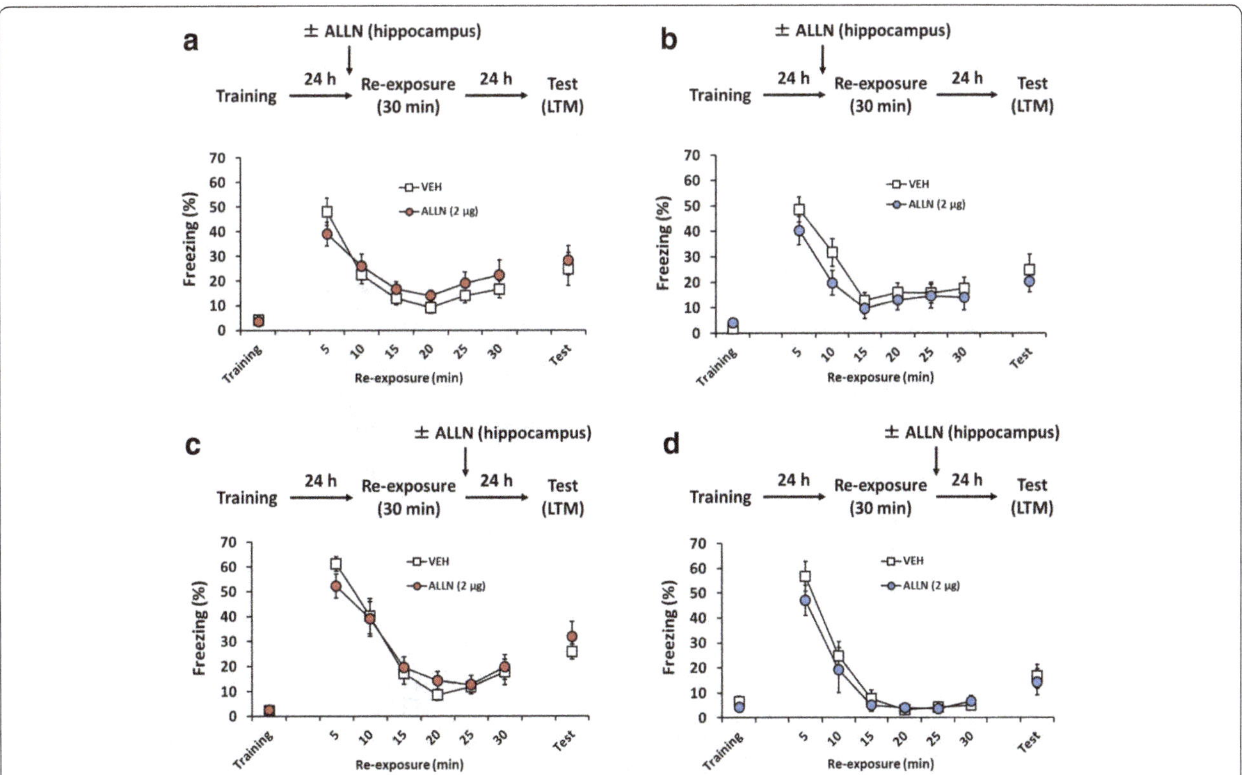

Fig. 3 Inhibition of hippocampal calpain does not affect the long-term extinction of contextual fear memory. Effects of a microinfusion of ALLN into the dorsal hippocampus at 10 min before (**a** and **b**) or immediately after (**c** and **d**) the 30-min re-exposure on long-term extinction in female (**a** and **c**) or male (**b** and **d**) mice (**a**: VEH, $n = 13$; ALLN, $n = 13$; **b**: VEH, $n = 10$; ALLN, $n = 11$; **c**: VEH, $n = 13$; ALLN, $n = 15$; **d**: VEH, $n = 10$; ALLN, $n = 11$). Error bars indicate SEM

affected the induction of c-fos expression, which depends on neuronal activity [59–61].

We first examined the effects of a systemic injection of ALLN on the LTM of contextual fear at the behavioral level. We performed similar experiments to those outlined in Fig. 1, except the male mice were systemically injected with ALLN (low-dose, 30 mg/kg; high-dose, 70 mg/kg) or VEH immediately after the training. A one-way ANOVA revealed a significant drug effect ($F(2,27) = 4.662$, $p < 0.05$; Fig. 4a). Post-hoc Newman-Keuls analysis revealed that ALLN-treated mice froze significantly less, compared to VEH-treated mice, in a dose-dependent manner (low-dose, $p > 0.05$; high-dose, $p < 0.05$; Fig. 4a). Similar to Fig. 1, these observations indicated that the inhibition of calpain by ALLN inhibited the formation of contextual fear memory.

Next, we measured the number of c-fos-positive cells in the hippocampus (CA1, CA3, and dentate gyrus [DG]) of male mice at 90 min after the training using immunohistochemistry (IHC). Two groups were trained with a footshock (shock groups), while the remaining two groups did not receive a footshock (no-shock groups). These groups were systemically injected with ALLN (70 mg/kg) or VEH immediately after the training (the groups were as follows: shock/ALLN, shock/VEH, no-shock/ALLN, and no-shock/VEH groups; Fig. 4b). A two-way ANOVA revealed a significant shock × drug interaction in the CA1 and CA3 regions (CA1, shock, $F(1,32) = 5.314$, $p < 0.05$; drug, $F(1,32) = 10.119$, $p < 0.05$; interaction, $F(1,32) = 10.862$, $p < 0.05$; CA3, shock, $F(1,32) = 2.208$, $p > 0.05$; drug, $F(1,32) = 5.23$, $p < 0.05$; interaction, $F(1,32) = 5.003$, $p < 0.05$; Fig. 4c and d), but

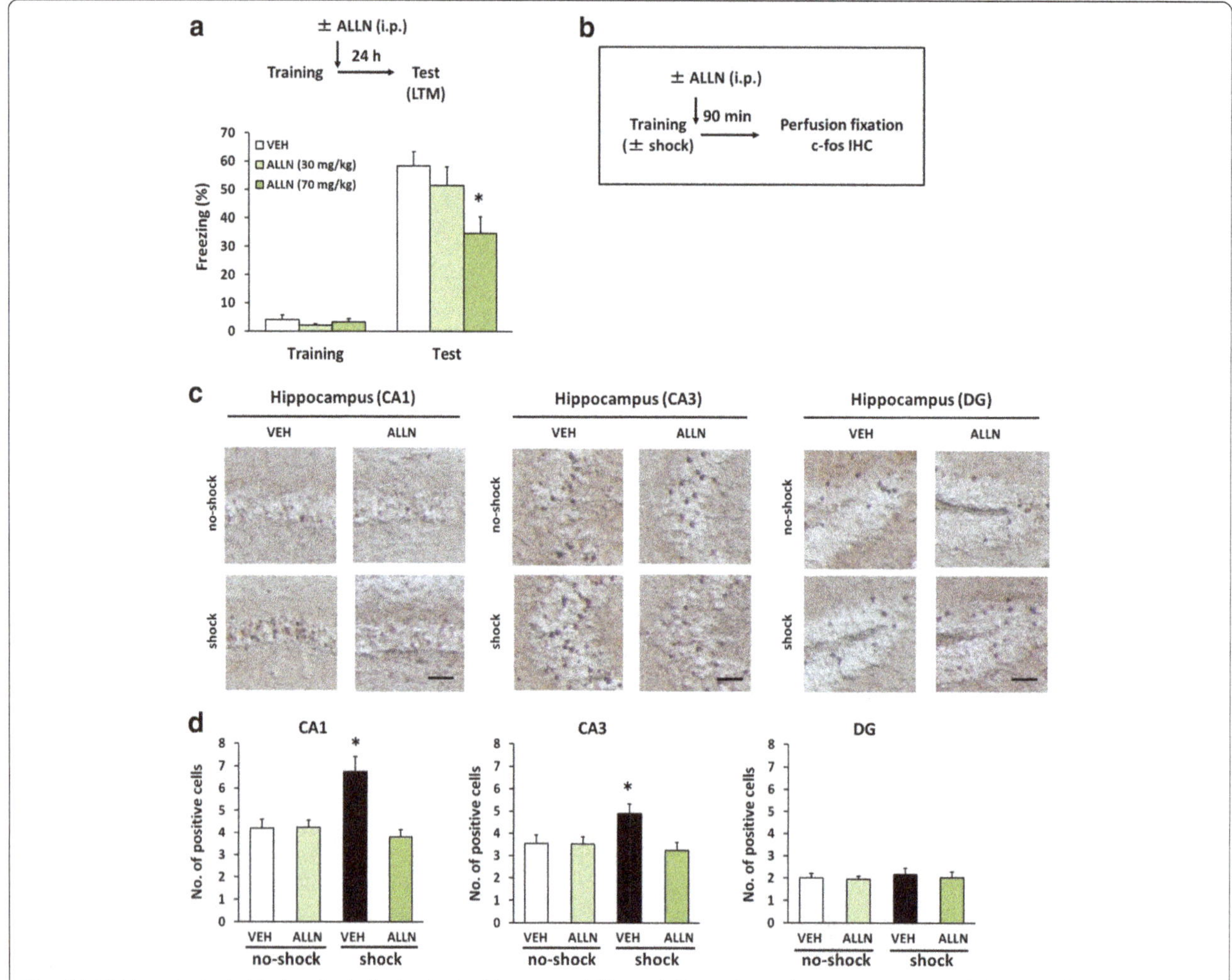

Fig. 4 Inhibition of calpain blocks c-fos induction in the hippocampal CA1 and CA3 regions when memory is consolidated. **a** Effects of a systemic injection of a low- or high-dose of ALLN immediately after the training on LTM (VEH, $n = 13$; ALLN 30 mg/kg, $n = 8$; ALLN 70 mg/kg, $n = 9$). *$p < 0.05$, compared with the VEH group at the test. **b** Experimental design for IHC. **c** Representative immunohistochemical staining of c-fos-positive cells in the CA1, CA3, and DG regions of the indicated groups. Scale bar, 50 μm. **d** The number of c-fos-positive cells in the CA1, CA3, and DG regions of no-shock/VEH, no-shock/ALLN, shock/VEH, and shock/ALLN groups ($n = 9$ for each group). *$p < 0.05$, compared with the other groups. Error bars indicate SEM

not in the DG region (shock, $F(1,32) = 0.275$, $p > 0.05$; drug, $F(1,32) = 0.254$, $p > 0.05$; interaction, $F(1,32) = 0.03$, $p > 0.05$; Fig. 4c and d). The shock/VEH group had significantly more c-fos-positive cells in the hippocampal CA1 and CA3 regions compared with the other groups, including the shock/ALLN group ($p < 0.05$; Fig. 4c and d). These results indicated that inhibition of calpain by ALLN blocked the c-fos induction in the hippocampus when memory is generated. This suggested that hippocampal calpain contributes to the activity–dependent gene expression when contextual fear memory is consolidated.

Discussion

In the present study, we examined the roles of hippocampal calpain in the consolidation, reconsolidation, and extinction of contextual fear memory. Inhibiting hippocampal calpain by a local infusion of the calpain inhibitor ALLN blocked the formation of LTM, without affecting STM. Moreover, the inhibition of hippocampal calpain immediately after memory retrieval disrupted reactivated memory. Conversely, the inhibition of hippocampal calpain had no effect on long-term extinction. Therefore, these observations demonstrated that hippocampal calpain is required for the consolidation and reconsolidation, but not extinction, of contextual fear memory.

Importantly, previous studies showed that protein degradation is involved in the molecular processes necessary for synaptic plasticity and learning and memory [16–20]. Calpain is Ca^{2+}-dependent cysteine protease involved in Ca^{2+} signaling pathway [21, 22]. Calpain specifically cleaves substrates in neurons, including synaptic proteins such as NMDA receptors subunits GluN2A and GluN2B, p35, calcineurin, alpha calcium/calmodulin-dependent protein kinase II (αCaMKII), spectrin, beta-catenin, and MAP2 [25, 26, 28–30, 32, 35, 36, 62–65]. Calpain is activated by NMDA receptor stimulation [30, 36, 66]. Activated calpain specifically cleaves the C-terminal of GluN2B, leading to degradation of NMDA receptors, which possibly modulates learning and synaptic plasticity [26, 30, 67, 68]. Activated calpain generates p25 by cleaving the N-terminal of the Cdk5 activator p35 [41]. Importantly, previous mouse genetic studies demonstrated that genetic deletion of p35 impaired hippocampus-dependent spatial learning and memory [39], whereas the transient or prolonged overexpression of p25 enhanced or impaired hippocampus dependent memory, respectively [42, 43]. Interestingly, Cdk5 facilitates the degradation of GluN2B by directly interacting with both it and calpain, suggesting crosstalk among calpain, NMDAR, and Cdk5 [40]. Taken together with our finding that hippocampal calpain is required for contextual fear memory consolidation and reconsolidation, it is possible that calpain in the hippocampus contributes to memory consolidation and reconsolidation through the functional modification of GluN2B and p35 by cleaving them.

Calpains, which are localized in spines [69, 70], have been suggested to mediate changes in the cytoskeletal structure and organization [42, 71] by cleaving substrate proteins [60, 61]. The genetic deletions of the calpain 1 / calpain 2 genes resulted in the decline in spine density and dendritic branching complexity in hippocampal CA1 pyramidal neurons, which further impaired the induction of LTP by theta burst stimulation in the CA1 area of the hippocampus [44, 72, 73]. Interestingly, recent studies have suggested distinct roles of calpain 1 and 2 in synaptic plasticity [45]; calpain 1 is required for the induction of LTP while calpain 2 is necessary for this maintenance. Moreover, deletions of calpain genes impaired hippocampus-dependent spatial learning in the Morris water maze [44]. In the current study, we extended these findings and demonstrated that hippocampal calpain is required for the consolidation and reconsolidation of contextual fear memory, but not for learning, short-term memory, and extinction memory. Further studies are required to understand the molecular mechanisms by which calpain contributes to the consolidation and reconsolidation by cleaving target substrates, and to compare and clarify roles of calpain 1 and 2 in these memory processes.

Additionally, we suggested that hippocampal calpain is not required for extinction of contextual fear memory, similarly with previous findings that long-term extinction does not require hippocampal gene expression. It is necessary to examine roles of calpain in the amygdala and mPFC in memory extinction since a previous study showed that extinction of contextual fear memory requires gene expression in these brain regions [48].

The activation of gene expression is necessary for the consolidation and reconsolidation of contextual fear memory [7, 15, 46–49, 58]. Interestingly, we showed that inhibiting calpain not only disrupted the consolidation of contextual fear memory, but also blocked the induction of c-fos expression that was observed following training. Calpains have been suggested to contribute to neuronal processes, including gene transcription and synaptic plasticity [32–34]. Therefore, it is possible that blocking the calpain inhibited the activation of gene expression, including the induction of c-fos expression, which is required for memory consolidation, since c-fos induction in hippocampal neurons is dependent on the activation of NMDA receptors [74–76]. Further studies are important to examine changes in cleavages of calpain targets such as beta-catenin following contextual fear conditioning to understand mechanisms for gene expression activation by calpain when memory is consolidated [65].

Sex differences had been observed in the molecular mechanisms that underlie the learning and memory process [50, 51]. However, the results of the current study did not demonstrate any sex differences in the role of hippocampal calpain in memory consolidation, reconsolidation, and extinction of contextual fear. This suggested that calpain is not involved in sex-specific molecular processes for memory performance.

Overall, the current study demonstrated that hippocampal calpain is necessary for both the consolidation and reconsolidation of contextual fear memory. Our findings suggested that calpain contributes to gene expression-dependent memory processes as a downstream regulator of the Ca^{2+}-signal transduction pathway.

Methods

Mice

All experiments were conducted according to the *Guide for the Care and Use of Laboratory Animals* (Japan Neuroscience Society and Tokyo University of Agriculture). The Animal Care and Use Committee of Tokyo University of Agriculture (authorization #280020) approved all the animal experiments that were performed in this study. All surgical procedures were performed under Nembutal anesthesia, with every effort to minimize suffering. Male and female C57BL/6 N mice were obtained from Charles River (Yokohama, Japan). The mice were housed in cages of 5 or 6, maintained on a 12-h light/dark cycle, and allowed ad libitum access to food and water. The mice were at least 8 weeks of age at the start of the experiments, and all behavioral procedures were conducted during the light phase of the cycle. All experiments were conducted by researchers who were blinded to the treatment condition of the mice.

Surgery for drug microinfusion

Surgeries were performed as described previously [56, 60, 61, 77–80]. Stainless-steel guide cannulae (22 gauge) were implanted into the dorsal hippocampus (−1.8 mm, ±1.8 mm, −1.9 mm), under Nembutal anesthesia, using standard stereotaxic procedures. The mice were allowed a recovery period of at least 1 week after surgery. Bilateral infusions into the dorsal hippocampus (0.5 μL/side) were made at a rate of 0.25 μL/min. The injection cannula was left in place for 2 min after infusion. Only mice with cannulation tips within the boundaries of the bilateral dorsal hippocampus were included in the data analysis. Cannulation tip placements are shown in Fig. 5.

Drugs

The calpain inhibitor N-Acetyl-Leu-Leu-norleucinal (ALLN; 0.4, 2, or 4 μg/μL; Millipore, MA, USA) was

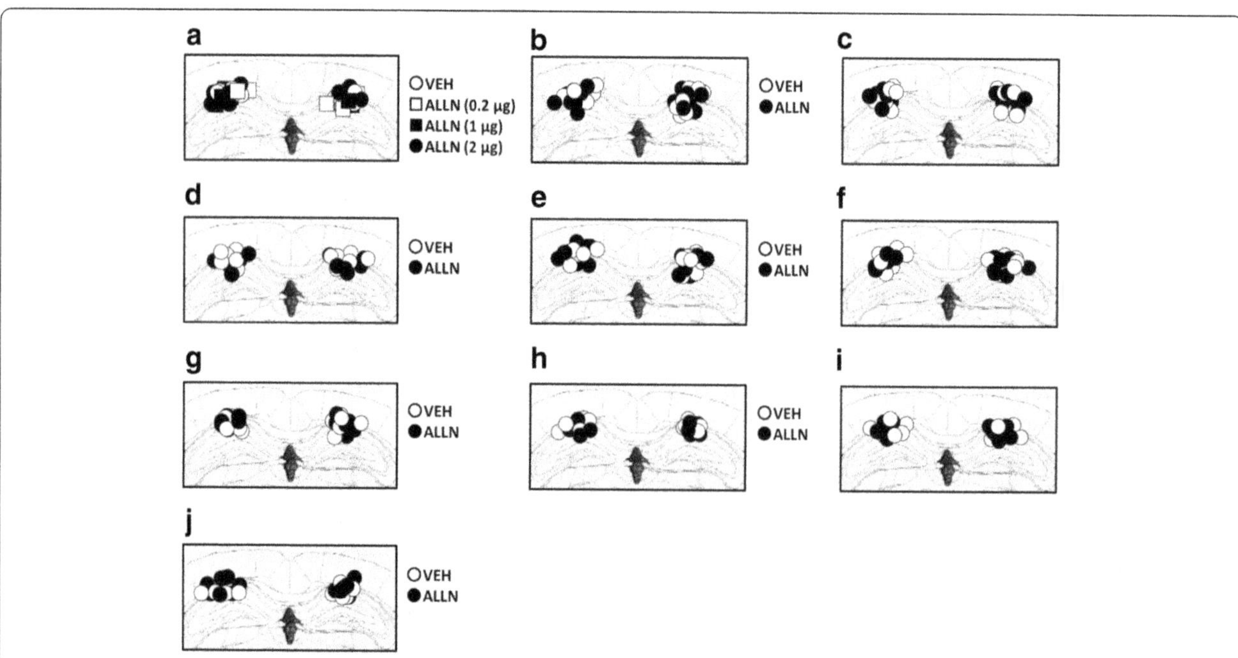

Fig. 5 Cannula tip placements in the dorsal hippocampus. Cannula tip placements from mice infused with each drug shown in Fig. 1a (**a**), Fig. 1b (**b**), Fig. 1c (**c**), Fig. 1d (**d**), Fig. 2a (**e**), Fig. 2b (**f**), Fig. 3a (**g**), Fig. 3b (**h**), Fig. 3c (**i**), Fig. 3d (**j**). Schematic drawing of coronal sections from all micro-infused animals (dorsal hippocampus, 1.94 mm posterior to the bregma). Only mice with needle tips within the boundaries of the dorsal hippocampus were included in the data analysis

dissolved in dimethyl sulfoxide with a final concentration that was less than 1% [81].

Contextual fear conditioning task

The mice were handled for 5 consecutive days prior to the commencement of contextual fear conditioning. The mice were trained and tested in conditioning chambers (17.5 × 17.5 × 15 cm; O'HARA & Co., Ltd., Tokyo, Japan) that had a stainless-steel grid floor through which the footshock could be delivered [15, 48, 60, 61, 78, 82, 83]. Training consisted of placing the mice in the chamber and delivering an unsignaled footshock (2 s duration, 0.4 mA) 148 s later. Then, the mice were returned to their home cage at 30 s after the footshock (training).

For the experiments examining the effects of drug treatment on memory consolidation, the mice received a microinfusion of ALLN or vehicle (VEH) into the dorsal hippocampus immediately after training (see Fig. 1). At 2 h or 24 h after training, the mice were placed back in the training context for 5 min and freezing was assessed (test). For the experiments examining the effects of drug treatment on memory reconsolidation or extinction, the mice were trained and placed back in the training context 24 h later (re-exposure) for 3 min (reconsolidation) or 30 min (extinction). The mice received a microinfusion of ALLN or VEH into the dorsal hippocampus at 10 min before or immediately after re-exposure (as indicated in Figs. 2 and 3). At 24 h after the re-exposure, the mice were once again placed back in the training context for 5 min and freezing was assessed (test). Memory was assessed as the percentage of time spent freezing in the training context. Freezing behavior (defined as complete lack of movement, except for respiration) was measured automatically as described previously [84]. ALLN or VEH was systemically injected (an i.p. injection) immediately after training (see Fig. 4).

Immunohistochemistry

Immunohistochemistry was performed as described previously [60, 61, 77–80, 85]. After anesthetization, all mice were perfused with 4% paraformaldehyde. Brains were then removed, fixed overnight, transferred to 30% sucrose, and stored at 4 °C. Coronal sections (30 μm) were cut using a cryostat. The sections were pretreated with 4% paraformaldehyde for 20 min and 3% H_2O_2 in methanol for 1 h, followed by incubation in blocking solution (phosphate-buffered saline [PBS] plus 1% goat serum albumin, 1 mg/mL bovine serum albumin, and 0.05% Triton X-100) for 3 h at 4 °C. Consecutive sections were incubated using a polyclonal rabbit primary antibody for anti-c-fos (1:5000; Millipore catalog #PC38, RRID: AB_2106755) in the blocking solution for 2 nights at 4 °C. Subsequently, the sections were washed with PBS and incubated for 4 h at room temperature with biotinylated goat anti-rabbit IgG (SAB-PO Kit; Nichirei Biosciences, Tokyo, Japan). Thereafter, the sections were incubated with streptavidin- biotin-peroxidase complex (SAB-PO Kit) for 1 h at room temperature. Immunoreactivity was detected using a DAB substrate kit (Nichirei Biosciences). Structures were anatomically defined according to the Paxinos and Franklin atlas [86]. Quantification of c-fos-positive cells in sections (100 × 100 μm) of the dorsal hippocampus (bregma between −1.46 and −1.82 mm) was performed using a computerized image analysis system (WinROOF version 5.6 software; Mitani Corporation, Fukui, Japan). Immunoreactive cells were counted bilaterally with a fixed sample window across at least 3 sections by an experimenter who was blinded to the treatment condition.

Data analysis

One-way or two-way factorial analysis of variance (ANOVA) followed by post hoc Newman-Keuls comparisons were used to analyze the effects of drug, time, and shock. A two-way repeated ANOVA followed by a post hoc Bonferroni's comparison was used to analyze the effects of drug and time. All values in the text and figure legends represent the mean ± standard error of the mean (SEM).

Abbreviations

ALLN: N-Acetyl-Leu-Leu-norleucinal; Cdk5: Cyclin-dependent kinase 5; GluN2B: NMDA receptor 2B subunits; IHC: Immunohistochemistry; LTM: Long-term memory; LTP: Long-term potentiation; STM: Short-term memory; VEH: Vehicle; DG: Dentate gyrus; αCaMKII: Alpha calcium/calmodulin-dependent protein kinase II

Acknowledgements

We thank Satoshi Kida's lab members for critical discussion for this manuscript.

Funding

SK was supported by The Science Research Promotion Fund, The Promotion and Mutual Aid Corporation for Private Schools of Japan, Grant-in-Aids for Scientific Research (A) [15H02488], Scientific Research (B) [23300120, 20380078], and Challenging Exploratory Research [24650172, 26640014, 17 K19464], Grant-in-Aids for Scientific Research on Priority Areas - Molecular Brain Science- [18022038, 22022039], Grant-in-Aid for Scientific Research on Innovative Areas (Research in a proposed research area) [24116008, 24116001, 23115716, 17H06084, 17H05961, 17H05581], Core Research for Evolutional Science and Technology (CREST), Japan, The Sumitomo Foundation, The Naito Foundation, The Uehara Memorial Foundation and the Takeda Science Foundation, Japan.

Authors' contributions

SK is responsible for the hypothesis development and overall design of the research and experiment, and supervised the experimental analyses. SK and TN co-wrote the manuscript. TN and KI performed all experiments. NM performed preliminary experiments. All authors read and approved this manuscript.

Competing interests

The authors declare that they have no competing interests.

References

1. Abel T, Lattal KM. Molecular mechanisms of memory acquisition, consolidation and retrieval. Curr Opin Neurobiol. 2001;11:180–7.
2. McGaugh JL. Memory–a century of consolidation. Science. 2000;287:248–51.
3. Silva AJ, Kogan JH, Frankland PW, Kida S. CREB and memory. Annu Rev Neurosci. 1998;21:127–48.
4. Bozon B, Davis S, Laroche S. A requirement for the immediate early gene zif268 in reconsolidation of recognition memory after retrieval. Neuron. 2003;40:695–701.
5. Kelly Á, Laroche S, Davis S. Activation of mitogen-activated protein kinase/ extracellular signal-regulated kinase in hippocampal circuitry is required for consolidation and reconsolidation of recognition memory. J Neurosci. 2003; 12:5354–60.
6. Kida S, Josselyn SA, Peña de Ortiz S, Kogan JH, Chevere I, Masushige S, et al. CREB required for the stability of new and reactivated fear memories. Nat Neurosci. 2002;5:348–55.
7. Nader K, Schafe GE, Le Doux JE. Fear memories require protein synthesis in the amygdala for reconsolidation after retrieval. Nature. 2000;406:722–6.
8. Pavlov I. Conditioned reflexes: an investigation of the physiological activity of the cerebral cortex. London: Oxford University Press; 1927.
9. Myers KM, Davis M. Behavioral and neural analysis of extinction. Neuron. 2002;36:567–84.
10. Myers KM, Davis M. Mechanisms of fear extinction. Mol Psychiatry. 2007;12: 120–50.
11. Delamater AR. Experimental extinction in Pavlovian conditioning: behavioural and neuroscience perspectives. Q J Exp Psychol B. 2004;57:97–132.
12. Davis HP, Squire LR. Protein synthesis and memory: a review. Psychol Bull. 1984;96:518–59.
13. Debiec J, LeDoux JE, Nader K. Cellular and systems reconsolidation in the hippocampus. Neuron. 2002;36:527–38.
14. Flexner LB, Flexner JB, Stellar E. Memory and cerebral protein synthesis in mice as affected by graded amounts of puromycin. Exp Neurol. 1965;13: 264–72.
15. Suzuki A, Josselyn SA, Frankland PW, Masushige S, Silva AJ, Kida S. Memory reconsolidation and extinction have distinct temporal and biochemical signatures. J Neurosci. 2004;24:4787–95.
16. Lee SH, Choi JH, Lee N, Lee HR, Kim JI, Yu NK, Choi SL, Lee SH, Kim H, Kaang BK. Synaptic protein degradation underlies destabilization of retrieved fear memory. Science. 2008;319(5867):1253–6.
17. Lee SH, Kwak C, Shim J, Kim JE, Choi SL, Kim HF, Jang DJ, Lee JA, Lee K, Lee CH, Lee YD, Miniaci MC, Bailey CH, Kandel ER, Kaang BK. A cellular model of memory reconsolidation involves reactivation-induced destabilization and restabilization at the sensorimotor synapse in Aplysia. Proc Natl Acad Sci U S A. 2012;109(35):14200–5.
18. Fioravante D, Byrne JH. Protein degradation and memory formation. Brain Res Bull. 2011;85(1–2):14–20.
19. Kaang BK, Choi JH. Protein degradation during reconsolidation as a mechanism for memory reorganization. Front Behav Neurosci. 2011;5:2.
20. Fonseca R, Vabulas RM, Hartl FU, Bonhoeffer T, Nägerl UV. A balance of protein synthesis and proteasome-dependent degradation determines the maintenance of LTP. Neuron. 2006;52(2):239–45.
21. Blanchard H, Grochulski P, Li Y, Arthur JS, Davies PL, Elce JS, Cygler M. Structure of a calpain ca(2+)-binding domain reveals a novel EF-hand and ca(2+)-induced conformational changes. Nat Struct Biol. 1997;4(7):532–8.
22. Goll DE, Thompson VF, Li H, Wei W, Cong J. The calpain system. Physiol Rev. 2003;83(3):731–801. Review
23. Lynch G, Baudry M. The biochemistry of memory: a new and specific hypothesis. Science. 1984;224:1057–63.
24. Wu HY, Lynch DR. Calpain and synaptic function. Mol Neurobiol. 2006;33:215–36.
25. Baudry M, Chou MM, Bi X. Targeting calpain in synaptic plasticity. Expert Opin Ther Targets. 2013;17(5):579–92.
26. Guttmann RP, Baker DL, Seifert KM, Cohen AS, Coulter DA, Lynch DR. Specific proteolysis of the NR2 subunit at multiple sites by calpain. J Neurochem. 2001;78: 1083–93.
27. Guttmann RP, Sokol S, Baker DL, Simpkins KL, Dong Y, Lynch DR. Proteolysis of the N-methyl-d-aspartate receptor by calpain in situ. J Pharmacol Exp Ther. 2002; 302(3):1023–30.
28. Lu X, Rong Y, Baudry M. Calpain-mediated degradation of PSD-95 in developing and adult rat brain. Neurosci Lett. 2000;286(2):149–53.
29. Wu HY, Tomizawa K, Oda Y, Wei FY, Lu YF, Matsushita M, Li ST, Moriwaki A, Matsui H. Critical role of calpain-mediated cleavage of calcineurin in excitotoxic neurodegeneration. J Biol Chem. 2004;279(6):4929–40.
30. Wu HY, Yuen EY, Lu YF, Matsushita M, Matsui H, Yan Z, Tomizawa K. Regulation of N-methyl-D-aspartate receptors by calpain in cortical neurons. J Biol Chem. 2005;280(22):21588–93.
31. Croall DE, DeMartino GN. Calcium-activated neutral protease (calpain) system: structure, function, and regulation. Physiol Rev. 1991;71(3):813–47.
32. Lee MS, Kwon YT, Li M, Peng J, Friedlander RM, Tsai LH. Neurotoxicity induces cleavage of p35 to p25 by calpain. Nature. 2000;405(6784):360–4.
33. Nixon RA. The calpains in aging and aging-related diseases. Ageing Res Rev. 2003;2(4):407–18. Review
34. Li J, Grynspan F, Berman S, Nixon R, Bursztajn S. Regional differences in gene expression for calcium activated neutral proteases (calpains) and their endogenous inhibitor calpastatin in mouse brain and spinal cord. J Neurobiol. 1996;30(2):177–91.
35. Kusakawa G, Saito T, Onuki R, Ishiguro K, Kishimoto T, Hisanaga S. Calpain-dependent proteolytic cleavage of the p35 cyclin-dependent kinase 5 activator to p25. J Bio Chem. 2000;275(22):17166–72.
36. Simpkins KL, Guttmann RP, Dong Y, Chen Z, Sokol S, Neumar RW, Lynch DR. Selective activation induced cleavage of the NR2B subunit by calpain. J Neurosci. 2003;23(36):11322–31.
37. Vianna MR, Alonso M, Viola H, Quevedo J, de Paris F, Furman M, de Stein ML, Medina JH, Izquierdo I. Role of hippocampal signaling pathways in long-term memory formation of a nonassociative learning task in the rat. Learn Mem. 2000;7(5):333–40.
38. Cammarota M, Bevilaqua LR, Bonini JS, Rossatto JI, Medina JH, Izquierdo N. Hippocampal glutamate receptors in fear memory consolidation. Neurotox Res. 2004;6(3):205–12.
39. Mishiba T, Tanaka M, Mita N, He X, Sasamoto K, Itohara S, Ohshima T. Cdk5/p35 functions as a crucial regulator of spatial learning and memory. Mol Brain. 2014;7:82.
40. Hawasli AH, Benavides DR, Nguyen C, Kansy JW, Hayashi K, Chambon P, Greengard P, Powell CM, Cooper DC, Bibb JA. Cyclin-dependent kinase 5 governs learning and synaptic plasticity via control of NMDAR degradation. Nat Neurosci. 2007;10(7):880–6.
41. Patrick GN, Zukerberg L, Nikolic M, de la Monte S, Dikkes P, Tsai LH. Conversion of p35 to p25 deregulates Cdk5 activity and promotes neurodegeneration. Nature. 1999;402(6762):615–22.
42. Fischer A, Sananbenesi F, Pang PT, Lu B, Tsai LH. Opposing roles of transient and prolonged expression of p25 in synaptic plasticity and hippocampus-dependent memory. Neuron. 2005;48(5):825–38.
43. Engmann O, Hortobágyi T, Thompson AJ, Guadagno J, Troakes C, Soriano S, Al-Sarraj S, Kim Y, Giese KP. Cyclin-dependent kinase 5 activator p25 is generated during memory formation and is reduced at an early stage in Alzheimer's disease. Biol Psychiatry. 2011;70(2):159–68.
44. Amini M, Ma CL, Farazifard R, Zhu G, Zhang Y, Vanderluit J, Zoltewicz JS, Hage F, Savitt JM, Lagace DC, Slack RS, Beique JC, Baudry M, Greer PA, Bergeron R, Park DS. Conditional disruption of calpain in the CNS alters dendrite morphology, impairs LTP, and promotes neuronal survival following injury. J Neurosci. 2013;33(13):5773–84.
45. Baudry M, Bi X. Calpain-1 and Calpain-2: the yin and Yang of synaptic plasticity and Neurodegeneration. Trends Neurosci. 2016;39(4):235–45.
46. Athos J, Impey S, Pineda VV, Chen X, Storm DR. Hippocampal CRE-mediated gene expression is required for contextual memory formation. Nat Neurosci. 2002;5:1119–20.

47. Lee JLC, Everitt BJ, Thomas KL. Independent cellular processes for hippocampal memory consolidation and reconsolidation. Science. 2004; 304:839–43.
48. Mamiya N, Fukushima H, Suzuki A, Matsuyama Z, Homma S, Frankland PW, et al. Brain region-specific gene expression activation required for reconsolidation and extinction of contextual fear memory. J Neurosci. 2009;29:402–13.
49. Trifilieff P, Herry C, Vanhoutte P, Caboche J, Desmedt A, Riedel G, et al. Foreground contextual fear memory consolidation requires two independent phases of hippocampal ERK/CREB activation. Learn Mem. 2006; 13:349–58.
50. Mizuno K, Giese KP. Towards a molecular understanding of sex differences in memory formation. Trends Neurosci. 2010;33(6):285–91.
51. Koss WA, Frick KM. Sex differences in hippocampal function. J Neurosci Res. 2017;95(1–2):539–62.
52. Anagnostaras SG, Gale GD, Fanselow MS. Hippocampus and contextual fear conditioning: recent controversies and advances. Hippocampus. 2001;11(1): 8–17. Review
53. Kim JJ, Rison RA, Fanselow MS. Effects of amygdala, hippocampus, and periaqueductal gray lesions on short- and long-term contextual fear. Behav Neurosci. 1993;107(6):1093–8.
54. Phillips RG, LeDoux JE. Differential contribution of amygdala and hippocampus to cued and contextual fear conditioning. Behav Neurosci. 1992;106(2):274–85.
55. Suzuki A, Mukawa T, Tsukagoshi A, Frankland PW, Kida S. Activation of LVGCCs and CB1 receptors required for destabilization of reactivated contextual fear memories. Learn Mem. 2008;15:426–33.
56. Frankland PW, Ding HK, Takahashi E, Suzuki A, Kida S, Silva AJ. Stability of recent and remote contextual fear memory. Learn Mem. 2006;13:451–7.
57. Santini E, Ge H, Ren K, Peña de Ortiz S, Quirk GJ. Consolidation of fear extinction requires protein synthesis in the medial prefrontal cortex. J Neurosci. 2004;24:5704–10.
58. Hall J, Thomas KL, Everitt BJ. Rapid and selective induction of BDNF expression in the hippocampus during contextual learning. Nat Neurosci. 2000;3:533–5.
59. Frankland PW, Bontempi B, Talton LE, Kaczmarek L, Silva AJ. The involvement of the anterior cingulate cortex in remote contextual fear memory. Science. 2004;304:881–3.
60. Inaba H, Tsukagoshi A, Kida S. PARP-1 activity is required for the reconsolidation and extinction of contextual fear memory. Mol Brain. 2015;8:63.
61. Inaba H, Kai D, Kida S. N-glycosylation in the hippocampus is required for the consolidation and reconsolidation of contextual fear memory. Neurobiol Learn Mem. 2016;135:57–65.
62. Fischer I, Romano-Clarke G, Grynspan F. Calpain-mediated proteolysis of microtubule associated proteins MAP1B and MAP2 in developing brain. Neurochem Res. 1991;16(8):891–8.
63. Zadran S, Bi X, Baudry M. Regulation of calpain-2 in neurons: implications for synaptic plasticity. Mol Neurobiol. 2010;42(2):143–50.
64. Hajimohammadreza I, Raser KJ, Nath R, Nadimpalli R, Scott M, Wang KK. Neuronal nitric oxide synthase and calmodulin-dependent protein kinase IIalpha undergo neurotoxin-induced proteolysis. J Neurochem. 1997;69(3): 1006–13.
65. Abe K, Takeichi M. NMDA-receptor activation induces calpain-mediated beta-catenin cleavages for triggering gene expression. Neuron. 2007;53(3): 387–97.
66. Dong YN, Waxman EA, Lynch DR. Interactions of postsynaptic density-95 and the NMDA receptor 2 subunit control calpain-mediated cleavage of the NMDA receptor. J Neurosci. 2004;24(49):11035–45.
67. Bi R, Rong Y, Bernard A, Khrestchatisky M, Baudry M. Src-mediated tyrosine phosphorylation of NR2 subunits of N-methyl-D-aspartate receptors protects from calpain-mediated truncation of their C-terminal domains. J Biol Chem. 2000;275(34):26477–83.
68. Plattner F, Hernández A, Kistler TM, Pozo K, Zhong P, Yuen EY, Tan C, Hawasli AH, Cooke SF, Nishi A, Guo A, Wiederhold T, Yan Z, Bibb JA. Memory enhancement by targeting Cdk5 regulation of NR2B. Neuron. 2014; 81(5):1070–83.
69. Baudry M, Lynch G. Remembrance of arguments past: how well is the glutamate receptor hypothesis of LTP holding up after 20 years? Neurobiol Learn Mem. 2001;76(3):284–97.
70. Zadran S, Jourdi H, Rostamiani K, Qin Q, Bi X, Baudry M. Brain-derived neurotrophic factor and epidermal growth factor activate neuronal m-calpain via mitogen-activated protein kinase-dependent phosphorylation. J Neurosci. 2010;30(3):1086–95.
71. Wilson MT, Kisaalita WS, Keith CH. Glutamate-induced changes in the pattern of hippocampal dendrite outgrowth: a role for calcium-dependent pathways and the microtubule cytoskeleton. J Neurobiol. 2000;43(2):159–72.
72. Wang Y, Zhu G, Briz V, Hsu YT, Bi X, Baudry M. A molecular brake controls the magnitude of long-term potentiation. Nat Commun. 2014;5:3051.
73. Liu Y, Sun J, Wang Y, Lopez D, Tran J, Bi X, Baudry M. Deleting both PHLPP1 and CANP1 rescues impairments in long-term potentiation and learning in both single knockout mice. Learn Mem. 2016;23(8):399–404.
74. Cole AJ, Saffen DW, Baraban JM, Worley PF. Rapid increase of an immediate early gene messenger RNA in hippocampal neurons by synaptic NMDA receptor activation. Nature. 1989;340(6233):474–6.
75. Lerea LS, Butler LS, McNamara JO. NMDA and non-NMDA receptor-mediated increase of c-fos mRNA in dentate gyrus neurons involves calcium influx via different routes. J Neurosci. 1992;12(8):2973–81.
76. Xia Z, Dudek H, Miranti CK, Greenberg ME. Calcium influx via the NMDA receptor induces immediate early gene transcription by a MAP kinase/ERK-dependent mechanism. J Neurosci. 1996;16(17):5425–36.
77. Fukushima H, Zhang Y, Archbold G, Ishikawa R, Nader K, Kida S. Enhancement of fear memory by retrieval through reconsolidation. elife. 2014;3:e02736.
78. Ishikawa R, Fukushima H, Frankland PW, Kida S. Hippocampal neurogenesis enhancers promote forgetting of remote fear memory after hippocampal reactivation by retrieval. Elife. 2016;5:e17464.
79. Tanimizu T, Kenney JW, Okano E, Kadoma K, Frankland PW, Kida S. Functional connectivity of multiple brain regions required for the consolidation of social recognition memory. J Neurosci. 2017;37(15):4103–16.
80. Tanimizu T, Kono K, Kida S. Brain networks activated to form object recognition memory. Brain Res Bull. 2017.
81. Rami A, Krieglstein J. Protective effects of calpain inhibitors against neuronal damage caused by cytotoxic hypoxia in vitro and ischemia in vivo. Brain Res. 1993;609(1–2):67–70.
82. Fujinaka A, Li R, Hayashi M, Kumar D, Changarathil G, Naito K, Miki K, Nishiyama T, Lazarus M, Sakurai T, Kee N, Nakajima S, Wang SH, Sakaguchi M. Effect of context exposure after fear learning on memory generalization in mice. Mol Brain. 2016;9:2.
83. Yokota S, Suzuki Y, Hamami K, Harada A, Komai S. Sex differences in avoidance behavior after perceiving potential risk in mice. Behav Brain Funct. 2017;13(1):9.
84. Anagnostaras SG, Josselyn SA, Frankland PW, Silva AJ. Computer-assisted behavioral assessment of Pavlovian fear conditioning in mice. Learn Mem. 2000;7:58–72.
85. Zhang Y, Fukushima H, Kida S. Induction and requirement of gene expression in the anterior cingulate cortex and medial prefrontal cortex for the consolidation of inhibitory avoidance memory. Mol Brain. 2011;4:4.
86. Paxinos G, Franklin KBJ. The mouse brain in stereotaxic coordinates. San Diego: Academic; 1997.

11

The ERM protein Moesin is essential for neuronal morphogenesis and long-term memory in *Drosophila*

Patrick S. Freymuth and Helen L. Fitzsimons*

Abstract

Moesin is a cytoskeletal adaptor protein that plays an important role in modification of the actin cytoskeleton. Rearrangement of the actin cytoskeleton drives both neuronal morphogenesis and the structural changes in neurons that are required for long-term memory formation. Moesin has been identified as a candidate memory gene in *Drosophila*, however, whether it is required for memory formation has not been evaluated. Here, we investigate the role of Moesin in neuronal morphogenesis and in short- and long-term memory formation in the courtship suppression assay, a model of associative memory. We found that both knockdown and overexpression of Moesin led to defects in axon growth and guidance as well as dendritic arborization. Moreover, reduction of Moesin expression or expression of a constitutively active phosphomimetic in the adult *Drosophila* brain had no effect on short term memory, but prevented long-term memory formation, an effect that was independent of its role in development. These results indicate a critical role for *Moesin* in both neuronal morphogenesis and long-term memory formation.

Keywords: Moesin, Ezrin, Radixin, ERM, Cytoskeleton, Actin, *Drosophila*, Memory, Neuron, Courtship, Synaptic plasticity

Introduction

Moesin belongs to the ERM (Ezrin/Radixin/Moesin) family of proteins, a group of adaptor molecules that are essential organizers of specialized membrane domains, which have been implicated in various fundamental physiological processes including the regulation of cell shape, motility and signaling. For review, see [1, 2]. ERMs maintain the structural stability of the cell cortex by linking transmembrane proteins to the actin cytoskeleton via an N-terminal FERM domain and a C-terminal actin-binding domain [1, 3]. Regulation of ERM activity is facilitated through head to tail folding in which an intramolecular association between the N- and C-terminal domains results in a "closed", inactive conformation. Phosphorylation of a conserved threonine residue in the C-terminal actin-binding domain relieves this intermolecular association resulting in an "open", active conformation and the unmasking of ligand-binding sites [3].

* Correspondence: h.l.fitzsimons@massey.ac.nz
Institute of Fundamental Sciences, Massey University, Palmerston North, New Zealand

ERMs play a critical role in regulation of the cytoskeletal rearrangements that lead to changes in cell shape [4–10]. Activation of ERMs occurs via phosphorylation of threonine 558 through activation of kinases such as Rho-kinase [11]. Constitutive activation of RhoA, which activates Rho-kinase, induces the formation of microvilli-like structures at the apical membrane of fibroblasts, and this is enhanced on co-expression of T559D, a constitutively active phosphomimetic of Moesin. However co-expression of the non-phosphorylatable mutant T559A inhibits formation of the RhoA-induced microvilli-like structures, indicating that phosphorylation of Moesin is essential for this growth process [11]. Similarly, in epithelial cells, the constitutively active form of Ezrin, T567D, associates with the actin-rich plasma membrane and induces the growth of actin-rich projections, but the inactive form, T567A, does not [12]. In *Drosophila*, Moesin is required for photoreceptor morphogenesis where it facilitates normal assembly of the apical membrane skeleton of the rhabdomere. When expressed during photoreceptor morphogenesis, the constitutively active mutant T559D concentrates at the apical membrane, resulting in a profusion of irregular microvilli [7].

In neurons, rearrangements in the actin cytoskeleton underpin neuronal morphogenesis and synaptic plasticity [13–16]. A key process driving neuronal morphogenesis is the guidance of the growing axons toward synaptic targets [17] and the dynamic activity of the growth cone is characterized by persistent extension and withdrawal of actin-rich membrane protrusions, which bear membrane receptors that detect extrinsic guidance cues [18, 19]. Moesin and Radixin have been identified as prominent components of axonal growth cones of cultured rat hippocampal pyramidal neurons, with the double suppression of their expression leading to disorganization of F-actin and defects in morphology and motility [20]. Phosphorylation of Moesin is required for nerve growth factor-mediated outgrowth of PC12 cell neurites [21], and exposure of hippocampal neurons to glutamate induces activation of Moesin and is associated with an increase in the number of active synaptic boutons, the presynaptic axon terminals that contact dendritic spines to form a synapse [22]. This increase is diminished by Moesin knockdown as well as impairment of ERM phosphorylation, indicating that ERMs may be involved in the synaptic response to activity [22].

Rearrangement of the actin cytoskeleton also drives the structural changes that occur in dendritic spines, which are believed to underlie memory formation and maintenance [15, 16, 23, 24]. Progestogen and estrogen both induce cytoskeletal remodeling in cortical neurons, which is coincident with phosphorylation of Moesin via a signaling cascade involving RhoA and the Rho-associated kinase, ROCK-2 [25, 26]. These hormones are critical modulators of neuronal morphology and function and have been demonstrated to play a critical role not only in brain development but also learning and memory [27–29]. Activation of this pathway is associated with increased dendritic spine density and a redistribution of Moesin to membrane sites where spines are formed, while shRNA-mediated silencing of Moesin abrogates this spine growth [25, 26]. These data together indicate that Moesin regulates activity-dependent cytoskeletal rearrangements and dendritic spine growth, suggesting a potential role in the structural changes that are thought to underpin memory formation. Indeed, Moesin has been identified as a candidate memory gene through DNA microarray analysis of the *Drosophila* transcriptional response following training in the olfactory conditioning paradigm, which found that Moesin transcription was induced after spaced relative to massed training [30]. Since spaced but not massed training leads to the formation of protein synthesis-dependent long-term memory [31], this transcriptional response suggests that Moesin may be involved in long-term memory formation.

Despite this accumulating evidence, there have been no studies to date examining whether ERMs play a specific role in memory. As *Drosophila* has a single ERM orthologue *Moesin*, sharing 58% amino acid identity with its human counterpart, analyses are not hindered by the functional redundancy of the ERMs that has been previously observed in vertebrate studies [32]. This advantage, combined with *Drosophila*'s amenability to genetic manipulation and the well-established memory assays that have been developed, provides an informative means for investigation of the role of ERMs in learning and memory. Here, we found that knockdown of Moesin as well as its constitutive activation in the adult *Drosophila* brain prevented long-term memory formation, indicating an essential role in this process, which was independent of its role in development. Moreover, knockdown of Moesin impaired dendritic arborization, whereas constitutive activation appeared to increase the intensity of dendritic protrusions, suggesting Moesin may promote memory formation through facilitation of cytoskeletal rearrangements at synapses.

Results

Characterization of Moesin expression in the *Drosophila* brain

We first sought to characterize the expression pattern of Moesin in the *Drosophila* brain, which has not been previously examined. Immunohistochemical staining of whole mount brains revealed widespread expression of Moesin throughout all regions of the brain (Fig. 1a, h). The subcellular distribution of Moesin was non-nuclear and predominantly cytoplasmic, as observed by the lack of colocalization with ELAV, a marker of neuronal nuclei (Fig. 1b–j) and the Moesin-positive cytoplasmic haloes surrounding the ELAV-positive nuclei (Fig. 1d–g). In the mushroom body, a region of the brain critical for memory formation and recall [33, 34], Moesin was not observed in the lobes (axons) of the Kenyon cells, the intrinsic neurons of the mushroom body (Fig. 1a; see Additional file 1: Figure S1B to visualize the location of the lobes in the brain), however magnification of the cell bodies of the Kenyon cells revealed cytoplasmically localized Moesin (Fig. 1m, n).

In order to investigate the importance of Moesin in neuronal development as well as in learning and memory in adult flies, we genetically manipulated the level of Moesin expression in the brain via the UAS/GAL4 system combined with the pan-neuronal elav-GAL4 driver. The resulting expression patterns of the transgenic constructs were then examined via immunohistochemistry on whole mount brains. As overexpression of Moesin could potentially affect neuronal development, expression was induced in adulthood via the TARGET system, which utilizes a temperature-sensitive repressor of GAL4

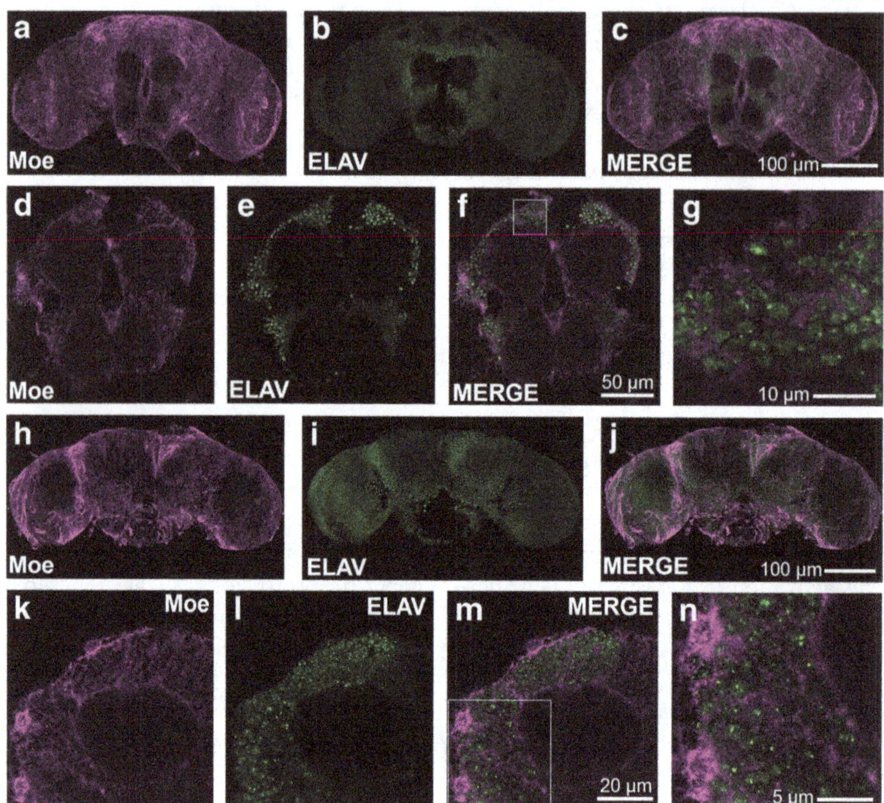

Fig. 1 Expression and subcellular localization of Moesin in the brain. Whole mount brains were subjected to immunohistochemistry with anti-Moesin (magenta) and anti-ELAV (green) antibodies. **a–c**. frontal confocal projection through the brain illustrating widespread Moesin expression. **d–f**. One micron optical slice through the central lobes of the brain illustrating non-nuclear Moesin expression, appearing as a cytoplasmic halo around the ELAV stained nuclei. **g**. Magnification of area surrounded by the white square in **f**. **h–j**. Posterior confocal projection through the brain. **k–m**. One micron optical slice through the calyx illustrating non-nuclear Moesin expression in Kenyon cells. **n**. Magnification of area surrounded by the white square in **m**

transcription, GAL80ts. Flies were raised at a GAL80 permissive temperature (19 °C) until two days after eclosion, at which time expression was induced at the restrictive temperature (30 °C) for 48 h as expected. The expression pattern of a Myc-tagged wild-type Moesin transgene (Myc-Moe) was very similar to that of endogenous Moesin (Fig. 2a–f). Expression of the phosphomimetic Myc-MoeT559D, a constitutively active mutant of Moesin [7] also resulted in robust expression throughout the brain (Fig. 2g–i). However, unlike Myc-Moe, Myc-MoeT559D was targeted to the mushroom body lobes (compare Fig. 2j and k) and also displayed a stronger presence in the calyx (compare Fig. 2e and h). This pattern mimics that of Lifeact, a GFP-tagged actin-binding peptide (Additional file 1: Figure S1) [35], indicating that on activation, Moesin redistributes from the cytoplasm to actin-rich regions of the neuron.

Appropriate overexpression and knockdown of Moesin was also confirmed via western blot. A specific band of approximately 75 kDa, the estimated molecular weight of *Drosophila* Moesin, was detected in whole-cell lysates of wild-type *Drosophila* heads (Fig. 2l), whereas expression of each RNAi resulted in a reduced signal, confirming that each targeted Moesin. Expression of Myc-Moe was detected as a slightly higher molecular weight band in addition to endogenous Moesin, as was Myc-MoeT559D. In the two strains co-expressing Myc-Moe and a Moesin RNAi construct, the levels of both endogenous Moesin and Myc-Moe proteins are reduced, which is expected as both endogenous Moesin and the Myc-Moe constructs contain the mRNA sequences targeted by RNAi.

Altered Moesin expression disrupts mushroom body development

In light of the demonstrated role of Moesin in neuronal morphogenesis [7], we first investigated the impact of Moesin knockdown and overexpression on mushroom body development. Immunohistochemical staining for the neuronal marker FasII strongly labels the α and β lobes of the mushroom body and weakly labels the γ lobe enabling the visualization of mushroom body lobes

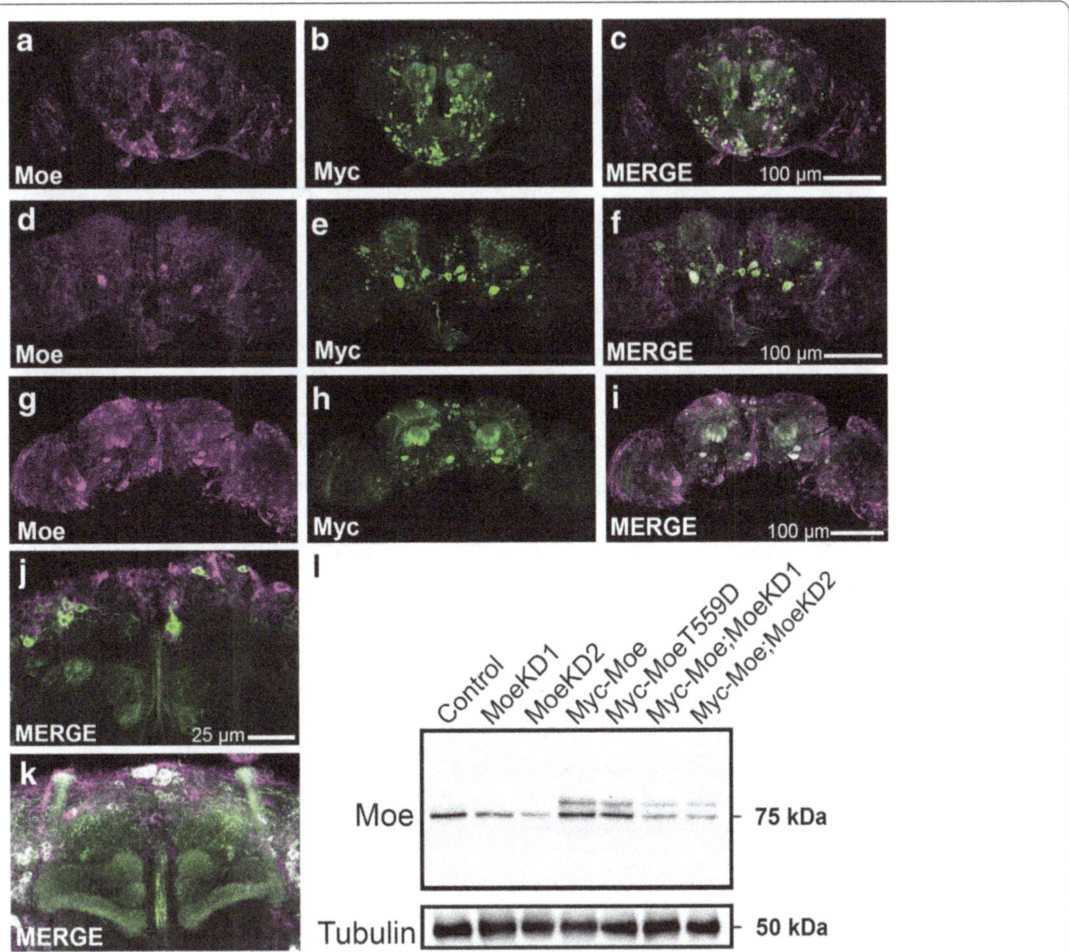

Fig. 2 Characterisation of *Moesin* knockdown and overexpression. **a**–**k**. Immunohistochemistry with anti-Moesin (magenta) and anti-Myc (green) antibodies on whole mount brains. In all brains, elav-GAL4-mediated expression was restricted to the adult brain with the TARGET system. **a**–**c**. frontal confocal projection through a brain expressing Myc-Moe. **d**–**f**. Posterior confocal projection through a brain expressing Myc-Moe. **g**–**i**. Posterior confocal projection through a brain expressing Myc-MoeT559D. **j**, **k**. Confocal projection through a mushroom body expressing Myc-Moe (**j**) and Myc-Moe T559D (**k**). **l**. Western blot shows the expression of Moesin in head lysates of flies in which *Moesin* is overexpression or knocked down. The wild-type strain *w1118* was also crossed to elav-GAL4 as a control genotype. Blots were probed with anti-Moesin to detect endogenous Moesin as well as Myc-Moe and Myc-MoeT559D. Anti-α-tubulin antibody was used as a loading control

[36]. In the wild-type brain, the axons of the α and β neurons each project from the cell bodies in a bundled fiber termed the peduncle, and then bifurcate to form the vertical and horizontal α and β lobes (Fig. 3a). Both elav-GAL4 driven overexpression of Myc-Moe and RNAi-mediated knockdown of Moesin resulted in clear disruption of mushroom body development (Table 1). Given that RNAi can have off target effects, we wished to determine whether the RNAi phenotypes were a specific result of a decrease in Moesin, therefore we reintroduced wild-type Moesin into both of the Moesin RNAi lines. Knockdown of Moesin resulted in an obvious deficit in α/β lobe development in an average of 85% of brains, which was reduced to 23% in brains of flies in which Moesin was co-expressed.

Mushroom body defects ranged from misdirected or malformed lobes to the complete absence of α/β lobes, as well as axon arrest/stalling, in which the projection of α/β neurons from the peduncle is halted, resulting in partially formed lobes (Fig. 3). Additional defects in α/β lobe morphology included lobes that were thin or diminished, misdirected, misoriented, and those with defects in branching. Gamma lobe phenotypes were mild and observed as thinner lobes that were often distorted. Together these data demonstrate that wild-type levels of Moesin are required for normal axon outgrowth and guidance.

While generating the above-mentioned flies, we noticed that elav > Myc-MoeT559D resulted in photoreceptor deficits, displaying a rough eye phenotype, which is indicative of malformed or missing photoreceptor clusters,

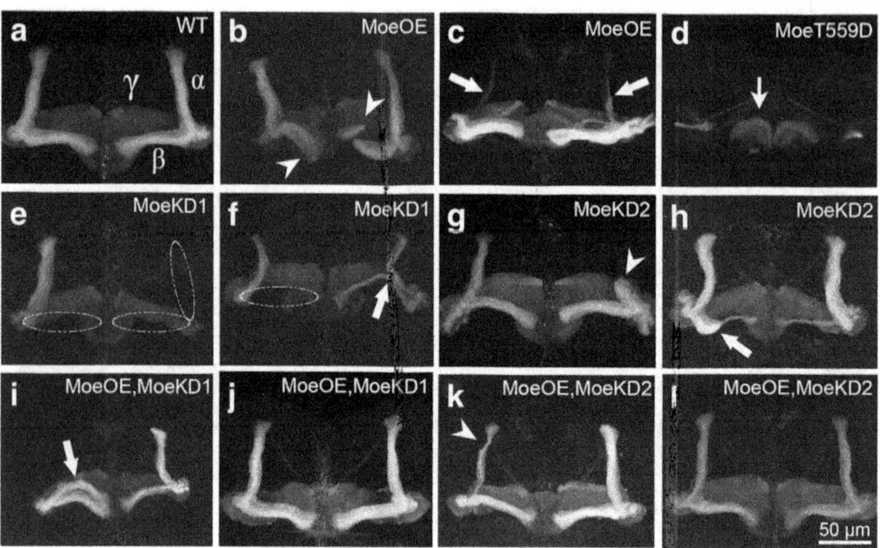

Fig. 3 Altered Moesin expression disrupts mushroom body development. **a**–**h**. Immunohistochemistry with anti-FasII antibody on whole mount brains reveals mushroom body defects resulting from elav-GAL4 driven expression of UAS-Moe constructs. All images are frontal confocal projections through the mushroom body region of the brain. Scale bar = 50 μm. **a**. Wild-type mushroom body. α, β and γ lobes of the mushroom body are labeled in white. **b**. Misoriented β lobes (arrowheads) in a fly expressing Myc-Moe. **c**. Thin, reduced, α lobe projections in a fly expressing Moe-KD2. **d**. Complete disruption of mushroom body development in a fly expressing Myc-MoeT559D, with thin, distorted γ lobes (arrow). **e**. Missing α and β lobes (dashed lines) in a fly expressing Moe-KD1. **f**. Missing β lobe (dashed line) and α/β branching defect (arrow) in a fly expressing Moe-KD1. **g**. Axon stalling defect characterized by a partially formed α lobe (arrowhead) in a fly expressing Moe-KD2. **h**. β lobe outgrowth defect (arrow) in a fly expressing Moe-KD2. **i**. Misdirected α lobe (arrow) in a fly co-expressing Myc-Moe and Moe-KD2. **j**. Rescue of mushroom body development through coexpression of Myc-Moe with Moe-KD1. **k**. Thin α lobe (arrowhead) in a fly co-expressing Myc-Moe and Moe-KD1. **l**. Rescue of mushroom body development through coexpression of Myc-Moe with Moe-KD2

producing a rough, glassy look to the eye [37]. As *elav* is expressed in cells of neuronal progenitor origin including photoreceptors, the elav-GAL4 driver induces target gene expression in the eye as well as the brain [38]. The discovery of this eye development phenotype led to the examination of each of our transgenic Moesin expression lines by scanning electron microscopy to identify if altered Moesin expression resulted in visible disruption of photoreceptor development in the adult. SEM analysis revealed that expression of Myc-MoeT559D resulted in severe disorganization of bristles and ommatidia (Additional file 2: Figure S2A–E). We also observed that elav-GAL4 > Myc-MoeT559D flies lacked stereotypical climbing behavior, with all unable to climb and congregating at the bottom of vials (Additional file 2: Figure S2F), highlighting the importance of Moesin phosphoregulation in neurological function.

Moesin regulates dendrite arborization and spine-like protrusion growth

In vertebrates, actin remodeling by Moesin has been shown to be crucial to dendritic spine growth and development [25, 26], therefore we next sought to interrogate

Table 1 Summary of mushroom body defects resulting from elav-GAL4 driven expression of UAS-Moe constructs

	Myc-Moe	Myc-MoeT559D	Moe-KD1	Moe-KD2	Myc-Moe; MoeKD1	Myc-Moe; MoeKD2
α/β lobes number[a]	104	70	84	88	84	74
Axon stalling[b] (%)	21	4	10	5	12	11
Lobe missing[c] (%)	35	89	67	70	5	5
Abnormal morphology[d] (%)	2	7	10	11	5	8
Normal morphology (%)	52	0	14	16	79	76
γ lobes number	38	40	37	42	37	39
Thinner (%)	11	100	8	14	3	5
Normal morphology (%)	89	0	92	86	97	95

[a]The percentage of each lobe phenotype was calculated from the total number of brain hemispheres analyzed for each genotype (n). [b]Brain hemispheres were scored as "axon stalling" when one or more partially elongated α/β lobes were present. [c]The complete absence of one or more α/β lobes in a hemisphere was scored as "lobes missing". [d]Brain hemispheres presenting any other defects of lobe morphology were scored as "abnormal morphology"

whether Moesin is required for this process in the adult *Drosophila* central nervous system. The vertical system (VS) of lobula plate tangential cells (LPTCs), a group of visual system interneurons in the optic lobe, represent a model system particularly suited to the study of dendritic growth as these neurons display complex but stereotypical dendritic arborization [39]. In addition, dendrites in LPTCs have been shown to bear vertebrate spine-like protrusions that are actin-enriched [40]. To visualize dendritic morphology, the LPTC driver 3A–GAL4 was used to express Lifeact, which labels the dendrites of LPTCs with a particular concentration in the actin-rich dendritic protrusions. The characteristic arborization pattern of the six neurons, which form the VS of the LPTCs, is not altered by expression of Lifeact [40] (Fig. 4a, b). However, co-expression of Moesin RNAi with Lifeact revealed severely reduced dendritic projections (Fig. 4c, d, Table 2). Myc-Moe localized to primary branches and its expression also resulted in notable deficits in projections (Fig. 4e–g). Consistent with localization to actin-rich regions of the mushroom body, Myc-MoeT559D localized not only to the dendrite branches but also was strongly concentrated in branchlets and protrusions (Fig. 4i–k) with an apparent increase in the intensity of Lifeact, suggesting an increase in protrusion density (compare Fig. 4e to i and h to l). These data suggest that wild-type levels of Moesin are required for normal dendrite branching and arborization in *Drosophila* LPTCs, and activation of Moesin via phosphorylation may promote growth of dendritic spine-like protrusions.

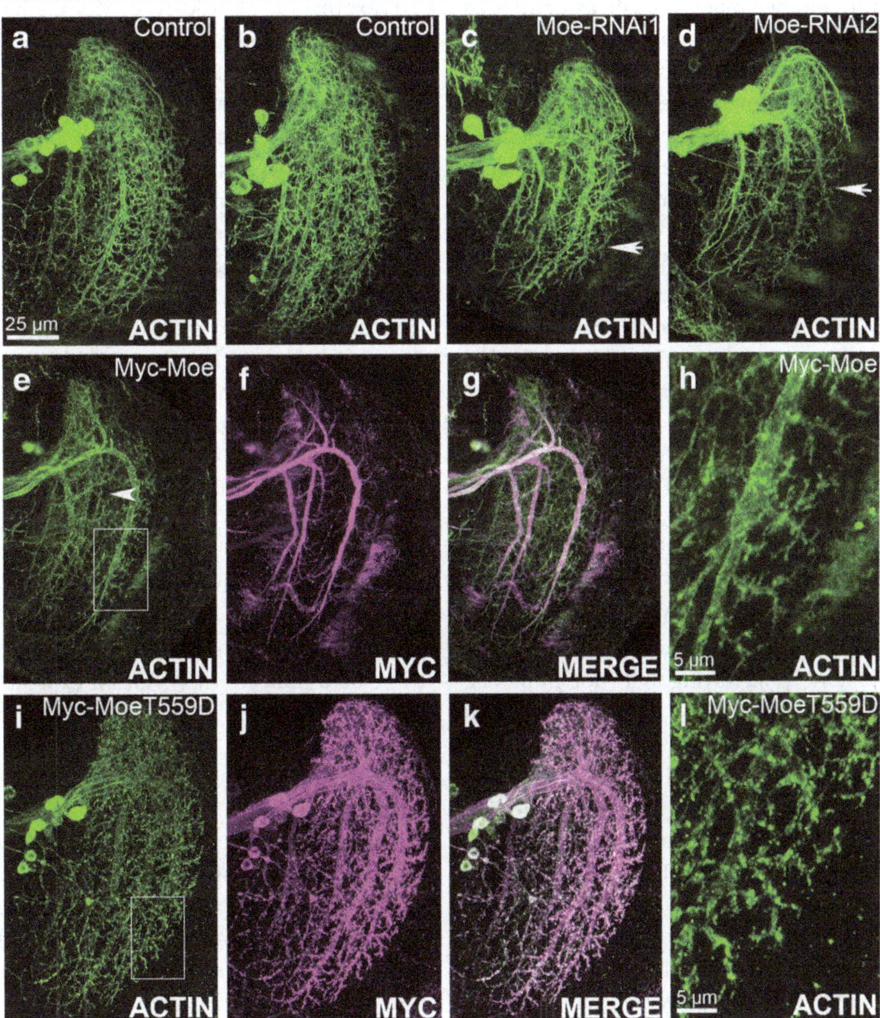

Fig. 4 Altered Moesin expression disrupts dendritic arborization. Immunohistochemistry with anti-GFP (green) antibody on whole mount brains. All images are confocal projections through the optic lobe of the brain. **a**, **b**. 3A–GAL4 > Lifeact labels the dendritic arbor of the six neurons comprising the vertical system of LPTCs. **c**, **d**. Knockdown of *Moesin* results in defects in dendritic branching; arrows show stunted growth of VS branches. **e–g**. Overexpression of *Moesin* disrupts dendritic branching; arrow points to stunted VS branch. Anti-Myc staining (magenta) reveals that it localizes to the primary branches of the vertical system. **i–k**. Myc-MoeT559D distributes throughout the VS neurons, including the branchlets and spines. **l**. Expression of Myc-MoeT559D results in increased Lifeact staining the VS1 branch in comparison to expression of Myc-Moe (**h**)

Table 2 Summary of LPTC defects resulting from elav-GAL4 driven expression of UAS-Moe constructs

	Control	MoeKD	Myc-Moe	Myc-MoeT559D
Number[a]	19	21	15	18
Abnormal morphology[b] (%)	0	76	40	22
Increased intensity of Lifeact in VS1 dendritic protrusions[c] (%)	0	n/a[d]	0	44

[a]The percentage of each lobe phenotype was calculated from the total number of brain hemispheres analyzed for each genotype (n). [b]Brain hemispheres were scored as "abnormal morphology" when one or more branches were missing, reduced in length or thinner than controls. [c]The relative intensity of Lifeact in the dendritic protrusions was visually compared to that of the branch. If the protusion/branch intensity appeared higher than control brains, it was scored as "increased". [d]MoeKD was unable to be scored due to the severe branching defects. All analyses were performed by a blinded observer

Moesin is required for long-term memory formation

We next investigated the role of Moesin in memory formation in the repeat training courtship suppression assay [41–44]. In this assay, a male trained with a mated, unreceptive female will learn to recognize the rejection behavior of a mated female and therefore court less when presented with another mated female as compared to a male lacking this training. Pan-neuronal knockdown of Moesin had no significant impact on courtship of sham-trained Moesin knockdown males (Additional file 3: Figure S3), indicating that reduction of Moesin does not alter courtship behavior and any observed memory deficits would not be simply due to decreased courtship in this group. Pan-neuronal knockdown of Moesin resulted in a significant defect in 24-h long-term memory (Fig. 5a). As an intact mushroom body is critical for formation of courtship memory, the memory deficits observed were unsurprising. Therefore, in order to establish whether Moesin also plays a non-developmental role in long-term memory, the TARGET system was utilized to restrict Moesin knockdown to the adult brain. Flies were raised to adulthood at 19 °C (GAL4 repressed) then switched to 30 °C (GAL4 active) three days prior to testing to allow induction of RNAi expression. Tight induction of expression and negligible leakiness of the TARGET system was confirmed by western blotting (Additional file 4: Figure S4). Assessment of 24-h memory revealed a significant impairment in long-term memory, signifying that Moesin plays a non-developmental role in memory (Fig. 5b). We also assessed the integrity of short-term memory one hour after a one-hour training session, and found that knockdown of Moesin in the adult brain had no impact on short-term memory (Fig. 5c). As long-term courtship memory is mushroom body-dependent [34], we examined the specific requirement for Moesin in the mushroom body by restricting knockdown primarily to the α/β and γ neurons with the MB247-GAL4 driver [45]. This also resulted in impaired 24-h memory (Fig. 5d), and similarly short-term memory was unaffected (Fig. 5e). The requirement for Moesin in mushroom body neurons for normal long-term memory formation led us to investigate the effect of Moesin overexpression on long-term memory. MB247-driven expression of Myc-Moe in the adult mushroom body resulted in robust long-term memory, therefore elevated levels of Moesin had no significant effect on long-term courtship memory (Fig. 5f). In addition, co-expression of Myc-Moe rescued the long-term memory defect caused by knockdown of Moesin in the mushroom body (Fig. 5g), confirming that the memory deficit was specifically caused by a reduction in Moesin. While overexpression of wild-type Moesin had no impact, expression of constitutively active Moesin abolished long-term memory (Fig. 5h).

The three Kenyon cell types, α/β, α'/β' and γ, differ in connectivity and have been previously shown to be functionally distinct with respect to their roles in long-term memory. We examined the spatial requirements for Moesin in the mushroom body by knocking down expression in each Kenyon cell subtype in the mature brain. The GAL4 drivers c739 and c305a drive expression in the α/β and α'/β' Kenyon cell subtypes, respectively [46–48], and knockdown of Moesin with either of these drivers did not have a significant effect on long-term memory (Fig. 5i, j). Knockdown of Moesin in γ neurons with the 1471 and NP1131 drivers [49] recapitulated the impairment of long-term memory that was observed with elav and MB247 (Fig. 5k, l). Lastly, as an additional control, anti-FasII immunohistochemistry was performed on brains of flies of the genotypes that resulted in memory impairments to confirm normal mushroom body morphology (Fig. 5m). Taken together, these data indicate that Moesin expression is required in the γ neurons in order to form long-term courtship memory.

Discussion

Here, we describe an essential role for Moesin in morphogenesis of mushroom body axons as well as a distinct non-developmental role in long-term memory. The examination of developmental deficits in the mushroom body of flies with reduced Moesin indicates an integral role for Moesin in axon projection, targeting, and branching. Increased Moesin expression also perturbed normal axonal outgrowth, but generally resulted in less severe developmental phenotypes, most likely because the majority of Moesin exists in an inactive conformation. However, the expression of the constitutively active Moesin resulted in complete disruption of

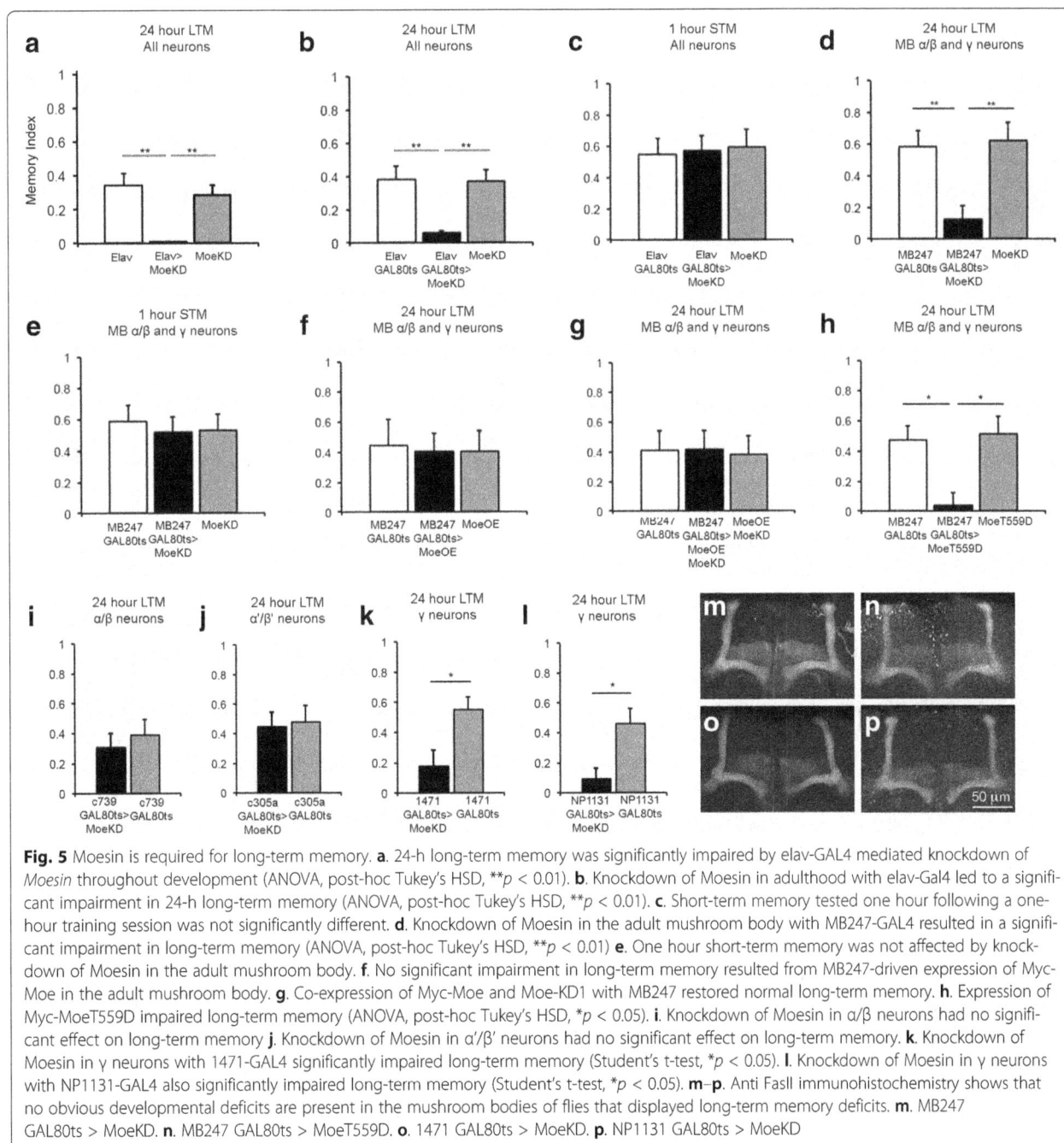

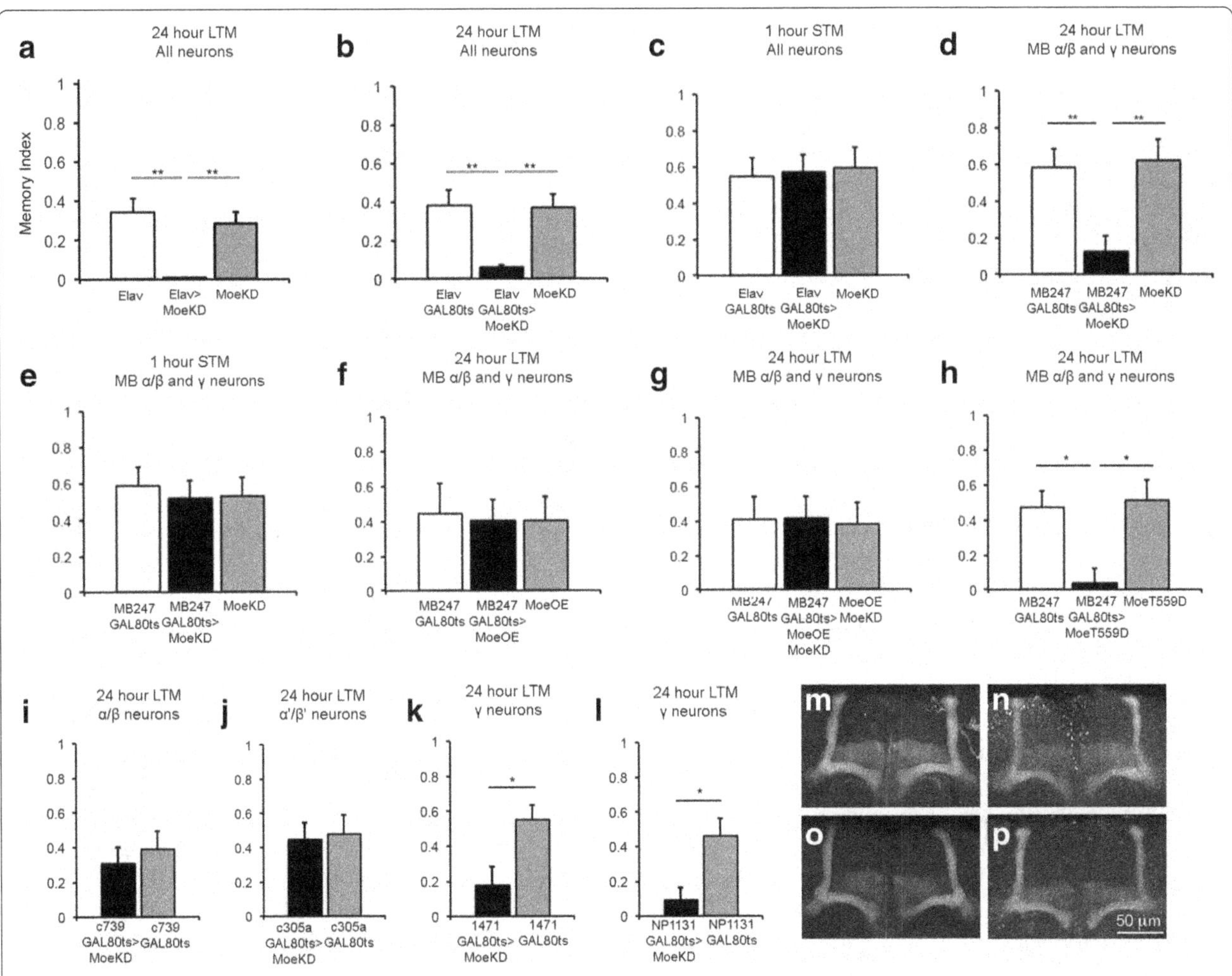

Fig. 5 Moesin is required for long-term memory. **a**. 24-h long-term memory was significantly impaired by elav-GAL4 mediated knockdown of *Moesin* throughout development (ANOVA, post-hoc Tukey's HSD, $**p < 0.01$). **b**. Knockdown of Moesin in adulthood with elav-Gal4 led to a significant impairment in 24-h long-term memory (ANOVA, post-hoc Tukey's HSD, $**p < 0.01$). **c**. Short-term memory tested one hour following a one-hour training session was not significantly different. **d**. Knockdown of Moesin in the adult mushroom body with MB247-GAL4 resulted in a significant impairment in long-term memory (ANOVA, post-hoc Tukey's HSD, $**p < 0.01$) **e**. One hour short-term memory was not affected by knockdown of Moesin in the adult mushroom body. **f**. No significant impairment in long-term memory resulted from MB247-driven expression of Myc-Moe in the adult mushroom body. **g**. Co-expression of Myc-Moe and Moe-KD1 with MB247 restored normal long-term memory. **h**. Expression of Myc-MoeT559D impaired long-term memory (ANOVA, post-hoc Tukey's HSD, $*p < 0.05$). **i**. Knockdown of Moesin in α/β neurons had no significant effect on long-term memory **j**. Knockdown of Moesin in α'/β' neurons had no significant effect on long-term memory. **k**. Knockdown of Moesin in γ neurons with 1471-GAL4 significantly impaired long-term memory (Student's t-test, $*p < 0.05$). **l**. Knockdown of Moesin in γ neurons with NP1131-GAL4 also significantly impaired long-term memory (Student's t-test, $*p < 0.05$). **m**–**p**. Anti FasII immunohistochemistry shows that no obvious developmental deficits are present in the mushroom bodies of flies that displayed long-term memory deficits. **m**. MB247 GAL80ts > MoeKD. **n**. MB247 GAL80ts > MoeT559D. **o**. 1471 GAL80ts > MoeKD. **p**. NP1131 GAL80ts > MoeKD

mushroom body assembly, highlighting a critical role for phosphoregulation of Moesin in this developmental process.

Moesin was recently found to interact with the cell adhesion molecule Neuroglian, the sole *Drosophila* L1CAM [50]. Mutational analysis of Neuroglian identified a requirement for the ERM-interaction domain, to which Moesin binds, in the establishment of the mushroom body's highly organized architecture [51]. *Neuroglian* mutants display severe mushroom body phenotypes including growth and guidance errors, missing lobes and branching defects [50, 51], similar to those herein that result from the modulation of Moesin expression. The deletion of the ERM interaction domain of Neuroglian, however, results in a phenotype in which aberrant axonal projections form a ball-like structure from continuous circular growth in the posterior of the brain [50, 51]. This phenotype has been described previously as axon stalling, however, it was subsequently characterized as a guidance error following the discovery that the defect results from a failure of axons to enter the peduncle [50, 51]. In contrast, our data reveal an axon stalling phenotype in which axon growth is arrested subsequent to branching from the peduncle and is observed in both *Moesin k*nockdown and overexpression brains. Additionally, the lack of any aberrant axonal accumulations in the posterior of brain hemispheres with missing mushroom body lobes indicates that these defects are likely the result of branching errors as axons either fail to bifurcate or subsequently segregate into vertical and medial lobes. The prevalence of this lobe formation defect in Neuroglian knockdown mushroom bodies and the importance of the ERM protein interaction domain to L1CAM-mediated axon branching in vertebrates suggests that reduction of Moesin expression may impair branching in part due to a reduced interaction with Neuroglian [50, 52]. The range of mushroom body defects resulting from the modulation of Moesin expression and activation highlights a central role for Moesin in axon growth and guidance.

Our data also reveal the importance of phosphoregulation of Moesin in photoreceptor and mushroom body development, as evidenced by the severe defects that result from the pan-neuronal expression of phosphomimetic Moesin. While the modulation of Moesin expression also led to serious defects in mushroom body assembly, no defect was observed in photoreceptors in which wild-type Moesin was knocked down or overexpressed. This finding is consistent with previous reports in which reduction of *Moesin* dosage by up to half did not impair photoreceptor development and only overexpression of Myc-MoeT559D led to guidance defects [53].

We also examined the role of Moesin in dendritic development and found that modulation of Moesin expression resulted in a disruption of the stereotypical dendritic arborization of the LPTC VS. Knockdown of Moesin resulted in a reduced dendritic field with fewer projections from multiple VS neurons, as did overexpression of wild-type Moesin. Constitutive activation of Moesin resulted in fewer branching deficits, but there was an increase in the density of dendritic protrusions on the VS1 branch. The complex phenotypes emerging from the modulation of Moesin suggest that it may be involved in multiple aspects of dendritic arborization. Previously characterized regulators of dendritic arborization in *Drosophila* include the Rho GTPases Rac1 and Rho1, which have opposing effects on the growth and complexity of dendrites. Rac1 promotes dendritic branching and extension while Rho1 restricts both branching and branch length [54–56]. Moesin has been shown to negatively regulate Rho1 activity in *Drosophila* epithelial cells [57, 58] and neurons [59], therefore, the lack of dendritic projections in some Moesin-knockdown neurons may be the result of Rho1 hyperactivity. *Rho1* null MB neurons display increased dendritic volume, whereas constitutively active Rho1 results in reduced dendritic volume in the mushroom body [55], which is consistent with the hypothesis that Moesin negatively regulates Rho1. However, the regulatory interaction may be more complex, as Rho1 has also been demonstrated to act upstream of Moesin [11]. In addition, expression of constitutively active Moesin and overexpression of wild-type Rac1 in LPTCs [40] both result in an increased number of dendritic protrusions, suggesting that Moesin may interact with both Rac1 and Rho1 to regulate growth of dendritic protrusions.

While we found that expression of constitutively active Moesin resulted in severely reduced and malformed mushroom body axons, most dendrites displayed arbors with typical field coverage. The molecular pathways for axon and dendritic morphogenesis are distinct, and insight into some of the molecular mechanisms that are responsible have been provided by Lee and colleagues who demonstrated that Rho GTPases play contrasting molecular roles in axon and dendrite morphogenesis [55]. For example, although they display altered dendritic development, *Rho1* null flies develop normal mushroom body axons. *Rac1* mutants, on the other hand, display severe defects in mushroom body axon growth and guidance but display far milder phenotypes in mushroom body dendrites [60] and do not disrupt dendritic branching in LPTCs [40]. Interestingly, the defects in mushroom body axon morphogenesis and the increase in dendritic protrusions in the LPTC visual system that we observed on expression of constitutively active Moesin are both similar phenotypes to those that result from increased Rac1 activity [40, 55]. *Rac1* and *Neuroglian* also interact genetically in mushroom body axons, with a *Rac1* mutant exacerbating the growth and guidance deficits resulting from both loss and gain of function of *Neuroglian,* suggesting *Rac1* may act both up and downstream [51]. Assays for Rac1 and Rho1 activity in presence of WT and mutant forms of Moesin (i.e. knockdown, and expression of T559A and T559D), in combination with analysis of Moesin phosphorylation in the presence of *Rac1* and *Rho1* mutants will be valuable in determining whether Moesin acts upstream and/or downstream of Rho GTPases.

We also provide evidence for an adult-specific role of Moesin in long-term memory formation. We found that pan-neuronal knockdown of Moesin throughout development had no effect on courtship activity, with males displaying the full repertoire of courtship behaviors and no difference in the amount of time spent in courtship behavior between sham control and Moesin knockdown flies. Thus wild-type levels of Moesin are not required in the brain for normal courtship activity. Long-term courtship memory was impaired, as would be expected since formation of this memory is dependent on an intact mushroom body [34]. However, conditional knockdown of Moesin in all neurons of the adult brain led to similar defects in long-term memory. This argues strongly for a post-developmental role for Moesin in long-term memory, which is not attributable to a non-specific disruption of cellular function or role in general neurotransmission, as one-hour short-term memory, which is also dependent on an intact mushroom body [34] was not affected. By targeting Moesin knockdown in the adult specifically to the neurons that comprise the mushroom body, the requirement for Moesin in long-term memory was traced to the γ neurons of the mushroom body. While the precise molecular mechanisms behind courtship learning are still largely unresolved, several steps in the acquisition and consolidation of memory have been elucidated. Loss of the cytoplasmic polyadenylation element–binding protein Orb2 results in a specific impairment in long-term memory formation, and restoration of Orb2 in the γ neurons during or immediately after a training session is sufficient to rescue this long-term memory deficit [44]. The activation of Orb2 requires input to the mushroom body from aSP13 dopaminergic neurons during both acquisition and consolidation, which is dependent on the presence of the dopamine receptor DopR1 in γ neurons [61]. During consolidation, this activation results in the formation of a complex between the two Orb2 isoforms, Orb2A and Orb2B at synapses. This Orb2 complex then induces translation of CaMKII [61], a protein critical for persistence of memory [62]. Transcriptional modulators have also been found to act in the γ neurons to facilitate normal long-term memory. Overexpression of the histone deacetylase HDAC4 specifically in the γ neurons of adult flies impairs long-term memory [42], as does knockdown of *Rpd3 (HDAC1)* [43]. Together these data are consistent with the synapses of mushroom body γ neurons being a likely site of the protein synthesis-dependent plastic modifications that underpin long-term courtship memory in *Drosophila*. These plastic changes at synapses are highly contingent upon actin remodeling within particular compartments to enable the dynamic structural modifications in neuronal morphology [13, 15, 16]. As a key regulator of the actin cytoskeleton in neurons, we hypothesize that training results in activation of Moesin, which promotes actin rearrangements that underpin the morphological changes at specific synapses. This is consistent with the lack of an effect from the overexpression of wild-type Moesin, which was largely cytoplasmic and inactive.

Conclusions

In summary, we provide evidence that the actin-binding protein Moesin is necessary for both normal development of the mushroom body as well as a mushroom body-dependent post-developmental role in long-term memory. These data, taken together with the evidence that Moesin regulates cytoskeletal rearrangement and promotes the growth of dendritic spine-like protrusions in *Drosophila* and spine growth in mammals [25, 26], suggest that Moesin may be a key facilitator of the morphological changes in neurons that occur during long-term memory consolidation.

Methods

Fly strains

All flies were cultured on standard medium on a 12-h light/dark cycle and maintained at a temperature of 25 °C unless otherwise indicated. Canton S flies were used as wild-type controls. *P{w[+mW.hs] = GawB}elav[C155]* (elav-GAL4, #458); *w[1118];P{w[+mC] = UASMoe.IR.327–775}3* (MoeKD2, #8629); *w[1118];P{w[+mC] = UASMoe.MYC.K}2* (Myc-Moe, #8631); *w[1118];P{w[+mC] = UAS MoeT559D.MYC}2* (Myc-MoeT559D, #8630); y [1] w[67c23]; P{w[+mW.hs] = GawB}Hr39[c739], (c739-GAL4, #7362); *w[1118];P{w + mW.hs = GawB}c305a* (c305a-GAL4); *w[1118];P{w + mW.hs = GawB}1471* (1471-GAL4, #9465); *y* [1] *w[*]; P{w[+mW.hs] = GawB}3A* (3A–GAL4, #51629) and *y* [1] *w[*]; P{y[+t*] w[+mC] = UAS-Lifeact-GFP}VIE-260B* (Lifeact, #35544) were obtained from the Bloomington *Drosophila* Stock Center, stock numbers indicated in brackets. w^*; *P{w + mC = tubP-GAL80ts}10* (tubP-GAL80^{ts}), *w[*];P{w[+m*] = Mef2-GAL4.247}3* [63] (MB247-GAL4) and *w(CS10)* strains were kindly provided by R. Davis (The Scripps Research Institute, Jupiter, FL). *w[1118]; P{w[+mC] (UASMoe IR.528–897}2* (MoeKD1, Transformant ID110654) was obtained from the Vienna Drosophila Resource Center. All strains used for behavioral testing and analysis of brain development were outcrossed for a minimum of five generations to *w(CS10)* flies. Homozygous lines harbouring *w(CS10); P{w + mC = tubP-GAL80ts}10* and the appropriate GAL4 drivers were generated by standard genetic crosses.

Immunohistochemistry

Whole flies were fixed in PFAT/DMSO (4% paraformaldehyde in 1X phosphate buffered saline + 5% dimethyl sulfoxide + 0.1% Triton X-100) for one hour then washed in PBT (1Xphosphate buffered saline + 0.5% Triton X-100). Brains were microdissected in PBT then post fixed in PFAT/DMSO for 20 min and stored in methanol at −20 °C. Following rehydration in PBT, brains were blocked in immunobuffer (5% normal goat serum in PBT) for >2 h at room temperature. They were then incubated overnight at room temperature with primary antibody and subsequently incubated overnight at 4 °C with secondary antibody (goat anti-mouse Alexa488, goat anti-mouse Alexa555, goat anti-rabbit Alexa488, or goat anti-rabbit Alexa555, Molecular Probes, 1:200) and mounted with Antifade mounting medium (4% n-propyl gallate in 90% glycerol + 10%

phosphate buffered saline). The following antibodies were used: Anti-Moesin (1:5000) kind gift from D. Kiehart [6]; anti-Myc (1:50) developed by J. M. Bishop and anti-ELAV 9F89A clone (1:100) developed by G.M. Rubin, both of which were obtained from the Developmental Studies Hybridoma Bank developed under the auspices of the NICHD and maintained by The University of Iowa, Department of Biology, Iowa City, IA. For confocal microscopy, optical sections were taken with a Leica TCS SP5 DM6000B Confocal Microscope. Image stacks taken at intervals of 1 µm (whole brain) or 0.5 µm (MB and LPTCs) and were processed with Leica Application Suite Advanced Fluorescence (LAS AF) and ImageJ software.

Western blot

Flies were collected in tubes and frozen in a dry ice/ ethanol bath. The tubes were vortexed to snap the heads from the bodies, and the heads were collected. Cytoplasmic extracts were prepared by homogenizing heads with a disposable mortar and pestle in RIPA buffer (150 mM sodium chloride, 1% Triton X-100, 1% sodium deoxycholate, 0.1% sodium dodecyl sulfate, 25 mM Tris, pH 8.0). Following centrifugation at 13,000 g for 2 min at 4 °C, the supernatant was retained as the cytoplasmic fraction. Protein concentration was then determined with the Pierce BCA Protein Assay Kit (ThermoFisher Scientific). 20 µg of each sample was loaded onto a 10% sodium dodecyl sulfate-polyacrylamide gel electrophoresis gel and resolved at 200 V. Protein was transferred onto nitrocellulose and blocked for >2 h in 5% skim milk powder in TBST (50 mM Tris, 150 mM NaCl, 0.05% Tween-20, pH 7.6). The membrane was incubated overnight at 4 °C in primary antibody and one hour in secondary antibody. Antibodies used were anti-Moesin (D. Kiehart, Duke University, 1:50,000), anti-Myc (1:100) and anti α-tubulin (12G10 clone, developed by J. Frankel and *M. nelson*, Developmental Studies Hybridoma Bank, 1:500). Detection was performed with ECL Plus (GE).

Behavioral analyses

The repeat training courtship suppression assay [37, 41–44] was used to assess one-hour and 24-h memory. In this assay, a male trained with a mated, unreceptive female will learn the rejection behavior of a mated female and therefore court less when presented with a mated female in the future as compared to an untrained male. All behavioral assays and statistical analyses were performed as previously described [43]. A training session consists of pairing a virgin male with a female who was mated the previous night for 1 to 7 h. The male is left to court the mated female for the duration of the training session, after which time the female was removed. A one-hour training session was administered for the analysis of short-term memory, while a seven-hour training session was applied in long-term memory assessment. In parallel, a naïve "sham" male of the same genotype was housed alone. Long-term memory was measured 24 h after training by pairing each male with another freshly mated female and scoring his courtship activity (licking, chasing, or orienting toward the female, wing extension and vibration) over a ten-minute period. Short-term memory was assessed in the same manner one hour after the training session. In order to generate a memory score from this courtship data a memory index was calculated by comparing the percentage of the ten-minute period spent engaging in courtship behavior (courtship index) against the mean of the sham flies of its genotype (n≥16/ group). Memory was measured on a scale of 0 to 1, with 1 being the highest memory score possible, and a score of 0 indicating memory is no different than untrained sham controls.

Additional files

Additional file 1: Figure S1. Confocal projections of brains expressing Lifeact and counterstained with the neuropil marker nc82. A-C. *frontal* confocal projection showing localization of Lifeact (green) primarily to the mushroom body lobes and glomeruli. D-F. Posterior confocal projection showing localisation of Lifeact to the optic lobes and calyx of the mushroom body. Abbreviations: MB, mushroom body lobes; G, glomeruli; C, calyx; OL, optic lobe. (PDF 4815 kb)

Additional file 2: Figure S2. Eye and locomotor phenotypes resulting from elav-GAL4-driven knockdown and overexpression of Moesin. A-E. Scanning electron micrographs of the Drosophila eye. A. elav/+ control. B elav > MoeKD1. C. elav > MoeKD2. D. elav > Myc-Moe. E. elav > Myc-MoeT559D. F. Left vial, elav/+ control. Right vial, elav > Myc-Moe. (PDF 2264 kb)

Additional file 3: Figure S3. Courtship activity of sham trained flies from each of the courtship suppression assays. Sham controls were exposed to the same training procedure as the trained flies but were not exposed to a female. The lack of significant difference in courtship activity between the genotypes indicates that courtship activity itself was not affected by genetic manipulation of Moesin. (PDF 1007 kb)

Additional file 4: Figure S4. Temperature sensitive regulation of Moesin RNAi and transgene expression. A. Whole cell lysates were prepared from heads from *elav-GAL4/+; tub-GAL80ts/+* and *elav-GAL4/+; tub-GAL80ts/UAS-MoeRNAi* flies that were raised and maintained at 19°C, or raised at 19°C then switched to 30°C for three days prior to harvest. The blot was probed with anti-Moesin and anti-α-tubulin antibody was used as a loading control. B. Whole cell lysates were prepared from heads from *elav-GAL4/+; tub-GAL80ts/+* and *elav-GAL4/+; tub-GAL80ts/UAS-Myc-Moe* and *elav-GAL4/+; tub-GAL80ts/UAS-Myc-MoeT559D* flies that were raised and maintained at 19°C, or raised at 19°C then switched to 30°C for three days prior to harvest. The blot was probed with anti-Myc and anti-α-tubulin antibody was used as a loading control. (PDF 849 kb)

Acknowledgements

We thank Matthew Savoian and Niki Murray and the Manawatu Microscopy and Imaging Centre for scanning electron microscopy and assistance with confocal microscopy. Professor Dan Kiehart for the gift of the anti-Moesin antibody. Stocks obtained from the Bloomington Drosophila Stock Center (NIH P40OD018537) and the Vienna *Drosophila* Resource Center were used in this study.

Funding

This work was supported by a grant from the Palmerston North Medical Research Foundation and a Health Research Council of New Zealand Sir

Charles Hercus Health Research Fellowship to HLF. The funding bodies had no role in the design of the study and collection, analysis, interpretation of data, or in writing the manuscript.

Authors' contributions

HLF conceived the study, analyzed and interpreted the data and wrote the manuscript. PSF conceived the study, performed the experiments, analyzed and interpreted the data and wrote the manuscript. Both authors read and approved the final manuscript.

Competing interests

The authors declare they have no competing interests.

References

1. Bretscher A, Edwards K, Fehon RG. ERM proteins and merlin: integrators at the cell cortex. Nat Rev Mol Cell Biol. 2002;3:586–99.
2. Mangeat P, Roy C, Martin M. ERM proteins in cell adhesion and membrane dynamics. Trends Cell Biol. 1999;9:187–92.
3. Tsukita S, Yonemura S. ERM (ezrin/radixin/moesin) family: from cytoskeleton to signal transduction. Curr Opin Cell Biol. 1997;9:70–5.
4. Mackay DJ, Esch F, Furthmayr H, Hall A. Rho- and rac-dependent assembly of focal adhesion complexes and actin filaments in permeabilized fibroblasts: an essential role for ezrin/radixin/moesin proteins. J Cell Biol. 1997;138:927–38.
5. Manchanda N, Lyubimova A, Ho HY, James MF, Gusella JF, Ramesh N, Snapper SB, Ramesh V. The NF2 tumor suppressor Merlin and the ERM proteins interact with N-WASP and regulate its actin polymerization function. J Biol Chem. 2005;280:12517–22.
6. Edwards KA, Demsky M, Montague RA, Weymouth N, Kiehart DP. GFP-moesin illuminates actin cytoskeleton dynamics in living tissue and demonstrates cell shape changes during morphogenesis in drosophila. Dev Biol. 1997;191:103–17.
7. Karagiosis SA, Ready DF. Moesin contributes an essential structural role in drosophila photoreceptor morphogenesis. Development. 2004;131:725–32.
8. Kunda P, Pelling AE, Liu T, Baum B. Moesin controls cortical rigidity, cell rounding, and spindle morphogenesis during mitosis. Current biology : CB. 2008;18:91–101.
9. Seabrooke S, Stewart BA. Moesin helps to restrain synaptic growth at the drosophila neuromuscular junction. Developmental neurobiology. 2008;68: 379–91.
10. Jankovics F, Sinka R, Lukacsovich T, Erdelyi M. MOESIN crosslinks actin and cell membrane in drosophila oocytes and is required for OSKAR anchoring. Current biology : CB. 2002;12:2060–5.
11. Oshiro N, Fukata Y, Kaibuchi K. Phosphorylation of moesin by rho-associated kinase (rho-kinase) plays a crucial role in the formation of microvilli-like structures. J Biol Chem. 1998;273:34663–6.
12. Gautreau A, Louvard D, Arpin M. Morphogenic effects of ezrin require a phosphorylation-induced transition from oligomers to monomers at the plasma membrane. J Cell Biol. 2000;150:193–203.
13. Matus A. Actin-based plasticity in dendritic spines. Science. 2000;290:754–8.
14. Cingolani LA, Goda Y. Actin in action: the interplay between the actin cytoskeleton and synaptic efficacy. Nat Rev Neurosci. 2008;9:344–56.
15. Ramachandran B, Frey JU. Interfering with the actin network and its effect on long-term potentiation and synaptic tagging in hippocampal CA1 neurons in slices in vitro. The Journal of neuroscience : the official journal of the Society for Neuroscience. 2009;29:12167–73.
16. Lamprecht R, LeDoux J. Structural plasticity and memory. Nat Rev Neurosci. 2004;5:45–54.
17. Gomez TM, Letourneau PC. Actin dynamics in growth cone motility and navigation. J Neurochem. 2014;129:221–34.
18. Dent EW, Gertler FB. Cytoskeletal dynamics and transport in growth cone motility and axon guidance. Neuron. 2003;40:209–27.
19. Lowery LA, Van Vactor D. The trip of the tip: understanding the growth cone machinery. Nat Rev Mol Cell Biol. 2009;10:332–43.
20. Paglini G, Kunda P, Quiroga S, Kosik K, Caceres A. Suppression of radixin and moesin alters growth cone morphology, motility, and process formation in primary cultured neurons. J Cell Biol. 1998;143:443–55.
21. Jeon S, Park JK, Bae CD, Park J. NGF-induced moesin phosphorylation is mediated by the PI3K, Rac1 and Akt and required for neurite formation in PC12 cells. Neurochem Int. 2010;56:810–8.
22. Kim HS, Bae CD, Park J. Glutamate receptor-mediated phosphorylation of ezrin/radixin/moesin proteins is implicated in filopodial protrusion of primary cultured hippocampal neuronal cells. J Neurochem. 2010;113:1565–76.
23. Matsuzaki M, Honkura N, Ellis-Davies GC, Kasai H. Structural basis of long-term potentiation in single dendritic spines. Nature. 2004;429:761–6.
24. Okamoto K, Nagai T, Miyawaki A, Hayashi Y. Rapid and persistent modulation of actin dynamics regulates postsynaptic reorganization underlying bidirectional plasticity. Nat Neurosci. 2004;7:1104–12.
25. Sanchez AM, Flamini MI, Fu XD, Mannella P, Giretti MS, Goglia L, Genazzani AR, Simoncini T. Rapid signaling of estrogen to WAVE1 and moesin controls neuronal spine formation via the actin cytoskeleton. Mol Endocrinol. 2009; 23:1193–202.
26. Sanchez AM, Flamini MI, Genazzani AR, Simoncini T. Effects of progesterone and medroxyprogesterone on actin remodeling and neuronal spine formation. Mol Endocrinol. 2013;27:693–702.
27. Baudry M, Bi X, Aguirre C. Progesterone-estrogen interactions in synaptic plasticity and neuroprotection. Neuroscience. 2013;239:280–94.
28. Foy MR, Akopian G, Thompson RF. Progesterone regulation of synaptic transmission and plasticity in rodent hippocampus. Learn Mem. 2008;15: 820–2.
29. Foy MR, Baudry M, Akopian GK, Thompson RF. Regulation of hippocampal synaptic plasticity by estrogen and progesterone. Vitam Horm. 2010;82:219–39.
30. Dubnau J, Chiang AS, Grady L, Barditch J, Gossweiler S, McNeil J, Smith P, Buldoc F, Scott R, Certa U, et al. The staufen/pumilio pathway is involved in drosophila long-term memory. Current biology : CB. 2003;13:286–96.
31. Tully T, Preat T, Boynton SC, Del Vecchio M. Genetic dissection of consolidated memory in drosophila. Cell. 1994;79:35–47.
32. Doi Y, Itoh M, Yonemura S, Ishihara S, Takano H, Noda T, Tsukita S. Normal development of mice and unimpaired cell adhesion/cell motility/actin-based cytoskeleton without compensatory up-regulation of ezrin or radixin in moesin gene knockout. J Biol Chem. 1999;274:2315–21.
33. Heisenberg M. Mushroom body memoir: from maps to models. Nat Rev Neurosci. 2003;4:266–75.
34. McBride SM, Giuliani G, Choi C, Krause P, Correale D, Watson K, Baker G, Siwicki KK. Mushroom body ablation impairs short-term memory and long-term memory of courtship conditioning in Drosophila Melanogaster. Neuron. 1999;24:967–77.
35. Riedl J, Crevenna AH, Kessenbrock K, Yu JH, Neukirchen D, Bista M, Bradke F, Jenne D, Holak TA, Werb Z, et al. Lifeact: a versatile marker to visualize F-actin. Nat Methods. 2008;5:605–7.
36. Crittenden JR, Skoulakis EM, Han K-A, Kalderon D, Davis RL. Tripartite mushroom body architecture revealed by antigenic markers. Learn Mem. 1998;5:38–51.
37. Schwartz S, Truglio M, Scott MJ, Fitzsimons HL. Long-term memory in drosophila is influenced by histone deacetylase HDAC4 interacting with SUMO-conjugating enzyme Ubc9. Genetics. 2016;203:1249–64.
38. Robinow S, White K. The locus elav of Drosophila Melanogaster is expressed in neurons at all developmental stages. Dev Biol. 1988;126: 294–303.
39. Scott EK, Raabe T, Luo L. Structure of the vertical and horizontal system neurons of the lobula plate in drosophila. J Comp Neurol. 2002;454:470–81.
40. Leiss F, Koper E, Hein I, Fouquet W, Lindner J, Sigrist S, Tavosanis G. Characterization of dendritic spines in the drosophila central nervous system. Developmental neurobiology. 2009;69:221–34.

41. Ejima A, Griffith LC: Assay for courtship suppression in Drosophila. *Cold Spring Harbor protocols* 2011, 2011:pdb prot5575.
42. Fitzsimons HL, Schwartz S, Given FM, Scott MJ. The histone deacetylase HDAC4 regulates long-term memory in drosophila. PLoS One. 2013;8:e83903.
43. Fitzsimons HL, Scott MJ. Genetic modulation of Rpd3 expression impairs long-term courtship memory in drosophila. PLoS One. 2011;6:e29171.
44. Keleman K, Kruttner S, Alenius M, Dickson BJ. Function of the drosophila CPEB protein Orb2 in long-term courtship memory. Nat Neurosci. 2007;10:1587–93.
45. Schwaerzel M, Heisenberg M, Zars T. Extinction antagonizes olfactory memory at the subcellular level. Neuron. 2002;35:951–60.
46. Aso Y, Grubel K, Busch S, Friedrich AB, Siwanowicz I, Tanimoto H. The mushroom body of adult drosophila characterized by GAL4 drivers. J Neurogenet. 2009;23:156–72.
47. Krashes MJ, Keene AC, Leung B, Armstrong JD, Waddell S. Sequential use of mushroom body neuron subsets during drosophila odor memory processing. Neuron. 2007;53:103–15.
48. Yang MY, Armstrong JD, Vilinsky I, Strausfeld NJ, Kaiser K. Subdivision of the drosophila mushroom bodies by enhancer-trap expression patterns. Neuron. 1995;15:45–54.
49. Isabel G, Pascual A, Preat T. Exclusive consolidated memory phases in drosophila. Science. 2004;304:1024–7.
50. Siegenthaler D, Enneking EM, Moreno E, Pielage J. L1CAM/Neuroglian controls the axon-axon interactions establishing layered and lobular mushroom body architecture. J Cell Biol. 2015;208:1003–18.
51. Goossens T, Kang YY, Wuytens G, Zimmermann P, Callaerts-Vegh Z, Pollarolo G, Islam R, Hortsch M, Callaerts P. The drosophila L1CAM homolog Neuroglian signals through distinct pathways to control different aspects of mushroom body axon development. Development. 2011;138:1595–605.
52. Cheng L, Itoh K, Lemmon V. L1-mediated branching is regulated by two ezrin-radixin-moesin (ERM)-binding sites, the RSLE region and a novel juxtamembrane ERM-binding region. The Journal of neuroscience : the official journal of the Society for Neuroscience. 2005;25:395–403.
53. Ruan W, Unsain N, Desbarats J, Fon EA, Barker PA. Wengen, the sole tumour necrosis factor receptor in drosophila, collaborates with moesin to control photoreceptor axon targeting during development. PLoS One. 2013;8: e60091.
54. Iyer SC, Wang D, Iyer EP, Trunnell SA, Meduri R, Shinwari R, Sulkowski MJ, Cox DN. The RhoGEF trio functions in sculpting class specific dendrite morphogenesis in drosophila sensory neurons. PLoS One. 2012;7:e33634.
55. Lee T, Winter C, Marticke SS, Lee A, Luo L. Essential roles of drosophila RhoA in the regulation of neuroblast proliferation and dendritic but not axonal morphogenesis. Neuron. 2000;25:307–16.
56. Lee A, Li W, Xu K, Bogert BA, Su K, Gao FB. Control of dendritic development by the Drosophila Fragile X-related gene involves the small GTPase Rac1. Development. 2003;130:5543–52.
57. Neisch AL, Formstecher E, Fehon RG. Conundrum, an ARHGAP18 orthologue, regulates RhoA and proliferation through interactions with Moesin. Mol Biol Cell. 2013;24:1420–33.
58. Speck O, Hughes SC, Noren NK, Kulikauskas RM, Fehon RG. Moesin functions antagonistically to the rho pathway to maintain epithelial integrity. Nature. 2003;421:83–7.
59. Hsieh HH, Chang WT, Yu L, Rao Y. Control of axon-axon attraction by Semaphorin reverse signaling. Proc Natl Acad Sci U S A. 2014;111:11383–8.
60. Ng J, Nardine T, Harms M, Tzu J, Goldstein A, Sun Y, Dietzl G, Dickson BJ, Luo L. Rac GTPases control axon growth, guidance and branching. Nature. 2002;416:442–7.
61. Kruttner S, Traunmuller L, Dag U, Jandrasits K, Stepien B, Iyer N, Fradkin LG, Noordermeer JN, Mensh BD, Keleman K. Synaptic Orb2A bridges memory acquisition and late memory consolidation in drosophila. Cell Rep. 2015;11: 1953–65.
62. Mehren JE, Griffith LC. Cholinergic neurons mediate CaMKII-dependent enhancement of courtship suppression. Learn Mem. 2006;13:686–9.
63. Anderson DB, Wilkinson KA, Henley JM. Protein SUMOylation in neuropathological conditions. Drug news & perspectives. 2009;22:255–65.

12

Multiple myosin motors interact with sodium/potassium-ATPase alpha 1 subunits

Bhagirathi Dash[1,2,3], Sulayman D. Dib-Hajj[1,2,3] and Stephen G. Waxman[1,2,3*]

Abstract

The alpha1 (α1) subunit of the sodium/potassium ATPase (i.e., Na^+/K^+-ATPase α1), the prototypical sodium pump, is expressed in each eukaryotic cell. They pump out three sodium ions in exchange for two extracellular potassium ions to establish a cellular electrochemical gradient important for firing of neuronal and cardiac action potentials. We hypothesized that myosin (myo or myh) motor proteins might interact with Na^+/K^+-ATPase α1 subunits in order for them to play an important role in the transport and trafficking of sodium pump. To this end immunoassays were performed to determine whether class II non-muscle myosins (i.e., NMHC-IIA/myh9, NMHC-IIB/myh10 or NMHC-IIC/myh14), myosin Va (myoVa) and myosin VI (myoVI) would interact with Na^+/K^+-ATPase α1 subunits. Immunoprecipitation of myh9, myh10, myh14, myoVa and myoVI from rat brain tissues led to the co-immunoprecipitation of Na^+/K^+-ATPase α1 subunits expressed there. Heterologous expression studies using HEK293 cells indicated that recombinant myh9, myh10, myh14 and myoVI interact with Na^+/K^+-ATPase α1 subunits expressed in HEK293 cells. Additional results indicated that loss of tail regions in recombinant myh9, myh10, myh14 and myoVI did not affect their interaction with Na^+/K^+-ATPase α1 subunits. However, recombinant myh9, myh10 and myh14 mutants having reduced or no actin binding ability, as a result of loss of their actin binding sites, displayed greatly reduced or null interaction with Na^+/K^+-ATPase α1 subunits. These results suggested the involvement of the actin binding site, but not tail regions, of NMHC-IIs in their interaction with Na^+/K^+-ATPase α1 subunits. Overall these results suggest a role for these diverse myosins in the trafficking and transport of sodium pump in neuronal and non-neuronal tissues.

Keywords: Myosins, Class II non-muscle myosins, myh9, myh10, myh14, Myosin Va, Myosin VI, Sodium/potassium ATPase, Sodium pump, Na^+/K^+-ATPase α1 subunits

Introduction

The sodium pump (sodium/potassium ATPase; Na^+/K^+-ATPase) is an integral membrane protein found in the cells of all higher eukaryotes [1]. It utilizes ATP as a driving force to pump out three sodium ions in exchange for two extracellular potassium ions which establishes both a chemical and an electrical gradient across the cell membrane. The electrical gradient is essential for maintaining cellular resting potential and excitability of myocytes (skeletal and cardiac) and neurons. The sodium gradient helps drive various transport processes such as the fluid reabsorption and translocation of glucose, amino acids, and other nutrients into the cells [1, 2]. Sodium/potassium-ATPase also function as a signaling molecule and is shown to regulate MAPK pathway, reactive oxygen species (ROS) formation as well as intracellular calcium [2–4]. It is principally composed of two subunits, an alpha-subunit (α; ≈100 kDa) and a beta-subunit (β; ≈40 kDa). The α subunit (i.e., catalytic subunit) has four isoforms: α1 (*Atp1a1*), α2 (*Atp1a2*), α3 (*Atp1a3*) and α4 (*Atp1a4*). The β subunits has four isoforms as well: β1 (*Atp1b1*), β2 (*Atp1b2*), β3 (*Atp1b3*) and β4 (*Atp1b4*). These α and β subunits admix to form a minimal functional sodium pump. The minimal functional unit of the Na^+/K^+-ATPase can be further modified by a third FXYD subunit (also known as gamma-subunit (γ)) [5]. Mammals express seven FXYD proteins. Na^+/K^+-ATPase α1 subunits in association with its β1 subunit is found in nearly every tissue [5] . The α2 subunits are predominantly expressed in adipocytes,

* Correspondence: stephen.waxman@yale.edu
[1]Department of Neurology, Yale University Schoolof Medicine, New Haven, CT 06510, USA
[2]Center for Neuroscience & Regeneration Research, Yale University School of Medicine, New Haven, CT 06510, USA
Full list of author information is available at the end of the article

muscle, heart, and brain (i.e., mostly glial cells). The α3 subunits are abundant in nervous tissues (i.e., mostly neurons). The α4 subunits are a testis-specific isoform [6]. Ablation of Na^+/K^+-ATPase α1, α2 or α3 subunits result in the death of the animal [7].

The mechanisms by which Na^+/K^+-ATPase α and β subunits are trafficked to the cell surface are not well understood. Generally, vesicles carrying membrane proteins traffic from the intracellular pools to the plasma membranes. This involves their transport by kinesin family of motor proteins (KIF) along the microtubules and/or by myosin (myo or myh) family of motor proteins (myo or myh) along the actin filaments. Kinesin light chain 2 (KLC2) of kinesin-1 heavy chain (KIF5B) has been shown to be involved in the trafficking of Na^+/K^+-ATPase α1 subunits in alveolar epithelial cells [8]. In the same cell types, myosin Va (myoVa), a member of the myosin family of actin-based motor proteins, is shown to be involved in the trafficking of Na^+/K^+-ATPase α1 subunits [9].

Class II non-muscle myosins (NM-II), like class II muscle myosins, are hexameric molecules comprising of two heavy chains (HC), two myosin essential light chains (ELCs) and two regulatory light chains (RLCs or MRLCs). The non-muscle myosin heavy chain (NMHC) is comprised of a globular head/motor domain (the site for interaction with actin and adenosine triphosphate (ATP)); a neck region (site for interaction with ELCs and RLCs); and a tail region which homodimerizes in a helical fashion (and possibly the site for interaction with the cargo) [10]. By contrast, myoVI is a monomeric heavy chain that consists of a head domain, a neck region (that contains converter/reverse gear domain, IQ motif/domain and site for interaction with calmodulin light chain) and a tail domain that contains a cargo-binding domain (CBD, the site for association with cargo adaptors). MyoVI moves toward the slow-growing (minus) ends of the actin filaments contrary to all other native myosins that move toward the fast-growing (plus) ends of F-actin [11]. We hypothesized that myosins (myh or myo), particularly class II non-muscle myosins (NM-II; myh9, myh10 and myh14) and myosin VI (myoVI) in addition to myoVa, might play an important role in the trafficking of Na^+/K^+-ATPase α1 subunits to cell membranes.

Methods

Bioinformatics analyses

Mammalian non-muscle myosin II isoforms were aligned using ClustalO program (https://www.ebi.ac.uk/Tools/msa/clustalo/). The 3-D coordinates of human myh14 (PDB: 5I4E) was retrieved from protein data bank [12]. Structural features of myh14 was visualized and analyzed using UCSF Chimera (http://www.cgl.ucsf.edu/chimera/).

Antibodies

Various polyclonal (rabbit or goat) antibodies and monoclonal (mouse) antibodies used for immunoprecipitation (IP) and/or immunoblotting (IB) are provided in the supporting information section (Additional file 1: Tables S1 and S2). Antibody dilutions and/or concentrations used for IP and/or IB assays along with the molecular weight (~kDa) of the antigens detected by these antibodies are also provided (Additional file 1: Table S2). Immunoblots were incubated with monoclonal antibodies against myh9 (1:500; Abcam), myh10 (1:1000; Abcam), myosin regulatory light chain (MRLC) (1:200; Santa Cruz Biotechnology), Na^+/K^+-ATPase α1 (0.5 μg/mL; DSHB), Na^+/K^+-ATPase α1 (1:1000; EMD Millipore), Na^+/K^+-ATPase α (1:200; Santa Cruz Biotechnology), GFP (1:1000, NeuroMab), myosin VI (1:500; Sigma), voltage gated sodium channel α subunits (pan-Na_vα; 1:1000; Sigma) and β-actin (1:10000; Sigma). Polyclonal antibodies against GFP (1:2000; Abcam), mCherry (1:1000; Abcam) and myosin Va (1:500; Cell Signaling Technology) were also used for immunoblotting.

Na^+/K^+ ATPase α antibody obtained from Santa Cruz Biotechnology (sc-58,628; clone M7-PB-E9) is considered as a pan-Na^+/K^+ ATPase α antibody in some quarters as it detects Na^+/K^+ ATPase α subunits (i.e., α1, α2 and α3) from human, mouse, sheep, dog, pig and chicken. It also detects rat Na^+/K^+ ATPase α3 but not rat Na^+/K^+ ATPase α1 or α2 subunits. The monoclonal antibody against Na^+/K^+ ATPase α1 (α6F) was developed by Dr. D.M. Fambrough. It was obtained from the Developmental Studies Hybridoma Bank (DSHB) and was developed under the auspices of NIHCD and maintained by the University of Iowa, Department of Biological Sciences, Iowa City, IA 52242.

The MRLC antibody used in this study (sc-28,329; clone E4; SCBT) is already shown to detect various MRLCs and hence considered as a pan-MRLC in some quarters [13]. It is claimed to recognize the MRLCs from human (i.e., MRCL3, MRLC2, MYL9 and LOC391722: myosin regulatory light chain 12B-like), mouse (i.e., Mylc2b, Myl9 and Myl12a) and rat (i.e., Mrlcb and Myl9) tissues. In our hand, it poorly detects the MRLCs from HEK293 cell lysates, but it detects the MRLCs as a co-immunoprecipitate from precipitation of NMHC-IIs very well (Additional file 2: Figure S1).

Molecular cloning

Standard molecular cloning or fast cloning methods [14] were followed for sub-cloning. Details about the various cDNA constructs (i.e., species, isoform, amino acid length; etc.) used in this study are provided in the supporting information section (Additional file 1: Table S3).

Myosin constructs

CMV-GFP-NMHC II-A (i.e., GFP-myh9), CMV-GFP -NMHC II-B (i.e., GFP-myh10) and EGFP-NMHC II-C (i.e., myh14-GFP) were gifts from Robert Adelstein (Additional file 1: Table S3) [15, 16]. Like myh14-GFP, myh9 and myh10 were sub-cloned to have GFP fused to their C-termini (i.e., myh9-GFP and myh10-GFP). The tail regions of myh9 (i.e., AAs:1928–1960), myh10 (i.e., AAs:1934–1976) and myh14 (i.e., AAs:1946–1992) were deleted to make myh9-Δatil-GFP, myh10-Δtail-GFP and myh14-Δtail-GFP constructs respectively following the work of others [17]. The actin binding sites (ABS) of myh9 (i.e., AAs:654–676), myh10 (i.e., 661–683) and myh14 (i.e., 674–696) were also deleted to make myh9-ΔABS-GFP, myh9-ΔABS-GFP and myh9-ΔABS-GFP constructs respectively. Information about the actin binding sites and/or tail regions of NMHC-IIs were obtained from literature and/or UniProt site [17–19].

The human myosin Va (myoVa) and myosin VI (myoVI) cDNA clones were obtained from Dharmacon (Lafayette, CO, USA) (Additional file 1: Table S3). Both myoVa and myoVI were sub-cloned to have GFP fused to their C-termini (i.e., myoVa-GFP and myoVI-GFP, respectively). MyoVI was also tagged with mCherry in the N-terminus (i.e., mCherry-MyoVI). Twenty two (22), 60 and 120 AAs were deleted from the C-terminal end of mCherry-MyoVI to make mCherry-Myo6-ΔT1, mCherry-Myo6-ΔT2 and mCherry-Myo6-ΔT3 constructs respectively following the work of others [20].

Non-myosin constructs

A mouse Na^+/K^+-ATPase α1 cDNA clone was obtained from Dharmacon (Lafayette, CO, USA). Na^+/K^+-ATPase α1 subunits were sub-cloned to have mCherry fused into their C-terminus (i.e., Na^+/K^+-ATPase α1-mCherry). The ankyrin-G-270-mCherery (i.e., AnkG270-mCherry) construct was a gift from Benedicte Dargent [21] (Additional file 1: Table S3). The $Na_v1.6$ (i.e., voltage gated sodium channel alpha 6 subunit/SCN8A) construct was available in our laboratory. It harbors a mutation [Tyr371Ser] that renders it resistant to tetrodotoxin (TTX).

Cell culture and transfection

HEK293 cells were cultured according to standard procedures and were transfected with desired cDNA constructs using Optifect (Thermo Fisher Scientific, Waltham, MA) or LipoJet™ transfection reagent (SignaGen Laboratories, Rockville, MD) according to manufacturer's instructions.

Preparation of cell and tissues lysates

All animal care and experimental studies were approved by the Veterans Administration Connecticut Healthcare System Institutional Animal Care and Use Committee. We followed the protocols published elsewhere [22] with some modifications to prepare the adult rat (Sprague--Dawley) brain tissue or HEK293 cell lysates for IP and immunoblotting. The lysis or IP buffer was made of 20 mM Tris-Cl (pH 7.4), 150 mM NaCl, 1% Triton X-100, 1 mM DTT, 10 mM EGTA and 2× Complete protease inhibitor cocktail (Roche Diagnostics Corporation, Indianapolis, IN). An adult whole rat (male or female) brain was homogenized in pieces in a tissue grinder (Qiagen, Valencia, CA) to a final volume ~ 50 mL lysis buffer. Homogenates were solubilized for 2 h at 4 °C, and centrifuged at 50,000 g for 30 min at 4 °C using a Beckman Coulter Optima® ultra-centrifuge to collect the supernatants for immunoprecipitation (IP) and immunoblotting.

Non-transfected HEK293 cells (control) or those transiently transfected with plasmid constructs were collected by centrifugation at 500 g for 5 min at 4 °C upon trypsinization. These pellets were washed twice with ice cold PBS by centrifugation at 500 g for 5 min at 4 °C before lysis using the IP buffer. Cell supernatants were obtained by centrifugation at 15,000 g for 20 min at 4 °C for IP and immunoblotting.

Protein concentration in the tissue lysates was determined using the Bradford reagent (Bio-Rad, Hercules, CA).

Immunoprecipitation

For IP experiment, HEK293 cell or rat brain tissue supernatants containing 1–4 mg protein (in ~ 1 mL lysate) was pre-cleared (PC) for 1–4 h at 4 °C with 5–10 μg of suitable mouse antibody isotypes, rabbit immunoglobulins or goat immunoglobulins, and 80–100 μl of Dynabead® protein G (Thermo Fisher Scientific). Precleared supernatants were incubated (overnight, 4 °C) with 5–10 μg of desired IP antibody (Additional file 1: Table S1) and 80–100 μl of Dynabead® protein G. Dynabead® Protein G beads bound to control antibody isotypes (i.e., PC complexes) or desired primary antibodies (i.e., IP complexes) were washed for 5 times with IP buffer or wash buffer supplied by the vendor (Thermo Fisher Scientific) and eluted with NuPAGE® LDS Sample Buffer (Thermo Fisher Scientific) in the presence of NuPAGE® Sample Reducing Agent (Thermo Fisher Scientific).

Western blotting

About 30–50 μg of HEK293 cell or rat brain tissue lysates were denatured using NuPAGE® Sample Reducing Agent in the presence of NuPAGE® LDS Sample Buffer to serve as input (In) sample for western blotting. The input samples, PC complexes, IP complexes and/or at times denatured depleted supernatants (DS) were resolved on NuPAGE® Novex® 4–12% Bis-Tris Gels (1.0 mm, 12 well) and transferred to a nitrocellulose membrane. Membranes were blocked using a blocking buffer (5% non-fat dry milk and 1% BSA in 0.1% TBST or 5% BSA in 0.1% TBST) for 1 h, washed and incubated overnight with desired primary antibodies (Additional file 1: Table S2) diluted in the blocking buffer. The blots were washed and incubated in horseradish peroxidase-conjugated goat anti-mouse (1:10000; Dako, Santa Clara, CA), goat anti-rabbit (1:10000; Dako, Santa Clara, CA) or donkey anti-goat (1:5000) immunoglobulins for 1 h. The blots were washed extensively and developed for 1 to 10 min with the Perkin Elmer Western Lightning Plus-enhanced chemiluminescence (ECL) kit using a Bio-Rad ChemiDoc XRS+ or ChemiDoc Imaging System. At times immunoblots were stripped using a stripping buffer (Thermo Fisher Scientific) to re-probe with another primary antibody.

We usually cut through the IgG-HC and/or IgG-LC regions of the Ponceau S (Sigma) stained nitrocellulose membranes for probing different section of the membrane with different antibodies. Therefore, cut marks could be seen in some images.

Results

Antibody characterization

Antibodies already known to be suitable for immunoprecipitation (IP) were used. Antibodies, for which such information is not available, were considered suitable for IP assays when they would precipitate their cognate antigen and/or co-immunoprecipitate a known partner protein of their cognate antigens. Hence, for myosin antibodies we evaluated their ability to immunoprecipitate their respective cognate antigens and/or co-immunoprecipitate β-actin and/or MRLCs. This is because class II myosins (such as myh9, myh10, myh14; etc.) invariably interact with actins and MRLCs (Figs. 1, 2, 3 and Additional file 2: Figure S1).

First, we tested the ability of the myh9 (Abcam: ab55456) and myh10 (Abcam: ab684/3H2) antibodies to immunoprecipitate their cognate antigens and co-immunoprecipitate β-actin and/or MRLCs from HEK293 cells (Additional file 2: Figure S1). Both myh9 and myh10 antibodies immunoprecipitated their respective cognate antigens and co-immunoprecipitated β-actin and MRLCs from HEK293 cells. Myh9 appeared to co-immunoprecipitate β-actin better than myh10 from HEK293 cells which could be due to many factors [23] including the fact that myh10 antibodies are available as ascites and their use was determined empirically. However, both myh9 and myh10 antibodies pulled down β-actin from rat brain tissues very well (Fig. 1a). We also assessed the ability of myh14 (a close homolog of myh9 and myh10 and the 3rd member of the class II NMHC), myoVa and myoVI to immunoprecipitate their respective cognate antigens and/or co-immunoprecipitate β-actin (Figs. 1b and 4). β-actin was co-immunoprecipitated with myh14, myoVa and myoVI to various degrees from rodent brain tissues (Fig. 1). We also observed that myoVa and myoVI antibodies would not or very poorly co-immunoprecipitate β-actin from HEK293 cells (Figs. 4 and 5). As expected the microtubule-based kinesin motor, KIF5B, did not co-immunoprecipitate β-actin from rat brain tissue lysates (Fig. 1a).

We also immunoprecipitated recombinant myh9 (Fig. 6, Additional file 3: Figure S2, Additional file 4: Figure S3B, Additional file 5: Figure S4 and Additional file 6: Figure S5), myh10 (Additional file 3: Figure S2, Additional file 4: Figure S3 and Additional file 6: Figure S5), myh14

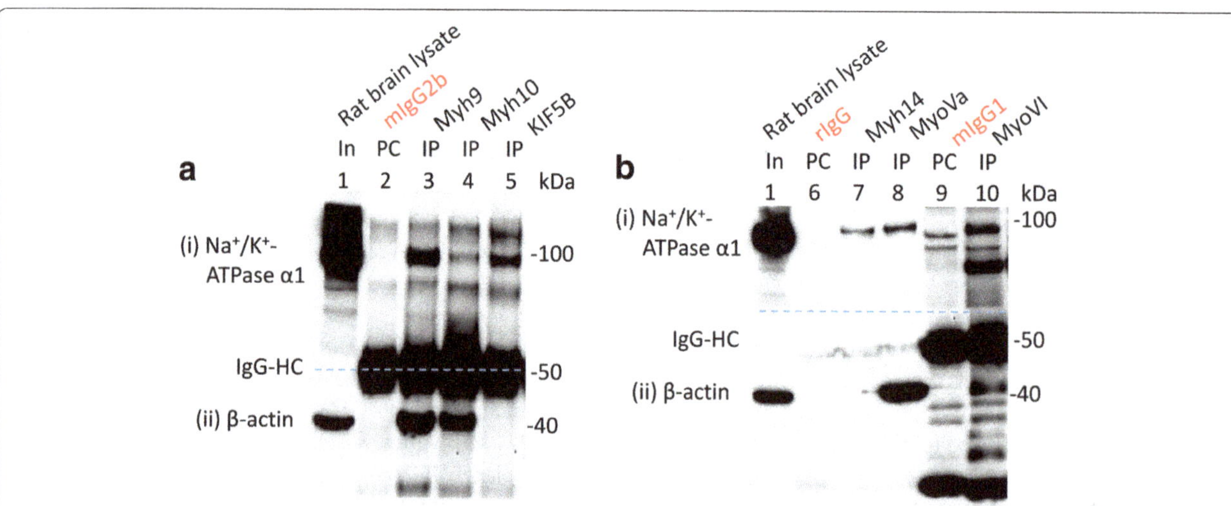

Fig. 1 Interaction of multiple myosins with Na^+/K^+-ATPase α1 subunits expressed in rat brain. WT adult rat brain lysates (In, lane 1 in **a** and **b**) were precleared (PC) with indicated immunoglobulin isotypes (PC; lane2 = mIgG2b, lane 6 = rIgG and lane 9 = mIgG1) prior to immunoprecipitation (IP) using indicated antibodies (IP; lane 3 = myh9, lane 4 = myh10, lane 5 = KIF5B, lane 7 = Myh14, lane 8 = myoVa and lane 10 = myoVI). Loading of PC complexes in the gel preceded those of the IP complexes. Na^+/K^+-ATPase α1 subunits (i) were co-immunoprecipitated with myh9, myh10, KIF5B, myh14, myoVa and myoVI expressed in rat brain tissues. Co-immunoprecipitation of Na^+/K^+-ATPase α1 subunits by KIF5B served as a positive control. All the myosins assayed co-immunoprecipitated β-actin (ii). Denatured mouse IgG-HC (i.e., lanes 2–5, 9 and 10; panel (ii)), but not those of rabbit IgG (i.e., lanes 6–8) separated from their intact immunoglobulins (that is used for PC or IP) could be seen as this section was probed with mouse anti-β-actin antibodies

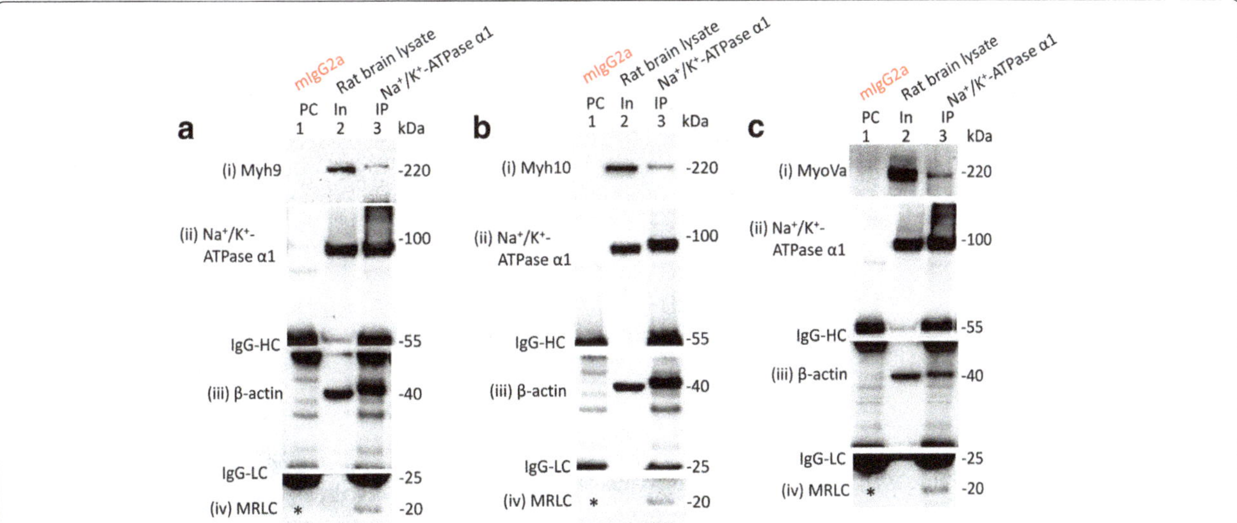

Fig. 2 Na^+/K^+-ATPase α1 subunits co-immunoprecipitate multiple myosins expressed in adult rat brain. WT adult rat brain lysates (In, lane 2 in **a**, **b** and **c**) were precleared (PC) with mouse IgG1 antibodies (PC, lane 1 in **a**, **b** and **c**) prior to immunoprecipitation (IP) using mouse anti-Na^+/K^+-ATPase α1 antibodies of the IgG1 isotypes (IP, lane 3 in **a**, **b** and **c**). Loading of PC complexes in the gel preceded those of the lysate inputs (In). Na^+/K^+-ATPase α1 subunits co-immunoprecipitated myh9 (**a** (i)), myh10 (**b**, (i)), myoVa (**c** (i)), β-actin ((iii) in **a**, **b** and **c**) and myosin regulatory light chain (MRLC) ((iv) in **a**, **b** and **c**) from rat brain. An asterisk ('*'; (iv) in **a**, **b** and **c**) indicates lack of detection of the input signal for the MRLCs. As expected anti-Na^+/K^+-ATPase α1 antibodies immunoprecipitated Na^+/K^+-ATPase α1 subunits expressed in brain tissues ((ii) in **a**, **b** and **c**)

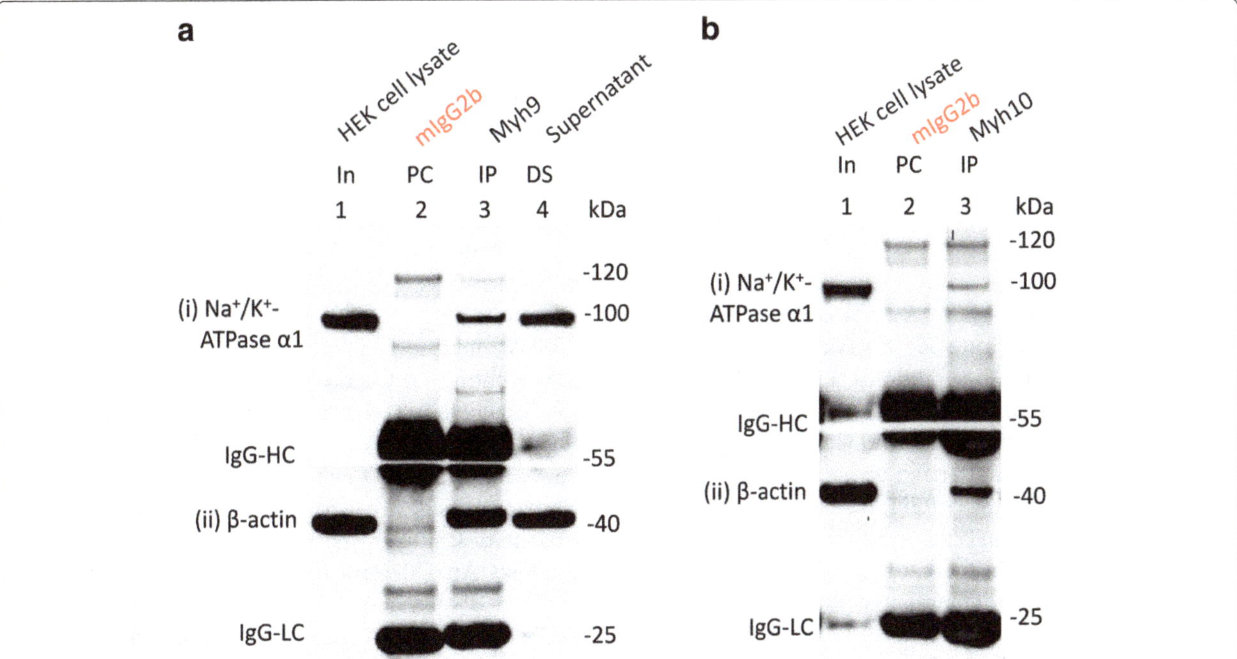

Fig. 3 Interaction of non-muscle myosin heavy chains with Na^+/K^+-ATPase α1 subunits endogenously expressed in HEK293 cells. HEK293 cell lysates (In, lane 1 in **a** and **b**) were precleared (PC) with mouse IgG2b (PC, lane 2 in **a** and **b**) prior to immunoprecipitation (IP, lane 3) using antibodies for myh9 (**a**) and myh10 (**b**). Loading of PC complexes in the gel preceded those of the IP complexes. Immunoprecipitation of myh9 (**a**) and myh10 (**b**) led to the co-immunoprecipitation of Na^+/K^+ ATPase α1 subunits ((i) in **a** and **b**) and β-actin ((ii) in **a** and **b**) expressed in HEK293 cells. Na^+/K^+-ATPase α1 and β-actin immunoreactive signals in the depleted supernatant lane (DS, lane 4 in **a**) indicates that the ATPase survives the IP procedure. Denatured mouse IgG-HC and IgG-LC separated from their intact immunoglobulins (that is used for PC or IP) are seen in (**a** and **b**) as those blot sections were probed with mouse anti-β-actin antibodies

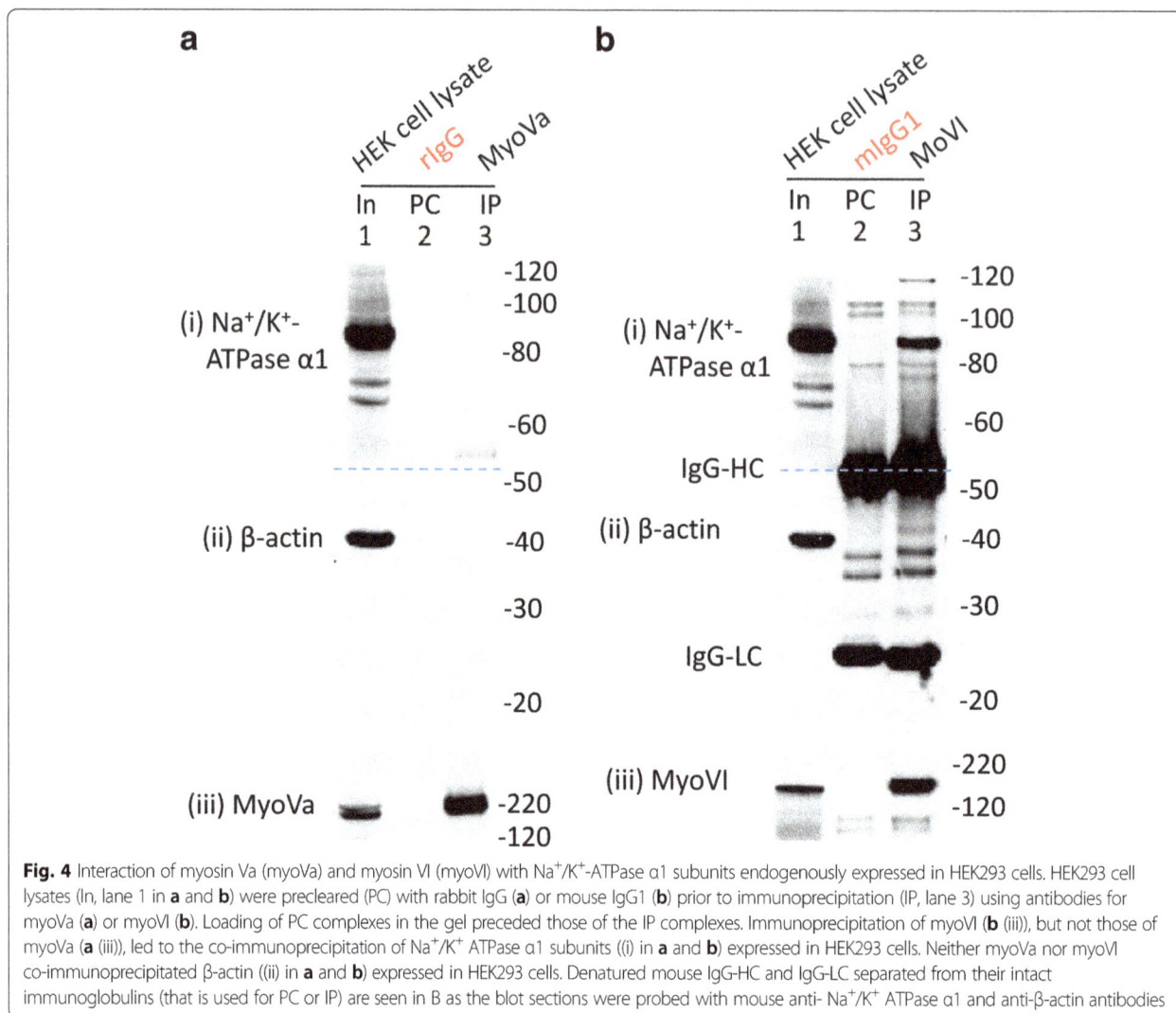

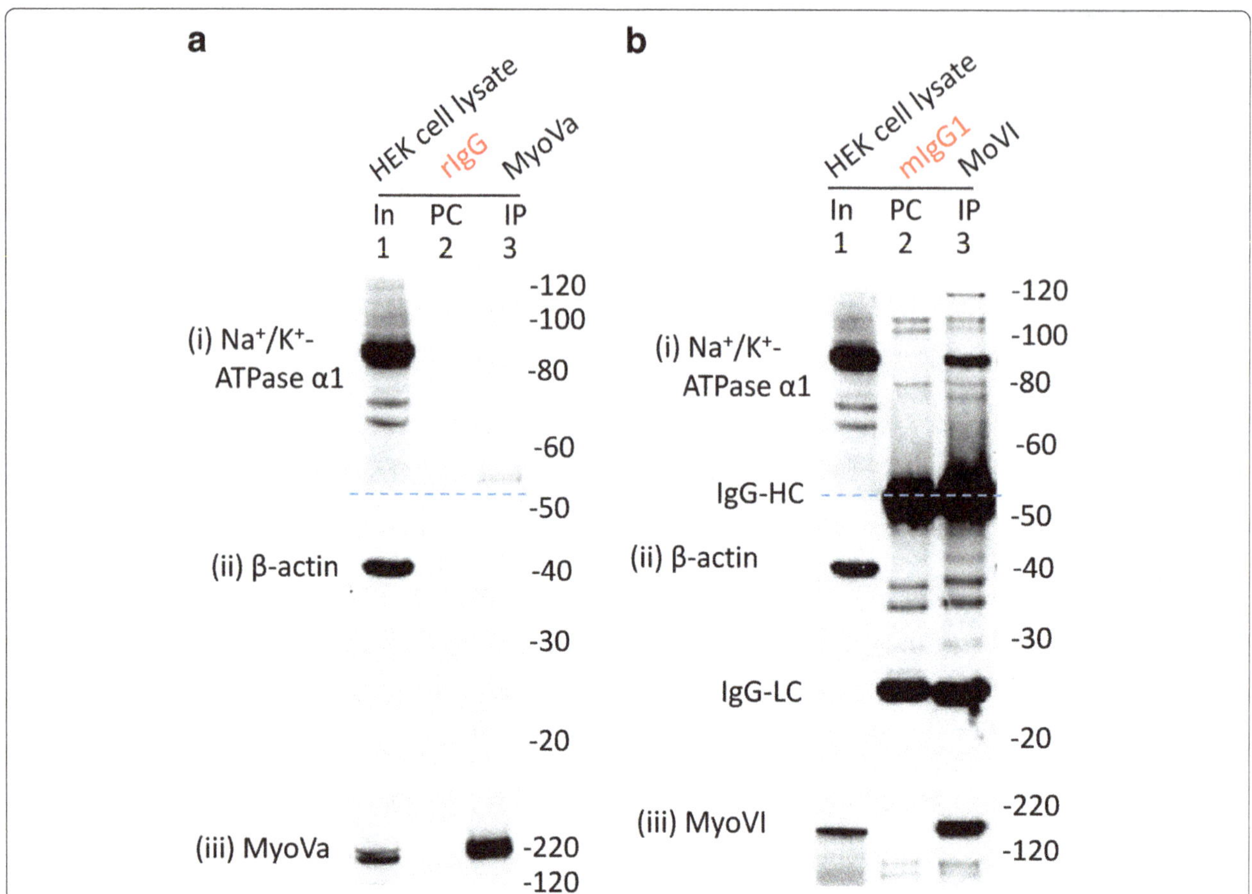

Fig. 4 Interaction of myosin Va (myoVa) and myosin VI (myoVI) with Na^+/K^+-ATPase α1 subunits endogenously expressed in HEK293 cells. HEK293 cell lysates (In, lane 1 in **a** and **b**) were precleared (PC) with rabbit IgG (**a**) or mouse IgG1 (**b**) prior to immunoprecipitation (IP, lane 3) using antibodies for myoVa (**a**) or myoVI (**b**). Loading of PC complexes in the gel preceded those of the IP complexes. Immunoprecipitation of myoVI (**b** (iii)), but not those of myoVa (**a** (iii)), led to the co-immunoprecipitation of Na^+/K^+ ATPase α1 subunits ((i) in **a** and **b**) expressed in HEK293 cells. Neither myoVa nor myoVI co-immunoprecipitated β-actin ((ii) in **a** and **b**) expressed in HEK293 cells. Denatured mouse IgG-HC and IgG-LC separated from their intact immunoglobulins (that is used for PC or IP) are seen in B as the blot sections were probed with mouse anti- Na^+/K^+ ATPase α1 and anti-β-actin antibodies

(Additional file 4: Figure S3A, Additional file 5: Figure S4 and Additional file 7: Figure S6), myoVa (Additional file 8 Figure S7) and myoVI (Additional file 9: Figure S8) expressed in HEK293 cells to determine whether they would reflect the β-actin and/or MRLC binding abilities of myosins antibodies characterized earlier. Immunoprecipitation of recombinant myh9 (GFP tag either in the N- or C-terminus), myh10 (GFP tag either in the C-terminus) and myh14 (GFP tag in the C-terminus) using anti-GFP antibodies led to the co-immunoprecipitate β-actin and/or MRLCs from HEK293 cells. Neither recombinant myoVa nor myoVI (tagged with GFP in the C-terminus) would co-immunoprecipitate β-actin from HEK293 cells. These results recaptured the findings from myosin antibody-based assays that NMHC-IIs, but not myoVa nor myoVI, co-immunoprecipitate β-actin from HEK293 cells. These results also demonstrated that the GFP antibodies are suitable for use in IP assays.

The suitability of the mCherry antibodies (Abcam: ab183628) for use in IP assays was evaluated by immunoprecipitating mCherry tagged ankyrin-G (AnkG) (Additional file 10: Figure S9). Immunoprecipitation of AnkG-mCherry (i.e. AnkG tagged with mCherry in their C-terminus: AnkG270-mCherry = AnkG-mCherry) using mCherry antibodies led to the co-IP of Na^+/K^+-ATPase α1 subunits (a known partner of AnkG) from HEK293 cells. Also, AnkG270-mCherry, but not mCherry, IP led to the co-IP of $Na_v1.6$ subunits (a known partner of AnkG) and Na^+/K^+-ATPase α1 subunits when HEK293 cells were co-expressing both AnkG270-mCherry and $Na_v1.6$ subunits. These results also suggested that the mCherry antibodies are suitable for use in IP assays.

The suitability of anti-Na^+/K^+-ATPase α1 antibodies for use in IP assays was evaluated by determining their ability to immunoprecipitate their cognate antigens and/or co-immunoprecipitate β-actin (as Na^+/K^+-ATPase α1

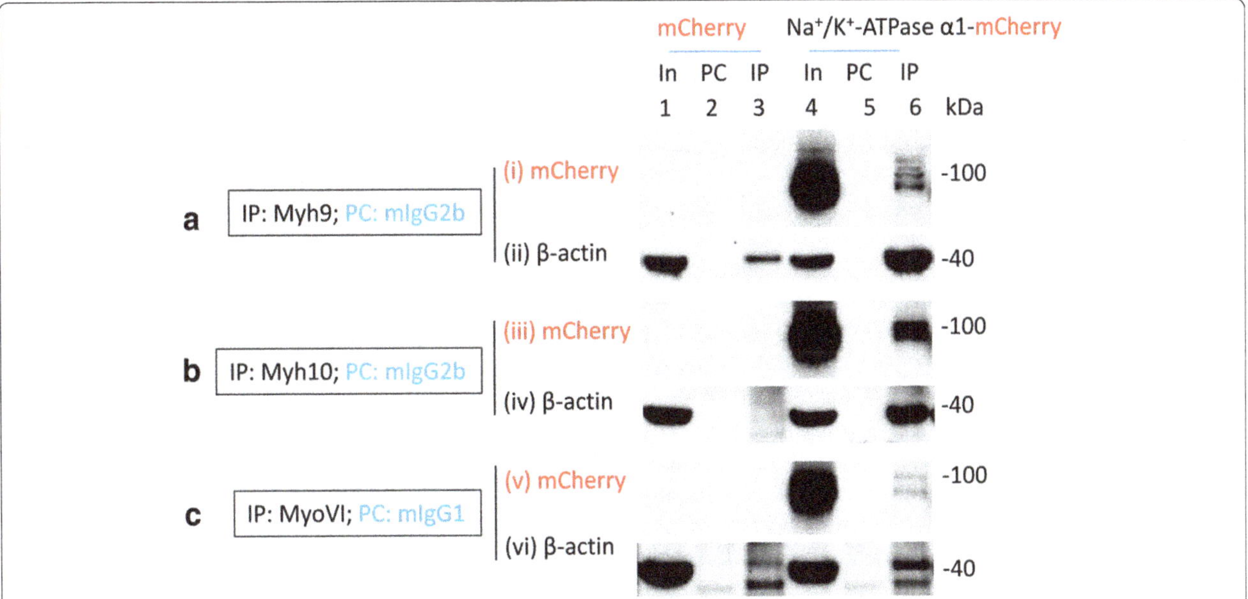

Fig. 5 Multiple myosins co-immunoprecipitate recombinant Na^+/K^+-ATPase α1 subunits expressed in HEK293 cells. Lysates of HEK293 cells transiently transfected with mCherry (In, lane 1) or Na^+/K^+-ATPase α1 tagged with mCherry in the C-terminus (In, lane 4; Na^+/K^+ ATPase α1-mCherry) were precleared (PC) with mouse IgG2b antibodies (**a** and **b**; lanes 2 and 5) or mouse IgG1 antibodies (**c**; lanes 2 and 5) prior to immunoprecipitation (IP) using mouse anti-myh9 antibodies of the IgG2b isotypes (**a**; lanes 3 and 6), mouse anti-myh10 antibodies of the IgG2b isotypes (**b**; lanes 3 and 6) or mouse anti-myoVI antibodies of the IgG1 isotypes (**c**; lanes 3 and 6). Loading of PC complexes in the gel preceded those of the IP complexes. mCherry immunoreactive bands in lanes 4 and 6 but not in any other lanes indicated co-immunoprecipitation of recombinant Na^+/K^+-ATPase α1 subunits by myh9 (lane 6, panel (i)), myh10 (lane 6, panel (iii)) and myoVI (lane 6, panel (v)) from HEK293 cells transfected with Na^+/K^+-ATPase α1-mCherry plasmids but not from those transfected with mCherry. As expected β-actin (lanes 3 and 6 in panels (ii)) was co-immunoprecipitated with myh9. Myh10 and myoVI noticeably co-immunoprecipitated β-actin (lane 6 in (iv) and (vi)) from HEK293 cells overexpressing Na^+/K^+-ATPase α1 subunits but not from those overexpressing mCherry. Full length images of western blots are presented in Additional file 12: Figure S11, Additional file 13: Figure S12, Additional file 14: Figure S13)

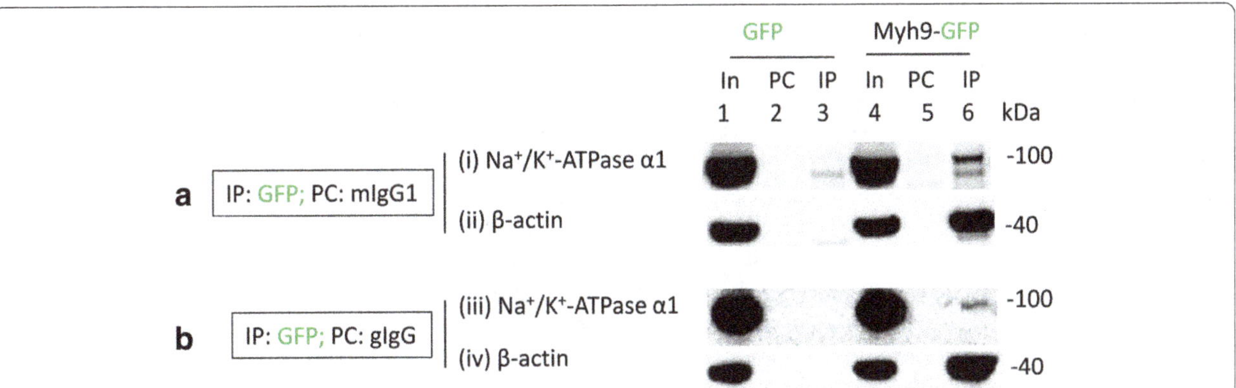

Fig. 6 Recombinant myh9 co-immunoprecipitate Na^+/K^+-ATPase α1 subunits expressed in HEK293 cells. Lysates of HEK293 cells transiently transfected with GFP (In, lane 1) or myh9 tagged with GFP in the C-terminus (In, lane 4; myh9-GFP) were precleared (PC) with mouse IgG1 antibodies (**a**, lanes 2 and 5) or goat immunoglobulins (gIgG) (**b**, lanes 2 and 5) prior to immunoprecipitation (IP) using mouse anti-GFP antibodies of the IgG1 isotypes (**a**, lanes 3 and 6) or goat anti-GFP antibodies (**b**, lanes 3 and 6). Loading of PC complexes in the gel preceded those of the IP complexes. Na^+/K^+-ATPase α1 immunoreactive bands in lanes 1, 4 and 6 but not in any other lanes ((i) and (iii)) indicated co-immunoprecipitation of Na^+/K^+-ATPase α1 subunits from HEK293 cells transfected with myh9-GFP plasmids but not from those transfected with GFP plasmids. As expected immunoprecipitation using anti-GFP antibodies led to the co-immunoprecipitation of β-actin (lane 6 in (ii) and (iv)) from HEK293 cells transfected with myh9-GFP plasmids but not from those transfected with GFP plasmids. Immunoprecipitation using goat anti-GFP antibodies (**b**) led to a cleaner co-IP of Na^+/K^+-ATPase α1 subunits from HEK293 cells expressing myh9-GFP. Full length images of western blots are presented in Figure Additional file 4: Figure S3B (for part **a**) and Additional file 5: Figure S4B (for part **b**)

subunits are known to interact with β-actin) (Figs. 2 and Additional file 11: Figure S10) [24]. As expected immunoprecipitation using Na^+/K^+-ATPase α1 antibodies (DSHB: a6F or Millipore: 05–369) led to the precipitation of its cognate antigens and co-IP of β-actin.

Thus, all the antibodies used in IP assays appeared to suitable for such purposes.

Interaction of myosins with Na^+/K^+-ATPase α1 subunits expressed in the rodent brain or HEK293 cells

In this work we largely focus on the interaction of NMHC-IIs, myoVa and myoVI with Na^+/K^+-ATPase α1 subunits. It is because these myosins are well studied and heavily involved in the transport and trafficking of various cellular cargoes [11]. Non-muscle myosin II isoforms (i.e., myh9, myh10 and myh14), myoVa and myoVI were immunoprecipitated from adult rat brain tissue lysates to ascertain the potential in vivo interaction of these myosin motors with Na^+/K^+-ATPase α1 subunits (Fig. 1). Sodium/potassium ATPase α1 subunits were co-immunoprecipitated with myh9, myh10, myh14, myoVa and myoVI expressed in adult rat brain tissues (Fig. 1a and b). Kinesin-1 heavy chain (KIF5B) was immunoprecipitated to control for the co-IP Na^+/K^+-ATPase α1 subunits. Immunoprecipitation of KIF5B led to the co-immunoprecipitation of Na^+/K^+-ATPase α1 subunits expressed in rat brain tissues (Fig. 1a). This was not surprising given that kinesin light chain 2 (KLC2) is involved in the movement of Na^+/K^+-ATPase-containing vesicles [8].

We also investigated whether the cell background would have any effect on the interaction of NMHC-IIs, myoVa and myoVI with Na^+/K^+-ATPase α1 subunits. To this end we immunoprecipitated these myosins from HEK293 cells and probed for the co-immunoprecipitation Na^+/K^+-ATPase α1 subunits expressed there. Na^+/K^+-ATPase α1 subunits were co-immunoprecipitated with myh9, myh10, myh14 and myoVI expressed in HEK293 cells (Figs. 3 and 4). However, myoVa did not co-immunoprecipitate Na^+/K^+-ATPase α1 subunits expressed in HEK293 cells. These results are in agreement with the findings from the brain tissues except that myoVa could not co-immunoprecipitate Na^+/K^+-ATPase α1 subunits expressed in HEK293 cells.

Reciprocally, we also wanted to determine whether the immunoprecipitation of Na^+/K^+-ATPase α1 subunits from adult rat brain tissues would lead to the co-immunoprecipitation of any of the myosins targeted in this study (Fig. 1b). Results indicated that Na^+/K^+-ATPase α1 subunits expressed in the rat brain could co-immunoprecipitate myh9, myh10 and myoVa but not myoVI (Fig. 2). We also observed that IP of Na^+/K^+-ATPase α1 subunits led to the co-IP of MRLCs expressed in rat brain tissues (Fig. 2; panel (iv)). MRLCs are associated with NMHC-IIs and other myosins (smooth muscle myosin/Myh11, myosin 15/Myo15, myosin 18A/Myo18A, myosin 19/Myo19) expressed in the nervous tissues [25–27]. It is possible that co-IP of MRLCs with Na^+/K^+-ATPase α1 subunits is as a result of Na^+/K^+-ATPase α1 subunits pulling down class NMHC-IIs and other myosins expressed in rat brain tissues. Alternatively, it is plausible that Na^+/K^+-ATPase α1 subunits might be interacting with MRLCs directly or indirectly via other proteins.

Similarly, we wanted to know whether the immunoprecipitation of Na^+/K^+-ATPase α1 subunits from HEK293 cells would lead to the co-immunoprecipitation of any of the myosins targeted in this study (Additional file 11: Figure S10). To our surprise, Na^+/K^+-ATPase α1 subunits could not co-immunoprecipitate myh9, myh10, myoVa or myoVI expressed in HEK293 cells though anti-Na^+/K^+-ATPase α1 antibodies immunoprecipitated Na^+/K^+-ATPase α1 subunits and co-immunoprecipitated β-actin from HEK293 cells (not all data are shown; Additional file 11: Figure S10).

Interaction of myosins with recombinant Na^+/K^+-ATPase α1 subunits

Based on our earlier findings we investigated whether myh9, myh10 or myoVI would co-immunoprecipitate recombinant Na^+/K^+-ATPase α1 subunits expressed in HEK293 cells. To this end, we overexpressed mCherry (as a control) and Na^+/K^+-ATPase α1 subunits tagged with mCherry in their C-terminus (i.e., Na^+/K^+-ATPase α1-mCherry) in HEK293 cells (Fig. 5, Additional file 12: Figure S11, Additional file 13: Figure S12 and Additional file 14: Figure S13). Both myh9 and myh10 co-immunoprecipitated recombinant Na^+/K^+-ATPase α1 subunits (i.e., Na^+/K^+-ATPase α1-mCherry), but not mCherry, expressed in HEK293 cells. Similarly, myoVI also co-immunoprecipitated Na^+/K^+-ATPase α1-mCherry, but not mCherry, expressed in HEK293 cells (Fig. 5c). The co-immunoprecipitation signals for Na^+/K^+-ATPase α1-mCherry subunits by myh9, myh10 or myoVI revealed multiple mCherry immunoreactive bands which could be, among others, as a result of overexpression, degradation, propeptide cleavage and post-translational modifications of recombinant Na^+/K^+-ATPase α1 subunits expressed in HEK293 cells [28]. We also observed significant co-immunoprecipitation of β-actin by myh10 and myoVI (lane 6, panel (vi), Fig. 5c) only in the presence of heterologously expressed Na^+/K^+-ATPase α1 subunits in HEK293 cells. This was surprising as myh10 and myoVI antibodies poorly co-immunoprecipitate β-actin from HEK293 cells. Hence, the β-actin co-immunoprecipitation seen in lane 6 of panels (iv) and (vi) (Fig. 5c) appears to be as a result of overexpression of Na^+/K^+-ATPase α1 subunits.

Interaction of recombinant myosins with Na^+/K^+-ATPase α1 subunits

We also determined whether recombinant myosins would co-immunoprecipitate Na^+/K^+-ATPase α1 subunits expressed in HEK293 cells. To this end, we overexpressed GFP (as a control), GFP-myh9 and GFP-myh10 (GFP tag in their N-terminus) in HEK293 cells (Additional file 3: Figure. S2). Results indicated a lack of or very poor co-immunoprecipitation of endogenous Na^+/K^+-ATPase α1 subunits as a result of immunoprecipitation of GFP-myh9 or GFP-myh10 heterologously expressed in HEK293 cells (Additional file 3: Figure S2). As expected GFP-myh9, not GFP, co-immunoprecipitated β-actin expressed in HEK293 cells. However, immunoprecipitation of GFP-myh10 using mouse anti-GFP antibodies did not lead to co-immunoprecipitation of β-actin expressed in HEK293 cells. Use of a pan-Na^+/K^+-ATPase α subunit antibody (Santa Cruz Biotechnology: sc-58,628/clone M7-PB-E9) for immunoblotting did not alter the outcome seen with the use of anti-Na^+/K^+-ATPase α1 subunit antibodies (DSHB) (Additional file 3: Figure S2B). We reasoned the fusion of the GFP tag in the N-terminus of myh9 and myh10 could be partly responsible for this outcome.

Next, we immunoprecipitated myh9, myh10 or myh14 tagged with GFP in the C-terminus (i.e., myh9-GFP, myh10-GFP or myh14-GFP respectively) using anti-GFP antibodies of mouse, rabbit and/or goat origin to investigate whether these recombinant myosins, not GFP, upon heterologous expression would co-immunoprecipitate Na^+/K^+-ATPase α1 subunits expressed in HEK293 cells (Figs. 6, 7 and Additional file 4: Figure S3, Additional file 5: Figure S4, Additional file 6: Figure S5 and Additional file 7: Figure S6). Immunoprecipitation of myh9-GFP or myh14-GFP using the same mouse anti-GFP antibodies led to the co-immunoprecipitation of Na^+/K^+-ATPase α1 subunits and β-actin (Additional file 4: Figure S3). However, immunoprecipitation of myh9-GFP (Fig. 6b and Additional file 5: Figure S4), myh10-GFP (Additional file 6: Figure S5) and myh14-GFP (Fig. 7 and Additional file 7: Figure S6) using goat anti-GFP antibodies or rabbit anti-GFP antibodies led to a much cleaner co-immunoprecipitation of Na^+/K^+-ATPase α1 subunits expressed in HEK293 cells.

We employed an approach similar to the one described above to study the interaction of recombinant myoVI with Na^+/K^+-ATPase α1 subunits expressed in HEK293 cells. Hence, we tagged myoVI with GFP in the C-terminus (i.e., myoVI-GFP) and expressed them in HEK293 cells (Additional file 9: Figure S8). Surprisingly, immunoprecipitation of recombinant myoVI using rabbit or goat anti-GFP antibodies did not lead to the co-immunoprecipitation of Na^+/K^+-ATPase α1 subunits expressed in HEK293 cells (Additional file 9: Figure S8). As a recourse, we tagged myoVI with mCherry in the N-terminus (i.e., mCherry-myoVI) and expressed them in HEK293 cells. mCherry-myoVI, but not mCherry, immunoprecipitation led to the co-immunoprecipitation of Na^+/K^+-ATPase α1 subunits expressed in HEK293 cells (Fig. 8).

Tail-less myosins interact with Na^+/K^+-ATPase α1 subunits

Myosins employ various adaptor proteins to transport their cargoes (i.e., myosin-adaptor-cargo) [29, 30]. The adaptor proteins typically interact with the tail regions of various myosins. Hence myosins possess cargo binding domains (CBD) in their tail regions. Therefore, we wanted to know whether the tail regions of NMHC-IIs (i.e., myh9, myh10, myh14) and myoVI are involved in their interaction with Na^+/K^+-ATPase α1 subunits.

We deleted the tail regions of NMHC-IIs (i.e., 33, 43 and 47 AAs from their C-terminal ends in myh9, myh10 and myh14 respectively) to make myh9-Δtail-GFP, myh10-Δtail-GFP or myh14-Δtail-GFP (Fig. 7a). Then we overexpressed and immunoprecipitated tail-less (Δtail) recombinant NMHC-IIs (i.e., myh9-Δtail-GFP, myh10-Δtail-GFP or myh14-Δtail-GFP) and probed for their ability to interact with Na^+/K^+-ATPase α1 subunits expressed in HEK293 cells. Tail-less myh9 (i.e., myh9-Δtail-GFP), myh10 (i.e., myh10-Δtail-GFP) or myh14 (i.e., myh14-Δtail-GFP) were able to co-immunoprecipitate Na^+/K^+-ATPase α1 subunits expressed in HEK293 cells (Fig. 7d and Additional file 5: Figure S4, Additional file 6: Figure S5 and Additional file 7: Figure S6). These results indicated that regions other than the tail ends are probably involved in the interaction of NMHC-IIs with Na^+/K^+-ATPase α1 subunits expressed in HEK293 cells.

Next, we wanted to know whether tail-less (ΔT) myoVI would interact with Na^+/K^+-ATPase α1 subunits expressed in HEK293 cells (Fig. 8). The C-terminal end (or tail region) of myoVI possesses many sites for interaction with various adaptor proteins and/or cargoes [29, 30]. Hence, first we made and expressed a recombinant myoVI that lacked 22 AAs (i.e., i.e., mCherry-Myo6-ΔT1) from its C-terminal end and examined its ability to interact with Na^+/K^+-ATPase α1 subunits expressed in HEK293 cells (Fig. 8). Immunoprecipitation of mCherry-myoVI-ΔT1, but not mCherry, led to the co-immunoprecipitation of Na^+/K^+-ATPase α1 subunits expressed in HEK293 cells (Fig. 8c). Then we made two additional myoVI deletion constructs which lacked either 60 AAs (i.e., mCherry-Myo6-ΔT2) or 120 AAs (i.e., mCherry-Myo6-ΔT3) from their C-terminal ends. Like mCherry-Myo6-ΔT1, both mCherry-Myo6-ΔT2 and mC herry-Myo6-ΔT3 co-immunoprecipitated Na^+/K^+-ATPase α1 subunits expressed in HEK293 cells (Fig. 8c). Hence, tail-less myo6, like those of tail-less NMHC-IIs, interact with Na^+/K^+-ATPase α1 subunits and regions aside their tail regions appear to be involved in the interaction of myoVI with Na^+/K^+-ATPase α1 subunits.

The actin binding sites (ABS) of NMHC-IIs influence their interaction with Na^+/K^+-ATPase α1 subunits

Previous results indicated that tail-less NMHC-IIs interact with Na^+/K^+-ATPase α1 subunits. These results indicated that region(s) other than the C-terminal tail ends

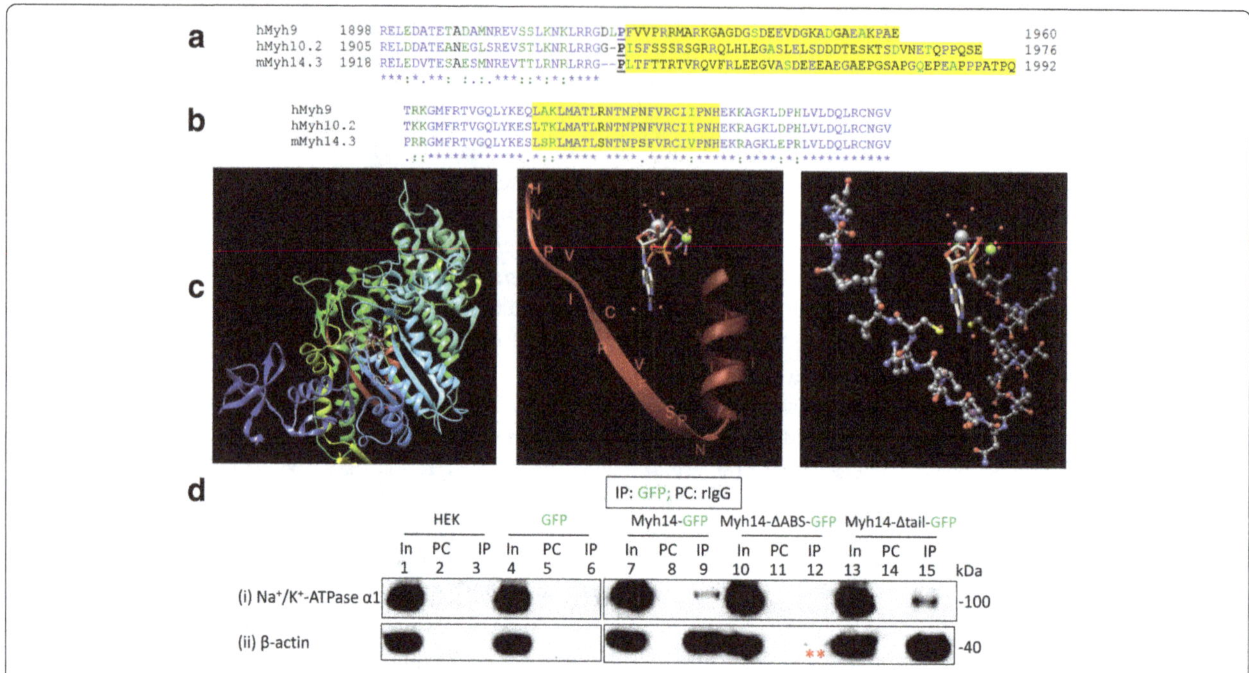

Fig. 7 Interaction of actin-binding-site-less (ΔABS) and tail-less (Δtail) NMHC-IIs with Na^+/K^+-ATPase α1 subunits expressed in HEK293 cells. **a** Tail-less NMHC-IIs were made by deleting the tail regions, yellow shaded, of human (h) myh9 (i.e., hMyh9 AAs: 1928–1960), human (h) myh10 isoform 2 (i.e., hMyh10.2 AAs: 1934–1976) and mouse (m) myh14 isoform 3 (i.e., mMyh14.3 AAs:1946–1992) following a conserved proline residue (bold and underlined) where the numbers indicate the position of the amino acids in the WT constructs. **b** Actin-binding-site-less (ΔABS) NMHC-IIs were made by deleting a 23 amino acids (AAs) segment, yellow shaded, of hMyh9 (i.e., AAs: 654–676), hMyh10.2 (i.e., AAs: 661–683) and mMyh14.3 (i.e., AAs: 674–696). For both (**a**) and (**b**) symbols below sequences indicate fully (*), strongly (:) or weakly (.) conserved residues, and the lack of a symbol indicates amino acid divergence. **c** The actin binding site (ABS) of human myh14. The 3-D coordinates of human myh14 was retrieved from protein data bank (PDB: 5I4E). Structural features of myh14 was visualized and analyzed using UCSF Chimera (http://www.cgl.ucsf.edu/chimera/). Left panel shows the relative position of the ABS (red ribbon), nucleotide analog (adenosine diphosphate vanadate (ADP.VO4): ball and stick model) binding site and N-terminal SH3 domain (deep blue) in the motor domain of human myh14 (5I4E.pdb). The center and right panel show the relative position of the ABS (red ribbon; and ball and stick model) with respect to the position of the adenosine diphosphate vanadate (ADP.VO4) and magnesium co-factor (green ball) in the motor domain of myh14. **d** Tail-less (Δtail) but not actin-binding-site-less (ΔABS) myh14 co-immunoprecipitate Na^+/K^+-ATPase α1 subunits expressed in HEK293 cells. Lysates of non-transfected HEK293 cells (In; 1) or HEK293 cells transiently transfected with GFP (In; 4), myh14-GFP (In; 7), myh14-ΔABS-GFP (In; 10), or myh14-Δtail-GFP (In; 13) plasmids (where the GFP tag is in their C-terminus) were precleared with rabbit IgG (PC; lanes 2, 5, 8, 11 and 14) prior to immunoprecipitation using rabbit anti-GFP antibodies (IP; lanes 3, 6, 9, 12 and 15). Loading of PC complexes in the gel preceded those of the IP complexes. Presence of Na^+/K^+-ATPase α1 immunoreactive bands in lanes 1, 4, 7, 9, 10, 13 and 15 and absence of any Na^+/K^+-ATPase α1 immunoreactive bands in lanes 2, 3, 5, 6, 8, 11, 12 and 14 (in (i)) indicated co-immunoprecipitation of Na^+/K^+-ATPase α1 subunits from HEK293 cells transfected with myh14-GFP or myh14-Δtail-GFP plasmids but not from non-transfected HEK293 cells or those transfected with GFP or myh14-ΔABS-GFP plasmids. While myh14-ΔABS-GFP showed almost complete loss of actin binding (indicated with double asterisk '*'; lane 12, panel (ii)) both myh14-GFP and myh14-Δtail-GFP co-immunoprecipitated β-actin (lane 9 and lane 15 in panel (ii) respectively). Full length images of western blots are presented in Additional file 7: Figure S6 B

in NMHC-IIs is/are important for their interaction with Na^+/K^+-ATPase α1 subunits. Hence a non-tail region such as motor domain (site for ATP and actin binding), neck region (the site for light chain binding) or a conserved AA motif in these domains could be involved in the interaction of NMHC-IIs with Na^+/K^+-ATPase α1 subunits. This is plausible as the tails are divergent and a common or conserved mechanism appear to be involved in the interaction of NMHC-IIs with Na^+/K^+-ATPase α1 subunits. Additionally, we knew (and observed) that Na^+/K^+-ATPase α1 subunits co-immunoprecipitate β-actin [24] and NMHC-IIs (i.e., myh9, myh10 or myh14), native or recombinant, also co-immunoprecipitate β-actin. Hence, we wanted to determine whether the conserved actin binding site (ABS) of NMHC-IIs (Fig. 7b) are important in their interaction with Na^+/K^+-ATPase α1 subunits.

To this end, we made and expressed recombinant myh9, myh10 or myh14 lacking 22 AAs (involved in actin binding) from their motor head regions (i.e., myh9-ΔABS-GFP, myh10-ΔABS-GFP and myh14-ΔABS-GFP) in HEK293 cells (Fig. 7b and Additional file 5: Figure S4, Additional file 6: Figure S5 and Additional file 7: Figure S6) [18, 19]. Immunoprecipitation of myh9-ΔABS-GFP (Additional file 5: Figure S4), myh10-ΔABS-GFP (Additional file 6: Figure S5) or myh14-ΔABS-GFP (Fig. 7d and Additional file 7: Figure S6) led to reduced or complete lack of co-IP of Na^+/K^+-ATPase α1 subunits from HEK293 cells. As expected,

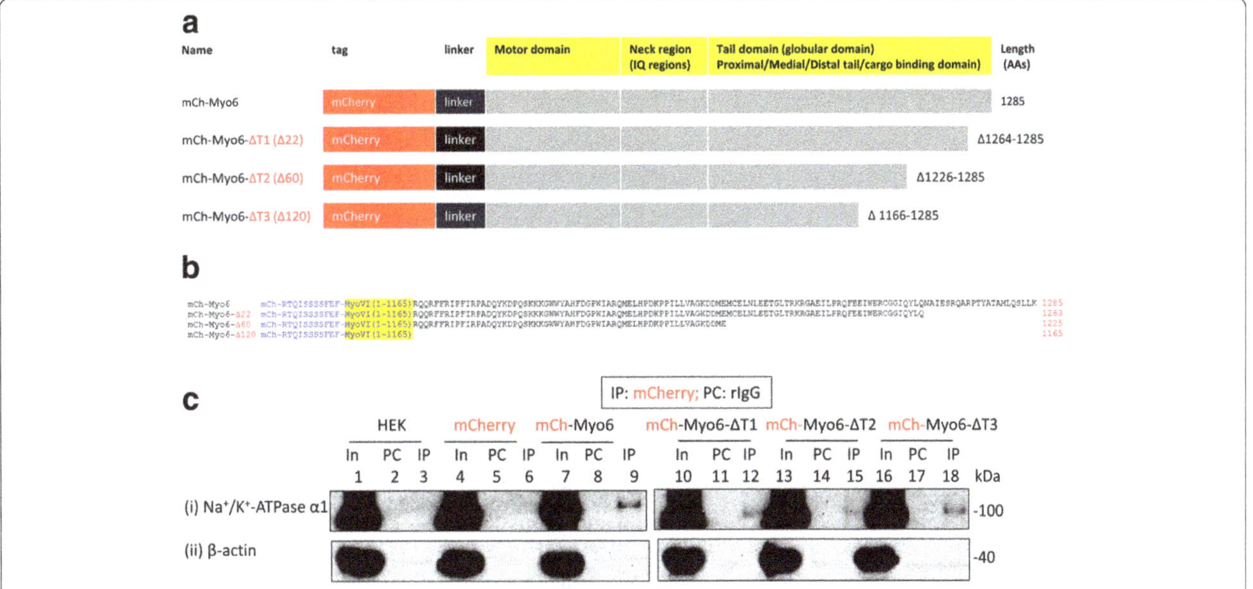

Fig. 8 Interaction of full length or tail-less (ΔT) recombinant myo6 with Na⁺/K⁺-ATPase α1 subunits expressed in HEK293 cells. **a** and **b** Schematic representation of myo6 constructs. All the myo6 constructs possessed a short amino acid linker of 11 AAs (shown in blue colored letters in **b**) between the mCherry tag (N-terminal) and coding sequences for myo6. mCherry tagged full length myo6 constructs (i.e., mCherry-Myo6) were truncated by 22 AAs (i.e., Δ1264–1285 = mCherry-myoVI-ΔT1), 60 AAs (i.e., Δ1226–1285 = mCherry-myoVI-ΔT2) and 120 AAs (i.e., Δ1166–1285 = mCherry-myoVI-ΔT3) from the C-terminal end where the numbers indicate the amino acid positions in the WT myo6. **c** Lysates of non-transfected HEK293 cells (In; 1) or HEK293 cells transiently transfected with mCherry (In; 4), mCherry-myo6 (In; 7), mCherry-myo6-ΔT1 (In; 10), mCherry-myo6-ΔT2 (In; 13) or mCherry-myo6-ΔT3 (In; 16) plasmids (where mCherry tag is in the N-terminus) were precleared with rabbit IgG (PC; lanes 2, 5, 8, 11, 14 and 17) prior to immunoprecipitation using rabbit anti-mCherry antibodies (IP; lanes 3, 6, 9, 12, 15 and 18). Loading of PC complexes in the gel preceded those of the IP complexes. Presence of Na^+/K^+-ATPase α1 immunoreactive bands in lanes 1, 4, 7, 9, 10, 12, 13, 15, 16 and 18 in (i) and absence of any Na^+/K^+-ATPase α1 immunoreactive bands in lanes 2, 3, 5, 6, 8, 11, 14 and 17 in (i) indicated co-immunoprecipitation of Na^+/K^+-ATPase α1 subunits from the IP of recombinant mCherry-myo6, mCherry-myo6-ΔT1, mCherry-myo6-ΔT2 or mCherry-myo6-ΔT3 but not from those of mCherry thus confirming interaction between myo6 and Na^+/K^+-ATPase α1 subunits which is not perturbed due to loss of tail regions in myo6. Recombinant mCherry-Myo6, mCherry-myo6-ΔT1, mCherry-myo6-ΔT2 or mCherry-myo6-ΔT3 could not co-immunoprecipitate β-actin (i.e., lanes 9, 12, 15 and 18 in (ii)) from HEK293 cells. Full length images of western blots are presented in Additional file 15: Figure S14

β-actin co-IP was drastically reduced or eliminated from these ABS-less recombinant NMHC-IIs. Hence it appears that the ABS in NMHC-IIs is involved in the interaction of NMHC-IIs with Na^+/K^+-ATPase α1 subunits.

Discussion

Class II myosins, traditionally known as conventional myosins, are expressed in striated muscles (i.e., myh1, myh2, myh3, myh4; etc.), cardiac muscles (i.e., myh6, myh7, and myh7B), smooth muscles (myh11) and non-muscles (i.e., myh9, myh10, and myh14) [31]. The non-muscle myosin II heavy chains (NMHC-IIs) (i.e., three of them: NMHC-IIA/myh9, NMHC-IIB/myh10, and NMHC-IIC/myh14) are widely expressed, as their name suggests, in non-muscle cells including neurons, microglia, podocytes; etc. [32–35]. They are also expressed in cardiomyocytes and at low levels in muscle cells [32, 34]. In this work we show that all the three NMHC-IIs (i.e., myh9, myh10 and myh14) interact with Na^+/K^+-ATPase α1 subunits expressed in the rodent brain and HEK293 cells (Table 1). These results may not be surprising as NMHC-IIs are homologous protein molecules possibly possessing similar structural and functional features for their interaction with Na^+/K^+-ATPase α1 subunits although they are engaged in unique biological functions at distinct cellular locations [36–40]. The interaction of NMHC-IIs with Na^+/K^+-ATPase α1 subunits are consistent with previous findings that NMHC-IIs interact with various proteins such as C-X-C chemokine receptor type 4 (CXCR4) [41], collagen receptor DDR1 (discoidin domain receptor 1) [42], Ins (1,4,5)P_3 receptor [43], epidermal growth factor receptor (EGFR) [44], N-Methyl-d-aspartate (NMDA) receptors [45], α-amino-3-hydroxy-5-methyl-4-isoxazolepropionic acid (AMPA) receptor [46], the pore-forming subunit of P/Q-type calcium channels ($Ca_v2.1$) [47], battenin/juvenile Batten disease protein (Cln3: a lysosomal membrane protein) [48]; etc. A recent report implicates non-muscle myosin II (NM-II) in the sorting and post-Golgi dendritic trafficking of Kv2.1 channels [49]. Hence our results possibly indicate that NMHC-IIs could be involved in the trafficking of Na^+/K^+-ATPase α1 subunits. These results are also suggesting that other class II myosins (such as myh1, myh3, myh6, myh7, myh14; etc.), which are similar to NMHC-IIs in their structural configurations, could be

Table 1 Summary of interaction of various myosins with Na^+/K^+-ATPase α1 subunits obtained via immunoprecipitation (IP) and co-IP assay

	Immunoprecipitation (IP) of native myosins		IP of recombinant myosins	IP of native Na^+/K^+ -ATPase α1	
Interaction/Tissue or cell types	Brain tissues	HEK293 cells	HEK293 cells	Brain tissues	HEK293 cells
Myh9:: Na^+/K^+-ATPase α1	Yes	Yes	Yes	Yes	No
Myh10::Na^+/K^+-ATPase α1	Yes	Yes	Yes	Yes	No
Myh14::Na^+/K^+-ATPase α1	Yes	–	Yes	–	No
MyoVa::Na^+/K^+-ATPase α1	Yes	No	No	Yes	No
MyoVI::Na^+/K^+-ATPase α1	Yes	Yes	Yes	No	No

'-'indicates unavailability of data

involved in the transport and/or trafficking of Na^+/K^+-ATPase α1 subunits in cells (such as cardiomyocytes, skeletal muscles, smooth muscles; etc.) where both molecules are expressed.

Positive interaction of NMHC-IIs with Na^+/K^+-ATPase α1 subunits prompted us to investigate whether non-class II myosins (i.e., unconventional myosins) would interact with Na^+/K^+-ATPase α1 subunits. Myosin Va (myoVa) immediately caught our attention. In alveolar epithelial cells it is involved in restraining Na^+/K^+-ATPase-containing vesicles within intracellular pools and overexpression of dominant-negative myoVa or knockdown with specific shRNA increased the average speed and distance traveled by the Na^+/K^+-ATPase-containing vesicles [9]. These results suggested that myoVa might be interacting with Na^+/K^+-ATPase α1 subunits expressed in alveolar epithelial cells. Our data indicate that myoVa interact with Na^+/K^+-ATPase α1 subunits expressed in the brain tissues (Figs. 1 and 2, Table 1) but not in HEK293 cells. This is possibly an indication that myoVa interact with Na^+/K^+-ATPase α1 subunits in a tissue specific manner and one or more molecular components required for their interaction in native tissues might not be present in HEK293 cells. Nonetheless our results are consistent with earlier observation that myoVa is involved in the trafficking of membrane proteins such as AMPA receptors; glucose transporter type 4 (GLUT-4); etc. [9, 50, 51]. These results also suggest that myoVa might be involved in the anterograde trafficking of Na^+/K^+-ATPase α1 subunits because of its known role in such processes [9, 51–56].

Our results also indicated that myoVI, another unconventional myosin, interact with Na^+/K^+-ATPase α1 subunits (Table 1). It is consistent with previous reports that myoVI interact or associate with various proteins and is involved in their transport and trafficking [9, 20, 57–60]. For example, myoVI is implicated in the trafficking and sorting of a transmembrane receptor (PlexinD1), transporter (GLUT1), cotransporters (NaPi2a and NaPi2c), transmembrane conductance regulator (CFTR); etc. [58]. It is possible that myoVI might be involved in the retrograde trafficking of Na^+/K^+-ATPase α1 subunits because of its known role in endocytosis, autophagy and trafficking of ubiquitinated cargoes [57, 58].

We observed that Na^+/K^+-ATPase α1 subunits interact with the myosin regulatory light chains (MRLCs; also known as regulatory light chain 20 (RLC20)). This is consistent with previous observations that myosin light chains are important for interaction of NMHC-IIs with their partner proteins. Both the heavy and light chains of NMHC-IIB interact with the cytoplasmic C-terminal region of the Ca(v)2.1 subunit of P/Q-type calcium channels [47]. Similarly, the interaction of NMHC-IIs and EGFR requires the regulatory light chain 20 (RLC20) of NMHC-IIs [44]. These results indicate that the neck region, the site for MRC or RLC20 binding, of NMHC-IIs could be important for their interaction with partner proteins including Na^+/K^+-ATPase α1 subunits. As a whole the observations that Na^+/K^+-ATPase α1 subunits interact with multiple myosins and MRLCs are consistent with earlier observations that they interact and/or co-localize with various proteins including atypical sodium channel (Na_x: SCN7A, SCN6A), water channel aquaporin 4 (AQP4), ionotropic glutamatergic AMPA receptors (AMPARs), glutamate transporter (GLAST and GLT-1), glycine transporter (GlyT2), STIM1(-stromal interaction molecule 1)-POST (partner of STIM1) complex, follistatin-like 1 (FSTL1), Polycystin-1 (PC-1); etc. [61–69].

We observed that tail-less NMHC-IIs and myoVI interact with Na^+/K^+-ATPase α1 subunits. These results indicated that region(s) other than the C-terminal tail ends in NMHC-IIs is/are important for their interaction with Na^+/K^+-ATPase α1 subunits. Hence a non-tail region such as motor domain, neck region or a conserved AA motif in these domains could be involved in the interaction of NMHC-IIs with Na^+/K^+-ATPase α1 subunits. Consistent with these ideas we show that NMHC-IIs lacking their actin binding sites, which are conserved in myosins, show reduced or null interaction with Na^+/K^+-ATPase α1 subunits. Hence, actin binding sites of NMHC-IIs are possibly involved in their interaction with Na^+/K^+-ATPase α1 subunits. These results also indicate that actin might be involved in the interaction of NMHC-IIs with Na^+/K^+-ATPase α1 subunits. Moreover, both NMHC-IIs and Na^+/K^+-ATPase α1 subunits directly interact with actin. Therefore, it is plausible that a tripartite interaction of Na^+/K^+-ATPase, β-actin and myosin could be occurring where (monomeric or polymeric) actin might serve as a link between Na^+/K^+-ATPase α1 subunits and myosin (i.e., Na^+/K^+-ATPase::actin:myosin complex).

Alternatively, it is possible that myosins (such as myh9, myh10, myh14, myoVa and myoVI) are interacting with Na^+/K^+-ATPase α1 subunits using adaptor or partner proteins. This idea of a myosin-adaptor- Na^+/K^+-ATPase complex may not be farfetched as Na^+/K^+-ATPase α1 subunits contain multiple structural motifs that enable them to interact with various soluble, membrane and structural proteins such as ankyrins, BiP, calnexin, cofilin, adducin, actin; etc. [2, 3, 70–73]. It appears that NMHC-IIs could be using a common set of adaptors for their interaction with Na^+/K^+-ATPase α1 subunits though alternative use of unique adaptors can't be discounted.

In this work we provide evidence that actins and myosins interact with Na^+/K^+-ATPase α1 subunits. The actin-myosin network is involved in short range trafficking whereas the microtubule-kinesin network is involved in long range cellular trafficking [52]. Moreover, in neurons microtubules extend along the full length of the axon and transect actins both in the soma and axon. Hence it appears that kinesins could play a role in concert with myosins to localize Na^+/K^+-ATPase α1 subunits (sodium pump) to far off places from the cell body. Overall, our data support a model in which the actin-myosin network is involved in the trafficking of sodium pumps in neuronal and non-neuronal tissues.

Additional files

Additional file 1: Table S1. Antibodies used for immunoprecipitation (IP) assays. **Table S2.** Antibodies used for immunoblotting. **Table S3.** Various features of the cDNA constructs used in the study. (DOCX 21 kb)

Additional file 2: Figure S1. Anti-myh9 and anti-myh10 antibodies immunoprecipitate their cognate antigens and/or co-immunoprecipitate partner proteins (such as β-actin and/or MRLCs) of their cognate antigens from HEK293 cells. Lysates of non-transfected HEK293 cells (In, lane 1 in A and B) were precleared (PC) with mouse IgG2b isotypes (mIgG2b; lane 2 in A and B) prior to immunoprecipitation (IP) using antibodies for myh9 (lane 3 in A) and myh10 (lane 3 B) of mIgG2b isotypes. IP complexes in the gel were loaded following the loading of their respective PC complexes. Myh9 immunoreactive bands in lane 3 of panel (i) in A and myh10 immunoreactive bands in lane 3 of panel (i) in B indicated immunoprecipitation of myh9 and myh10 by their respective antibodies. Presence of β-actin immunoreactive bands in the IP lanes of A (ii) and B (ii) indicated co-immunoprecipitation of it by myh9 and myh10 from non-transfected HEK293 cells. Both myh9 and myh10 also co-immunoprecipitated MRCLs (panel (iii) of A and B) from HEK293 cells. An asterisk ('*') in A and B indicates lack of detection of MRLCs in the input samples. Myh9 or myh10 immunoreactive bands in the depleted supernatant lanes (DS, lane 4 in panel (i) in A and B) indicate that both Mg^{2+}-ATPases survive the IP procedure. Mouse IgG-HC and IgG-LC (panel (ii) in A and B) separated from their intact immunoglobulins (that is used for PC or IP) upon denaturation could be seen as this section of the blot is probed with mouse anti-β-actin antibodies. (TIF 1319 kb)

Additional file 3: Figure S2. Lack of co-immunoprecipitation of Na^+/K^+-ATPase α1 subunits by recombinant myh9 or myh10 tagged with GFP-in their N-termini. Lysates of non-transfected HEK293 cells (In; lane 1 in B) or HEK293 cells transiently transfected with GFP (In; lane 4 in A and B), GFP-myh9 (In; lane 7 in A and B) or GFP-myh10 (In; lane 10 in A and B) plasmids were precleared with mouse IgG1 isotypes (PC; lanes 2, 5, 8 and 11 in A or B) prior to immunoprecipitation using mouse anti-GFP antibodies (IP; lanes 3, 6, 9 and 12; Abcam: ab1218) of the IgG1 isotypes. Loading of PC complexes in the gel preceded those of the IP complexes. Na^+/K^+-ATPase α1 (Abcam: ab7671) immunoreactive bands in the input lanes 4, 7 and 10 but not in the PC or IP lanes 5, 6, 8, 9, 11 and 12 (A (i)) or Na^+/K^+-ATPase α (pan- Na^+/K^+-ATPase α) immunoreactive bands (Santa Cruz Biotechnology: sc-58,628) in the input lanes 1, 4, 7 and 10 but not in the PC or IP lanes 2, 3, 5, 6, 8, 9, 11 and 12 (B (ii)) indicated lack of co-immunoprecipitation of Na^+/K^+-ATPase α (or α1) subunits by N-terminally GFP tagged myh9 or myh10 expressed in HEK293 cells. GFP-myh9 (but not GFP-myh10) co-immunoprecipitated β-actin (lanes 9 vs. 12 in panel (ii) of A and B). Stripping and staining the uppermost section of the blot with rabbit anti-GFP antibodies indicated successful immunoprecipitation of GFP-myh9 (lane 9 in (iii) in A) and GFP-myh10 (lane 12 in (iii) in A) from HEK293 cell lysates. Denatured mouse IgG-HC and/or IgG-LC (iii) separated from their intact immunoglobulins (used in PC or IP reactions) are seen as the blot section is probed with mouse anti-β-actin antibodies. (TIF 2367 kb)

Additional file 4: Figure S3. Co-immunoprecipitation of Na^+/K^+-ATPase α1 subunits by C-terminally GFP tagged myh14 or myh9. Lysates of non-transfected HEK293 cells (In; lane 1 in A) or HEK293 cells transiently transfected with GFP (In; lane 4 in A and B), myh14-GFP (In; lane 7 in A) or myh9-GFP (In; lane 7 in B) plasmids were precleared with mouse IgG1 isotypes (PC; lanes 2, 5 and 8 in A and B) prior to immunoprecipitation using mouse anti-GFP antibodies (IP; lanes 3, 6 and 9 in A and B; Abcam: ab1218) of the IgG1 isotypes. Loading of PC complexes in the gel preceded those of the IP complexes. Na^+/K^+-ATPase α1 (Abcam: ab7671) immunoreactive bands in IP lane 9 (denoted by asterisk "*" in (i) in A and B) but not in any other IP or PC lanes indicated co-immunoprecipitation of Na^+/K^+-ATPase α1 subunits by C-terminally GFP tagged myh14 or myh9 expressed in HEK293 cells. Both myh14-GFP and myh9-GFP (but not GFP) co-immunoprecipitated β-actin (lane 9 in (ii) in A and B). Myh9-GFP (but not GFP) also co-immunoprecipitated MRLC (lane 9 in (iii) in B). Denatured mouse IgG-HC and/or IgG-LC separated from their intact immunoglobulins (used in PC or IP reactions) are observed as those blot sections are probed with mouse antibodies (for Na^+/K^+-ATPase α1, β-actin and/or MRLCs). Part of S3B is presented in Fig. 6a. (TIF 2846 kb)

Additional file 5: Figure S4. Interaction of full length, actin binding site less (ΔABS) or tail-less (Δtail) recombinant myh9 with Na^+/K^+-ATPase α1 subunits and β-actin expressed in HEK293 cells. Lysates of non-transfected HEK293 cells (In; lane 1 in A, B and C) or HEK293 cells transiently transfected with GFP (In; lane 4 in A, B and C), myh9-GFP (In; lane 7 in A, B and C), myh9-ΔABS-GFP (In; lane 10 in C) or myh9-Δtail-GFP (In; lane 13 in C) plasmids (where the GFP tag is in their C-terminus) were precleared with rabbit IgG (PC; lanes 2, 5 and 8 in A) or goat IgG (PC; lanes 2, 5, 8, 11 and 14 in B or C) prior to immunoprecipitation using rabbit anti-GFP antibodies (IP; lanes 3, 6 and 9 in A) or goat anti-GFP antibodies (IP; lanes 3, 6, 9, 12 and 15 in B or C). Presence of obvious Na^+/K^+-ATPase α1 immunoreactive bands in lanes 1, 4, 7, 9, 10, 13 and 15 in A, B or C; greatly reduced Na^+/K^+-ATPase α1 immunoreactive bands in lane 12 in C; and absence of any Na^+/K^+-ATPase α1 immunoreactive bands in lanes 2, 3, 5, 6, 8, 11 and 14 in A, B or C indicated co-immunoprecipitation of Na^+/K^+-ATPase α1 subunits (panel (i)) from HEK293 cells transfected with myh9-GFP, myh9-ΔABS-GFP or myh9-Δtail-GFP plasmids thus confirming interaction between myh9 and Na^+/K^+-ATPase α1 subunits which is almost abrogated due to loss of actin binding site but not the tail regions in myh9. Myh9-GFP and myh9-Δtail-GFP, but not GFP, co-immunoprecipitated β-actin (lanes 9 and 15 respectively in panel (ii)). There was almost total loss of actin binding upon deletion of the actin binding site in myh9 (panel (ii), lane 12). Part of S4B is presented in Fig. 6b. (TIF 4636 kb)

Additional file 6: Figure S5. Interaction of full length, actin-binding-site-less (ΔABS) or tail-less (Δtail) recombinant myh10 with Na^+/K^+-ATPase α1 subunits and β-actin expressed in HEK293 cells. Lysates of HEK293 cells transiently transfected with myh10-GFP (In; lane 1 in A, B and C), myh10-

ΔABS-GFP (In; lane 4 in A, B and C) or myh10-Δtail-GFP (In; lane 7 in A, B and C) plasmids (where the GFP tag is in their C-terminus) were precleared with rabbit IgG (PC; lanes 2, 5 and 8 in A) or goat IgG (PC; lanes 2, 5 and 8 in B and C) prior to immunoprecipitation using rabbit anti-GFP antibodies (IP; lanes 3, 6 and 9 in A) or goat anti-GFP antibodies (IP; lanes 3, 6 and 9 in B and C). Loading of PC complexes in the gel preceded those of the IP complexes. Presence of Na^+/K^+-ATPase α1 immunoreactive bands in lanes 1, 3, 4, 7 and 9 (panel (i) in A, B and C) and greatly reduced or lack of presence of Na^+/K^+-ATPase α1 immunoreactive bands in lane 5 (panel (i) in A, B and C) indicated co-immunoprecipitation of Na^+/K^+-ATPase α1 subunits from HEK293 cells transfected with myh10-GFP or myh10-Δtail-GFP plasmids but not from those transfected with myh10-ΔABS-GFP plasmids thus confirming interaction between myh10 and Na^+/K^+-ATPase α1 subunits which is eliminated due to loss of actin binding site but not the tail regions in myh10. Myh10-GFP co-immunoprecipitated β-actin (lane 3 in (ii) in A, B and C) and there was complete loss of actin binding upon deletion of its actin binding site (lane 6 in (ii) in A, B and C). Tail-less myh10 also co-immunoprecipitated β-actin (lane 9 in (ii) in A, B and C). Control experiments for non-transfected HEK293 cells or HEK293 cells transiently transfected with GFP are done previously. (TIF 3566 kb)

Additional file 7: Figure S6. Interaction of full length, actin binding site less (ΔABS) or tail-less (Δtail) recombinant myh14 with Na^+/K^+-ATPase α1 subunits and β-actin expressed in HEK293 cells. Lysates of non-transfected HEK293 cells (In; lane 1 in A and B) or HEK293 cells transiently transfected with GFP (In; lane 4 in A and B), myh14-GFP (In; lane 7 in A and B), myh14-ΔABS-GFP (In; lane 10 in A and B) or myh14-Δtail-GFP (In; lane 13 in A and B) plasmids (where the GFP tag is in their C-terminus) were precleared with rabbit IgG (PC; lanes 2, 5, 8 11 and 14 in A) or goat IgG (PC; lanes 2, 5, 8, 11 and 14 in B) prior to immunoprecipitation using rabbit anti-GFP antibodies (IP; lanes 3, 6, 9, 12 and 15 in A) or goat anti-GFP antibodies (IP; lanes 3, 6, 9, 12 and 15 in B). Presence of obvious Na^+/K^+-ATPase α1 immunoreactive bands in lanes 1, 4, 7, 9, 10, 13 and 15 in A or B; absence of Na^+/K^+-ATPase α1 immunoreactive bands in lane 12 in A or B; and absence of any Na^+/K^+-ATPase α1 immunoreactive bands in lanes 2, 3, 5, 6, 8, 11 and 14 in A or B indicated co-immunoprecipitation of Na^+/K^+-ATPase α1 subunits (panel (i)) from HEK293 cells transfected with myh14-GFP, myh14-ΔABS-GFP or myh14-Δtail-GFP plasmids thus confirming interaction between myh14 and Na^+/K^+-ATPase α1 subunits which is abrogated due to loss of actin binding site but not the tail regions in myh14. Myh14-GFP and myh14-Δtail-GFP co-immunoprecipitated β-actin (lanes 9 and 15 respectively in panel (ii) in A and B). There was almost total loss of actin binding upon deletion of the actin binding site in myh14 (panel (ii), lane 12 in A and B). Part of S6B is presented in Fig. 7d. (TIF 4560 kb)

Additional file 8: Figure S7. Lack of co-immunoprecipitation of Na^+/K^+-ATPase α1 subunits and β-actin by recombinant myoVa. Lysates of HEK293 cells transiently transfected with GFP or myoVa-GFP plasmids were precleared with rabbit IgG (PC; lanes 2 and 5 in A) or goat IgG (PC; lanes 2 and 5 in B) prior to immunoprecipitation using rabbit anti-GFP antibodies (IP; lanes 3 and 6 in A) or goat rabbit anti-GFP antibodies (IP; lanes 3 and 6 in B). Loading of PC complexes in the gel preceded those of the IP complexes. Presence of Na^+/K^+-ATPase α1 immunoreactive bands in lanes 1 and 4, and absence of any Na^+/K^+-ATPase α1 immunoreactive bands in lanes 2, 3, 5 and 6 (panel (i) in A and B) indicated lack of co-immunoprecipitation of Na^+/K^+-ATPase α1 subunits from HEK293 cells transfected with myoVa-GFP. MyoVa-GFP did not co-immunoprecipitate β-actin (lane 6 in (ii) in A and B) from HEK293 cells. Staining the blots with mouse anti-GFP antibodies (NeuroMab: 75–131) indicated successful immunoprecipitation of GFP (lane 3 in (iii) in A and B) and myoVa-GFP (lane 6 in (iv) in B) from HEK293 cell lysates. (TIF 1906 kb)

Additional file 9: Figure S8. Lack of co-immunoprecipitation of Na^+/K^+-ATPase α1 subunits and β-actin by recombinant myoVI. Lysates of HEK293 cells transiently transfected with GFP or myoVI-GFP plasmids were precleared with rabbit IgG (PC; lanes 2 and 5 in A) or goat IgG (PC; lanes 2 and 5 in B) prior to immunoprecipitation using rabbit anti-GFP antibodies (IP; lanes 3 and 6 in A) or goat anti-GFP antibodies (IP; lanes 3 and 6 in B). Loading of PC complexes in the gel preceded those of the IP complexes. Presence of Na^+/K^+-ATPase α1 immunoreactive bands in lanes 1 and 4, and absence of any Na^+/K^+-ATPase α1 immunoreactive bands in lanes 2, 3, 5 and 6 (panel (i) in A and B) indicated lack of co-immunoprecipitation of Na^+/K^+-ATPase α1 subunits from HEK293 cells transfected with myoVI-GFP. MyoVI-GFP did not co-immunoprecipitate β-actin (lane 6 in (ii) in A and B) from HEK293 cells. Staining the blots with mouse anti-GFP antibodies (NeuroMab: 75–131) indicated successful immunoprecipitation of GFP (lane 3 in (iii) in A and B) and myoVI-GFP (lane 6 in (iv) in A and B) from HEK293 cell lysates. The input signal for myoVI-GFP (indicated with an asterisk '*') appears to be lost during stripping and/or staining with anti-GFP antibodies (lane 4 in (iv)). (TIF 2117 kb)

Additional file 10: Figure S9. mCherry antibodies are suitable for use in IP assay. Lysates of HEK293 cells transiently transfected with mCherry plasmids (In, lane 1) or ankyrin-G-mCherry plasmids (mCherry fused to the C-terminus: AnkG-mCh) (In, lane 4) or co-transfected with both AnkG-mCherry and $Na_v1.6$ plasmids (In, lane 7) were precleared (PC) with rabbit IgG (PC; lanes 2, 5 and 8) prior to immunoprecipitation using rabbit anti-mCherry antibodies (IP; lanes 3, 6 and 9). Loading of PC complexes in the gel preceded those of the IP complexes. Pan-$Na_v\alpha$ immunoreactive bands (panel (i)) in IP lane 9 but not in other IP (i.e., 3 and 6) or PC lanes (2 and 5) indicated co-IP of $Na_v1.6$ subunits (IP, lane 9) by recombinant ankyrin-G from HEK293 cells co-transfected with both ankyrin-G and $Na_v1.6$ subunits but not from HEK293 cells transfected with mCherry or AnkG-mCherry. Similarly, Na^+/K^+-ATPase α1 immunoreactive bands (panel (ii)) in lanes 1, 4, 6, 7 and 9 (but not in lanes 2, 3, 5 and 8) indicated co-IP of Na^+/K^+-ATPase α1 subunits (i.e., lanes 6 and 9) by recombinant ankyrin-G from HEK293 cells transfected with recombinant AnkG alone or along with $Na_v1.6$ subunits but not from HEK293 cells transfected with mCherry thus confirming interaction between AnkG and Na^+/K^+-ATPase α1 subunits. Also, mCherry immunoreactive bands in lanes 4, 6, 7 and 9 (panel (iii)) indicated IP of AnkG-mCherry by mCherry antibodies. (TIF 1055 kb)

Additional file 11: Figure S10. Na^+/K^+-ATPase α1 subunits could not co-immunoprecipitate myh9 expressed in HEK293 cells. (A) Immunoprecipitation of Na^+/K^+-ATPase α1 subunits expressed in HEK293 cells. HEK293 cell lysates (In, lane 1) were precleared (PC, lane 2) with mouse IgG2a isotypes prior to immunoprecipitation (IP, lane 3) using mouse anti-Na^+/K^+-ATPase α1 antibodies (DSHB: a6F) of the IgG2a isotypes. Na^+/K^+ ATPase α1 immunoreactive bands in lanes 1, 3 and 5 but not in lane 2 (i) indicated immunoprecipitation of Na^+/K^+-ATPase α1 subunits expressed in HEK293 cells by the antibody in use. Na^+/K^+-ATPase α1 immunoreactive band was also observed in the depleted supernatant lane (DS, lane 4). As expected Na^+/K^+-ATPase α1 subunits also co-immunoprecipitated β-actin from HEK293 cells (iii). Denatured mouse IgG-HC (ii) and IgG-LC (iv) separated from their intact immunoglobulins (that is used for PC or IP) are seen as the blot was probed with mouse antibodies (for Na^+/K^+-ATPase α1 or β-actin). (B) and (C). Lack of co-immunoprecipitation of myh9 by Na^+/K^+-ATPase α1 subunits. HEK293 cell lysates (In, lane 1) were precleared (PC, lane 2) with indicated immunoglobulin isotypes (PC; mIgG2a in B and mIgG1 in C) prior to immunoprecipitation (IP, lane 3) using mouse anti-Na^+/K^+-ATPase α1 antibodies (DSHB: a6F in B and EMD Millipore; clone C464.6 in C). Antibodies for Na^+/K^+-ATPase α1 subunits could not co-immunoprecipitate myh9 (lane 3, panel (i) in B or C) though they could co-immunoprecipitate β-actin (lane 3, panel (iii) in B or C) and immunoprecipitate their cognate antigens (lane 3, panel (ii) in B or C) from HEK293 cells. (TIF 2570 kb)

Additional file 12: Figure S11. Myh9 co-immunoprecipitate recombinant Na^+/K^+-ATPase α1 subunits expressed in HEK293 cells. Part of S11 is presented in Fig. 5a. (TIF 2388 kb)

Additional file 13: Figure S12. Myh10 co-immunoprecipitate recombinant Na^+/K^+-ATPase α1 subunits expressed in HEK293 cells. Part of S12 is presented in Fig. 5b. (TIF 2619 kb)

Additional file 14: Figure S13. MyoVI co-immunoprecipitate recombinant Na^+/K^+-ATPase α1 subunits expressed in HEK293 cells. Part of S13 is presented in Fig. 5c. (TIF 2302 kb)

Additional file 15: Figure S14. Interaction of full length or tail-less (ΔT) recombinant myo6 with Na^+/K^+-ATPase α1 subunits expressed in HEK293 cells. Part of S14 is presented in Fig. 8c. (TIF 6409 kb)

Abbreviations

AA: Amino acid; DS: Depleted supernatant; ELC: Essential light chain; GFP: Green fluorescent protein; gIgG: Goat immunoglobulins; HEK293 cells: Human embryonic 293 cells; IB: Immunoblot; IgG: Immunoglobulin; IgG-HC: Immunoglobulin heavy chain; IgG-LC: Immunoglobulin light chain; In: Lysate input; IP: Immunoprecipitation; KIF5B: kinesin family member 5B = kinesin-1 heavy chain; mCh: mCherry; mIgG1: Mouse immunoglobulin isotype 1; mIgG2a: Mouse immunoglobulin isotype 2a; mIgG2b: Mouse immunoglobulin isotype 2b; MM: Protein molecular weight marker; Myh: Myosin heavy chain; Myh10: Myosin heavy chain 10; Myh14: Myosin heavy chain 14; Myh9: Myosin heavy chain 9; MyoVa: Myo5a = Myosin Va; MyoVI: Myo6 = Myosin VI; Na^+/K^+-ATPase alpha 1: Sodium/potassium ATPase α1; NMHC: Non-muscle myosin heavy chain; PC: Pre-clear/immunoprecipitation using an isotype antibody; rIgG: Rabbit immunoglobulins; RLC: Regulatory light chain; WT: Wild type

Acknowledgements
We thank Fadia Dib-Hajj and Palak Shah for molecular biology support. We also thank Shujun Liu, Peng Zhao and Lawrence J Macala for animal tissue collection. The Center for Neuroscience and Regeneration Research is a Collaboration of the Paralyzed Veterans of America with Yale University. This material is the result of work supported with resources and the use of facilities at VA Medical Center, West Haven, CT. Portions of this work has been presented in abstract form: B. Dash, C. Han, E. J. Akin, S. D. Dib-Hajj, S. G. Waxman (2017). Myosins interact with voltage gated sodium channels, sodium calcium exchangers and sodium potassium ATPases. *Soc. Neurosci. Abst.* 288.11/D32.

Funding
This work was supported in part by grants from the Rehabilitation Research Service and Medical Research Service, Department of Veterans Affairs (to S.D.D.-H. and S.G.W.).

Authors' contributions
BD, SDH and SGW conceived the idea for the project, designed the experiments and wrote the manuscript. BD conducted the experiments, analyzed the results, and wrote the first draft of the paper. All authors read and approved the final manuscript.

Competing interests
The authors declare that they have no competing interests.

Author details
[1]Department of Neurology, Yale University Schoolof Medicine, New Haven, CT 06510, USA. [2]Center for Neuroscience & Regeneration Research, Yale University School of Medicine, New Haven, CT 06510, USA. [3]Rehabilitation Research center, VA Connecticut Healthcare System, 950 Campbell Avenue, Bldg. 34, West Haven, CT 06516, USA.

References
1. Clausen MV, Hilbers F, Poulsen H. The structure and function of the Na,K-ATPase Isoforms in Health and Disease. Front Physiol. 2017;8:371.
2. Xie Z, Cai T. Na+-K+—-ATPase-mediated signal transduction: from protein interaction to cellular function. Mol Interv. 2003;3:157–68.
3. Tian J, Cai T, Yuan Z, Wang H, Liu L, Haas M, Maksimova E, Huang XY, Xie ZJ. Binding of Src to Na+/K+-ATPase forms a functional signaling complex. Mol Biol Cell. 2006;17:317–26.
4. Reinhard L, Tidow H, Clausen MJ, Nissen P. Na(+),K (+)-ATPase as a docking station: protein-protein complexes of the Na(+),K (+)-ATPase. Cell Mol Life Sci. 2013;70:205–22.
5. Blanco G, Mercer RW. Isozymes of the Na-K-ATPase: heterogeneity in structure, diversity in function. Am J Phys. 1998;275:F633–50.
6. Forrest MD. The sodium-potassium pump is an information processing element in brain computation. Front Physiol. 2014;5:472.
7. Ikeda K, Onimaru H, Kawakami K. Knockout of sodium pump alpha3 subunit gene (Atp1a3(−/−)) results in perinatal seizure and defective respiratory rhythm generation. Brain Res. 1666;2017:27–37.
8. Trejo HE, Lecuona E, Grillo D, Szleifer I, Nekrasova OE, Gelfand VI, Sznajder JI. Role of kinesin light chain-2 of kinesin-1 in the traffic of Na,K-ATPase-containing vesicles in alveolar epithelial cells. FASEB J. 2010;24:374–82.
9. Lecuona E, Minin A, Trejo HE, Chen J, Comellas AP, Sun H, Grillo D, Nekrasova OE, Welch LC, Szleifer I, et al. Myosin-Va restrains the trafficking of Na+/K+-ATPase-containing vesicles in alveolar epithelial cells. J Cell Sci. 2009;122:3915–22.
10. Hartman MA, Spudich JA. The myosin superfamily at a glance. J Cell Sci. 2012;125:1627–32.
11. Kneussel M, Wagner W. Myosin motors at neuronal synapses: drivers of membrane transport and actin dynamics. Nat Rev Neurosci. 2013;14:233–47.
12. Chinthalapudi K, Heissler SM, Preller M, Sellers JR, Manstein DJ. Mechanistic insights into the active site and allosteric communication pathways in human nonmuscle myosin-2C. Elife. 2017;6
13. Kondo T, Okada M, Kunihiro K, Takahashi M, Yaoita Y, Hosoya H, Hamao K. Characterization of myosin II regulatory light chain isoforms in HeLa cells. Cytoskeleton (Hoboken). 2015;72:609–20.
14. Li C, Wen A, Shen B, Lu J, Huang Y, Chang Y. FastCloning: a highly simplified, purification-free, sequence- and ligation-independent PCR cloning method. BMC Biotechnol. 2011;11:92.
15. Wei Q, Adelstein RS. Conditional expression of a truncated fragment of nonmuscle myosin II-A alters cell shape but not cytokinesis in HeLa cells. Mol Biol Cell. 2000;11:3617–27.
16. Golomb E, Ma X, Jana SS, Preston YA, Kawamoto S, Shoham NG, Goldin E, Conti MA, Sellers JR, Adelstein RS. Identification and characterization of nonmuscle myosin II-C, a new member of the myosin II family. J Biol Chem. 2004;279:2800–8.
17. Breckenridge MT, Dulyaninova NG, Egelhoff TT. Multiple regulatory steps control mammalian nonmuscle myosin II assembly in live cells. Mol Biol Cell. 2009;20:338–47.
18. Maruta S, Homma K. A unique loop contributing to the structure of the ATP-binding cleft of skeletal muscle myosin communicates with the actin-binding site. J Biochem. 1998;124:528–33.
19. Suzuki R, Nishi N, Tokura S, Morita F. F-actin-binding synthetic heptapeptide having the amino acid sequence around the SH1 cysteinyl residue of myosin. J Biol Chem. 1987;262:11410–2.
20. Arden SD, Tumbarello DA, Butt T, Kendrick-Jones J, Buss F. Loss of cargo binding in the human myosin VI deafness mutant (R1166X) leads to increased actin filament binding. Biochem J. 2016;473:3307–19.
21. Leterrier C, Vacher H, Fache MP, d'Ortoli SA, Castets F, Autillo-Touati A, Dargent B. End-binding proteins EB3 and EB1 link microtubules to ankyrin G in the axon initial segment. Proc Natl Acad Sci U S A. 2011;108:8826–31.
22. Barry J, Gu Y, Jukkola P, O'Neill B, Gu H, Mohler PJ, Rajamani KT, Gu C. Ankyrin-G directly binds to kinesin-1 to transport voltage-gated Na+ channels into axons. Dev Cell. 2014;28:117–31.
23. Kelley CA, Sellers JR, Gard DL, Bui D, Adelstein RS, Baines IC. Xenopus nonmuscle myosin heavy chain isoforms have different subcellular localizations and enzymatic activities. J Cell Biol. 1996;134:675–87.
24. Cantiello HF. Actin filaments stimulate the Na(+)-K(+)-ATPase. Am J Phys. 1995;269:F637–43.
25. Bird JE, Takagi Y, Billington N, Strub MP, Sellers JR, Friedman TB. Chaperone-enhanced purification of unconventional myosin 15, a molecular motor specialized for stereocilia protein trafficking. Proc Natl Acad Sci U S A. 2014; 111:12390–5.
26. Guzik-Lendrum S, Heissler SM, Billington N, Takagi Y, Yang Y, Knight PJ, Homsher E, Sellers JR. Mammalian myosin-18A, a highly divergent myosin. J Biol Chem. 2013;288:9532–48.
27. Lu Z, Ma XN, Zhang HM, Ji HH, Ding H, Zhang J, Luo D, Sun Y, Li XD. Mouse myosin-19 is a plus-end-directed, high-duty ratio molecular motor. J Biol Chem. 2014;289:18535–48.

28. Fuller W, Tulloch LB, Shattock MJ, Calaghan SC, Howie J, Wypijewski KJ. Regulation of the cardiac sodium pump. Cell Mol Life Sci. 2013;70:1357–80.
29. Li J, Lu Q, Zhang M. Structural basis of cargo recognition by unconventional Myosins in cellular trafficking. Traffic. 2016;17:822–38.
30. Buss F, Kendrick-Jones J. Multifunctional myosin VI has a multitude of cargoes. Proc Natl Acad Sci U S A. 2011;108:5927–8.
31. Sellers JR. Myosins: a diverse superfamily. Biochim Biophys Acta. 2000;1496: 3–22.
32. Redowicz MJ. Unconventional myosins in muscle. Eur J Cell Biol. 2007;86: 549–58.
33. Lofgren M, Ekblad E, Morano I, Arner A. Nonmuscle myosin motor of smooth muscle. J Gen Physiol. 2003;121:301–10.
34. Tullio AN, Accili D, Ferrans VJ, Yu ZX, Takeda K, Grinberg A, Westphal H, Preston YA, Adelstein RS. Nonmuscle myosin II-B is required for normal development of the mouse heart. Proc Natl Acad Sci U S A. 1997;94:12407–12.
35. Janssen S, Gudi V, Prajeeth CK, Singh V, Stahl K, Heckers S, Skripuletz T, Pul R, Trebst C, Tsiavaliaris G, Stangel M. A pivotal role of nonmuscle myosin II during microglial activation. Exp Neurol. 2014;261:666–76.
36. Ma X, Kawamoto S, Hara Y, Adelstein RS. A point mutation in the motor domain of nonmuscle myosin II-B impairs migration of distinct groups of neurons. Mol Biol Cell. 2004;15:2568–79.
37. Rubio MD, Johnson R, Miller CA, Huganir RL, Rumbaugh G. Regulation of synapse structure and function by distinct myosin II motors. J Neurosci. 2011;31:1448–60.
38. Rex CS, Gavin CF, Rubio MD, Kramar EA, Chen LY, Jia Y, Huganir RL, Muzyczka N, Gall CM, Miller CA, et al. Myosin IIb regulates actin dynamics during synaptic plasticity and memory formation. Neuron. 2010;67:603–17.
39. Ma X, Jana SS, Conti MA, Kawamoto S, Claycomb WC, Adelstein RS. Ablation of nonmuscle myosin II-B and II-C reveals a role for nonmuscle myosin II in cardiac myocyte karyokinesis. Mol Biol Cell. 2010;21:3952–62.
40. Vicente-Manzanares M, Ma X, Adelstein RS, Horwitz AR. Non-muscle myosin II takes Centre stage in cell adhesion and migration. Nat Rev Mol Cell Biol. 2009;10:778–90.
41. Rey M, Vicente-Manzanares M, Viedma F, Yanez-Mo M, Urzainqui A, Barreiro O, Vazquez J, Sanchez-Madrid F. Cutting edge: association of the motor protein nonmuscle myosin heavy chain-IIA with the C terminus of the chemokine receptor CXCR4 in T lymphocytes. J Immunol. 2002;169:5410–4.
42. Huang Y, Arora P, McCulloch CA, Vogel WF. The collagen receptor DDR1 regulates cell spreading and motility by associating with myosin IIA. J Cell Sci. 2009;122:1637–46.
43. Hours MC, Mery L. The N-terminal domain of the type 1 ins(1,4,5)P3 receptor stably expressed in MDCK cells interacts with myosin IIA and alters epithelial cell morphology. J Cell Sci. 2010;123:1449–59.
44. Kim JH, Wang A, Conti MA, Adelstein RS. Nonmuscle myosin II is required for internalization of the epidermal growth factor receptor and modulation of downstream signaling. J Biol Chem. 2012;287:27345–58.
45. Bu Y, Wang N, Wang S, Sheng T, Tian T, Chen L, Pan W, Zhu M, Luo J, Lu W. Myosin IIb-dependent regulation of actin dynamics is required for N-methyl-D-aspartate receptor trafficking during synaptic plasticity. J Biol Chem. 2015;290:25395–410.
46. Ryu J, Liu L, Wong TP, Wu DC, Burette A, Weinberg R, Wang YT, Sheng M. A critical role for myosin IIb in dendritic spine morphology and synaptic function. Neuron. 2006;49:175–82.
47. Marqueze-Pouey B, Martin-Moutot N, Sakkou-Norton M, Leveque C, Ji Y, Cornet V, Hsiao WL, Seagar M. Toxicity and endocytosis of spinocerebellar ataxia type 6 polyglutamine domains: role of myosin IIb. Traffic. 2008;9:1088–100.
48. Getty AL, Benedict JW, Pearce DA. A novel interaction of CLN3 with nonmuscle myosin-IIB and defects in cell motility of Cln3(−/−) cells. Exp Cell Res. 2011;317:51–69.
49. Jensen CS, Watanabe S, Rasmussen HB, Schmitt N, Olesen SP, Frost NA, Blanpied TA, Misonou H. Specific sorting and post-Golgi trafficking of dendritic potassium channels in living neurons. J Biol Chem. 2014;289:10566–81.
50. Correia SS, Bassani S, Brown TC, Lise MF, Backos DS, El-Husseini A, Passafaro M, Esteban JA. Motor protein-dependent transport of AMPA receptors into spines during long-term potentiation. Nat Neurosci. 2008;11:457–66.
51. Sun Y, Chiu TT, Foley KP, Bilan PJ, Klip A. Myosin Va mediates Rab8A-regulated GLUT4 vesicle exocytosis in insulin-stimulated muscle cells. Mol Biol Cell. 2014;25:1159–70.
52. Langford GM. Myosin-V, a versatile motor for short-range vesicle transport. Traffic. 2002;3:859–65.
53. Oberhofer A, Spieler P, Rosenfeld Y, Stepp WL, Cleetus A, Hume AN, Mueller-Planitz F, Okten Z. Myosin Va's adaptor protein melanophilin enforces track selection on the microtubule and actin networks in vitro. Proc Natl Acad Sci U S A. 2017;114:E4714–23.
54. Varadi A, Tsuboi T, Rutter GA. Myosin Va transports dense core secretory vesicles in pancreatic MIN6 beta-cells. Mol Biol Cell. 2005;16:2670–80.
55. Wada F, Nakata A, Tatsu Y, Ooashi N, Fukuda T, Nabetani T, Kamiguchi H. Myosin Va and endoplasmic reticulum Calcium Channel complex regulates membrane export during axon guidance. Cell Rep. 2016;15:1329–44.
56. Wagner W, Brenowitz SD, Hammer JA 3rd. Myosin-Va transports the endoplasmic reticulum into the dendritic spines of Purkinje neurons. Nat Cell Biol. 2011;13:40–8.
57. He F, Wollscheid HP, Nowicka U, Biancospino M, Valentini E, Ehlinger A, Acconcia F, Magistrati E, Polo S, Walters KJ. Myosin VI contains a compact structural motif that binds to ubiquitin chains. Cell Rep. 2016;14:2683–94.
58. Tumbarello DA, Kendrick-Jones J, Buss F. Myosin VI and its cargo adaptors - linking endocytosis and autophagy. J Cell Sci. 2013;126:2561–70.
59. Sweeney HL, Houdusse A. Myosin VI rewrites the rules for myosin motors. Cell. 2010;141:573–82.
60. Spudich JA, Sivaramakrishnan S. Myosin VI: an innovative motor that challenged the swinging lever arm hypothesis. Nat Rev Mol Cell Biol. 2010; 11:128–37.
61. Krapivinsky G, Krapivinsky L, Stotz SC, Manasian Y, Clapham DE. POST, partner of stromal interaction molecule 1 (STIM1), targets STIM1 to multiple transporters. Proc Natl Acad Sci U S A. 2011;108:19234–9.
62. de Juan-Sanz J, Nunez E, Villarejo-Lopez L, Perez-Hernandez D, Rodriguez-Fraticelli AE, Lopez-Corcuera B, Vazquez J, Aragon C. Na+/K+-ATPase is a new interacting partner for the neuronal glycine transporter GlyT2 that downregulates its expression in vitro and in vivo. J Neurosci. 2013;33:14269–81.
63. Shimizu H, Watanabe E, Hiyama TY, Nagakura A, Fujikawa A, Okado H, Yanagawa Y, Obata K, Noda M. Glial Nax channels control lactate signaling to neurons for brain [Na+] sensing. Neuron. 2007;54:59–72.
64. Berret E, Nehme B, Henry M, Toth K, Drolet G, Mouginot D. Regulation of central Na+ detection requires the cooperative action of the NaX channel and alpha1 isoform of Na+/K+-ATPase in the Na+–sensor neuronal population. J Neurosci. 2013;33:3067–78.
65. Li KC, Zhang FX, Li CL, Wang F, Yu MY, Zhong YQ, Zhang KH, Lu YJ, Wang Q, Ma XL, et al. Follistatin-like 1 suppresses sensory afferent transmission by activating Na+,K+-ATPase. Neuron. 2011;69:974–87.
66. Rose EM, Koo JC, Antflick JE, Ahmed SM, Angers S, Hampson DR. Glutamate transporter coupling to Na,K-ATPase. J Neurosci. 2009;29:8143–55.
67. Illarionova NB, Gunnarson E, Li Y, Brismar H, Bondar A, Zelenin S, Aperia A. Functional and molecular interactions between aquaporins and Na,K-ATPase. Neuroscience. 2010;168:915–25.
68. Zhang D, Hou Q, Wang M, Lin A, Jarzylo L, Navis A, Raissi A, Liu F, Man HY. Na,K-ATPase activity regulates AMPA receptor turnover through proteasome-mediated proteolysis. J Neurosci. 2009;29:4498–511.
69. Zatti A, Chauvet V, Rajendran V, Kimura T, Pagel P, Caplan MJ. The C-terminal tail of the polycystin-1 protein interacts with the Na,K-ATPase alpha-subunit. Mol Biol Cell. 2005;16:5087–93.
70. Beggah AT, Geering K. Alpha and beta subunits of Na,K-ATPase interact with BiP and calnexin. Ann N Y Acad Sci. 1997;834:537–9.
71. Lee K, Jung J, Kim M, Guidotti G. Interaction of the alpha subunit of Na,K-ATPase with cofilin. Biochem J. 2001;353:377–85.
72. Ferrandi M, Salardi S, Tripodi G, Barassi P, Rivera R, Manunta P, Goldshleger R, Ferrari P, Bianchi G, Karlish SJ. Evidence for an interaction between adducin and Na(+)-K(+)-ATPase: relation to genetic hypertension. Am J Phys. 1999;277:H1338–49.
73. Devarajan P, Scaramuzzino DA, Morrow JS. Ankyrin binds to two distinct cytoplasmic domains of Na,K-ATPase alpha subunit. Proc Natl Acad Sci U S A. 1994;91:2965–9.

13

Lentivirus-mediated expression of human secreted amyloid precursor protein-alpha prevents development of memory and plasticity deficits in a mouse model of Alzheimer's disease

Valerie T. Y. Tan[1,2], Bruce G. Mockett[1], Shane M. Ohline[1], Karen D. Parfitt[3], Hollie E. Wicky[2], Katie Peppercorn[2], Lucia Schoderboeck[2], Mohamad Fairuz bin Yahaya[1,2], Warren P. Tate[2], Stephanie M. Hughes[2] and Wickliffe C. Abraham[1*]

Abstract

Alzheimer's disease (AD) is a neurodegenerative disease driven in large part by accumulated deposits in the brain of the amyloid precursor protein (APP) cleavage product amyloid-β peptide (Aβ). However, AD is also characterised by reductions in secreted amyloid precursor protein-alpha (sAPPα), an alternative cleavage product of APP. In contrast to the neurotoxicity of accumulated Aβ, sAPPα has many neuroprotective and neurotrophic properties. Increasing sAPPα levels has the potential to serve as a therapeutic treatment that mitigates the effects of Aβ and rescue cognitive function. Here we tested the hypothesis that lentivirus-mediated expression of a human sAPPα construct in a mouse model of AD (APPswe/PS1dE9), begun before the onset of plaque pathology, could prevent later behavioural and electrophysiological deficits. Male mice were given bilateral intra-hippocampal injections at 4 months of age and tested 8–10 months later. Transgenic mice expressing sAPPα performed significantly better than untreated littermates in all aspects of the spatial water maze task. Expression of sAPPα also resulted in partial rescue of long-term potentiation (LTP), tested in vitro. These improvements occurred in the absence of changes in amyloid pathology. Supporting these findings on LTP, lentiviral-mediated expression of sAPPα for 3 months from 10 months of age, or acute sAPPα treatment in hippocampal slices from 18 to 20 months old transgenic mice, completely reversed the deficits in LTP. Together these findings suggest that sAPPα has wide potential to act as either a preventative or restorative therapeutic treatment in AD by mitigating the effects of Aβ toxicity and enhancing cognitive reserve.

Keywords: Amyloid precursor protein, Lentivirus, Hippocampus, Memory, Long-term potentiation, Amyloid, APP/PS1 mouse

* Correspondence: cabraham@psy.otago.ac.nz
Valerie T. Y. Tan and Bruce G. Mockett joint first authors
Stephanie M. Hughes and Wickliffe C. Abraham are joint senior authors
[1]Department of Psychology, University of Otago, Box 56, Dunedin 9054, New Zealand
Full list of author information is available at the end of the article

Introduction

Alzheimer's disease (AD) is a neurodegenerative condition resulting in part from increased β-secretase cleavage of amyloid precursor protein (APP) and a concomitant increase in amyloid-β (Aβ) over the alternative α-secretase cleavage products [1, 2]. A key α-secretase cleavage product is the neuroprotective protein termed secreted amyloid precursor protein-alpha (sAPPα). Since the α-secretase cleavage site lies within the Aβ sequence, production of Aβ and sAPPα are mutually exclusive from the same molecule of APP. In AD, the shift towards β-secretase cleavage and Aβ accumulation appears to be associated with reduced sAPPα production in the brain [3, 4].

The reduction in sAPPα levels could serve as a significant compounding factor in the disease process as sAPPα exerts beneficial physiological, biochemical and behavioural effects that may mitigate the detrimental effects of Aβ accumulation. These effects include neuroprotection [5, 6], enhanced neuronal development [7, 8], facilitated long-term potentiation (LTP; [9–11], enhanced protein synthesis [12], enhanced memory [13] and rescue of spatial memory deficits induced by α-secretase inhibition [10] or APP knockout [11]. In contrast, reduced cerebrospinal fluid sAPPα levels correlate with poor memory performance in both aged humans and rats [14, 15]. The consistent role that sAPPα plays in neuroprotection and memory formation raises the possibility that elevating sAPPα levels in the damaged or diseased brain may be a useful therapeutic approach [16–19].

The progressive nature of AD presents the opportunity to test the ability of therapies to prevent the initial onset and progression of cognitive impairments, versus reversing or ameliorating cognitive impairments associated with moderate to advanced AD. Using the latter approach, expression of rodent sAPPα via AAV9 in the hippocampus of 12–13 month old APPswe/PS1dE9 mice largely reversed observed impairments in LTP, partially reduced plaque load and rescued spatial reference memory [20]. This result provides hope for a sAPPα-based therapy commencing even after frank disease onset. Should predictive biomarkers become available, however, it would potentially be possible to deliver therapeutic solutions earlier, before any cognitive decline begins, and thus be of even more value. However, it is not yet known whether raising sAPPα concentrations prior to disease pathology becoming evident can prevent or ameliorate AD-like symptoms.

In the present study, we used a lentiviral vector to express human sAPPα in the hippocampus of young adult APPswe/PS1dE9 mice to evaluate the potential of sAPPα to prevent the age-related onset of AD-associated neuropathologies and cognitive deficits. We found that sAPPα expression prevented deficits in spatial reference and working memory, as well as a partial rescue of the LTP deficit, even in the absence of an effect on Aβ accumulation and plaque load. Chronic expression commencing later in life, or acute delivery of sAPPα in aged transgenic mice, also rescued LTP. These findings demonstrate that elevating sAPPα levels in the presymptomatic phase has therapeutic potential for AD, and extends previous data [20] that either chronic or acute delivery of sAPPα delivery after symptom development may also be efficacious.

Methods

Animals

Male B6C3-Tg (APPswe, PSEN1dE9)85Dbo/Mmjax transgenic hemizygous and wild-type (WT) littermates (The Jackson Laboratory, Bar Harbor, USA, https://www.jax.org/strain/004462) were maintained as a colony at the University of Otago. Animals were group-housed in standard caging until surgery at either 4 or 10 months of age. They were transferred to single housing at ~ 8 months of age to prevent injury from fighting between the males. Food and water were available ad libitum, and the cage contained one red plastic tube (approximately 5 cm in diameter, 10 cm long) and shredded paper bedding as standard housing. Animals were kept on a 12 h light:dark cycle (lights on at 7 am), and the room temperature was controlled via a thermostat set at 21 °C. All procedures were approved by the University of Otago Animal Ethics Committee and conducted in accordance with New Zealand Animal Welfare and Biosecurity Legislation.

Genotyping was carried out on tail tips which were lysed overnight at 55 °C in lysis buffer (100 mM Tris HCl pH 8.5, 5 mM EDTA, 0.2% (*w*/*v*) SDS, 20 mM NaCl) containing 20 μg/ml proteinase K. Isopropanol extracted DNA pellets were dissolved in TE buffer pH 8.0 (10 mM Tris, 1 mM EDTA). Polymerase chain reactions using two sets of primers that amplify the Psen transgene and mouse DNA as a positive control were carried out to distinguish between wild-type and transgenic animals. Primer sequences were obtained from the Jackson Laboratory (PsenTg_forward oIMR1644 AAT AGA GAA CGG CAG GAG CA, PsenTg_reverse oIMR1645 GCC ATG AGG GCA CTA ATC AT, control_forward oIMR7338 CTA GGC CAC AGA ATT GAA AGA TCT, control_reverse oIMR739 GTA GGT GGA AAT TCT AGC ATC ATC C). Agarose gel electrophoresis stained with ethidium bromide showed either one band that indicated a wildtype animal or two bands indicating a transgenic animal.

Lentivirus (LV)

Approval for the packaging and use of recombinant lentiviral vectors was obtained from the Environmental

Protection Agency, NZ (GMD03091). The HIV-1 derived lentiviral plasmid, pCDH-EF1-MCS-T2A-copGFP (CD521A-1, System Biosciences, Palo Alto, CA) was modified to replace EF1 with the rat neuron-specific synapsin 1 promoter (Syn) [21] to drive neuronal expression of either copGFP (LV-control) or human sAPPα [22] and copGFP, separated by a T2A cleavage signal (LV-sAPPα). Vectors were packaged in HEK293FT cells using a second-generation packaging system [23]. Viral particles were pseudotyped with either the vesicular stomatitis virus (VSVg) envelope, which has tropism for a wide variety of cells, but has limited spread from injection sites [24, 25] or a chimeric rabies/VSVg (RabB19) envelope (Addgene #88865) containing the SADB19 (B19) extra-virion and transmembrane domains and the intra-virion domain of VSVg, which by contrast can undergo retrograde transport [26]. Average viral genome titres, determined by quantitative RT-PCR [23], were 2×10^{10} and 2×10^{9} viral genomes/mL for VSVg and RabB19 pseudotyped LV, respectively.

Cell culture methods for detection of expressed sAPPa

Primary neuronal mouse cultures were prepared from postnatal day 2 C57BL/6 mouse pups. Animals were deeply anaesthetized with pentobarbital (150 mg/kg, s.c.) and decapitated. After removing meninges and cerebellum from the brains, tissue was diced finely and then digested for 15 min at 37 °C on a MACS-Mix (Miltenyi Biotec, DE) in Leibovitz's L-15 medium (Life Technologies, NZ) supplemented with 20 mM D-(+)-glucose (Sigma Aldrich, NZ), 0.8 mM kynurenic acid (Sigma Aldrich, NZ), 0.05 mM D(−)-2amino-5-phosphovaleric acid (AP5; Sigma Aldrich, NZ), 50 U/mL penicillin, 0.05 mg/mL streptomycin (penicillin-streptomycin; Life Technologies, NZ), 5.5 mM L-cysteine HCl (Sigma Aldrich, NZ), 12 U/ml Papain (Worthington Biochemical Corporation, NJ, US), 1 U/ml DNaseI (Life Technologies, NZ), 1.1 mM EDTA, 0.067 mM beta-mercaptoethanol, and 2% (*v*/v) B27 (Life Technologies, NZ). The enzymatic digest was stopped by blocking for 10 min at 37 °C on a MACS-Mix (Miltenyi Biotec, DE) in Leibovitz's L-15 medium supplemented with 20 mM D-(+)-glucose, 0.8 mM kynurenic acid, 0.05 mM AP5, 50 U/mL penicillin, 0.05 mg/mL streptomycin, 10 mg/mL BSA and 10 mg/mL ovomucoid (Sigma Aldrich, NZ). Tissue was then triturated in OptiMEM supplemented with 20 mM D-(+)-glucose, 0.4 mM kynurenic acid, 0.025 mM AP5, 10 mg/mL BSA and 2% B27, passed through a 100 μm cell strainer and cells pelleted by centrifugation. The cell pellet was resuspended in culture media (Neurobasal A (Life Technologies, NZ) supplemented with 35 mM D-(+)-glucose, 0.4 mM L-glutamine (Life Technologies, NZ), penicillin (50 U/mL) and streptomycin (50 mg/mL), and 2% B27). Cells were plated at a density of 200,000 cells / well of a 24-well plate containing poly-L-lysine hydrochloride (Sigma Aldrich, NZ) coated coverslips. Cells were maintained in culture media in a 37 °C/5% CO_2 incubator, with half of the volume replaced with fresh media every 3 days [27]. Cultures were transduced at 6 days in vitro (DIV) by adding 4 μl/well lentivirus expressing Syn.sAPPα-T2A-copGFP or Syn.T2A-copGFP, respectively. For immunocytochemistry, cells were fixed in 4% paraformaldehyde at 10 DIV and then stained with a MAP2 antibody (Millipore Cat# MAB3418 RRID:AB 11212326, 1:1000)/goat-anti-mouse Alexa488 (Cat# A-11001 RRID:AB_2534069, Life Technologies, NZ; 1:1000), and 4′, 6-diamindino-2phenylindole (DAPI; Life Technologies, NZ). For western blotting, media was replaced with culture media without B27 the day after transduction, and collected at 10 DIV.

Stereotaxic surgery

At 4 or 10 months of age (prevention and rescue studies, respectively), animals were anaesthetised with a subcutaneous injection of ketamine/domitor/atropine (75/1/0.05 mg/kg body weight), and placed into a stereotaxic frame (Kopf Instruments; California, USA). Vectors were bilaterally injected through a 33 ga needle into the hippocampus using 2 μL of viral preparation per hemisphere at a rate of 150 nL/min. Four injection sites per hippocampus were used to optimize virus spread. Stereotaxic coordinates from bregma were (in mm): AP -1.8, ML ±1.2, DV -1.25 and – 1.95; and AP -2.5; ML ±1.8, DV -1.25 and – 1.95. The needle was left in place for 3 min after each injection before moving to the next site.

For surgeries at 4 months of age, a total of 25 WT animals were injected with LV-control, 16 Tg animals injected with LV-control, and 28 Tg animals injected with LV-sAPPα. For surgeries at 10 months of age, 26 mice were injected for electrophysiological analysis of LTP (9 WT with LV-control, 7 Tg with LV-control, and 10 Tg with LV- sAPPα).

Behavioural testing

Behavioural testing commenced at 12 months of age, eight months after surgery in the 4 month age group. All behavioural testing and data analysis were conducted by an experimenter blind to the treatment conditions.

Open field

The open field test was conducted in a 40 × 40 × 25 cm opaque white plastic box. The mouse was placed in the middle of the box and its behaviour observed and recorded for 5 min with a ceiling-mounted video camera linked to a computer running Ethovision XT7 software. The centre zone was defined as the 24 cm × 24 cm area in the middle of the open field and the percentage time spent in the periphery or the centre of the field was measured. At the end of the trial, the mouse was removed from the box, fecal boli were removed and the box cleaned with 10% ethanol.

Morris water maze

The Morris watermaze testing was performed in a white plastic circular pool with a diameter of 100 cm and filled with water (20–22 °C) until 9 cm from the top. A small circular transparent Perspex platform (diameter 6 cm) stood 0.7 cm under the surface of the water and 21.5 cm from the pool wall. Prominent visible spatial cues with dissimilar features were located around the room at different heights. Performance was recorded using a ceiling mounted camera linked to the Ethovision XT7 program. Day 1 consisted of habituation by placing the mouse into the pool without the platform for 1 min. Days 2 and 3 comprised the cued learning phase, during which a visible flag was attached to the submerged platform (SE quadrant) and the mouse learned to seek out the platform. Each mouse underwent 6 trials/day with a maximum time in the pool of 60 s/trial and an inter-trial interval of 3 min. When the mouse reached the platform, it was allowed to remain on it for 15 s, and if the mouse did not reach the platform within 60 s, it was then gently placed on the platform and left there for 15 s.

The spatial reference memory acquisition phase was conducted on days 4–9, with 6 trials a day for 6 days, an inter-trial interval of 3 min, and the platform maintained in a fixed position different from during cued learning. The same platform was used for all sessions and each trial began from a different pseudo-randomly chosen start position with the mouse facing the wall. The mice were each allowed a maximum of 60 s in the pool, and if the mice did not arrive at the platform within the 60 s, they were then picked up and placed on the platform and allowed to remain there for 15 s. Total distance travelled (path length) and proximity data (calculated as the average distance from the platform during a trial and considered a sensitive measure of spatial learning [28, 29]), were measured.

Probe trials to test spatial reference memory were conducted just prior to training on the fourth day of reference memory acquisition (probe trial 1), and then 24 h after the last day of acquisition (probe trial 2). The mouse was placed in the pool for 60 s without the platform present and the number of platform crossings and proximity data were measured.

Immediately following probe trial 2, three days of spatial working memory testing were conducted. The experimental protocols were the same as for the reference memory acquisition testing except that the platform location was different for each day, although fixed for each day. The first day of testing was used for familiarizing the mice with the working memory task, and data were collected and analysed for the next two days of testing.

Object recognition

Following a rest day, the mice were re-habituated to the open field box for 5 min. The object recognition task began the next day and consisted of placing two distinctly different objects in the centre of two adjacent quadrants of the box. The objects used (consisting of a plastic cube [4 × 4 × 4 cm], a cylinder [4 × 4 cm diameter], and a pyramid [4 × 4 × 4 cm] had 1.5 cm holes drilled into its sides in order to increase exploration [30]. The following day, one of the objects was replaced with a novel object with a different shape in order to test novel object recognition; 24 h later, the familiar object was moved to another quadrant of the box to test novel object recognition. The objects replaced and displaced were counterbalanced between mice. Each mouse was placed in the box and allowed to explore for 5 min. Exploring was defined as the mouse's direct interaction with the object, such as nose and paw touching. Mice that did not achieve a total of 10 s of exploration within the given 5 min were excluded from the study. One WT-control, one Tg-control, and three Tg-sAPPα mice were excluded from the study based on these criteria. The trials were recorded by an overhead camera and mouse behaviour observed and analysed by the experimenter off-line. All objects and the exploration box were cleaned with 10% (*v*/v) ethanol solution between trials. For each object recognition task, the amount of time the animal spent exploring each object was measured. The data were then converted into a discrimination ratio, defined as:

$$\frac{\text{exploration time of novel object (or location)} - \text{exploration time of familiar object (or location)}}{\text{total exploration time}}$$

Post-mortem tissue preparation

Beginning at least one week after the end of the behavioral testing, animals were deeply anaesthetized with pentobarbital (200 mg/kg, s.c.) and a transcardial perfusion was conducted with an ice-cold sucrose dissection solution (mM: 210 sucrose, 26 $NaHCO_3$, 2.5 KCl, 1.25 NaH_2PO_4, 0.5 $CaCl_2$, 3 $MgCl_2$, 20 D-glucose) which had been bubbled with carbogen (95% O_2–5% CO_2). Following removal of the brain, one hemisphere was assigned for hippocampal slice electrophysiology and the other hemisphere for post-mortem analyses including western blots, ELISAs and histochemistry. The assigned hemisphere for each analysis alternated between left and right for successive mice.

Extracellular electrophysiology

After removing the frontal cortex and cerebellum, the selected hemisphere was sectioned transversely into 400 μm coronal slices using a Leica vibrotome (VT 1000). Slices were transferred to a Millipore cell culture insert (Millicell®, Millipore, MA, USA) housed in a custom built incubation chamber containing artificial cerebrospinal fluid (ACSF, mM: 124 NaCl, 3.2 KCl, 1.25 NaH_2PO_4, 26 $NaHCO_3$, 2.5 $CaCl_2$, 1.3 $MgCl_2$, 10 D-glucose) bubbled with carbogen. The slices were subsequently incubated at interface for 30 min at 32 °C and then at room temperature for at least 90 min. After this recovery period, slices were transferred to a recording chamber where they were gradually warmed to 32.5 °C while superfused (2 mL/min) with oxygenated (with carbogen) and humidified ACSF.

All recordings were made by an experimenter blind to the genotype and treatment condition of the mice. Field potentials were evoked using stimulating electrodes made from 50 μm Teflon-insulated tungsten monopolar electrodes placed in either the alveus or stratum radiatum and driven by custom constant-current stimulators controlled by custom Labview software. Evoked potentials were recorded using glass micropipettes (1.5–2.5 MΩ filled with ACSF), amplified (× 1000), filtered (0.3 Hz-3 kHz) and stored for later analysis using custom software. Population spikes were recorded in the stratum pyramidale in order to assess cell excitability across stimuli ranging from 10 to 200 μA (average of 3 responses at each stimulus intensity) to generate an input-output (I-O) curve, and then to assess recurrent inhibition by paired-pulse stimulation (PPI), where stimulation was first applied to the alveus to antidromically activate CA1 pyramidal cell axons (antidromic spike 75% of maximum amplitude), and then the stratum radiatum to evoke orthodromic population spikes (50% of maximum amplitude). Interpulse intervals ranged from 20 to 200 ms, with two pairs of stimuli at each pairing interval, followed by one orthodromic stimulus alone in association with each interval. PPI was expressed as the average of the two orthodromic responses for each pair at each interval divided by the average of all the orthodromic-only responses.

After PPI assessment, the recording electrode was moved to stratum radiatum where field excitatory postsynaptic potentials (fEPSPs) were recorded. Basal synaptic transmission was assessed by the input-output (I-O) measurements of fEPSPs by applying stimulation at increasing intensities as described above. Presynaptic paired-pulse facilitation (PPF) was tested by giving the slice three consecutive stimulations at interpulse intervals ranging from 20 to 200 ms. PPF was expressed as a ratio and was calculated as pulse 2 amplitude/pulse 1 amplitude. In LTP experiments, the stimulus current was set at a value that yielded half maximum fEPSP slope and the slice was stimulated every 30 s while a 30 min baseline was recorded. LTP was induced by giving either two (prevention study) or three (rescue study) theta-burst stimulation protocols (TBS) spaced 30 s apart. Each TBS protocol comprised 10 bursts at 5 Hz, with 5 pulses at 100 Hz per burst, at baseline stimulus intensity. After TBS, responses were recorded for a further 120 min. The initial slopes of the fEPSPs were measured, and each response expressed as a percentage change from baseline, which was defined as the average of the last 20 responses before TBS.

Histochemical analysis

Coronal sections (40 μm) from frozen tissue were mounted on slides and allowed to dry overnight. Congo-red was used to stain the sections to reveal amyloid plaques, with nuclei labelled with DAPI. Congo-red staining and DAPI were visualised on a Zeiss AX10 fluorescence microscope, attached to a Jenoptic camera and computer, and the percentage area covered by plaques was analysed using ImageJ. In short, images were converted to 8 bit, a threshold value was determined and maintained for all images, and the percentage area covered by plaques was calculated using the ImageJ algorithm.

Western blots

The hippocampi not used for electrophysiology were snap-frozen on dry ice and stored at − 80 °C until protein extraction. Protein was extracted in solubilisation buffer (5 mM phosphate buffer pH 7.4, 0.32 M sucrose, 0.5 mM phenylmethylsulfonyl fluoride [PMSF in ethanol], 1 mM EGTA, 1 mM EDTA, and a protease inhibitor (cOmplete Ultra Mini Tablet, Roche)) without detergent, homogenized by pestle 30× and supernatant collected by two centrifugation steps at 14,000 *g* for 10 min and 30 min respectively at 4 °C. The resulting supernatant was identified as the soluble fraction. The resulting pellets were solubilized in a second buffer containing Triton-X and SDS (EGTA 1 mM, EDTA 1 mM, PMSF 0.5 mM, cOmplete protease inhibitor, Triton-X (1% *v/v*), sodium dodecyl sulphate (0.1% *w/v*) in phosphate buffered saline pH 7.4) and proteins solubilised by probe sonication (10 pulses at 1 s each; Qsonica, CT, USA). The resultant fraction was identified as the insoluble fraction. A DC protein assay (Bio-Rad) was use to quantify protein concentrations in both fractions.

Protein samples were separated on 9 or 12% (*w/v*) bis-acrylamide gels before transferring to a nitrocellulose membrane. Blots were incubated in Odyssey blocking buffer (LI-COR) at room temperature for 1 h. The primary antibody (microglia: Iba-1, WAKO 019–19,741, RRID:AB_839504; astrocytes: GFAP, Abcam-AB10062, RRID:AB_296804; presynaptic boutons: synaptophysin,

Abcam-AB32127, RRID:AB_2286946; postsynaptic density: PSD-95, BD Transduction 610,496, RRID:AB_397862) or tubulin (Abcam-AB4074, RRID:AB_2288001) was prepared in phosphate buffered saline (PBS)-tween, 0.1% (w/v) BSA and 0.1% (v/v) NGS, overnight at 4 °C. The secondary antibody was either IRDye goat anti-rabbit680 or IRDye goat anti-mouse800 (LI-COR (1:10,000) in PBS/Tween), 1 h at room temperature. Blots were imaged on a LI-COR Odyssey imaging system, quantified using Image Studio 4 (LI-COR) after normalising to a loading control protein (tubulin).

Detection of sAPPα in the cell culture media was achieved by western blotting. Media was initially concentrated by ammonium sulfate precipitation (at 75% saturation). Proteins were then separated on a 10% (w/v) SDS-PAGE gel and transferred to a nitrocellulose membrane (100 V, 1 h). Blocking overnight in 1% (w/v) milk powder-PBS tween was followed by incubation for 2 h at room temperature with an N-terminal APP antibody (Cat# A8967 RRID:AB_258427, Sigma Aldrich, NZ; 1:1000), diluted in blocking solution (1% milk powder-PBS tween).. After three washes in PBS-0.3% Tween-20 (PBS-T), anti-rabbit-HRP secondary antibody (Cat# NA934, RRID:AB_772206, GE Healthcare Life Sciences) was applied for 2 h at room temperature (1:10,000 in PBS-T). Unbound secondary antibody was removed with three PBS-T washes and the blot was developed using Amersham ECL Prime Western Blotting Detection Reagent (GE Healthcare Life Sciences) and imaged using a Fuji LAS-3000 ECL imaging system.

Enzyme-linked immunosorbent assay (ELISA)

Aβ and sAPPα concentrations of the hippocampal samples were measured using four ELISA kits: Human amyloid β (1–42) Assay Kit (IBL, Hokkaido, Japan, 27,711), human amyloid β (1–40) Assay Kit (IBL, 27,713), human sAPPα high sensitive ELISA (IBL, JP27734), and Mouse/Rat sAPPα (highly sensitive) ELISA (IBL, JP27419). The procedures were performed according to the kit instructions. ELISA for mouse and human sAPPα were performed on the soluble fraction (as prepared for western blotting), and ELISA for human Aβ (1–42) and (1–40) were performed in both the soluble and insoluble fractions. Despite its ability to detect recombinant human sAPPα samples, the human sAPPα kit was not able to detect either native or virus-mediated sAPPα expression in the Tg mice, and thus we could not determine degree of up-regulation of sAPPα levels in the tissue. Therefore copGFP expression was used as the marker of successful transduction in the hippocampus.

Statistical analysis

Behavioural and electrophysiological statistical data were calculated in Microsoft Excel and SPSS v21 (IBM), and differences between groups were compared using one-way analysis of variance (ANOVA) or a mixed model two-way ANOVA with repeated measures on one factor with Lower-Bound corrected values. Post-hoc tests were conducted using Tukey's test, with significance set at $p < 0.05$. All group data are presented as mean ± SEM. Planned comparisons were conducted using Students t-tests comparing WT-control group with Tg-control group to examine genotype, and Tg-control group with Tg-sAPPα group to determine treatment effect. T-tests were conducted using SPSS version 21 software.

Results

Expression of sAPPα

In order to test whether transduction of cells with LV-sAPPα resulted in the expression from the viral vector and secretion of sAPPα, primary mouse neural cultures were transduced with LV-sAPPα or LV-control. GFP expression was localised to neurons as expected (Fig. 1a), whereas sAPPα was specifically secreted into the media from the transduced cultures (Fig. 1b). The persistence of cell transduction in vivo was assessed by expression of copGFP histologically, which was used as a surrogate marker given that the ELISA kit was not able to determine sAPPα levels per se. Ongoing expression was evident in area CA1 and often the dentate gyrus in animals even 10 months after surgery (Fig. 1c-e). Although the intensity of copGFP fluorescence was reduced in the Tg-sAPPα animals compared to the two other groups that received the copGFP-only vector, clear transduction in the CA1 pyramidal cell layer and neuropil was nonetheless still visible, as well as in the dentate gyrus and overlying neocortex in some animals. No animals were excluded from the study due to a lack of copGFP expression in the hippocampus, as observed in the post-mortem analysis.

Prevention study

In order to test whether human sAPPα expressed chronically from an early presymptomatic stage can act to delay or prevent the development of AD-like symptoms, we studied Tg mice injected with LV-sAPPα at 4 months of age, with behavioural testing commencing at 12 months of age. Control groups were Tg and WT mice injected with the LV-control virus. Because there were no significant differences in the LTP and reference memory data between the VSVg and rabies packaged sAPPα constructs, all data from the two packaging procedures were pooled in the analysis below.

Behavioural testing

In the open field test of exploration, animals in all groups generally spent more time in the periphery of the open field, compared to the centre. Tg-control animals

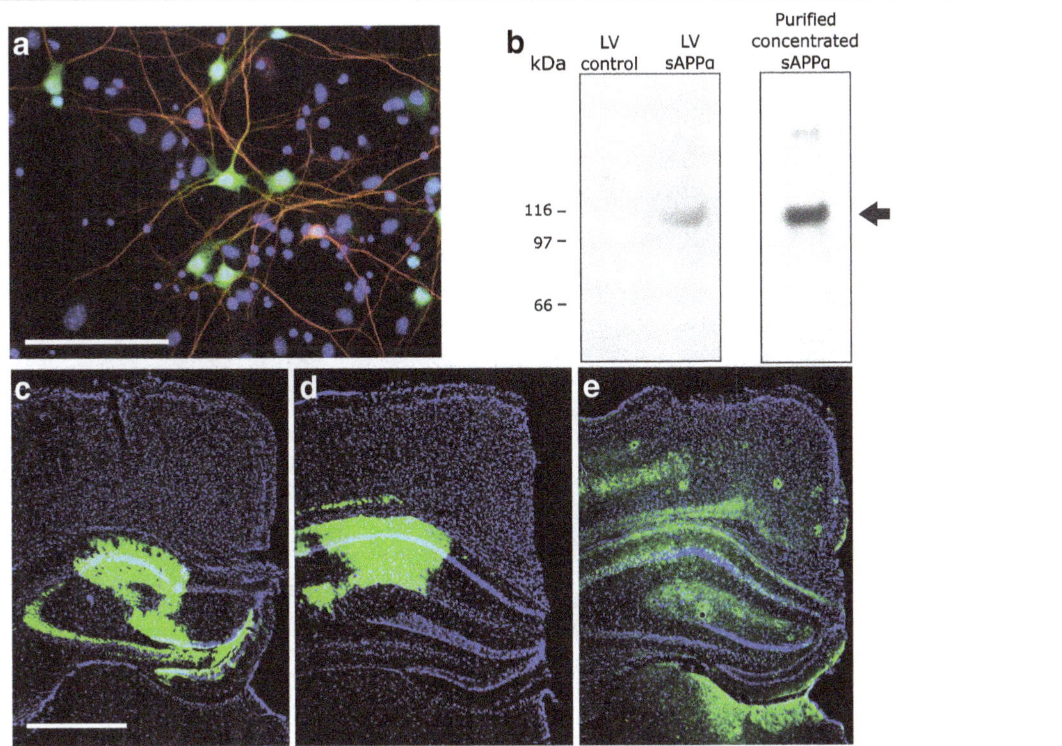

Fig. 1 In vitro and in vivo lentiviral transduction of hippocampal neurons with sAPPα-copGFP. **a** The transduction marker copGFP (green) was expressed in mouse primary hippocampal neurons co-labelled with the neuronal marker MAP2 (red) and the nuclear marker DAPI (blue). Scale bar, 50 μm. **b** Detection of sAPPα in media from primary mouse neural cultures transduced with LV-sAPPα, but not LV-control. The right-hand lane of the western blot illustrates the band from a sample fortified with purified sAPPα [22]. **c-e** Examples of in vivo copGFP expression (green) showing transduction of hippocampal regions containing LV-transduced neurons in slices from wild-type (**c**), transgenic-control (**d**) and transgenic-sAPPα (**e**) mice. Scale bar: 1 mm

spent significantly more time in the periphery of the open field compared to WT-control animals, suggesting a modest increase in anxiety in the Tg-control group. There was a trend for this genotype effect to be reversed in the Tg-sAPPα group compared to Tg-control animals ($p = 0.084$), such that there was no significant difference between the Tg-sAPPα group and the WT-controls (Fig. 2a). There was no difference in distance travelled between groups (Fig. 2b).

Water maze cue learning

There were no differences between groups in learning the cued phase of the water maze test (data not shown). However, based on the observations noted in this phase, two animals, one from the Tg-sAPPα group and one from the Tg-control group, were removed due to constantly swimming around the periphery of the water maze pool and thus not learning to use the platform as a goal.

Water maze spatial reference memory task

In the acquisition phase of the water maze spatial reference memory task, a mixed-model two-way ANOVA revealed a significant main effect of training days for the path-length taken to reach the platform, as well as for proximity, i.e. average distance from the platform. There was also a significant main effect of treatment group on proximity to the platform with Tukey post-hoc tests revealing a strong trend for an impairment in the Tg-control group relative to the WT-control group, and a significant enhancement of performance back to WT levels for the Tg-sAPPα group, compared to the Tg-control group (Fig. 2c, d). For the first probe trial (24 h after the first three days of training), there was a significant effect of group on proximity, with the Tg-control being impaired relative to the WT-control group ($p = 0.004$), with a partial rescue for the Tg-sAPPα group. By the second probe trial, there was a complete and significant rescue of memory in the Tg-sAPPα group compared to Tg-controls ($F_{(2,56)} = 4.69$, $p = 0.013$; Tukey's $p = 0.022$; Fig. 2e). The results were similar for platform crossings, where the Tg-control group showed fewer platform crossings than the WT-control group during probe trial 1 ($p = 0.037$), but no significant rescue for the Tg-sAPPα group ($p = 0.182$). However, by probe trial 2, there was both a genotype effect ($p = 0.006$), and a treatment difference such that the Tg-sAPPα group

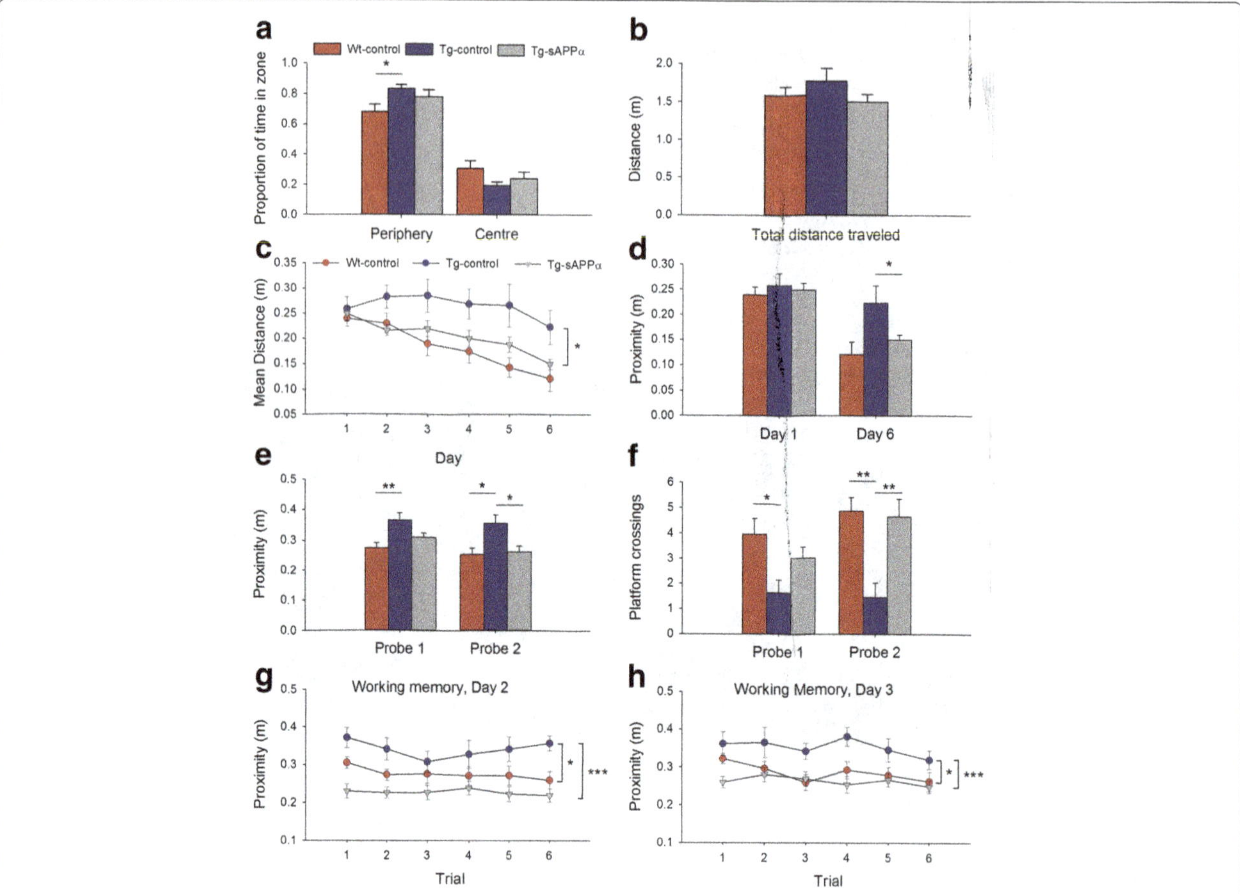

Fig. 2 sAPPα transduction rescued spatial learning and memory in the APP/PS1 mice. **a** In the open field all groups preferred the periphery ($p < 0.001$), but this preference was stronger in Tg-controls ($n = 11$) compared to WT-control ($n = 22$, $p < 0.05$, Students t-test). The Tg-sAPPa group showed a trend toward reduced time in the periphery ($n = 23$, $p = 0.084$) compared to Tg-controls. **b** Mean distances travelled by each group were not significantly different. **c** For spatial reference memory acquisition in the water maze, there was a significant group main effect ($F_{(1,54)} = 3.33$, $p = 0.043$) for proximity to the platform, with a strong trend for Tg-controls to be impaired relative to WT-control animals (Tukey $p = 0.071$), while Tg-sAPPα animals performed significantly better than Tg-control animals ($p = 0.046$). **d** There was a significant group main effect ($F_{(1,54)} = 3.33$, $p = 0.043$) with a strong trend for impaired performance on day 6 by the Tg-control group compared to WT-controls ($p = 0.068$) and by enhanced performance of the Tg-sAPPα group compared to Tg-controls ($p = 0.018$). **e, f** Tg-control mice had significantly poorer memory for the platform position than WT-controls (Probe 1: proximity $p = 0.004$, crossings $p = 0.037$; Probe 2: proximity $p = 0.016$, crossings $p = 0.006$). Tg-sAPPα mice exhibited a partial rescue in Probe 1 and a complete rescue in Probe 2 (proximity $p = 0.022$, crossings $p = 0.006$ compared to Tg-control). **g, h** Spatial working memory testing revealed a significant group main effect (G, Day 2: $p < 0.001$; H, Day 3: $p = 0.004$). On both days, Tg-controls performed significantly worse than WT-controls (Day 1: $p = 0.025$; Day 2: $p = 0.034$) while Tg-sAPPα animals were significantly better than Tg-controls (Day 1: $p < 0.001$; Day 2: $p = 0.003$). *$p < 0.05$, **$p < 0.01$, ***$p < 0.001$

showed significantly more crossings relative to the Tg-control group ($p = 0.006$), back to the level of the WT-control group (Fig. 2f).

Spatial working memory

The last three days of the water maze testing were used for working memory testing. The first day's training was used to teach the animals the new task. On each of days 2 and 3, there was a significant main effect of treatment group, whereby the Tg-controls performed more poorly than the WT-controls and the Tg-sAPPα group showed a virtually complete rescue of working memory performance to wildtype levels (Fig. 2g, h).

To summarize, the impairment in water maze learning by the Tg-control animals was completely prevented by sAPPα expression. Spatial memory retention, as evidenced during the probe trials, showed the same effects. Tg-control mice were also impaired on the spatial working memory task, and this was again prevented by sAPPα expression. Thus virus-mediated sAPPα expression was an effective treatment for both reference and working spatial memory tasks, even when commenced 8 months prior to behavioural testing.

Synaptic transmission and plasticity

To test for genotype and sAPPα effects on hippocampal electrophysiology in the same animals, we first undertook I/O curve and paired-pulse analyses of the Schaffer collateral input to area CA1, beginning at least one week after the end of behavioural testing. Mixed model ANOVA revealed that there was no main effect of group on the fEPSP initial slope ($p = 0.17$), nor a group x stimulus interaction ($p = 0.12$; Fig. 3a). Similarly, there was no group effect on population spike amplitude ($p = 0.14$, ns) nor group x stimulus interaction ($p = 0.63$; Fig. 3b). These data indicate that basal synaptic transmission and cell excitability were not affected by either the Tg genotype or the sAPPα (and copGFP) expression.

Paired-pulse stimulation was used to test for genotype or treatment effects on short-term plasticity of excitatory synaptic transmission. As expected, mixed-model ANOVA showed a main effect of inter-pulse interval ($F_{(1,48)} = 48.66$, $p < 0.001$), with longer intervals associated with less paired-pulse facilitation. However, there was no main effect of group (Fig. 3c), nor group x interval interaction. Thus there was no effect of viral transduction on short-term presynaptic plasticity mechanisms. To test for the strength of recurrent inhibition, a conditioning pulse was first delivered to the alveus in order to antidromically activate CA1 axons, and thus generate recurrent excitation of inhibitory interneurons, prior to a test pulse to the Schaffer collateral afferents that was above population spike threshold. Mixed-model ANOVA revealed a main effect of group (Fig. 3d), with Tg-controls showing less paired-pulse inhibition than WT-controls. The Tg-sAPPα group was not significantly different from either group, indicating a partial rescue of recurrent inhibition by sAPPα expression.

Long-term potentiation

Following theta-burst stimulation, all three groups showed a large initial potentiation that steadily decreased but without returning to baseline over the ensuing two hours (Fig. 3e). One-way ANOVAs revealed significant group differences at both 1 h and 2 h post-

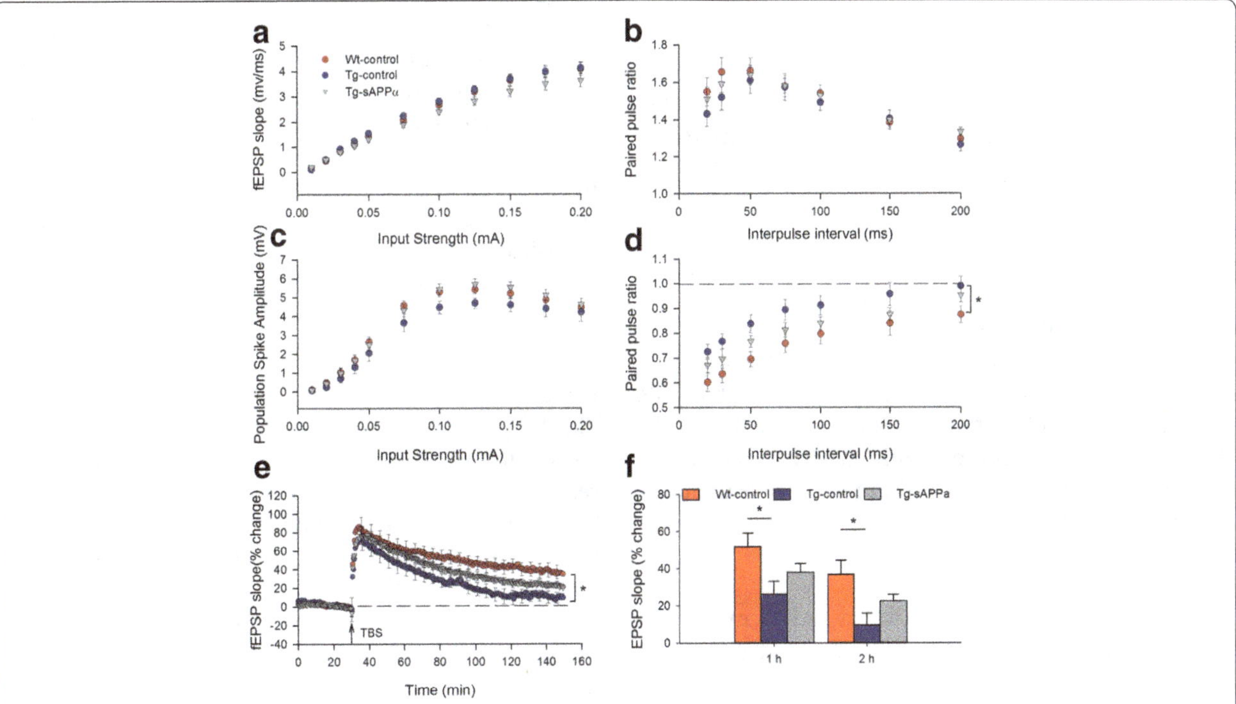

Fig. 3 Expression of sAPPα partially restored hippocampal LTP in transgenic mice. **a**, **b** There were no significant genotype or treatment effects on the I/O curves in CA1 for either the (**a**) EPSP slope, ($p = 0.17$ and 0.14, respectively) or (**b**) population spike amplitude ($p = 0.14$ and 0.63, respectively, indicating that basal synaptic transmission and cell excitability were unaffected in Tg mice and sAPPα over-expression. **c** There were no group differences in paired-pulse facilitation of the fEPSP (WT-control: n = 22; Tg-control: $n = 12$; Tg-sAPPα: $n = 17$, $F_{(2,48)} = 0.32$, $p = 0.73$), nor a group x interval interaction ($F_{(2,48)} = 0.96$, $p = 0.39$), indicating no difference in basal transmitter release probability. (**d**) Paired-pulse inhibition was reduced in Tg-controls compared to WT-controls (WT-control: $n = 16$; Tg-control: $n = 10$; $F_{(2,38)} = 4.18$, $p = 0.023$), indicating an impairment of recurrent inhibition. A partial rescue was produced by sAPPα expression. (**e**, **f**) TBS delivered to the Schaffer collaterals induced robust potentiation in all groups but which decayed at different rates between groups. Significant group differences were observed at both 1 h ($F_{(2,49)} = 4.20$, $p = 0.021$) and 2 h post-TBS ($F_{(2,49)} = 5.44$, $p = 0.007$) with Tg-controls significantly impaired (26.1 ± 6.9%, $n = 11$) compared to WT-controls (51.9 ± 7.4%, $n = 21$; $p < 0.05$) after 1 h. LTP in the Tg-sAPPα indicating a partial recovery of LTP expression. The partial recovery was still observed 2 h post-TBS (WT-controls: 36.8 ± 7.5%, $n = 21$; Tg-controls: 9.7 ± 6.2%, $n = 11$; Tg-sAPPα: 22.5 ± 3.5%, $n = 18$). *$p < 0.05$

TBS (Fig. 3f). At 1 h, Tg-controls showed significantly impaired LTP compared to WT-controls. The LTP for the Tg-sAPPα group occurred at an intermediate level that was not significantly different from either of the other groups, indicating a partial amelioration of the genotype effect on LTP. A similar pattern of results was found for the data at the 2 h time-point (Fig. 3f).

Amyloid-β load

To examine the effects of LV-sAPPα expression on amyloid-β load in the Tg mice, we examined a selection of hemispheres opposite to those used for the electrophysiology and stained with Congo red. There were no plaques observed in the hippocampus or overlying cortex of WT-control animals (Fig. 4a). In the Tg mice, there were large numbers of plaques, but no significant difference in the area of stained plaques between the Tg-sAPPα and Tg-control animals for either the hippocampus or the overlying cortex (Fig. 4b-e).

Human amyloid-β load was also assessed by ELISA for both soluble and insoluble fractions made from the hippocampus. A one-way ANOVA revealed an overall effect of group for soluble Aβ1–40 ($p < 0.001$), with a clear increase in the Tg-control animals compared to wild-type animals (post-hoc Tukey $p = 0.001$), but no effect on this elevated level by the expression of sAPPα ($p = 0.820$ compared to Tg-control; Fig. 4f). Aβ1–40 in the insoluble fraction showed a similar pattern of effects (ANOVA $p < 0.001$; Fig. 4g). Aβ1–42 levels in the insoluble fraction showed an overall effect of group (ANOVA $p < 0.001$) with Tg-controls showing the expected greater Aβ1–42 load compared to WT-controls (Tukey $p = 0.006$). Once again there was no significant effect of sAPPα expression on this elevated level (Tukey $p = 0.296$ compared to WT-control). A similar pattern of results was seen for soluble Aβ1–42 (Fig. 4h, i). Thus, the above-mentioned rescue of spatial memory and partial restoration of LTP was achieved in the absence of affecting amyloid load.

Western blot results

To assess the effect of genotype and sAPPα expression on inflammatory markers for microglia and astrocytes, we used western blot to determine the levels of markers for these cells, Iba-1 and GFAP, respectively, in the hippocampus. A one-way ANOVA comparing hippocampal Iba-1 levels between groups, normalised to WT-control, showed a significant effect of group ($p = 0.041$), indicating increased Iba1 in the transgenic mice but no significant difference between the Tg-control and the Tg-sAPPα groups (post-hoc Tukey $p = 0.991$; Fig. 5a). GFAP levels were also significantly different between groups ($p < 0.001$) with significantly higher levels in the Tg-control group compared to the WT group ($p = 0.007$) but once again this difference was also seen in the Tg-sAPPα group ($p = 0.001$; Fig. 5b).

To determine whether the occurrence of synaptic contacts was affected by genotype or sAPPα expression, we tested for expression of the presynaptic and postsynaptic proteins synaptophysin and PSD-95, respectively, in the hippocampus. There was no significant effect of group on the levels of presynaptic marker synaptophysin (Fig. 5c). There was also no group effect on the levels of the postsynaptic marker PSD-95 (Fig. 5d). The general lack of change in these synaptic protein markers was consistent with the lack of effects on the fEPSP I-O curve (cf. Fig. 3a).

Rescue of LTP deficits by LV-administered sAPPα

To address whether lentivirus-mediated expression of human sAPPα could also rescue hippocampal synaptic plasticity *after* plaque formation, a separate group of animals was transduced at 10 months of age, prior to in vitro electrophysiology beginning at ~ 13 months of age (the same age as for the prevention study). Characterization of the I-O curves for the fEPSP and population spike (data not shown) again revealed no main effect of treatment group, indicating that neither genotype nor sAPPα treatment affected basal synaptic transmission or cell excitability. Paired-pulse facilitation of the fEPSP was likewise unaffected (data not shown). In contrast, LTP was significantly impaired in the Tg-control group compared to the WT-control group, as described for the prevention study (cf. Fig. 3e, f). Notably, LTP was fully restored to control levels in the Tg-sAPPα group in this experiment (Fig. 6a).

Rescue of LTP deficits by acutely administered sAPPα

Finally, we asked whether even acute administration of sAPPα to the bathing medium would be sufficient to rescue LTP in slices prepared from Tg mice (18–20 months of age). Administration of recombinant human sAPPα_{1-612} (10 nM, [22] to the bathing solution 30 min prior to TBS caused no change in fEPSP slope as assessed by I-O curves for either genotype and no change to the baseline responses (data not shown). LTP induced by TBS was again significantly impaired in Tg slices compared to WT slices (Fig. 6b). Bath administration of sAPPα prior to and throughout the LTP protocol led to a complete rescue of LTP in Tg slices, without affecting LTP in the control slices. These data show that LTP is sensitive to the level of sAPPα available around the time of induction, and that long-term delivery is not required for LTP deficits to be reversed in this animal model of AD. It remains to be determined whether the concentration of sAPPα becomes critical for LTP just before, during or just after the induction protocol.

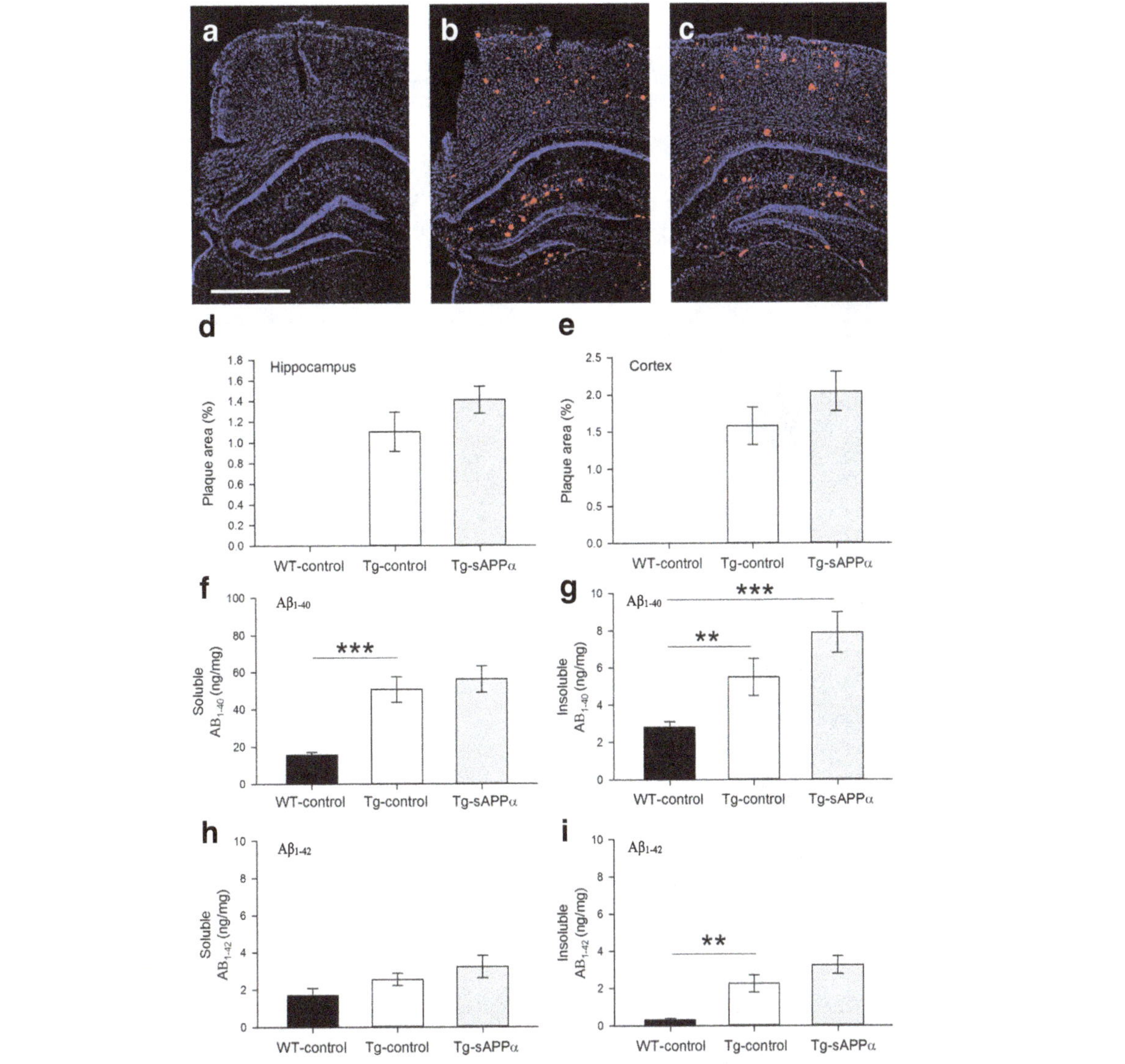

Fig. 4 Effect of sAPPα expression on the development of amyloid pathology. **a-c** Congo red staining of coronal brain sections from (**a**) WT-control, (**b**) Tg-sAPPα and (**c**) Tg-control animals revealed an absence of amyloid plaques in WT-control brains, but extensive plaque formation in Tg-sAPPα and Tg-control brains. **d-e** No significant differences in plaque density were observed between Tg- sAPPα and Tg-control in the hippocampus ($p = 0.316$, **d**) or overlying neocortex ($p = 0.297$, E). **f-i** Human amyloid-β load in the hippocampus. **f** Soluble Aβ1–40 levels differed between groups (one-way ANOVA $F(2,27) = 17.40$, $p < 0.001$), with higher levels in in Tg-control animals compared to wildtypes (WT-control: 15.6 ± 1.6 ng/mg, $n = 12$; Tg-control: 50.7 ± 6.9 ng/mg, $n = 6$, post-hoc Tukey $p = 0.001$), but no effect of sAPPα treatment compared to Tg-control (Tg-sAPPα: 56.1 ± 7.1 ng/mg, n = 12, Tukey = 0.820). **g** Insoluble Aβ1–40 levels showed a significant overall group effect (F(2,28 = 10.70) and while there was no significant difference between WT-control and Tg-control (WT-control, 2.8 ± 0.3 ng/mg, $n = 13$, Tg-control, 5.5 ± 1.0 ng/mg, $n = 6$, Tukey $p = 0.145$), the levels were elevated in the Tg-sAPPα group compared to WT-control (Tg-sAPPα 7.9 ± 1.1 ng/mg, Tukey $p < 0.001$) and they were not different to Tg-control (Tukey p + 0.194). (H) Soluble Aβ1–42 levels did not show any differences between groups. **i** For the insoluble fraction, there was an overall group effect (F(2,28) = 20.47, $p < 0.001$, whereby Tg-controls showed the expected greater Aβ1–42 load (2.26 ± 0.46 ng/mg, $n = 6$) compared to WT-controls (0.31 ± 0.077 ng/mg, $n = 13$; Tukey $p = 0.006$) and this level was not significantly affected by sAPPα over-expression (3.25 ± 0.48 ng/mg, $n = 12$, Tukey $p = 0.220$). $^{**}p < 0.01$, $^{***}p < 0.001$, Scale bar: 1 mm

Discussion

Our study has provided the first evidence that long-term expression (> 8 months) of the human form of sAPPα, beginning before development of the disease phenotype, can substantially mitigate the development of cognitive and synaptic deficits in a mouse model of AD. We observed that such treatment offered complete protection of spatial and working memory as measured by water maze performance 8 months after transduction. We further observed an apparent partial prevention of the deficit in LTP measured 9–10 months post-transduction that may in turn have contributed to the

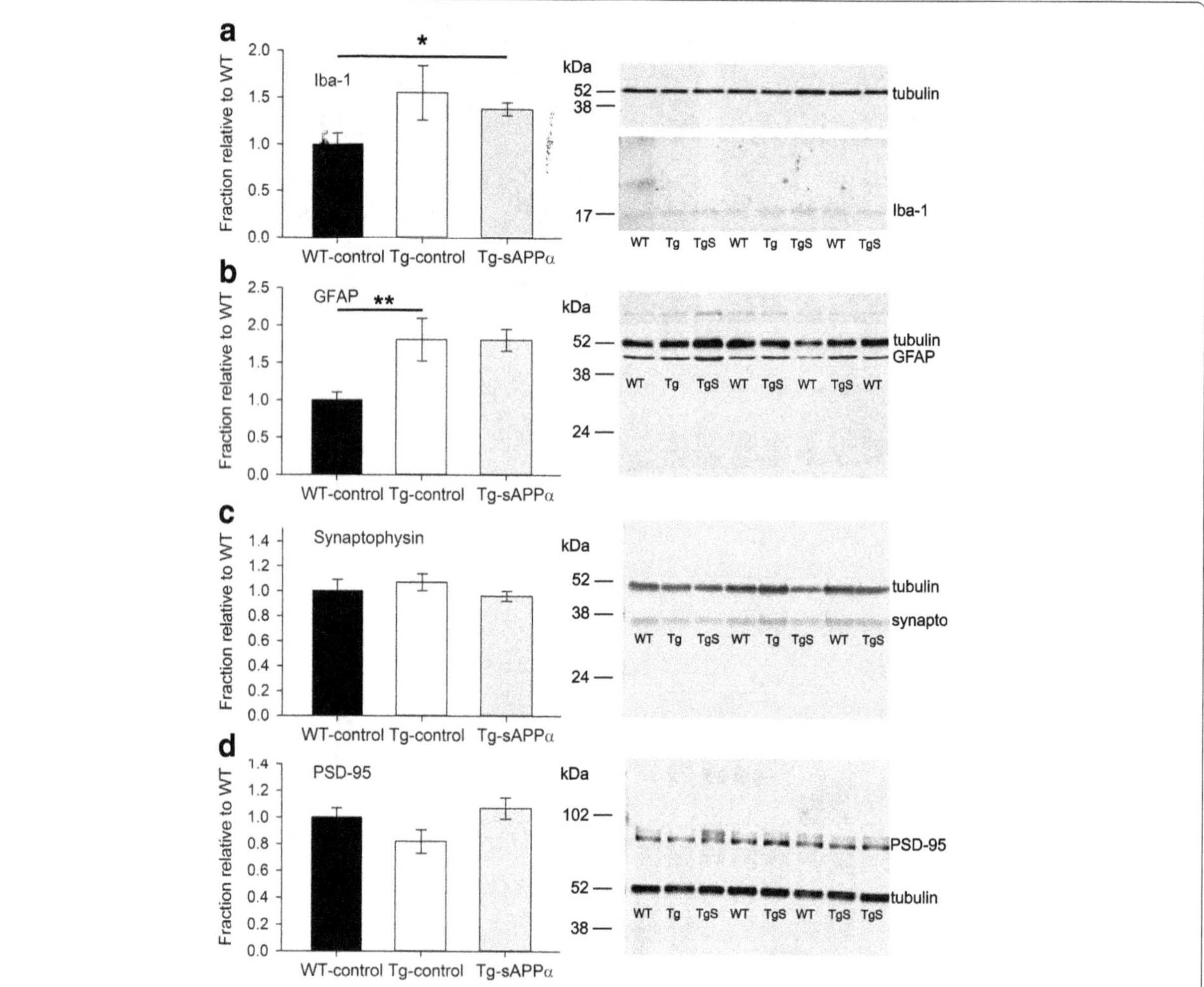

Fig. 5 Cellular markers for neuronal and non-neuronal cells. **a** Western blot analysis of the microglial marker Iba-1 (insoluble fraction), normalised to WT-control, showed an overall group effect (one-way ANOVA $F(2,28) = p = 0.041$) with a trend toward higher levels in Tg mice (WT-control: 1.0 ± 0.083, n = 12; Tg-control: 1.37 ± 0.299, n = 6), that was even more evident in the Tg-sAPPα group (Tg-sAPPα: 1.39 ± 0.065, $n = 13$; post-hoc Tukey $p = 0.046$). **b** GFAP levels (insoluble fraction) showed a significant overall group effect ($F(2,27) = 10.92$, $p < 0.001$), whereby there was significantly higher levels in the Tg-control group compared to the WT-control group (WT-control: 0.998 ± 0.105, $n = 13$; Tg-control: 1.81 ± 0.284, $n = 6$, Tukey $p = 0.007$) and expression of sAPPα did not alter this higher expression level (Tg-sAPPα: 1.86 ± 0.23, $n = 11$, Tukey $p = 0.974$). **c** Neither genotype (WT-control: 1 ± 0.02, n = 13; Tg-control: 1.07 ± 0.674, $n = 6$) nor sAPPα treatment (Tg-sAPPα: 0.96 ± 0.043, n = 12) affected the presynaptic marker synaptophysin (soluble fraction). **d** Levels of the postsynaptic marker PSD-95 (insoluble fraction) were also not affected by the APP/PS1 genotype (WT-control: 1.00 ± 0.072, $n = 13$; Tg-control: 0.82 ± 0.086, $n = 5$), although the PSD-95 levels tended to be higher for the Tg-sAPPα group compared to Tg-controls (Tg- sAPPα: 1.066 ± 0.082, $n = 12$, $t_{(17)} = -1.90$, $p = 0.074$. Representative western blots are presented. Note that in the case of Iba-1, its illustration and that of tubulin are from the same blot, but at different exposures. Tubulin was used as the loading control. *$p < 0.05$, **$p < 0.01$; synapto: synaptophysin; Lane labels: WT, WT-control; Tg, Tg-control; TgS, Tg-sAPPα

behavioural effect. Although the virus transductions targeted the hippocampus, expression in the overlying sensorimotor cortex was evidenced in at least some of the cases, and thus this brain region may have also contributed to the behavioural rescue. Collectively, these findings suggest that lasting restoration of sAPPα production beginning early in the disease process may be efficacious in preventing or at least delaying the later expression of the range of deficits that typically define the disease.

Given its neuroprotective, neurotrophic and plasticity enhancing properties, the therapeutic potential of sAPPα has been gaining considerable interest in recent years, particularly with respect to Alzheimer's disease but also for other neurological disorders [16, 18, 31, 32]. Indeed, acute intracerebroventricular administration of sAPPα shortly after traumatic head injury improved structural and functional outcomes in both normal [33] and APP knock-out mice [17]. Acute administration has also been used to ameliorate symptoms associated with ischemic

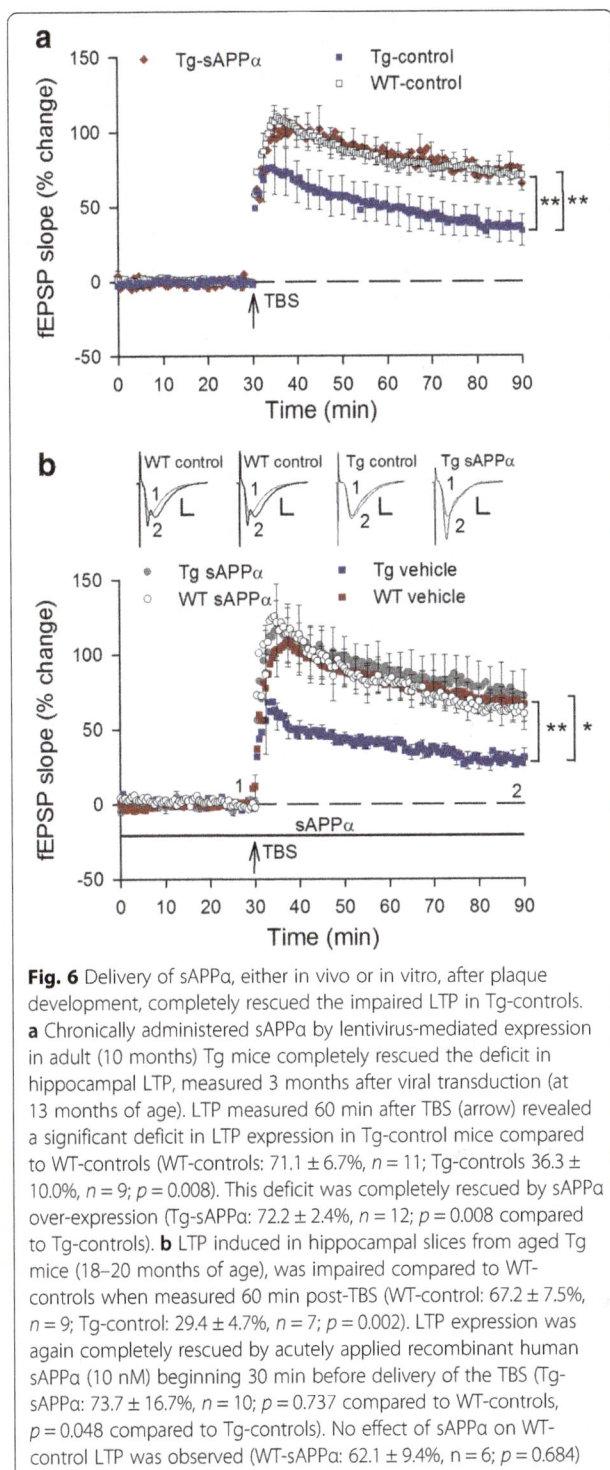

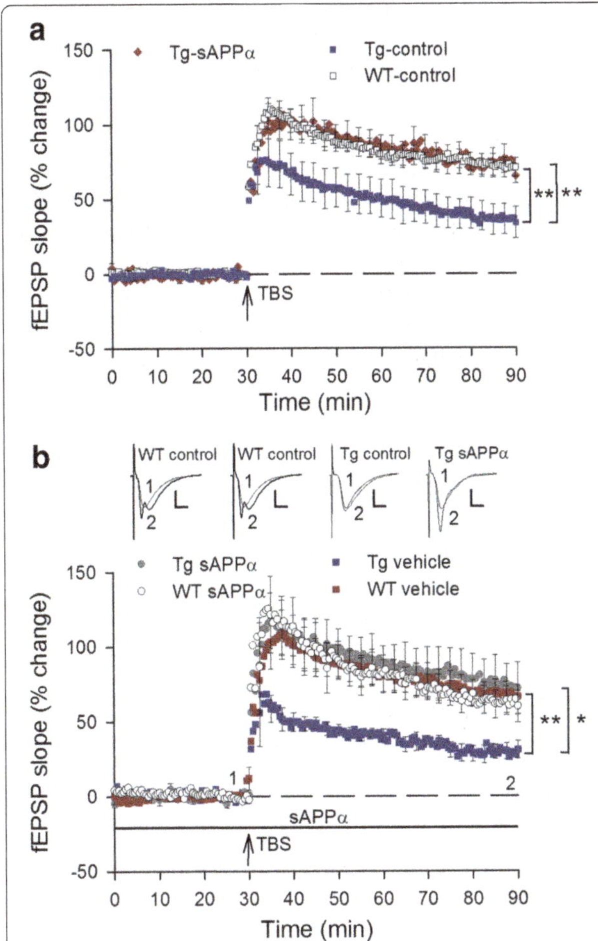

Fig. 6 Delivery of sAPPα, either in vivo or in vitro, after plaque development, completely rescued the impaired LTP in Tg-controls. **a** Chronically administered sAPPα by lentivirus-mediated expression in adult (10 months) Tg mice completely rescued the deficit in hippocampal LTP, measured 3 months after viral transduction (at 13 months of age). LTP measured 60 min after TBS (arrow) revealed a significant deficit in LTP expression in Tg-control mice compared to WT-controls (WT-controls: 71.1 ± 6.7%, $n = 11$; Tg-controls 36.3 ± 10.0%, $n = 9$; $p = 0.008$). This deficit was completely rescued by sAPPα over-expression (Tg-sAPPα: 72.2 ± 2.4%, $n = 12$; $p = 0.008$ compared to Tg-controls). **b** LTP induced in hippocampal slices from aged Tg mice (18–20 months of age), was impaired compared to WT-controls when measured 60 min post-TBS (WT-control: 67.2 ± 7.5%, $n = 9$; Tg-control: 29.4 ± 4.7%, $n = 7$; $p = 0.002$). LTP expression was again completely rescued by acutely applied recombinant human sAPPα (10 nM) beginning 30 min before delivery of the TBS (Tg-sAPPα: 73.7 ± 16.7%, $n = 10$; $p = 0.737$ compared to WT-controls, $p = 0.048$ compared to Tg-controls). No effect of sAPPα on WT-control LTP was observed (WT-sAPPα: 62.1 ± 9.4%, n = 6; $p = 0.684$)

brain injury [19] and normal aging [34, 35]. However, repeated acute administration of sAPPα would be problematic for AD patients, especially if intracerebral methods were to be required. Methods that engender longer term sAPPα up-regulation should therefore be advantageous. Recently, expression of mouse sAPPα in the hippocampus using a different viral vector (AAV), beginning well after strong phenotypic expression of AD-like symptoms, was found to rescue spatial memory and, as we observed, an associated substantial but not complete rescue of LTP measured several months after transduction [20]. Our study replicated the rescue of LTP using viral transduction of sAPPα that commenced at 10 months of age, even though a different viral vector (lentivirus), and a different sAPPα construct (human sAPPα) was used. Such studies show the effectiveness of sAPPα administration after disease onset. Importantly, we found that the same transduction procedure at 4 months of age rendered a long-term benefit lasting at least 9–10 months in protecting memory and LTP. The time of injection together with its long-lasting benefits suggests that, once predictive biomarkers for AD become readily available, a sAPPα-based therapy may be useful even in preventing or delaying the earliest onset of the disease, before individuals develop clinical symptoms. Together these studies make a strong statement about the therapeutic potential of sAPPα in AD.

Behavioural improvement in the absence of amyloid load reduction

It was notable in the present study that the memory and LTP improvements occurred in the absence of a decrease in amyloid load, as measured by either Congo red staining of plaques or by ELISA. This contrasts with the previous AAV study in which a partial reduction in amyloid levels and plaque load was evident [20]. The reasons for this difference are not clear, but may relate to differences in the expression system and thus level of sAPPα expression, or the difference in timing of the transduction event. However, in accord with the present study, a number of treatment approaches have generated improvements in cognitive performance but not Aβ pathology [36–40]. Interestingly, this could occur even with animals immunized with an Aβ peptide or an antibody against Aβ. These results may reflect the high degree of plaque load in some of the animal models used, including the APP/PS1 model that we used.

Because of the lack of effect by sAPPα on amyloid load in the present study, the effectiveness of sAPPα expression would appear to be due to increasing the functional capabilities of the diseased brain, rather than modifying the disease process per se, although this latter point merits further investigation. Therefore, the effect of sAPPα in our study could be characterized as increasing cognitive reserve, allowing the brain to function more normally despite the presence of clear pathology. Cognitive reserve has been hypothesized to account for the greater than expected functioning of humans despite a high plaque load as determined, for example, by positron emission tomography [41, 42]. Fol et al. [20] also showed changes in spine density supportive of neuronal plasticity and correlating with the LTP findings. We have not explored these local changes in spine densities, but did not see global increases in pre- or postsynaptic markers by western blot.

Immediacy of sAPPα's effects

It is clear from the studies cited above and the present experiments, that sAPPα can exert powerful effects on brain function and neural plasticity, whether administered acutely or by expression over extended periods of time. Insofar as its effects in AD models may not be due to modifying plaque pathology per se, the question can be asked whether long-term administration over months (whether delivered early or late in the disease process) is needed to cause LTP and memory rescue, or whether even acute administration can be effective in AD models, as shown in a study of aging-related memory decline [35]. Accordingly, we administered sAPPα to hippocampal slices from 18 to 20 mo APP/PS1 and wild-type mice and investigated its effect on LTP as induced by a strong TBS protocol. Interestingly, sAPPα completely rescued LTP induction and persistence in the transgenic mice, showing that raising sAPPα levels even acutely might have benefits for AD patients, albeit in a transient manner. The rescue was equally strong when viral transduction commenced just 3 months before the start of LTP testing. The reason for the differential effects on LTP in the prevention versus rescue experiments is not clear, although it may relate to the greater number of TBS trains used in the rescue experiments, which gave a larger and longer lasting form of LTP that may depend more on the protein synthesis mechanisms that sAPPα can trigger [12]. sAPPα administration did not however increase the already strong LTP exhibited by wild-type slices. This finding is consistent with our previous work in the dentate gyrus in vivo, where only a small improvement in a strongly induced control LTP could be elicited [10]. Thus, sAPPα appears to work optimally under conditions of either weakly induced LTP or LTP impairment, as suggested previously [10, 11, 18].

Mechanisms of sAPPα action

The mechanisms by which sAPPα enhances neural function in either AD models or normal animals are not clear. sAPPα is known to activate a number of signalling cascades involving mitogen-activated protein kinase, tyrosine kinases, cyclic GMP and protein kinase G (PKG), nuclear factor kappa-light-chain-enhancer of activated B cells (NFκB), PI3 kinase, and calcium/calmodulin-dependent protein kinase II (reviewed in [43, 44]. Downstream effects include increased gene expression [6, 45] and protein synthesis [12]. However, which if any of these cascades might be involved in the LTP rescue remains to be determined, although the activation of PKG has been suggested as one important signal transduction pathway for this purpose [9].

Conclusion

In summary, we have provided evidence that expression of human sAPPα in the mouse hippocampus can not only prevent the development of an AD-like phenotype, but also rescue synaptic plasticity once the phenotype has developed. Whether a sAPP-based gene therapy will be a viable treatment option for AD remains to be seen, although gene therapy trials have commenced for other therapeutic agents in AD, and for other degenerative neurological diseases [46, 47]. Scaling up the transduction to spread throughout the human brain, as likely will be needed for AD patients, will be a challenge for this approach. Nonetheless, this study together with that by Fol et al. [20] provides a basis for greater investigations into methods for up-regulating sAPPα for treating AD and possibly other degenerative neurological disorders. In particular, treatment regimens beginning early in the disease process, together with biomarkers for identifying those with a high risk of developing AD, should be able to offer the greatest quality of life benefits for patients.

Abbreviations

AAV: Adeno-associated virus; AD: Alzheimer's disease; ANOVA: Analysis of variance; APPswe/PS1dE9: Amyloid precursor protein (Swedish mutation)/ presenilin 1 (deleted exon 9); Aβ: Amyloid-beta; DIV: Days in vitro; ELISA: Enzyme-linked immunosorbent assay; FEPSP: Field excitatory postsynaptic potential; GFP: Green fluorescent protein; I-O: Input-output; LTP: Long-term potentiation; LV: Lentivirus; NFκB: Nuclear factor kappa-light-chain-enhancer of activated B; PKG: Protein kinase G; PMSF: Phenylmethylsulfonyl Fluoride; PPF: Paired-pulse facilitation; PPI: Paired-pulse inhibition; SAPPα: Secreted amyloid precursor protein-alpha; TBS: Theta-burst stimulation; Tg: Transgenic; VSVg: Vesicular stomatitis virus; WT: Wild-type

Acknowledgements

Not applicable

Funding

This research was supported by a grant from the Health Research Council of New Zealand to WCA, SMH, WPT, and BGM, and by a PhD scholarship from the Ministry of Education of Malaysia to MY. The granting agencies only provided funds for the experiments and had no involvement in project design, data collection and analysis, interpretation or writing of the manuscript.

Authors' contributions

WCA, SMH, WPT, BGM conceived and designed the experiments; VTYT, BGM, SMO, KP, LS, MFY, and KDP undertook the experiments; VTYT, SMO, BGM, KDP, LS, MFY analysed the data; BGM, VTYT, SMO, LS made the figures; BGM, VTYT, WCA wrote the manuscript; all authors contributed to the manuscript review and amendments, and agree to its submission. All authors read and approved the final manuscript.

Competing interests

The authors declare that they have no competing interests.

Author details

[1]Department of Psychology, University of Otago, Box 56, Dunedin 9054, New Zealand. [2]Department of Biochemistry, Brain Health Research Centre, Brain Research New Zealand, University of Otago, Box 56, Dunedin 9054, New Zealand. [3]Department of Neuroscience, Pomona College, Claremont, California 91711, USA.

References

1. Fukumoto H, Cheung BS, Hyman BT, Irizarry MC. B-secretase protein and activity are increased in the neocortex in Alzheimer disease. Arch Neurol. 2002;59:1381–9.
2. Ahmed RR, Holler CJ, Webb RL, Li F, Beckett TL, Murphy MP. BACE1 and BACE2 enzymatic activities in Alzheimer's disease. J Neurochem. 2010;112:1045–53.
3. Lannfelt L, Basun H, Wahlund LO, Rowe BA, Wagner SL. Decreased α-secretase-cleaved amyloid precursor protein as a diagnostic marker for Alzheimer's disease. Nat Med. 1995;1:829–32.
4. Sennvik K, Fastbom J, Blomberg M, Wahlund LO, Winblad B, Benedikz E. Levels of alpha- and beta-secretase cleaved amyloid precursor protein in the cerebrospinal fluid of Alzheimer's disease patients. Neurosci Lett. 2000;278:169–72.
5. Mattson MP, Cheng B, Culwell AR, Esch FS, Lieberburg I, Rydel RE. Evidence for excitoprotective and intraneuronal calcium-regulating roles for secreted forms of the β-amyloid precursor protein. Neuron. 1993;10:243–54.
6. Ryan MM, Morris GP, Mockett BG, Bourne K, Abraham WC, Tate WP, Williams JM. Time-dependent changes in gene expression induced by secreted amyloid precursor protein-alpha in the rat hippocampus. BMC Genomics. 2013;14:376.
7. Baratchi S, Evans J, Tate W, Abraham WC, Connor B. Secreted amyloid precursor proteins promote proliferation and glial differentiation of adult hippocampal neural progenitor cells. Hippocampus. 2012;22:1517–27.
8. Small D, Nurcombe V, Reed G, Clarris H, Moir R, Beyreuther K, Masters CA. Heparin-binding domain in the amyloid protein precursor of Alzheimer's disease is involved in the regulation of neurite outgrowth. J Neurosci. 1994;14:2117–27.
9. Ishida A, Furukawa K, Keller JN, Mattson MP. Secreted form of β-amyloid precursor protein shifts the frequency dependency for induction of LTD, and enhances LTP in hippocampal slices. Neuroreport. 1997;8:2133–7.
10. Taylor CJ, Ireland DR, Ballagh I, Bourne K, Marechal NM, Turner PR, Bilkey DK, Tate WP, Abraham WC. Endogenous secreted amyloid precursor protein-[alpha] regulates hippocampal NMDA receptor function, long-term potentiation and spatial memory. Neurobiol Dis. 2008;31:250–60.
11. Hick M, Herrmann U, Weyer S, Mallm J-P, Tschäpe J-A, Borgers M, Mercken M, Roth FC, Draguhn A, Slomianka L, et al. Acute function of secreted amyloid precursor protein fragment APPsα in synaptic plasticity. Acta Neuropathol. 2015;129:21–37.
12. Claasen AM, Guévremont D, Mason-Parker SE, Bourne K, Tate WP, Abraham WC, Williams JM. Secreted amyloid precursor protein-α upregulates synaptic protein synthesis by a protein kinase G-dependent mechanism. Neurosci Lett. 2009;460:92–6.
13. Meziane H, Dodart JC, Mathis C, Little S, Clemens J, Paul SM, Ungerer A. Memory-enhancing effects of secreted forms of the β-amyloid precursor protein in normal and amnestic mice. Proc Natl Acad Sci U S A. 1998;95:12683–8.
14. Almkvist O, Basun H, Wagner SL, Rowe BA, Wahlund L, Lannfelt L. Cerebrospinal fluid levels of α-secretase-cleaved soluble amyloid precursor protein mirror cognition in a Swedish family with Alzheimer disease and a gene mutation. Arch Neurol. 1997;54:641–4.
15. Anderson JJ, Holtz G, Baskin PP, Wang R, Mazzarelli L, Wagner SL, Menzaghi F. Reduced cerebrospinal fliud levels of à-secretase-cleaved amyloid precursor protein in aged rats: correlation with spatial memory deficits. Neuroscience. 1999;93:1409–20.
16. Habib A, Sawmiller D, Tan J. Restoring soluble amyloid precursor protein α functions as a potential treatment for Alzheimer's disease. J Neurosci Res. 2017;2017:973–91.
17. Corrigan F, Vink R, Blumbergs PC, Masters CL, Cappai R, van den Heuvel C. sAPPα rescues deficits in amyloid precursor protein knockout mice following focal traumatic brain injury. J Neurochem. 2012;122:208–20.
18. Mockett BG, Richter M, Abraham WC, Müller UC. Therapeutic potential of secreted amyloid precursor protein APPsα. Front Mol Neurosci. 2017;10(30)
19. Smith-Swintosky VL, Pettigrew LC, Craddock SD, Culwell AR, Rydel RE, Mattson MP. Secreted forms of β-amyloid precursor protein protect against ischemic brain injury. J Neurochem. 1994;63:781–4.
20. Fol R, Braudeau J, Ludewig S, Abel T, Weyer S, Roederer J-P, Brod F, Audrain M, Bemelmans A-P, Buchholz C, et al. Viral gene transfer of APPsα rescues synaptic failure in an Alzheimer's disease mouse model. Acta Neuropathol. 2016;131:247–66.
21. Dittgen T, Nimmerjahn A, Komai S, Licznerski P, Waters J, Margrie TW, Helmchen F, Denk W, Brecht M, Osten P. Lentivirus-based genetic manipulations of cortical neurons and their optical and electrophysiological monitoring in vivo. Proc Natl Acad Sci,USA. 2004;101:18206–11.
22. Turner PR, Bourne K, Garama D, Carne A, Abraham WC, Tate WP. Production, purification and functional validation of human secreted amyloid precursor proteins for use as neuropharmacological reagents. J Neurosci Meth. 2007;164:68–74.
23. Best HL, Neverman NJ, Wicky HE, Mitchell NL, Leitch B, Hughes SM. Characterisation of early changes in ovine CLN5 and CLN6 batten disease neural cultures for the rapid screening of therapeutics. Neurobiol Dis. 2017;100:62–74.
24. Desmaris N, Bosch A, Salaun C, Petit C, Prevost MC, Tordo N, Perrin P, Schwartz O, de Rocquigny H, Heard JM. Production and neurotropism of lentivirus vectors pseudotyped with lyssavirus envelope glycoproteins. Mol Ther. 2001;4:149–56.
25. Finkelshtein D, Werman A, Novick D, Barak S, Rubinstein M. LDL receptor and its family members serve as the cellular receptors for vesicular stomatitis virus. Proc Natl Acad Sci U S A. 2013;110:7306–11.
26. Schoderboeck L, Riad S, Bokor AM, Wicky HE, Strauss M, Bostina M, Oswald MJ, Empson RM, Hughes SM. Chimeric rabies SADB19-VSVg-pseudotyped lentiviral vectors mediate long-range retrograde transduction from the mouse spinal cord. Gene Ther. 2015;22:357–64.
27. Özdinler PH, Macklis JD. IGF-I specifically enhances axon outgrowth of corticospinal motor neurons. Nat Neurosci. 2006;9:1371.
28. Gallagher M, Burwell R, Burchinal M. Severity of spatial learning impairment in aging: development of a learning index for performance in the Morris water maze. Behav Neurosci. 1993;107:618–26.
29. Maei HR, Zaslavsky K, Teixeira CM, Frankland PW. What is the most sensitive measure of water maze probe test performance? Front Integr Neurosci. 2009;3:4.
30. Bevins RA, Besheer J. Object recognition in rats and mice: a one-trial non-matching-to-sample learning task to study 'recognition memory'. Nat Protocols. 2006;1:1306–11.
31. Hefter D, Draguhn A. APP as a protective factor in acute neuronal insults. Front Mol Neurosci. 2017;10(22)
32. Chasseigneaux S, Allinquant B. Functions of Aβ, sAPPα and sAPPβ: similarities and differences. J Neurochem. 2012;120:99–108.
33. Corrigan F, Vink R, Blumbergs PC, Masters CL, Cappai R, van den Heuvel C. Evaluation of the effects of treatment with sAPPα on functional and histological outcome following controlled cortical impact injury in mice. Neurosci Lett. 2012;515:50–4.
34. Moreno L, Rose C, Mohanraj A, Allinquant B, Billard JM, Dutar P. sAβPPα improves hippocampal NMDA-dependent functional alterations linked to healthy aging. J Alz Dis. 2015;48(4):927–35.
35. Xiong M, Jones OD, Peppercorn K, Ohline SM, Tate WP, Abraham WC. Secreted amyloid precursor protein-alpha can restore novel object location memory and hippocampal LTP in aged rats. Neurobiol Learn Mem. 2017;138:291–9.
36. Dodart J-C, Bales KR, Gannon KS, Greene SJ, DeMattos RB, Mathis C, DeLong CA, Wu S, Wu X, Holtzman DM, et al. Immunization reverses memory deficits without reducing brain a[beta] burden in Alzheimer's disease model. Nat Neurosci. 2002;5:452–7.

37. Heikkinen T, Kalesnykas G, Rissanen A, Tapiola T, Iivonen S, Wang J, Chaudhuri J, Tanila H, Miettinen R, Puoliväli J. Estrogen treatment improves spatial learning in APP + PS1 mice but does not affect beta amyloid accumulation and plaque formation. Exp Neurol. 2004;187:105–17.
38. Jankowsky JL, Melnikova T, Fadale DJ, Xu GM, Slunt HH, Gonzales V, Younkin LH, Younkin SG, Borchelt DR, Savonenko AV. Environmental enrichment mitigates cognitive deficits in a mouse model of Alzheimer's disease. J Neurosci. 2005;25:5217–24.
39. Morgan D, Diamond DM, Gottschall PE, Ugen KE, Dickey C, Hardy J, Duff K, Jantzen P, DiCarlo G, Wilcock D, et al. Aβ peptide vaccination prevents memory loss in an animal model of Alzheimer's disease. Nature. 2000;408:982–5.
40. Stackman RW, Eckenstein F, Frei B, Kulhanek D, Nowlin J, Quinn JF. Prevention of age-related spatial memory deficits in a transgenic mouse model of Alzheimer's disease by chronic Ginkgo Biloba treatment. Exp Neurol. 2003;184:510–20.
41. Bauckneht M, Picco A, Nobili F, Morbelli S. Amyloid positron emission tomography and cognitive reserve. World J Radiol. 2015;7:475–83.
42. Carapelle E, Serra L, Modoni S, Falcone M, Caltagirone C, Bozzali M, Specchio LM, Avolio C. How the cognitive reserve interacts with beta-amyloid deposition in mitigating FDG metabolism: an observational study. Medicine. 2017;96:e5876.
43. Turner PR, O'Connor K, Tate WP, Abraham WC. Roles of amyloid precursor protein and its fragments in regulating neural activity, plasticity and memory. Prog Neurobiol. 2003;70:1–32.
44. Kögel D, Deller T, Behl C. Roles of amyloid precursor protein family members in neuroprotection, stress signaling and aging. Exp Brain Res. 2012;217(3–4):471–9.
45. Stein TD, Anders NJ, DeCarli C, Chan SL, Mattson MP, Johnson JA. Neutralization of transthyretin reverses the neuroprotective effects of secreted amyloid precursor protein (APP) in APPSW mice resulting in tau phosphorylation and loss of hippocampal neurons: support for the amyloid hypothesis. J Neurosci. 2004;24:7707–17.
46. Choudhury SR, Hudry E, Maguire CA, Sena-Esteves M, Breakefield XO, Grandi P. Viral vectors for therapy of neurologic diseases. Neuropharmacology. 2017;120:63–80.
47. Joshi CR, Labhasetwar V, Ghorpade A. Destination brain: the past, present, and future of therapeutic gene delivery. J NeuroImmune Pharmacol. 2017;12:51–83.

14

Novel miR-b2122 regulates several ALS-related RNA-binding proteins

Zachary C. E. Hawley[1*], Danae Campos-Melo[1] and Michael J. Strong[1,2,3,4]

Abstract

Common pathological features of amyotrophic lateral sclerosis (ALS) include cytoplasmic aggregation of several RNA-binding proteins. Out of these RNA-binding proteins, TDP-43, FUS/TLS and RGNEF have been shown to co-aggregate with one another within motor neurons of sporadic ALS (sALS) patients, suggesting that there may be a common regulatory network disrupted. MiRNAs have been a recent focus in ALS research as they have been identified to be globally down-regulated in the spinal cord of ALS patients. The objective of this study was to identify if there are miRNA(s) dysregulated in sALS that are responsible for regulating the TDP-43, FUS/TLS and RGNEF network. In this study, we identify miR-194 and miR-b2122 to be significantly down-regulated in sALS patients, and were predicted to regulate *TARDBP*, *FUS/TLS* and *RGNEF* expression. Reporter gene assays and RT-qPCR revealed that miR-b2122 down-regulates the reporter gene through direct interactions with either the *TARDBP*, *FUS/TLS*, or *RGNEF* 3'UTR, while miR-194 down-regulates firefly expression when it contained either the *TARDBP* or *FUS/TLS* 3'UTR. Further, we showed that miR-b2122 regulates endogenous expression of all three of these genes in a neuronal-derived cell line. Also, an ALS-associated mutation in the *FUS/TLS* 3'UTR ablates the ability of miR-b2122 to regulate reporter gene linked to *FUS/TLS* 3'UTR, and sALS samples which showed a down-regulation in miR-b2122 also showed an increase in FUS/TLS protein expression. Overall, we have identified a novel miRNA that is down-regulated in sALS that appears to be a central regulator of disease-related RNA-binding proteins, and thus its dysregulation likely contributes to TDP-43, FUS/TLS and RGNEF pathogenesis in sALS.

Keywords: Amyotrophic lateral sclerosis (ALS), Motor neuron, miRNAs, TDP-43, FUS/TLS, RGNEF, mRNA stability, MotomiRs, Neurodegeneration

Background

Amyotrophic lateral sclerosis (ALS) is a progressive motor neurodegenerative disease resulting in paralysis and death within 2–5 years after diagnosis [1, 2]. 5–10% of ALS cases are familial (fALS), while the remaining are sporadic (sALS) although ~10–12% of these latter cases also have a genetic basis [1, 3, 4]. While our understanding of ALS pathogenesis has advanced significantly in recent years, this understanding, and in particular the relationship amongst the individual genetic defects and the associated formation of pathological intraneuronal inclusions, which are a hallmark of the disease, remains in its early phases [5–7].

Defects in mRNA metabolism has been suggested to be a major driver in the genesis of pathological inclusions within ALS [8–12]. Further, it has been shown that miRNAs, essential regulators of mRNA expression and protein synthesis, are globally down-regulated within the spinal cord tissue of sALS patients [13, 14]. This down-regulation of miRNA expression has been shown to be motor neuron specific [15], contributing to the concept that altered miRNA homeostasis is a major contributor to the pathogenesis of ALS [16, 17]. The finding of this global down-regulation of miRNAs within sALS patients is intriguing, as TDP-43 and FUS/TLS, two proteins often found to be dysregulated in sALS, are known to be essential components of miRNA biogenesis [18, 19]. Further, ALS mutations within the FUS/TLS 3′ untranslated region (UTR) have been shown to disrupt a negative feedback network between miR-141/200a and FUS/TLS, leading to

* Correspondence: zhawley@uwo.ca
[1]Molecular Medicine Group, Robarts Research Institute, Schulich School of Medicine and Dentistry, Western University, London, Ontario, Canada
Full list of author information is available at the end of the article

accumulation of FUS/TLS within the cell [20, 21]. This suggests that there may be a disruption in the feedback networks between miRNAs and RNA-binding proteins in ALS, including TDP-43 and FUS/TLS.

Beyond TDP-43 and FUS/TLS, we have described RGNEF, another RNA-binding protein, that forms pathological aggregates within motor neurons of sALS spinal cord and has mutations associated with ALS [6, 22–24]. Interestingly, we observed that TDP-43, FUS/TLS and RGNEF co-aggregate with each other within the motor neurons of sALS patients, suggesting a co-dysregulation of these three RNA-binding proteins [6]. While miRNA biogenesis has been clearly shown to be affected in sALS, it is unclear the consequence of this mass down-regulation, and how it may contribute to TDP-43, FUS/TLS and RGNEF pathogenesis.

In the current study, we describe two miRNAs, miR-194 and miR-b2122, that are predicted to regulate TDP-43, FUS/TLS and RGNEF. The novel miR-b2122 is expressed in human spinal motor neurons, is significantly down-regulated in sALS patients, and regulates the expression of all three of these RNA-binding proteins. Further, an ALS-associated mutation within the *FUS/TLS* 3'UTR is located in the miRNA recognition element (MRE) of miR-b2122 and disrupts its ability to suppress gene expression. Overall, our results suggest that the down-regulation of miR-b2122 within sALS cases could result in altered levels of all three of these RNA-binding proteins, contributing to the pathological state of TDP-43, FUS and RGNEF observed within motor neurons of sALS patients.

Methods

Tissue samples

Spinal cord tissue was obtained from sALS patients and age-matched, neurologically intact individuals. All ALS cases were both clinically and neuropathologically confirmed using the El Escorial Criteria (World Federation of Neurology Research Group on Neuromuscular Disease, 1994). All research was approved by "The University of Western Ontario Research Ethics Board for Health Sciences Research Involving Human Subjects (HSREB)". Written consent for autopsy was obtained from the next of kin at the time of death or from the patient antemortem in accordance with the London Health Sciences Centre consent for autopsy. Cases were genotyped and confirmed to have no known mutations in *SOD1, TARDBP, FUS/TLS, RGNEF* or expanded repeats in *C9orf72.*

3′ race

Total RNA extraction was performed on SH-SY5Y cells and spinal cord tissue from neurologically intact humans using TRIzol reagent (Life Technologies Inc., Ambion, Carlsbad, CA, USA). This was followed by cDNA synthesis and PCR with the SMARTer 5′/3′ RACE Kit (Takara Bio. Inc., Clontech, USA) to amplify the *TARDBP, FUS/TLS* and *RGNEF* 3'UTRs according to the manufactures instructions using the following forward primers: *TARDBP* 5′-TAG ACA GTG GGG TTG TGG TTG GTT GGT A-3′, *FUS/TLS* 5′- GCA GGG AGA GGC CGT ATT AAT TAG CCT-3′ and *RGNEF* 5′-GCC CCG AGG TAA TGG AAC TTA ATC G-3′. 3'UTRs were identified using a 1% agarose gel containing a SYBR Safe dye. 3'UTR bands were excised and extracted from the agarose gel, and then individually cloned into a pGEMT-easy vector according to manufactures instructions (Promega, Madison, WI, USA). All 3'UTRs were confirmed using Sanger sequencing.

MiRNA selection

MiRNAs predicted to target *TARDBP, FUS/TLS* and *RGNEF* 3'UTRs were selected using miRanda software. Further, the sequence of the miRNA had to be perfectly complementary to the miRNA recognition element (MRE) from +2 to +7. Novel miRNAs currently not found with the miRanda program were manually checked to see if their seed sequence had a MRE within the 3'UTR of *TARDBP, FUS/TLS* and *RGNEF.* We only considered those miRNAs for which we identified MREs within the 3'UTR isoforms of *TARDBP, FUS/TLS* and *RGNEF* within in the spinal cord tissue.

Real-time PCR

Total miRNA extractions were performed on ventral lumbar spinal cord tissue using the mirVana miRNA extraction kit according to manufactures instructions (Life Technologies Inc., Ambion, Carlsbad, CA, USA). Yield and purity of the miRNA extracts were measured using spectrophotometry (Nanodrop, ThermoFisher Scientific, Burlington, ON, Canada), while integrity was measured using Bioanalyzer (Aligent Technologies Canada Inc., Missasauga, ON, Canada) analysis. MiRNA extracts were reversed transcribed and then subjected to real-time PCR using miRCURY LNA™ Universal RT microRNA PCR (Exiqon, Woburn, MA, USA) and ExiLENT SYBR Green master mix (Exiqon, Woburn, MA, USA) kits, respectively, according to manufacturer's instructions. To detect novel miRNAs, miRNAs extracts went under reverse transcription using the Taqman microRNA reverse transcriptase kit (Life Technologies Inc., Applied Biosystems, Forest City, CA, USA), and then were pre-amplified using the Taqman PreAmp Master Mix Kit (Life Technologies Inc., Applied Biosystems, Forest City, CA, USA) followed by real-time PCR with the TaqMan Universal PCR Master Mix (×2) no AmpErase UNG (Life Technologies Inc., Applied Biosystems, Roche, Branchburg, NJ, USA). The 7900 HT Real Time PCR system was used to read PCR outputs. Relative expression of miRNAs was normalized to an internal control (miR-16-5p), followed by comparison of the relative expression of candidate miRNAs between ALS cases and a control population using the $2^{-\Delta\Delta CT}$ method. Negative values show down-regulation and positive values up-regulation of the expression. Statistical significance was determined using Student's t-test, and samples were considered significantly different if $p < 0.05$.

Fluorescent in situ hybridization (FISH)

Neuropathologically normal human lumbar spinal cord tissue was formalin-fixed paraffin-embedded and cut into 7 μm sections. Samples were UV treated overnight prior to the experiment to reduce lipofuscin-induced autofluorescent signaling. FISH of miRNAs was performed as described before [25]. Probes for miRNA detection were designed with double DIG labels (Exiqon, Woburn, MA, USA), and were targeted by a DIG-HRP secondary antibody (1:100; Roche, Indianapolis, IN, USA) and Tyramide Signal Amplification tagged with a Cy3 fluorophore (PerkinElmer, Waltham, MA, USA). Olympus FV1000 confocal microscope was used to observe miRNA expression within spinal motor neurons.

Cell culture and plasmid construction

HEK293T and SH-SY5Y cells were cultured in Dulbecco's Modified Eagle's Media (DMEM) containing 10% Fetal Bovine Serum (FBS). Cells were incubated at 37 °C with 5% CO_2.

3'UTR isoforms of RNA-binding proteins identified in the human spinal cord tissue were individually cloned into the pmirGLO vector in between SalI and NheI restriction enzyme sites and downstream from the firefly luciferase gene (Promega, Madison, WI, USA). Site-directed mutagenesis assays were done by adding a two-nucleotide mutation within the +2 and +3 positions of each miR-194 or miR-b2122 MRE using the Site-Directed Mutagenesis Kit II (Aligent Technologies Canada Inc., Missasauga, ON, Canada) according to the manufacturer's instructions. Primers used are showed in Additional file 1: Table S1. Mutations were carefully designed to ensure no changes to mRNA secondary structure using RNAfold WebServer (http://rna.tbi.univie.ac.at/cgi-bin/RNAfold.cgi).

Luciferase assay

HEK293T cells were seeded into 96 well plates (9000 cells per well) 24 h prior to transfection. Cells were co-transfected with 3.5 fmol of pmirGLO plasmid and 100 nM of miRNA mimics according to the Lipofectamine 2000 protocol (Life Technologies Inc., Invitrogen, Burlington, ON, Canada). Luciferase activity was measured 24 h post-transfection using the Dual-GLO Luciferase Assay System (Promega, Madison, WI, USA). Firefly activity was normalized to renilla activity. Experimental design and normalization of data was performed as previously described [26]. Data was quantified as relative difference from the control, and expressed as mean ± SEM. Statistical significance was determined by performing Student's t-test, and was considered significantly different if $p < 0.05$.

Relative quantitative RT-PCR

To determine the effects of miR-194 and miR-b2122 on the luciferase mRNA expression when it contained the 3'UTR of *TARDBP, FUS/TLS* or *RGNEF,* HEK293T cells were seeded into 24 well plates (20,000 cells per well) 48 h prior to transfection. Cells were co-transfected with 20.6 fmol of pmirGLO plasmid and 100 nM of miRNA mimics according to the Lipofectamine 2000 protocol (Life Technologies Inc., Invitrogen, Burlington, ON, Canada). 24 h after transfection, total RNA extraction was performed using TRIzol reagent (Life Technologies Inc., Ambion, Carlsbad, CA, USA) followed by first-strand cDNA synthesis (Life Technologies Inc., Invitrogen, Burlington, ON, Canada) and PCR amplification of firefly and renilla cDNA as previously described [13]. Data was quantified as relative difference from the control, and expressed as mean ± SEM. Statistical significance was determined by performing Student's t-test, and was considered significantly different if $p < 0.05$.

To identify whether miR-194 and miR-b2122 could regulate the endogenous mRNA expression of these three RNA-binding proteins within a neuronal-derived cell line, SH-SY5Y cells were seeded into 6-well plates (500,000 cells per well) 24 h prior to the transfection. 100 nM of miRNA mimics and anti-miRs were then either transfected individually or co-transfected. 24 h after transfection total RNA extraction was performed using TRIzol reagent (Life Technologies Inc., Ambion, Carlsbad, CA, USA) followed by cDNA synthesis (Life Technologies Inc., Invitrogen, Burlington, ON, Canada). Quantitative PCR (qPCR) to determine the relative change in endogenous mRNA expression of *TARDBP, FUS/TLS* and *RGNEF* was performed using following primers: TARDBP *for*: 5′-CAG GGT GGG TTT GGT AAC GT-3′ *rev*: 5′-AAA GCC CCC ATT AAA ACC AC-3′; FUS/TLS *for*: 5′-TCG GGA CCA AGG ATC ACG TC-3′ *rev*: 5′-ATC TGG TTT AGG GGC CTT ACA CTG-3′; RGNEF *for*: 5′-AGG AAC GCA ATA ACT GGA TGA GAC G-3′ *rev*: 5′-TTC CAC CTT CTC CCC TGC ATC AG-3′; 18S RNA *for*: 5′-AGT TGG TGG AGC GAT TTG TC-3′ *rev*: 5′-TTC CTC GTT CAT GGG GAA TA-3′. All expression profiles were normalized to 18S RNA levels prior to comparison. One-way ANOVA followed by a Tukey's post-hoc was used to determine statistical differences in endogenous mRNA expression, and samples were significantly different if $p < 0.05$.

Western blot analysis

SH-SY5Y cells were seeded into 6-well plates (500,000 cells per well) 24 h prior to the experiment. 100 nM of miRNA mimics and inhibitors were then either transfected individually or co-transfected. 48 h after transfection total protein extraction was performed using NP40 lysis buffer containing proteinase inhibitors (cOmplete, Roche, Indianapolis, IN, USA), followed by sonication. Samples were suspended in loading buffer and proteins were denatured at 90 °C for 5 min. Samples were run on a 12% SDS-gel, and transferred to a nitrocellulose membrane. To measure endogenous levels of TDP-43, FUS/TLS and RGNEF, the membrane was probed with either anti-TDP-43 (1:2500; Proteintech, 10,782–2-AP), anti-FUS/TLS (1:3000; Proteintech, 11,570–1-AP), or anti-RGNEF (1:1000; Abcam, ab157095) rabbit antibodies, respectively. Blots were then probed with a HRP-secondary antibody (goat anti-rabbit; 1:5000; Life Technologies Inc., Invitrogen, Burlington, ON, Canada). Blots were stripped using stripping buffer (2% SDS, 62.5 mM Tris-HCl, 100 mM β-mercaptoethanol, pH 6.8) and re-probed for GAPDH using anti-GAPDH rabbit antibody (1:2500; Abcam, ab9485). Relative protein expression of TDP-43, FUS/TLS and RGNEF were normalized to GAPDH expression levels. One-way ANOVA followed by a Tukey's post-hoc was used to determine statistical differences in endogenous protein expression, and samples were significantly different if $p < 0.05$.

Results

A small group of miRNAs contain MREs within the mRNA 3'UTR of *TARDBP, FUS/TLS,* and *RGNEF*

Spinal cord tissue from neurologically intact individuals was used to determine the 3'UTR isoform(s) of *TARDBP, FUS/TLS* and *RGNEF* being expressed. *TARDBP* consistently showed one 3'UTR isoform across all human samples with a length of 1398 bp (BC095435.1) (Fig. 1a) [27]. Subject two appeared to have a higher band, but we were unable to confirm a longer 3'UTR through sequencing, and for that reason, we focused only on the transcript that was consistently expressed across all samples.

FUS/TLS contained one 3'UTR isoform within three different control cases, which was 150 bp in length (Fig. 1a) (NM_004960). While *RGNEF* appeared to have three 3'UTR isoforms in each control case, we were only able to confirm the top and bottom bands through sequencing. The two *RGNEF* 3'UTR isoforms that were confirmed had a length of 177 bp and 981 bp, which we termed *RGNEF*-short and *RGNEF*-long, respectively (Fig. 1a). Both short and long 3'UTRs of *RGNEF* have been previously described (NM_001244364.1 and NM_0010804079.2, respectively).

Subsequently, we identified 5 miRNAs which had MREs within the 3'UTR of all three of these RNA-binding proteins. However, our previous work has indicated that miR-548d-3p was not dysregulated in sALS cases, and thus was eliminated from further analysis. We also previously observed that miR-194 is down-regulated in sALS patients [13], while miR-b2122, miR-sb659 and miR-548× have not been analyzed for dysregulation within sALS patients (Fig. 1b, c). The latter four miRNAs were thus of interest for further analysis.

MiR-194 and miR-b2122 are down-regulated in the spinal cord tissue of sALS patients

We characterized the relative expression of miR-194, miR-548×, miR-sb659 and miR-b2122 within the spinal cord tissue of sALS patients compared to control subjects. Using real-time PCR, we observed that miR-194 and miR-b2122 were significantly down-regulated in sALS patients (Fig. 2). The down-regulation of miR-194 is consistent with what we reported previously using TaqMan Array [13]. Using FISH, we confirmed that both miR-194 and miR-b2122 were strongly expressed within human spinal motor neurons of control samples with little to no non-motor neuronal expression, suggesting that the down-regulation of these two miRNAs is likely motor neuron specific (Fig. 3).

MiR-b2122 regulates a reporter linked to either *TARDBP, FUS/TLS,* or *RGNEF* 3'UTR

A reporter gene assay was used to examine the effect of miR-194 and miR-b2122 on the regulation of firefly luciferase protein when it contained the 3'UTR of either *TARDBP, FUS/TLS,* or *RGNEF* that we identified within the human spinal cord. MiR-b2122 significantly reduced firefly protein activity when it contained either the *TARDBP, FUS/TLS, RGNEF*-short, or *RGNEF*-long 3'UTR, whereas miR-194 down-regulated firefly protein activity only when it contained either the *TARDBP* or *FUS/TLS* 3'UTR, and had no effect when it contained the *RGNEF*-long 3'UTR (Fig. 4a). MiR-194 did not contain an MRE within the *RGNEF*-short 3'UTR and thus the interaction between these two components was not examined. Further, to determine if miR-194 and miR-b2122 could also alter luciferase mRNA levels, we performed RT-PCR analysis. The results in the RT-PCR analysis matched the down-regulation seen by these two mRNAs in the luciferase reporter gene assay, indicating that the effect of these miRNAs involves regulation of the levels of mRNA species (Fig. 4b).

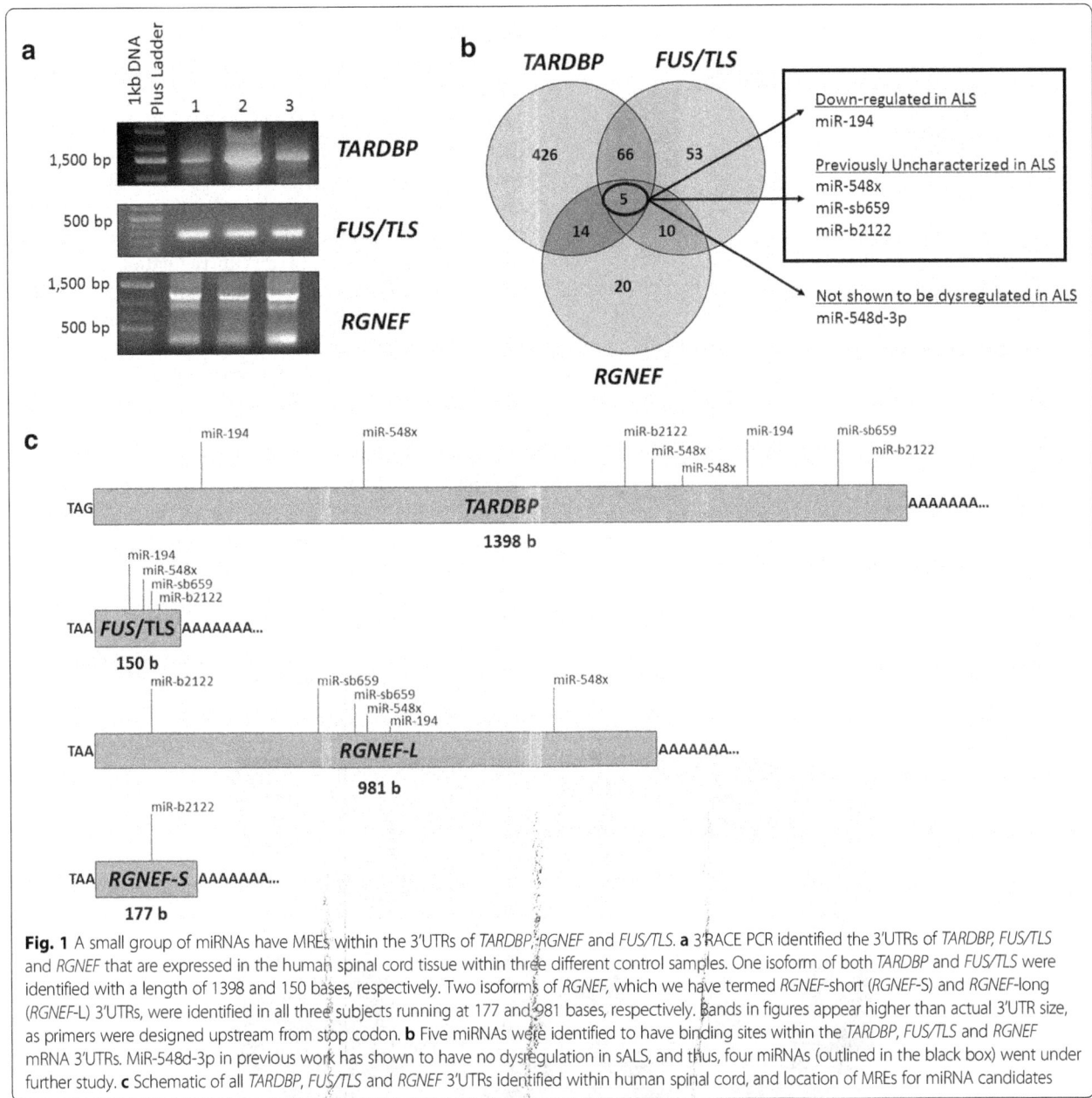

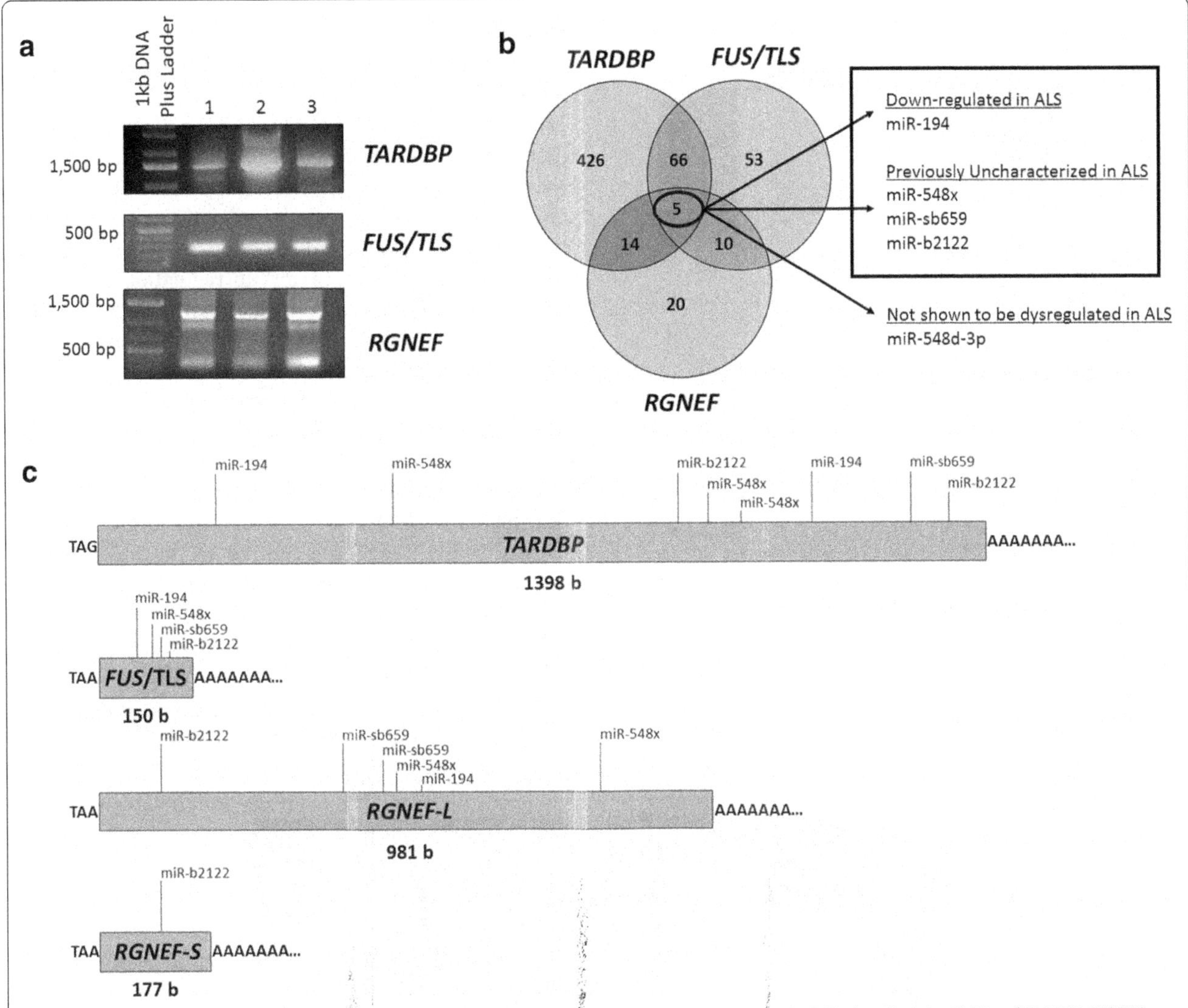

Fig. 1 A small group of miRNAs have MREs within the 3'UTRs of *TARDBP*, *RGNEF* and *FUS/TLS*. **a** 3'RACE PCR identified the 3'UTRs of *TARDBP*, *FUS/TLS* and *RGNEF* that are expressed in the human spinal cord tissue within three different control samples. One isoform of both *TARDBP* and *FUS/TLS* were identified with a length of 1398 and 150 bases, respectively. Two isoforms of *RGNEF*, which we have termed *RGNEF*-short (*RGNEF*-S) and *RGNEF*-long (*RGNEF*-L) 3'UTRs, were identified in all three subjects running at 177 and 981 bases, respectively. Bands in figures appear higher than actual 3'UTR size, as primers were designed upstream from stop codon. **b** Five miRNAs were identified to have binding sites within the *TARDBP*, *FUS/TLS* and *RGNEF* mRNA 3'UTRs. MiR-548d-3p in previous work has shown to have no dysregulation in sALS, and thus, four miRNAs (outlined in the black box) went under further study. **c** Schematic of all *TARDBP*, *FUS/TLS* and *RGNEF* 3'UTRs identified within human spinal cord, and location of MREs for miRNA candidates

To study if miR-194 and miR-b2122 were regulating firefly luciferase by directly interacting with the 3'UTR, we mutated two nucleotides within the MRE sites of miR-194 and miR-b2122. Mutating the miR-b2122 MRE sites within either the *TARDBP*, *FUS/TLS*, *RGNEF*-short, or *RGNEF*-long 3'UTR significantly abolished the ability of miR-b2122 to reduce firefly luciferase activity. Similarly, mutating the miR-194 MRE sites within either *TARDBP* or *FUS/TLS* ablated miR-194 down-regulation of the firefly protein (Fig. 5). These findings indicate that both miR-194 and miR-b2122 directly interact with their 3'UTR targets to regulate gene expression.

MiR-b2122 regulates endogenous TDP-43, FUS/TLS and RGNEF within a human neuronal cell line

Next, we decided to determine if miR-b2122 and miR-194 regulate the endogenous mRNA expression of *TARDBP*, *FUS/TLS* and *RGNEF* within a human neuronal-derived cell line – SH-SY5Y cells. SH-SY5Y cells express the *TARDBP*, *FUS/TLS* and *RGNEF* 3'UTR isoforms we identified with in the spinal cord. SH-SY5Y cells showed multiple bands in the *TARDBP* lane, but we were not able to confirm the top two bands through sequencing, only the 1398 b 3'UTR isoform identified in spinal cord, which also appears to be dominantly expressed in SH-SY5Y cells

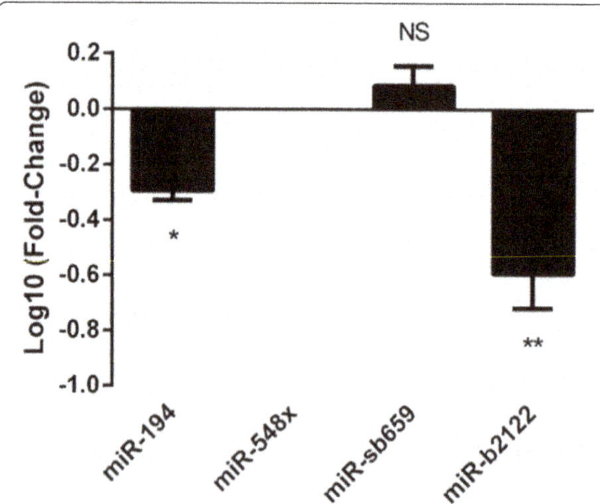

Fig. 2 Differential expression of candidate miRNAs within the spinal cord of sALS patients. Candidate miRNA expression was examined in ventral spinal cord tissue of sALS patients ($n = 8$) and control subjects ($n = 5$). MiR-194 and miR-b2122 were significantly down-regulated in sALS patients, while miR-sb659 showed no difference and miR-548x was not expressed in the spinal cord tissue. Data was expressed as Log10 (fold-change) ± SEM, and significance was determined using Students t-test (** = $p < 0.01$, *$p < 0.05$, NS = $p > 0.05$)

(Additional file 2: Figure S1a). Also, endogenous expression of miR-b2122 and miR-194 in SH-SY5Y cells was confirmed through real-time PCR (Additional file 2: Figure S1b).

Transfection of miR-b2122 lead to a significant down-regulation in *TARBDP*, *FUS/TLS* and *RGNEF* mRNA levels. Further, co-transfection of miR-b2122 with its anti-miR abrogates the down-regulation of these transcripts via miR-b2122. Transfection of the anti-miR of miR-b2122 alone lead to an up-regulation in mRNA levels of all three genes (Fig. 6a). The up-regulation observed with the addition of the anti-miR, suggests that miR-b2122 does regulate these RNA-binding proteins endogenously within this neuronal cell line. Let-7a was used as negative control, as we showed it has no effect on the endogenous mRNA and proteins levels of these three genes (Additional file 3: Figure S2).

Further, we also transfected miR-194 and/or its anti-miR within SH-SY5Y cells. Similar to the reporter gene assays, miR-194 only reduced *TARDBP* and *FUS/TLS* endogenous mRNA levels with no effect on *RGNEF* mRNA levels, which was abolished when co-transfecting miR-194 with its anti-miR (Fig. 6b). Also, only adding the anti-miR of miR-194 caused a strong trend towards up-regulation of *TARDBP* mRNA expression, but no

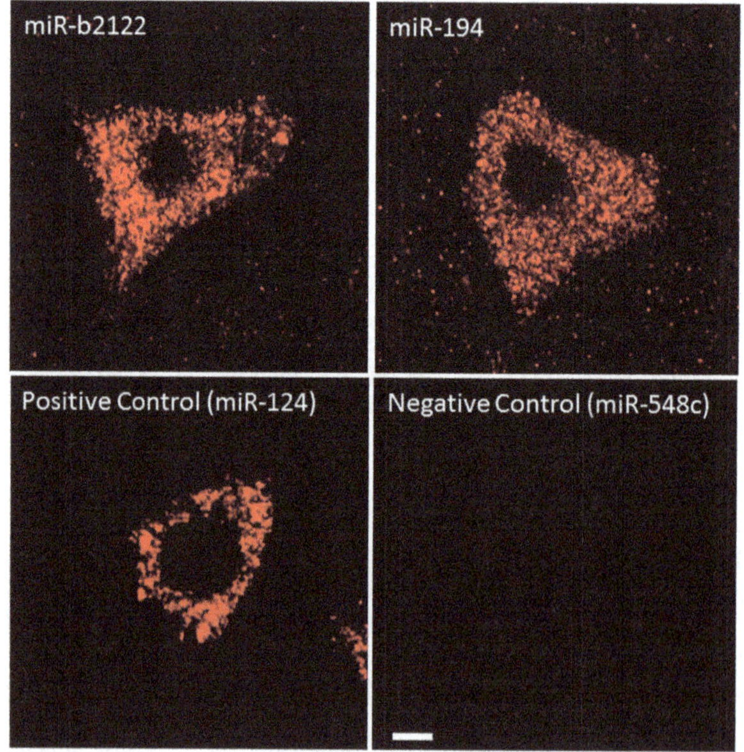

Fig. 3 MiR-194 and miR-b2122 are expressed in human spinal motor neurons. Ventral human spinal cord of control tissue was analyzed using FISH to determine the expression of miR-194 and miR-b2122 within motor neurons. Both miRNAs showed strong positive staining within motor neurons. MiR-124 and miR-548c were used as positive and negative controls, respectively. Scale bar represents 10 μm

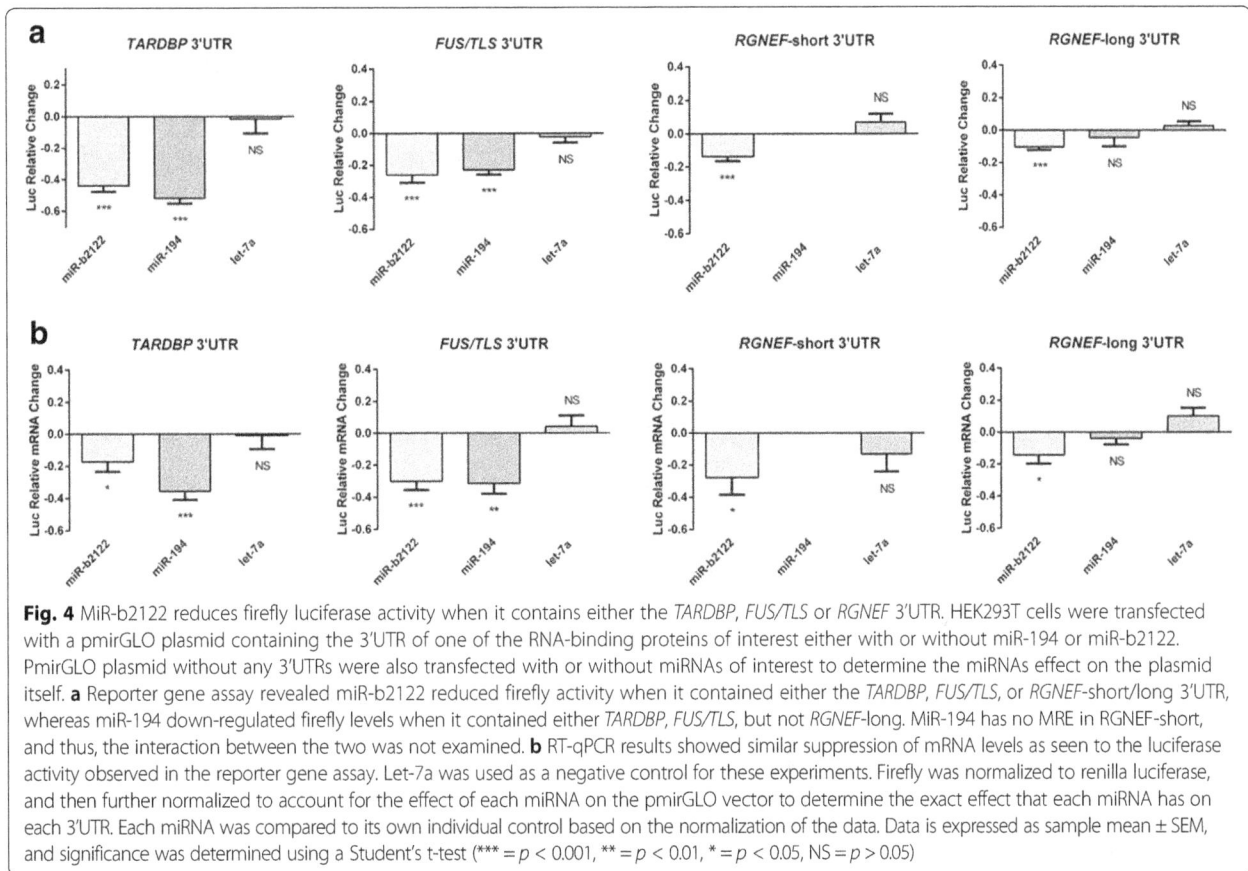

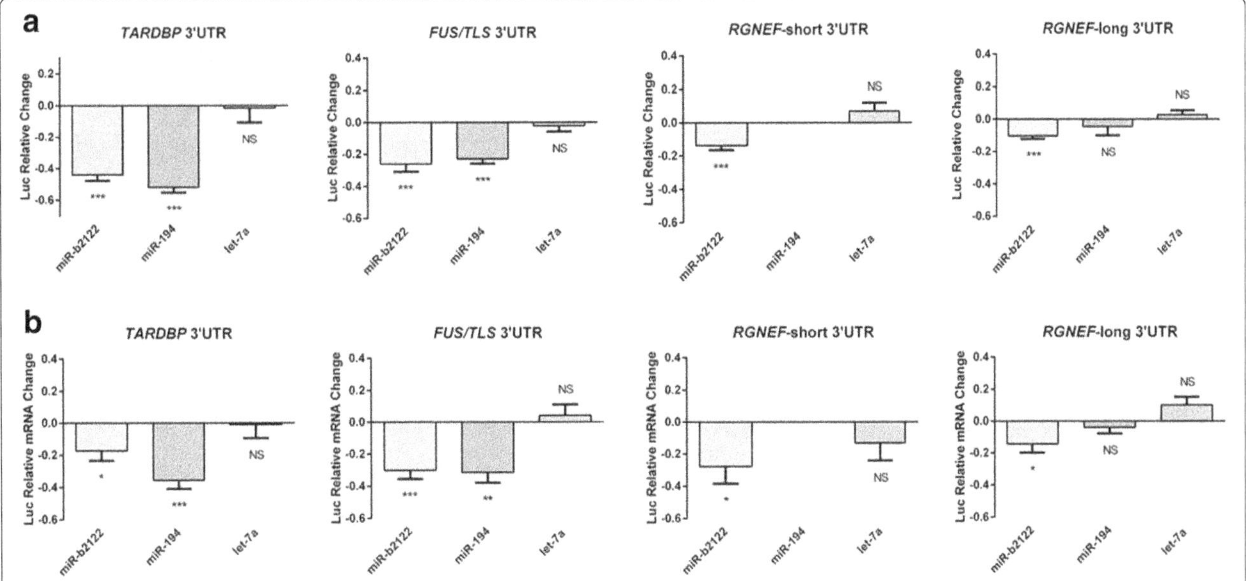

Fig. 4 MiR-b2122 reduces firefly luciferase activity when it contains either the *TARDBP*, *FUS/TLS* or *RGNEF* 3'UTR. HEK293T cells were transfected with a pmirGLO plasmid containing the 3'UTR of one of the RNA-binding proteins of interest either with or without miR-194 or miR-b2122. PmirGLO plasmid without any 3'UTRs were also transfected with or without miRNAs of interest to determine the miRNAs effect on the plasmid itself. **a** Reporter gene assay revealed miR-b2122 reduced firefly activity when it contained either the *TARDBP*, *FUS/TLS*, or *RGNEF*-short/long 3'UTR, whereas miR-194 down-regulated firefly levels when it contained either *TARDBP*, *FUS/TLS*, but not *RGNEF*-long. MiR-194 has no MRE in RGNEF-short, and thus, the interaction between the two was not examined. **b** RT-qPCR results showed similar suppression of mRNA levels as seen to the luciferase activity observed in the reporter gene assay. Let-7a was used as a negative control for these experiments. Firefly was normalized to renilla luciferase, and then further normalized to account for the effect of each miRNA on the pmirGLO vector to determine the exact effect that each miRNA has on each 3'UTR. Each miRNA was compared to its own individual control based on the normalization of the data. Data is expressed as sample mean ± SEM, and significance was determined using a Student's t-test (*** = $p < 0.001$, ** = $p < 0.01$, * = $p < 0.05$, NS = $p > 0.05$)

change in the *FUS/TLS* transcript levels, suggesting miR-194 might play a role in regulating *TARDBP* gene expression within SH-SY5Y cells. Overall, these results suggest that miR-b2122 is the central regulator of *TARDBP*, *FUS/TLS* and *RGNEF* mRNA expression.

To determine whether the alteration in mRNA levels was associated with alterations in protein expression, we examined protein levels of TDP-43, FUS/TLS and RGNEF post-transfection of miR-b2122 (Fig. 7a). MiR-b2122 alone had no significant effect on the protein levels of TDP-43 within the cell, but when the anti-miR alone was added, there was a strong trend towards up-regulation of TDP-43. This up-regulation was significantly different from when miR-b2122 was transfected alone, suggesting that endogenous miR-b2122 is likely participating keeping TDP-43 protein at steady-state levels, but loss of this miRNA leads to increase TDP-43 protein output (Fig. 7b). Transfection of miR-b2122 alone showed a strong trend towards the down-regulation in FUS/TLS protein levels, which was abrogated when the anti-miR was co-transfected with miR-b2122. The transfection of the anti-miR of miR-b2122 alone did lead to a significant up-regulation of FUS/TLS protein levels, indicating miR-b2122 regulates protein synthesis of FUS/TLS endogenously (Fig. 7b).

Interestingly, miR-b2122 had the reverse effect on the protein levels of RGNEF as compared to the changes observed at the mRNA level (Fig. 7b). Transfection of miR-b2122 alone lead to increased RGNEF protein levels, which was reduced to the control levels when miR-b2122 was co-transfected with its anti-miR. Transfection of the anti-miR alone lead to reduced levels of RGNEF compared with let-7a. While these results were not significantly different from the negative control, there was a significant difference in RGNEF protein levels between when either miR-b2122 or the anti-miR were transfected alone. All data was compared to let-7a (negative control), as we showed it, has no effect on the proteins levels of these three genes (Additional file 4: Figure S3). Overall, these results indicate that miR-b2122 can regulate FUS/TLS protein expression, while having minor changes on TDP-43 and RGNEF protein levels.

ALS mutation in *FUS/TLS* 3'UTR is located in miR-b2122 MRE

Previously, mutations within the *FUS/TLS* 3'UTR were found within ALS patients, all of which lead to the overexpression and increased cytoplasmic mislocalization of FUS/TLS protein [20]. Interestingly, one of these mutations (*c.108C > T) is located in the +2 position of the MRE for miR-b2122 (Fig. 8a), suggesting

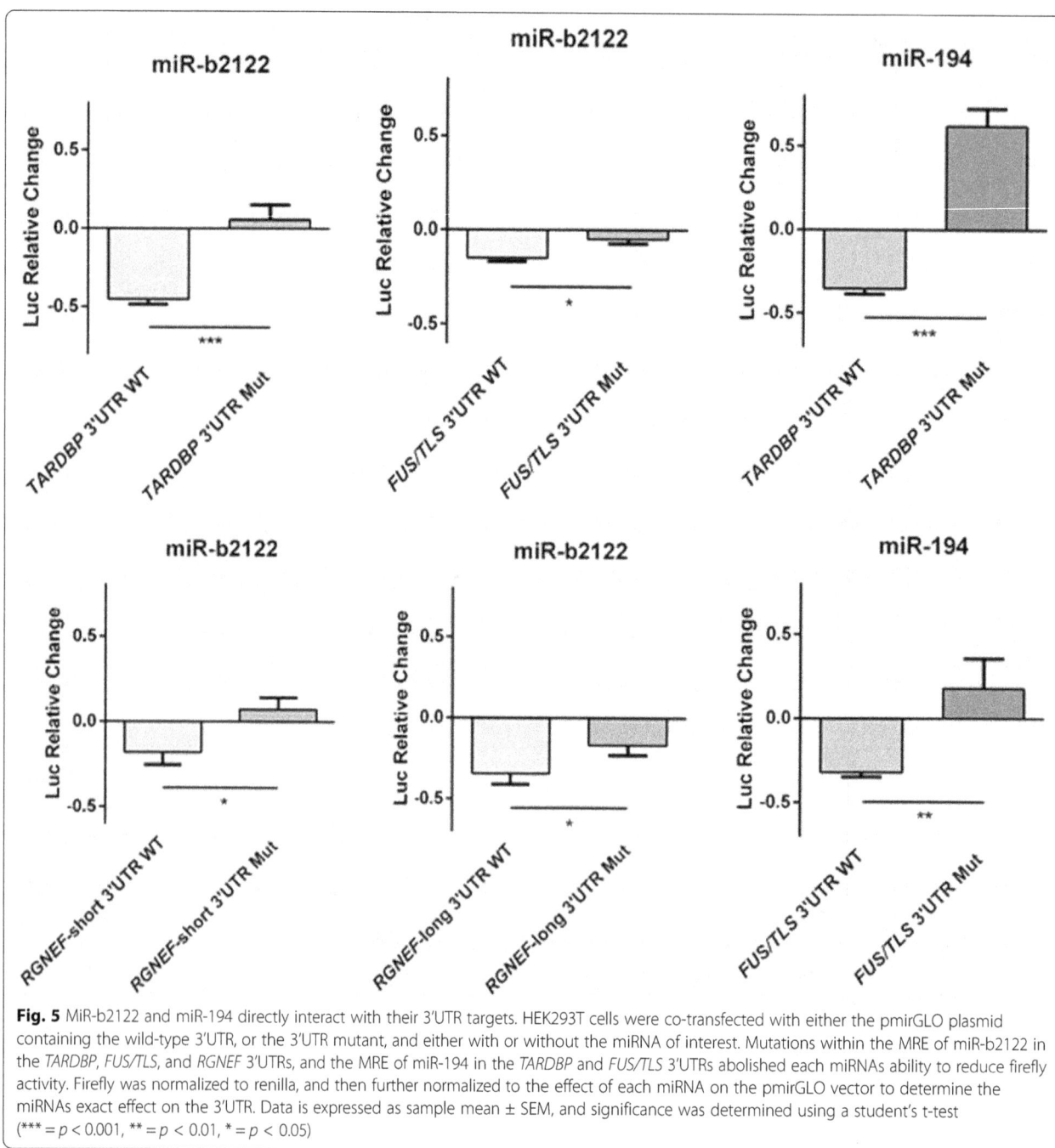

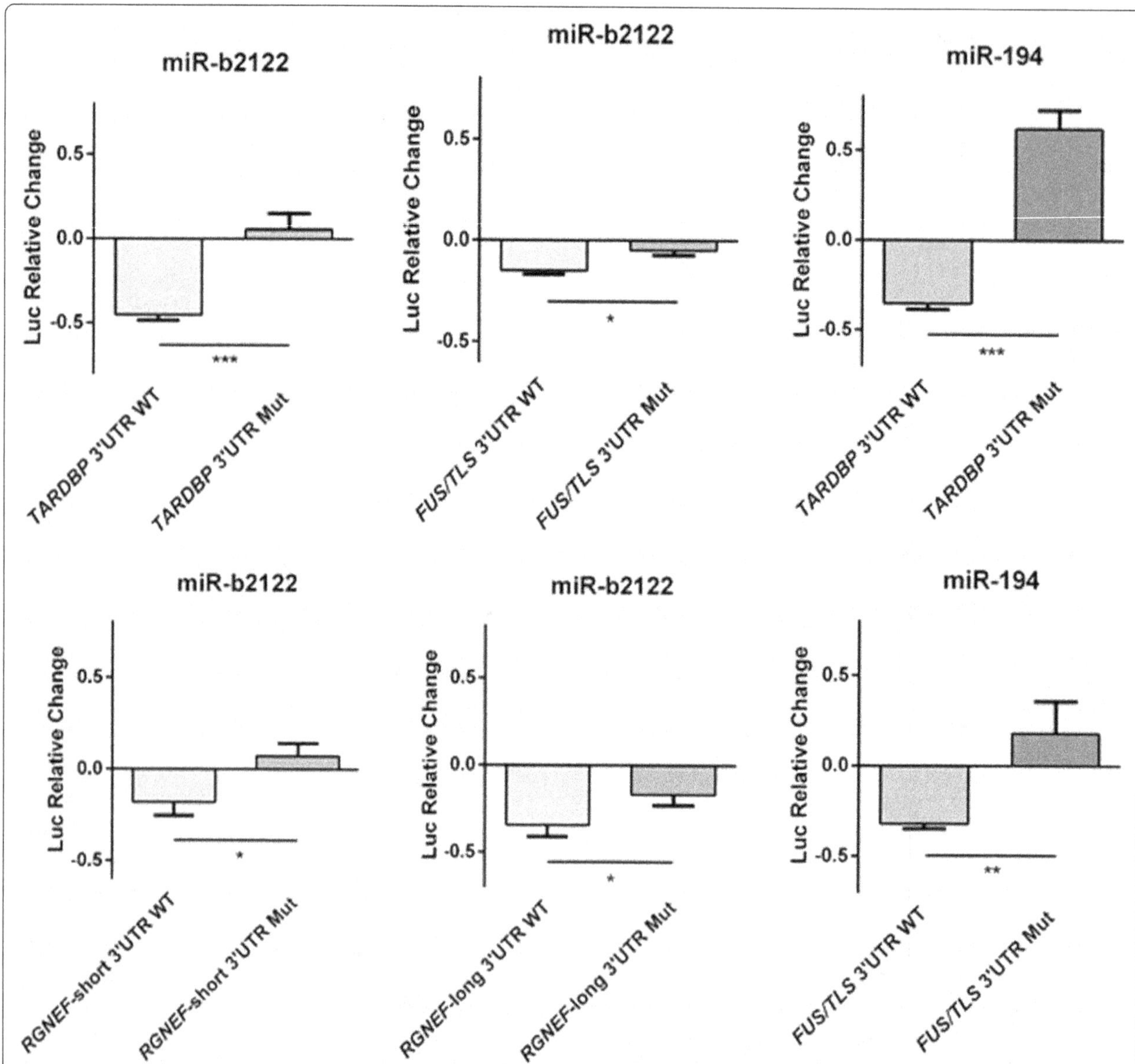

Fig. 5 MiR-b2122 and miR-194 directly interact with their 3'UTR targets. HEK293T cells were co-transfected with either the pmirGLO plasmid containing the wild-type 3'UTR, or the 3'UTR mutant, and either with or without the miRNA of interest. Mutations within the MRE of miR-b2122 in the *TARDBP*, *FUS/TLS*, and *RGNEF* 3'UTRs, and the MRE of miR-194 in the *TARDBP* and *FUS/TLS* 3'UTRs abolished each miRNAs ability to reduce firefly activity. Firefly was normalized to renilla, and then further normalized to the effect of each miRNA on the pmirGLO vector to determine the miRNAs exact effect on the 3'UTR. Data is expressed as sample mean ± SEM, and significance was determined using a student's t-test (*** = $p < 0.001$, ** = $p < 0.01$, * = $p < 0.05$)

this would critically affect the ability of miR-b2122 to bind and reduce *FUS/TLS* expression. We sought to investigate whether this mutation would affect the ability to regulate firefly expression when the firefly gene was linked to the *FUS/TLS* 3UTR that contained the *c.108C > T mutation. Indeed, this mutation significantly abolished the ability for miR-b2122 to reduce the firefly expression, compared to when the firefly gene contained the wild-type *FUS/TLS* 3UTR (Fig. 8b). This result implies that FUS/TLS would be overexpressed without proper regulation of miR-b2122 via direct interaction with the 3 UTR.

Based on the previous result, we decided to examine if sALS cases that showed a down-regulation in miR-b2122 have an increase in FUS/TLS expression. In sALS cases that showed a down-regulation of miR-b2122 there was a 3-fold increase in FUS/TLS protein expression (Fig. 8c, d), suggesting a relationship between reduced levels of miR-b2122 and increase FUS/TLS expression.

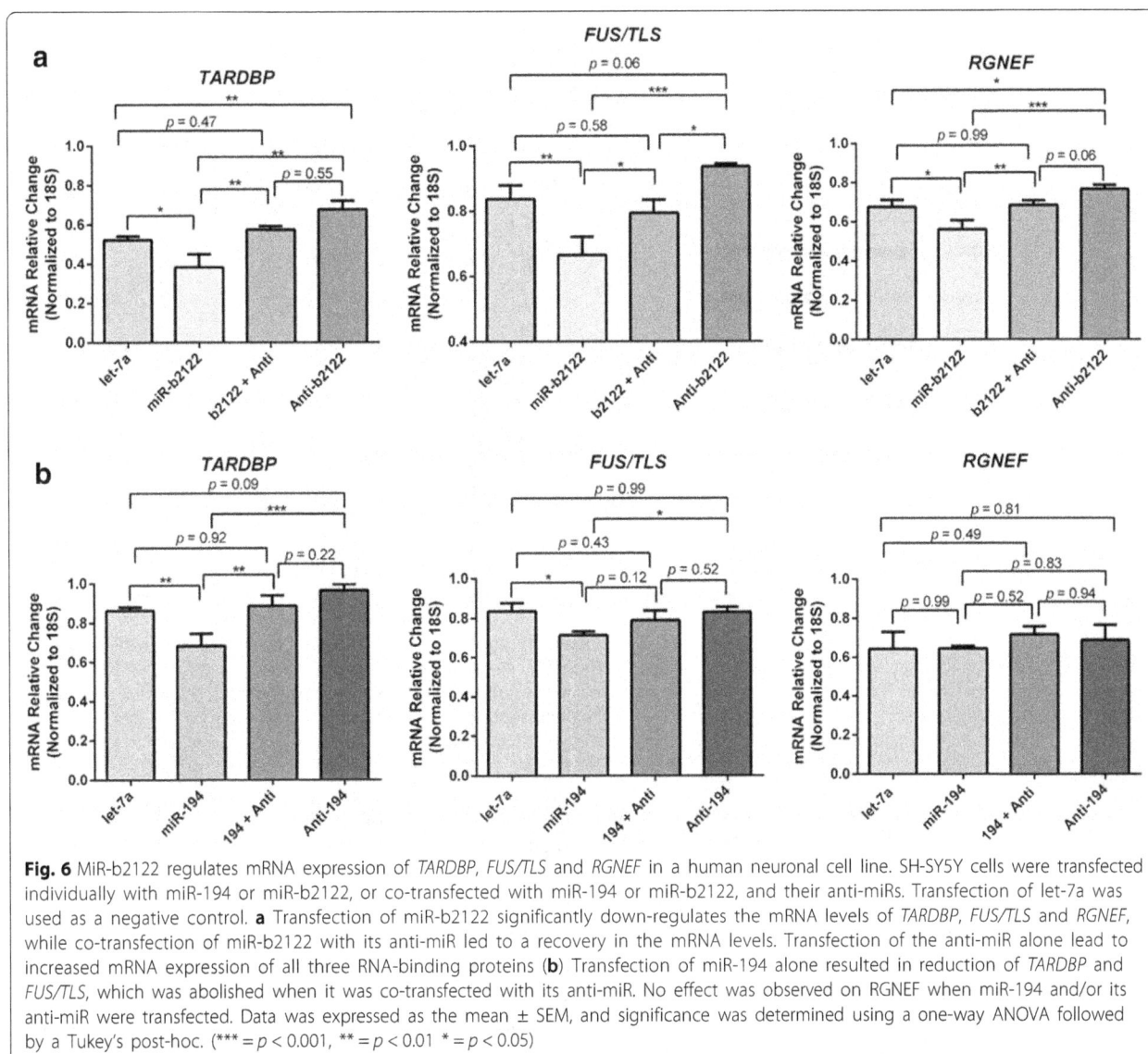

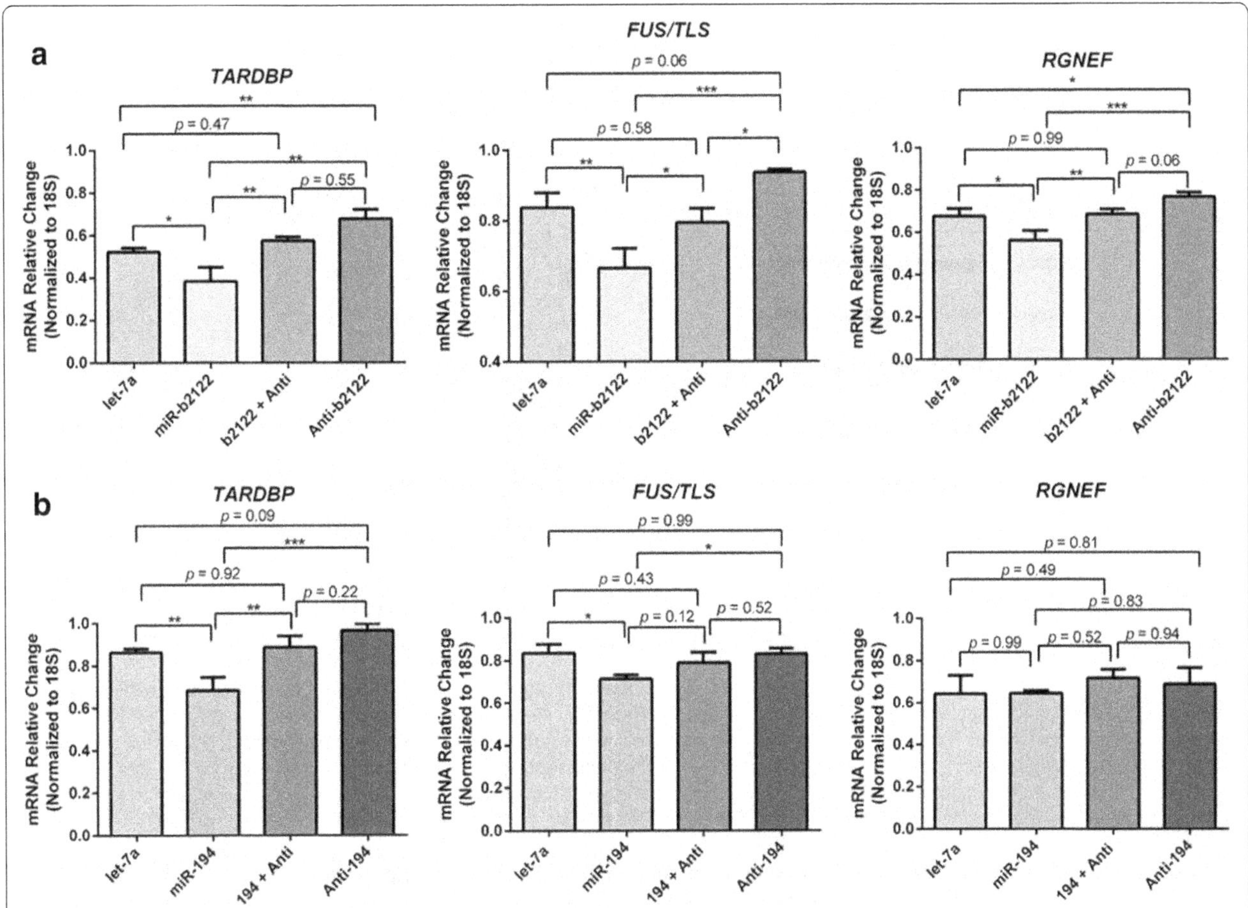

Fig. 6 MiR-b2122 regulates mRNA expression of *TARDBP*, *FUS/TLS* and *RGNEF* in a human neuronal cell line. SH-SY5Y cells were transfected individually with miR-194 or miR-b2122, or co-transfected with miR-194 or miR-b2122, and their anti-miRs. Transfection of let-7a was used as a negative control. **a** Transfection of miR-b2122 significantly down-regulates the mRNA levels of *TARDBP*, *FUS/TLS* and *RGNEF*, while co-transfection of miR-b2122 with its anti-miR led to a recovery in the mRNA levels. Transfection of the anti-miR alone lead to increased mRNA expression of all three RNA-binding proteins (**b**) Transfection of miR-194 alone resulted in reduction of *TARDBP* and *FUS/TLS*, which was abolished when it was co-transfected with its anti-miR. No effect was observed on RGNEF when miR-194 and/or its anti-miR were transfected. Data was expressed as the mean ± SEM, and significance was determined using a one-way ANOVA followed by a Tukey's post-hoc. (*** = $p < 0.001$, ** = $p < 0.01$ * = $p < 0.05$)

Discussion

In this study, we identified miR-b2122 to be a central regulator of ALS-linked RNA-binding proteins TDP-43, FUS/TLS and RGNEF. We showed that miR-b2122 was significantly down-regulated within the spinal cord tissue of sALS patients, and specifically expressed within motor neurons. MiR-194, which was also found be down-regulated in sALS patients, regulates the mRNA expression of *TARDBP* and *FUS/TLS*, but not *RGNEF*. Together, our data introduces a novel miRNA (miR-b2122) to sALS pathology, and indicates that the down-regulation of this miRNA in sALS could affect a regulatory network of RNA-binding proteins within motor neurons, contributing to the disease pathology.

The 3'UTRs for *TARDBP*, *FUS/TLS*, and *RGNEF* identified in spinal cord match those that have been previously described; however, for *TARDBP* we were only able to describe one 3'UTR isoform, while previous authors have described multiple. The *TARDBP* 3'UTR isoform we described matches the pA1 transcript isoform [27]. Whether this is the only isoform expressed in spinal cord, or a limitation of our technique, the pA1 isoform is known to be the dominant transcript expressed in steady-state conditions, and has been shown to be the main isoform for TDP-43 protein synthesis [28–30]. Further, it has been hypothesized that the pA1 isoform is the one overexpressed in ALS [28], providing another reason why we decided to focus on the pA1 isoform, and its interactions with miR-194 and miR-b2122.

MiR-194 is a well-known tumor suppressor, and reduced levels of miR-194 has been linked to both cancer and diabetes [31–36]. Interestingly, the dysfunctional pathways identified within both of these diseases relate

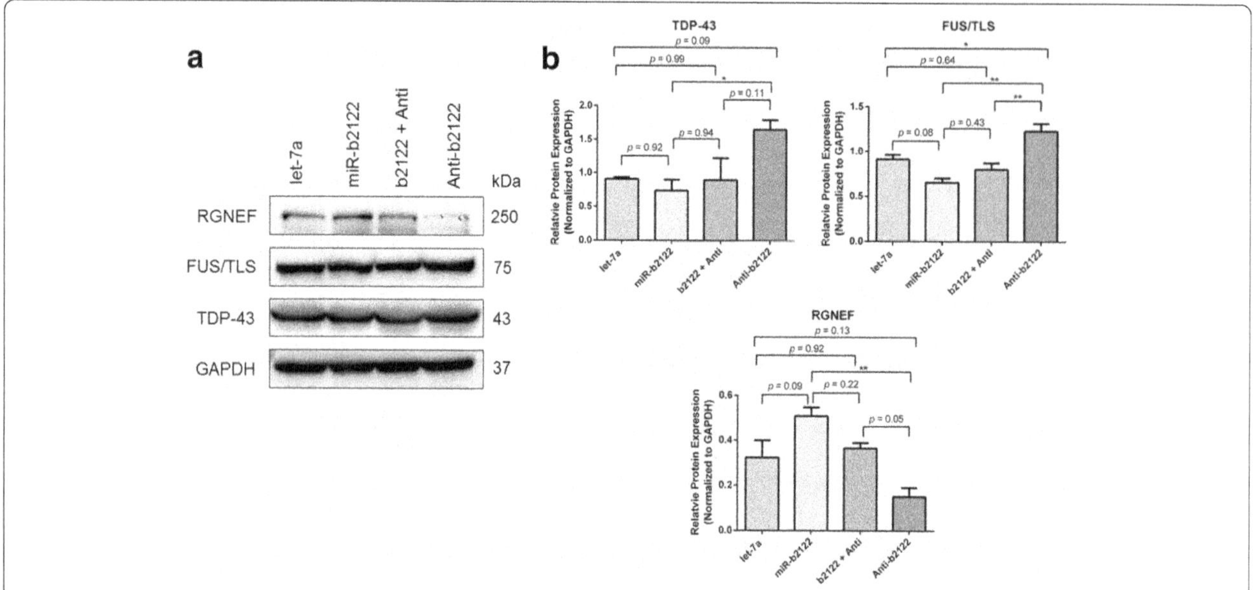

Fig. 7 MiR-b2122 alters protein levels of TDP-43, FUS/TLS and RGNEF within a human neuronal cell line. Changes in protein levels of TDP-43, FUS/TLS and RGNEF were studied when SH-SY5Y cells were transfected with either miR-b2122, miR-b2122 plus its anti-miR, or the anti-miR alone. Transfection of let-7a was used as a negative control. **a** Western blot showing expression of TDP-43, FUS/TLS, RGNEF, and GAPDH (**b**) Quantification of Western blots for TDP-43, FUS/TLS and RGNEF protein levels. TDP-43 and FUS/TLS show small reductions in protein levels when transfected with miR-b2122 alone, while their protein levels increased when the anti-miR is added. Differences in protein levels when miR-b2122 or the anti-miR are added alone are significantly different for both TDP-43 and FUS/TLS. RGNEF has increased and decreased protein levels when either miR-b2122 or its anti-miR are added alone, respectively, and these differences are significantly different from one another. Protein levels were normalized to GAPDH. Data was expressed as the mean ± SEM, and significance was determined using a one-way ANOVA followed by a Tukey's post-hoc (** = $p < 0.01$, * = $p < 0.05$)

to those described in ALS [33, 36]. For example, miR-194 expression has been shown to be switched off by NF-kB - a proinflammatory transcription factor that has been associated with ALS progression via increase activation in astrocytes and microglia [33, 37, 38]. Further, overexpression of TDP-43 has been related to an increase in NF-kB activation [38]. In this study, reduction of miR-194 leads to increased levels of *TARDBP* mRNA, and thus, through its regulation of TDP-43, miR-194 may be part of an inflammatory regulatory network that contributes to ALS progression.

Since miR-b2122 was a novel miRNA identified by our group previously [39], this is the first pathway in which this miRNA has been implicated. Our data suggests that the down-regulation of miR-b2122 would lead to a significant increase in *TARDBP, FUS/TLS* and *RGNEF* mRNA levels in sALS patients. This is consistent with the increase of *TARDBP* mRNA and protein levels observed in sALS patients [38]. Further, rodent models overexpressing wild-type human FUS/TLS and TDP-43 do develop age-related motor deficiencies and cytoplasmic protein aggregation in motor neurons similar to that seen in ALS cases [40–43]. However, the latter models look at the overexpression of a single gene, when it is the dysregulation of both expression and localization of multiple RNA-binding proteins which contributes to the disease progression. This makes miR-b2122 an intriguing miRNA, as its down-regulation in sALS would contribute to the overexpression and dysregulation of multiple RNA-binding proteins involved in its pathogenesis.

While TDP-43, FUS/TLS and RGNEF protein levels showed discrete changes when compared to the negative control, there were significant changes between when miR-b2122 and its anti-miR were transfected alone, suggesting that either overexpression, or reduced activity of miR-b2122, does in fact alter protein levels. These noticeable changes to the TDP-43, FUS/TLS and RGNEF protein levels when miR-b2122 levels are increased or decreased, suggests that chronic changes to miR-b2122 activity might have more drastic effects on protein levels within the cell over-time.

Interestingly, RGNEF protein levels went in the opposite direction of the mRNA levels within our study. While rare to see inverse correlations between mRNA and protein levels of a single gene, it is not unprecedented [44, 45]. This could imply when miR-b2122 binds to the *RGNEF* 3'UTR, its role is to maintain low levels of mRNA while keeping the transcript in a translationally stable state, and thus, loss of its binding stabilizes the mRNA molecule, but leaves the transcript in a translationally silent state. The latter phenomenon is a common one seen within stress and transport granules within neurons [46–48]. However, this would suggest

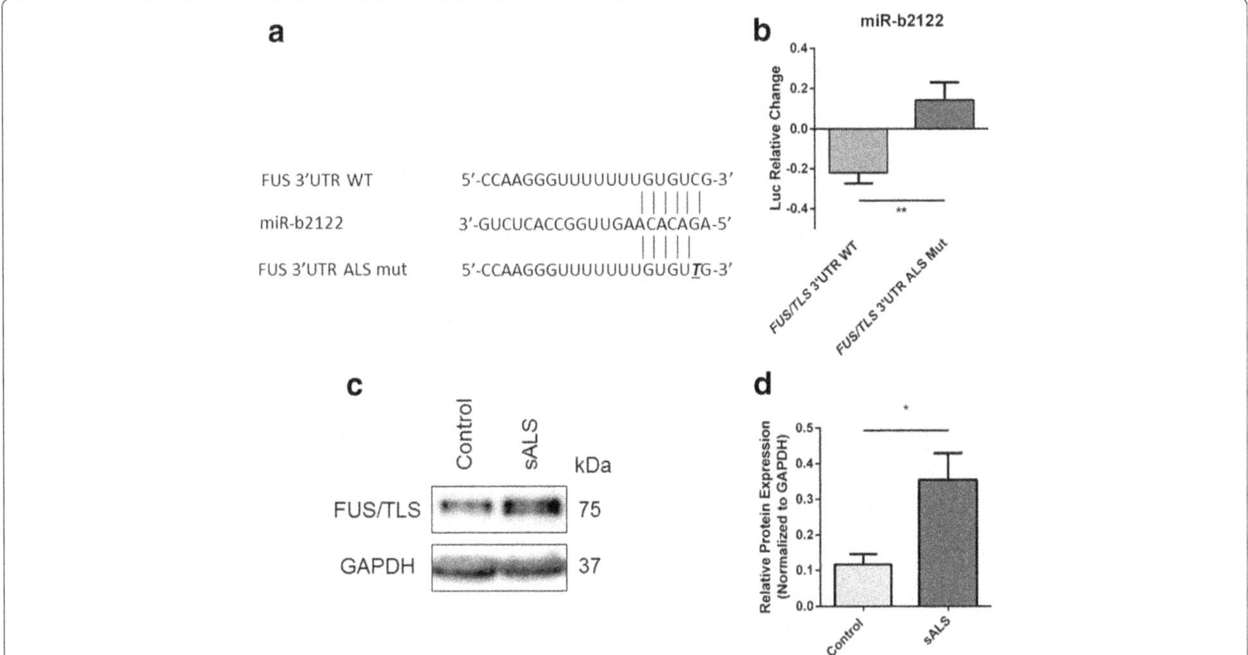

Fig. 8 ALS-associated mutation within *FUS/TLS* 3'UTR inhibits the ability for miR-b2122 to reduce firefly activity. HEK293T cells were co-transfected with either the pmirGLO plasmid containing the wild-type *FUS/TLS* 3'UTR, or the mutated form, and either with or without miR-b2122. **a** ALS-associated mutation (*c.108 C > T) affects the +2 binding site of the miR-b2122 MRE. **b** ALS-associated mutation within the *FUS/TLS* 3'UTR inhibits miR-b2122 from reducing firefly activity. Firefly expression was normalized to renilla expression, and then further normalized to account for the effect miR-b2122 on the pmirGLO vector itself to determine the miRNAs exact effect on the 3'UTR. **c** Western blot of FUS/TLS protein expression in the spinal cord of sALS cases versus control subjects. **d** Quantification of western blot. Data is expressed as sample mean ± SEM, and significance was determined using a Student's t-test (** = $p < 0.01$)

that there is competition between miR-b2122 and another miRNA, or RNA-binding protein at the *RGNEF* 3'UTR which would need further investigation.

We sought to determine whether an ALS mutation located in the MRE of miR-b2122 within the *FUS/TLS* 3'UTR effected the ability of miR-b2122 to reduce gene expression. Clinically, the patient identified with this FUS/TLS 3'UTR mutation (*c.108C > T) had limb onset ALS with severe limb weakness and respiratory difficulties. Previously, fibroblast cells cultured from the ALS patient with this mutation showed an overexpression of FUS/TLS mRNA and protein, and an increase in cytoplasmic localization – two factors believed to contribute to ALS development [20]. Despite identifying these phenotypes there was no clear mechanism to why this may happen. In this study, we showed that loss of direct interaction between miR-b2122 and the *FUS/TLS* 3'UTR may play a critical role in FUS/TLS overexpression. Further, we were able to show that reduced levels of miR-b2122 in sALS spinal cord seems to be related to an increase in FUS/TLS protein expression. In addition, reduction of the levels of miR-b2122 in a neuronal cell line (SH-SY5Y) using anti-b2122 hindered the ability for miR-b2122 to reduce endogenous *FUS/TLS* leading to an overall increase in both mRNA and protein levels.

In this study, we have not only provided an explanation of the significance for reduced levels of miR-b2122 in sALS, but provide a molecular link showing the importance of the interaction between miR-b2122 and the *FUS/TLS* 3'UTR. Thus, dysregulation of miR-b2122 either through reduce levels or mutations within the MRE could be a major contributing factor to FUS/TLS dysregulation and pathogenesis in ALS. In a different study, a group examined another ALS-related mutation within the *FUS/TLS* 3'UTR, which lead to an overexpression of FUS/TLS. This aberrant expression of FUS/TLS was attributed to the loss of its interaction with miR-141/200a due to the 3'UTR mutation [21]. These findings emphasize the importance of examining mutations outside of the coding regions, as alterations within the 3'UTR can have drastic effects on both protein expression and localization [49, 50].

While it is interesting to note the relationship between the dysregulation of RNA-binding proteins and miRNAs, it is still unclear how miRNAs, like miR-b2122 and miR-194, become reduced in sALS. However, there is strong evidence suggesting that the miRNA biogenesis pathway is disrupted in sALS, as both TDP-43 and FUS are crucial parts of miRNA production [18, 19]. More specifically, it appears that the dysregulation in miRNA biogenesis happens at the level of DICER, as it is the mature miRNA form, and not the pre-miRNA form, showing a global down-regulation in sALS [15]. Also, ALS-linked mutations in TDP-43 and FUS affect miRNA biogenesis specifically at the level DICER [15]. Thus, it is plausible that TDP-43 and/or FUS could regulate the biogenesis of miR-b2122 and miR-194, suggesting that a negative feedback loop between RNA binding proteins and miRNAs exists, and that it is the loss of this negative feedback loop that drives, at least in part, sALS disease progression.

Conclusions

It has been previously shown that the pathogenesis of sALS likely does not rely on the dysregulation of a single RNA-binding protein, but a combination of TDP-43, FUS/TLS and RGNEF, as they co-aggregate with each other in motor neurons of sALS patients [6]. In the current study, we have identified a single miRNA that regulates all three of these RNA-binding proteins. The observation that miR-b2122 is down-regulated in sALS suggests that this miRNA may play an essential role in the pathogenic mechanism of sALS. As we further look at those miRNAs related to ALS, we start developing an understanding of a miRNA network critical for motor neuron function, which we have termed MotomiRs [16]. Further, it would be intriguing to know whether these miRNAs play a role in closely related neurodegenerative diseases, including primary lateral sclerosis (PLS), spinal muscular atrophy (SMA), or frontotemporal dementia (FTD). Based on the current study, miR-b2122 should be added to the already established list of MotomiRs, as it regulates a network of RNA-binding proteins essential for motor neuron function, and its regulation could potentially contribute to motor neuron degeneration in ALS.

Additional files

Additional file 1: Table S1. Site-directed mutagenesis primers for *TARDBP*, *FUS/TLS* and *RGNEF* 3'UTRs. (DOCX 16 kb)

Additional file 2: Figure S1. 3'UTR isoforms of RNA-binding proteins, and miR-194 and miR-b2122 are expressed in SH-SY5Y cells. (A) 3'RACE PCR showing TARDBP, FUS/TLS and RGNEF 3'UTR isoforms expressed in SH-SY5Y cells. FUS/TLS and RGNEF isoforms match those expressed in human spinal cord. TARDBP showed multiple isoforms, but only the 1398b isoform identified in spinal cord could be confirmed by sequencing. (B) Real-time PCR indicating the expression of miR-194 and miR-b2122 in SH-SY5Y cells. (TIFF 171 kb)

Additional file 3: Figure S2. Let-7a has no effect on mRNA levels of TARDBP, FUS/TLS, or RGNEF within SH-SY5Y cells. Let-7a was transfected into SH-SY5Y cells to determine if it changed the basal mRNA levels of TARDBP, FUS/TLS or RGNEF, and was compared to a non-transfected control. The data indicated no significant change in the transcript levels of either TARDBP (p=0.64), FUS/TLS (p=0.51), or RGNEF (p=0.74) between the two conditions. Data is expressed as sample mean ± SEM, and significance was determined using a Student's t-test.(TIFF 160 kb)

Additional file 4: Figure S3. Let-7a has no effect on protein levels of TDP-43, FUS/TLS, or RGNEF within SH-SY5Y cells. Let-7a was transfected into SH-SY5Y cells to determine if it changed the basal protein levels of TDP-43, FUS/TLS or RGNEF, and was compared to a non-transfected control. The data indicated no significant change in the protein levels of either TDP-43 (p=0.71), FUS/TLS (p=0.28), or RGNEF (p=0.87) between the two conditions. Data is expressed as sample mean ± SEM, and significance was determined using a Student's t-test. (TIFF 215 kb)

Abbreviations

ALS: Amyotrophic lateral sclerosis; fALS: Familial ALS; FISH: Fluorescent in situ hybridization; FUS/TLS: Fused in sarcoma/translocation in liposarcoma; MRE: miRNA Recognition element; RACE: Rapid amplification of cDNA ends; RGNEF: Rho guanine nucleotide exchange factor; sALS: Sporadic ALS; TARDBP: TAR DNA-binding protein gene; TDP-43: TAR DNA-binding protein, 43 kDa; UTR: Untranslated region

Acknowledgements

Not applicable.

Funding

MJS research is supported by the European research projects of rare diseases (E-Rare), Ontario Neurodegeneration Diseases Research Initiative (ONDRI), ALS Society of Canada and Michael Halls Endowment.

Authors' contributions

ZCEH performed the experiments and data analysis, and contributed to the experimental design. DC-M conceived the experiments. MJS supervised the project with input from DC-M. ZCEH, DC-M and MJS wrote the manuscript. All authors read and approved the final manuscript.

Competing interests

The authors declare that this research in done in the absence of any financial and commercial relationships that could be interpreted as a potential competing interest.

Author details

[1]Molecular Medicine Group, Robarts Research Institute, Schulich School of Medicine and Dentistry, Western University, London, Ontario, Canada. [2]Department of Clinical Neurological Sciences, Schulich School of Medicine and Dentistry, Western University, London, Ontario, Canada. [3]Department of Pathology, Schulich School of Medicine and Dentistry, Western University, London, Ontario, Canada. [4]Rm C7-120 LHSC, University Hospital, 339 Windermere Road, London, Ontario N6A 5A5, Canada.

References

1. Taylor JP, Brown RH Jr. Cleveland DW: decoding ALS: from genes to mechanism. Nature. 539:197–206.
2. Zarei S, Carr K, Reiley L, Diaz K, Guerra O, Altamirano PF, Pagani W, Lodin D, Orozco G, Chinea A. A comprehensive review of amyotrophic lateral sclerosis. Surg Neurol Int. 2015;6:171.

3. Chen S, Sayana P, Zhang X, Le W. Genetics of amyotrophic lateral sclerosis: an update. Mol Neurodegener. 2013;8:28.
4. Al-Chalabi A, van den Berg LH, Veldink J. Gene discovery in amyotrophic lateral sclerosis: implications for clinical management. Nat Rev Neurol. 2017;13:96–104.
5. Blokhuis AM, Groen EJ, Koppers M, van den Berg LH, Pasterkamp RJ. Protein aggregation in amyotrophic lateral sclerosis. Acta Neuropathol. 2013;125:777–94.
6. Keller BA, Volkening K, Droppelmann CA, Ang LC, Rademakers R, Strong MJ. Co-aggregation of RNA binding proteins in ALS spinal motor neurons: evidence of a common pathogenic mechanism. Acta Neuropathol. 2012; 124:733–47.
7. Xiao S, McLean J, Robertson J. Neuronal intermediate filaments and ALS: a new look at an old question. Biochim Biophys Acta. 2006;1762:1001–12.
8. Cestra G, Rossi S, Di Salvio M, Cozzolino M. Control of mRNA translation in ALS Proteinopathy. Front Mol Neurosci. 2017;10:85.
9. Droppelmann CA, Campos-Melo D, Ishtiaq M, Volkening K, Strong MJ. RNA metabolism in ALS: when normal processes become pathological. Amyotroph Lateral Scler Frontotemporal Degener. 2014;15:321–36.
10. Tsuiji H, Iguchi Y, Furuya A, Kataoka A, Hatsuta H, Atsuta N, Tanaka F, Hashizume Y, Akatsu H, Murayama S, et al. Spliceosome integrity is defective in the motor neuron diseases ALS and SMA. EMBO Mol Med. 2013;5:221–34.
11. Hideyama T, Yamashita T, Aizawa H, Tsuji S, Kakita A, Takahashi H, Kwak S. Profound downregulation of the RNA editing enzyme ADAR2 in ALS spinal motor neurons. Neurobiol Dis. 2012;45:1121–8.
12. Freibaum BD, Chitta RK, High AA, Taylor JP. Global analysis of TDP-43 interacting proteins reveals strong association with RNA splicing and translation machinery. J Proteome Res. 2010;9:1104–20.
13. Campos-Melo D, Droppelmann CA, He Z, Volkening K, Strong MJ. Altered microRNA expression profile in amyotrophic lateral sclerosis: a role in the regulation of NFL mRNA levels. Molecular brain. 2013;6:26.
14. Figueroa-Romero C, Hur J, Lunn JS, Paez-Colasante X, Bender DE, Yung R, Sakowski SA, Feldman EL. Expression of microRNAs in human post-mortem amyotrophic lateral sclerosis spinal cords provides insight into disease mechanisms. Mol Cell Neurosci. 2016;71:34–45.
15. Emde A, Eitan C, Liou LL, Libby RT, Rivkin N, Magen I, Reichenstein I, Oppenheim H, Eilam R, Silvestroni A, et al. Dysregulated miRNA biogenesis downstream of cellular stress and ALS-causing mutations: a new mechanism for ALS. EMBO J. 2015;34:2633–51.
16. Hawley ZCE, Campos-Melo D, Droppelmann CA, Strong MJ. MotomiRs: miRNAs in motor neuron function and disease. Front Mol Neurosci. 2017;10:127.
17. Rinchetti P, Rizzuti M, Faravelli I, Corti S. MicroRNA metabolism and Dysregulation in amyotrophic lateral sclerosis. Mol Neurobiol. 2017;
18. Morlando M, Dini Modigliani S, Torrelli G, Rosa A, Di Carlo V, Caffarelli E, Bozzoni I. FUS stimulates microRNA biogenesis by facilitating co-transcriptional Drosha recruitment. EMBO J. 2012;31:4502–10.
19. Kawahara Y, Mieda-Sato A. TDP-43 promotes microRNA biogenesis as a component of the Drosha and Dicer complexes. Proc Natl Acad Sci U S A. 2012;109:3347–52.
20. Sabatelli M, Moncada A, Conte A, Lattante S, Marangi G, Luigetti M, Lucchini M, Mirabella M, Romano A, Del Grande A, et al. Mutations in the 3′ untranslated region of FUS causing FUS overexpression are associated with amyotrophic lateral sclerosis. Hum Mol Genet. 2013;22:4748–55.
21. Dini Modigliani S, Morlando M, Errichelli L, Sabatelli M, Bozzoni I. An ALS-associated mutation in the FUS 3′-UTR disrupts a microRNA-FUS regulatory circuitry. Nat Commun. 2014;5:4335.
22. Droppelmann CA, Keller BA, Campos-Melo D, Volkening K, Strong MJ. Rho guanine nucleotide exchange factor is an NFL mRNA destabilizing factor that forms cytoplasmic inclusions in amyotrophic lateral sclerosis. Neurobiol Aging. 2013;34:248–62.
23. Droppelmann CA, Wang J, Campos-Melo D, Keller B, Volkening K, Hegele RA, Strong MJ. Detection of a novel frameshift mutation and regions with homozygosis within ARHGEF28 gene in familial amyotrophic lateral sclerosis. Amyotroph Lateral Scler Frontotemporal Degener. 2013;14:444–51.
24. Ma Y, Tang L, Chen L, Zhang B, Deng P, Wang J, Yang Y, Liu R, Yang Y, Ye S, et al. ARHGEF28 gene exon 6/intron 6 junction mutations in Chinese amyotrophic lateral sclerosis cohort. Amyotroph Lateral Scler Frontotemporal Degener. 2014;15:309–11.
25. de Planell-Saguer M, Rodicio MC, Mourelatos Z. Rapid in situ codetection of noncoding RNAs and proteins in cells and formalin-fixed paraffin-embedded tissue sections without protease treatment. Nat Protoc. 2010;5: 1061–73.
26. Campos-Melo D, Droppelmann CA, Volkening K, Strong MJ. Comprehensive luciferase-based reporter gene assay reveals previously masked up-regulatory effects of miRNAs. Int J Mol Sci. 2014;15:15592–602.
27. Ayala YM, De Conti L, Avendano-Vazquez SE, Dhir A, Romano M, D'Ambrogio A, Tollervey J, Ule J, Baralle M, Buratti E, Baralle FE. TDP-43 regulates its mRNA levels through a negative feedback loop. EMBO J. 2011; 30:277–88.
28. Koyama A, Sugai A, Kato T, Ishihara T, Shiga A, Toyoshima Y, Koyama M, Konno T, Hirokawa S, Yokoseki A, et al. Increased cytoplasmic TARDBP mRNA in affected spinal motor neurons in ALS caused by abnormal autoregulation of TDP-43. Nucleic Acids Res. 2016;44:5820–36.
29. Avendano-Vazquez SE, Dhir A, Bembich S, Buratti E, Proudfoot N, Baralle FE. Autoregulation of TDP-43 mRNA levels involves interplay between transcription, splicing, and alternative polyA site selection. Genes Dev. 2012; 26:1679–84.
30. Bembich S, Herzog JS, De Conti L, Stuani C, Avendano-Vazquez SE, Buratti E, Baralle M, Baralle FE. Predominance of spliceosomal complex formation over polyadenylation site selection in TDP-43 autoregulation. Nucleic Acids Res. 2014;42:3362–71.
31. Zhang M, Zhuang Q, Cui L. MiR-194 inhibits cell proliferation and invasion via repression of RAP2B in bladder cancer. Biomed Pharmacother. 2016;80:268–75.
32. Zhou L, Di Q, Sun B, Wang X, Li M, Shi J. MicroRNA-194 restrains the cell progression of non-small cell lung cancer by targeting human nuclear distribution protein C. Oncol Rep. 2016;35:3435–44.
33. Bao C, Li Y, Huan L, Zhang Y, Zhao F, Wang Q, Liang L, Ding J, Liu L, Chen T, et al. NF-kappaB signaling relieves negative regulation by miR-194 in hepatocellular carcinoma by suppressing the transcription factor HNF-1alpha. Sci Signal. 2015;8:ra75.
34. Song Y, Zhao F, Wang Z, Liu Z, Chiang Y, Xu Y, Gao P, Xu H. Inverse association between miR-194 expression and tumor invasion in gastric cancer. Ann Surg Oncol. 2012;19(Suppl 3):S509–17.
35. Dong P, Kaneuchi M, Watari H, Hamada J, Sudo S, Ju J, Sakuragi N. MicroRNA-194 inhibits epithelial to mesenchymal transition of endometrial cancer cells by targeting oncogene BMI-1. Mol Cancer. 2011;10:99.
36. Latouche C, Natoli A, Reddy-Luthmoodoo M, Heywood SE, Armitage JA, Kingwell BA. MicroRNA-194 modulates glucose metabolism and its skeletal muscle expression is reduced in diabetes. PLoS One. 2016;11:e0155108.
37. Frakes AE, Ferraiuolo L, Haidet-Phillips AM, Schmelzer L, Braun L, Miranda CJ, Ladner KJ, Bevan AK, Foust KD, Godbout JP, et al. Microglia induce motor neuron death via the classical NF-kappaB pathway in amyotrophic lateral sclerosis. Neuron. 2014;81:1009–23.
38. Swarup V, Phaneuf D, Dupre N, Petri S, Strong M, Kriz J, Julien JP. Deregulation of TDP-43 in amyotrophic lateral sclerosis triggers nuclear factor kappaB-mediated pathogenic pathways. J Exp Med. 2011;208:2429–47.
39. Ishtiaq M, Campos-Melo D, Volkening K, Strong MJ. Analysis of novel NEFL mRNA targeting microRNAs in amyotrophic lateral sclerosis. PLoS One. 2014; 9:e85653.
40. Wils H, Kleinberger G, Janssens J, Pereson S, Joris G, Cuijt I, Smits V, Ceuterick-de Groote C, Van Broeckhoven C, Kumar-Singh S. TDP-43 transgenic mice develop spastic paralysis and neuronal inclusions characteristic of ALS and frontotemporal lobar degeneration. Proc Natl Acad Sci U S A. 2010;107:3858–63.
41. Xu YF, Gendron TF, Zhang YJ, Lin WL, D'Alton S, Sheng H, Casey MC, Tong J, Knight J, Yu X, et al. Wild-type human TDP-43 expression causes TDP-43 phosphorylation, mitochondrial aggregation, motor deficits, and early mortality in transgenic mice. J Neurosci. 2010;30:10851–9.
42. Mitchell JC, McGoldrick P, Vance C, Hortobagyi T, Sreedharan J, Rogelj B, Tudor EL, Smith BN, Klasen C, Miller CC, et al. Overexpression of human wild-type FUS causes progressive motor neuron degeneration in an age- and dose-dependent fashion. Acta Neuropathol. 2013;125:273–88.
43. Janssens J, Wils H, Kleinberger G, Joris G, Cuijt I, Ceuterick-de Groote C, Van Broeckhoven C, Kumar-Singh S. Overexpression of ALS-associated p.M337V human TDP-43 in mice worsens disease features compared to wild-type human TDP-43 mice. Mol Neurobiol. 2013;48:22–35.
44. Marinova Z, Monoranu CM, Fetz S, Walitza S, Grunblatt E. Region-specific regulation of the serotonin 2A receptor expression in development and ageing in post mortem human brain. Neuropathol Appl Neurobiol. 2015;41:520–32.
45. Xiu J, Zhang Q, Zhou T, Zhou TT, Chen Y, Hu H. Visualizing an emotional valence map in the limbic forebrain by TAI-FISH. Nat Neurosci. 2014;17:1552–9.
46. Panas MD, Ivanov P, Anderson P. Mechanistic insights into mammalian stress granule dynamics. J Cell Biol. 2016;215:313–23.

47. Buchan JR. mRNP granules. Assembly, function, and connections with disease. RNA Biol. 2014;11:1019–30.
48. Anderson P, Kedersha N. Stress granules: the Tao of RNA triage. Trends Biochem Sci. 2008;33:141–50.
49. Berkovits BD, Mayr C. Alternative 3' UTRs act as scaffolds to regulate membrane protein localization. Nature. 2015;522:363–7.
50. Mayr C. Evolution and biological roles of alternative 3'UTRs. Trends Cell Biol. 2016;26:227–37.

15

T-type calcium channels functionally interact with spectrin (α/β) and ankyrin B

Agustin Garcia-Caballero[1], Fang-Xiong Zhang[1], Victoria Hodgkinson[1], Junting Huang[1], Lina Chen[1], Ivana A. Souza[1], Stuart Cain[2], Jennifer Kass[2], Sascha Alles[2], Terrance P. Snutch[2] and Gerald W. Zamponi[1*]

Abstract

This study describes the functional interaction between the Cav3.1 and Cav3.2 T-type calcium channels and cytoskeletal spectrin (α/β) and ankyrin B proteins. The interactions were identified utilizing a proteomic approach to identify proteins that interact with a conserved negatively charged cytosolic region present in the carboxy-terminus of T-type calcium channels. Deletion of this stretch of amino acids decreased binding of Cav3.1 and Cav3.2 calcium channels to spectrin (α/β) and ankyrin B and notably also reduced T-type whole cell current densities in expression systems. Furthermore, fluorescence recovery after photobleaching analysis of mutant channels lacking the proximal C-terminus region revealed reduced recovery of both Cav3.1 and Cav3.2 mutant channels in hippocampal neurons. Knockdown of spectrin α and ankyrin B decreased the density of endogenous Cav3.2 in hippocampal neurons. These findings reveal spectrin (α/β) / ankyrin B cytoskeletal and signaling proteins as key regulators of T-type calcium channels expressed in the nervous system.

Keywords: T-type channels, Spectrin (α/β), Ankyrin B, Trafficking, Cav3.1, Cav3.2

Introduction

T-type calcium channels are important regulators of neuronal excitability and low threshold-mediated exocytosis [1, 2]. The mammalian genome encodes three different T-type calcium channels (Cav3.1, Cav3.2 and Cav3.3) [3]. The pore forming Cavα1 subunits of these channels are comprised of four homologous transmembrane domains linked by cytoplasmic segments and flanked by intracellular N- and C-terminus structures. T-type channels are highly expressed in the central nervous system including neocortex, cerebellum, thalamus and hippocampus [4] and have been linked to pathophysiologies such as idiopathic generalized epilepsies [5] and tremor [6]. The Cav3.2 subtype is expressed in dorsal root ganglion neurons and spinal cord where its dysregulation contributes to the development of inflammatory and neuropathic pain [7]. Notably, T-type calcium channel blockers are effective in attenuating absence seizures and chronic pain in rodent models [8, 9] and have also been shown efficacious in a human model of inflammatory pain. In this context, understanding how these channels are regulated and trafficked to the cell surface is of importance.

T-type channels are known to interact with numerous regulatory proteins including CamKII [10], G-proteins [11], calcineurin [12], calmodulin [13], syntaxin [1] and calnexin [14], and to form protein complexes with members of the potassium channel family such as Kv4, KCa3.1, and KCa1.1 [15–17]. Many of these interactions appear to involve the cytosolic carboxy-terminal region of Cav3.x proteins and here we utilized a proteomic approach to identify additional interacting partners. In particular, we focused on a stretch of conserved negatively charged residues located in the proximal carboxy-terminal regions of Cav3.1 and Cav3.2 channels. Mass spectrometry identified spectrins as Cav3.2 C-terminal interacting proteins. We further describe the interactions and functional regulation of Cav3.1 and Cav3.2 channels with spectrin (α/β) and ankyrin B in both exogenous expression and native systems, revealing that these interactions regulate whole cell current density. Together, the results indicate that cytoskeletal elements are important regulators of T-type calcium channel function and physiology.

* Correspondence: zamponi@ucalgary.ca
[1]Department of Physiology and Pharmacology, Hotchkiss Brain Institute and Alberta Children's Hospital Research Institute, Cumming School of Medicine, University of Calgary, 3330 Hospital Dr. NW, Calgary T2N 4N1, Canada
Full list of author information is available at the end of the article

Results

Spectrins interact with T-type calcium channels

The proximal C-terminus regions of Cav3.1 and Cav3.2 contain a conserved α-helical (http://bioinf.cs.ucl.ac.uk/psipred) stretch of charged amino acid residues (amino acids 1851–1875 in Cav3.1, and 1860–1884 in Cav3.2) (Fig. 1a). To determine whether this motif is a binding region for regulatory proteins, we used a proteomic approach with a corresponding Cav3.2 CT synthetic peptide conjugated with biotin as bait for interacting proteins in mouse brain lysates. Bound proteins were resolved in a denaturing Coomassie gel (Fig. 1b) and protein bands that appeared in samples incubated with the Cav3.2CT bait, but not in samples incubated with the control scramble peptide, were excised and analyzed by MALDI/TOF mass spectrometry. This analysis yielded hits for three cytoskeletal proteins: spectrin- αII (SPTAN1) and two isoforms of spectrin-β (SPTBN1 and SPTBN2) (Fig. 1c), with the former showing the highest score. Spectrin is a heterodimeric protein comprised of α- and β- subunits (280 and 246 kDa, respectively) that form a supercoiled triple-helix structure through 106 residue modules known as "spectrin repeats" [18]. This particular structural organization allows spectrin to expand and contract to remodel the cytoskeleton and, hence, cellular architecture [19]. In humans, there are two α and five β spectrin subunit genes. Spectrin-αI is expressed in erythroid cells whereas spectrin-αII is expressed in all nonerythroid cells, including the brain where it is important for synaptic transmission [20] and participates in neurotransmitter release [21]. Spectrins possess multiple interacting domains such as a pleckstrin homology domain, a Src homology 3 domain (SH3), a calcium binding EF hand domain, an ankyrin binding repeat and an actin binding domain, that interact with a diverse set of cell signaling proteins, receptors and ion channels [18]. To confirm SPTAN1-Cav3 interactions, we performed co-immunoprecipitations between SPTAN1 and either Cav3.1 or Cav3.2. Figure 1d and e show that SPTAN1 co-immunoprecipitated with both T-type channel isoforms from mouse brain lysates.

We next asked whether deletion of the helical region in the proximal C-terminus regions of Cav3.1 and Cav3.2 could alter their association with SPTAN1. For this purpose, we expressed GFP-tagged wild type or deletion-mutant channels in tsA-201 cells and performed co-immunoprecipitations between the exogenously expressed channels and endogenous spectrin. Consistent with the data in Fig. 1, both GFP-tagged Cav3.1 and Cav3.2 channels co-immunoprecipitated with SPTAN1 (Fig. 2a and b). Deleting the helical region (Cav3.1-GFP ΔCT (1851–1875), Cav3.2-GFP ΔCT

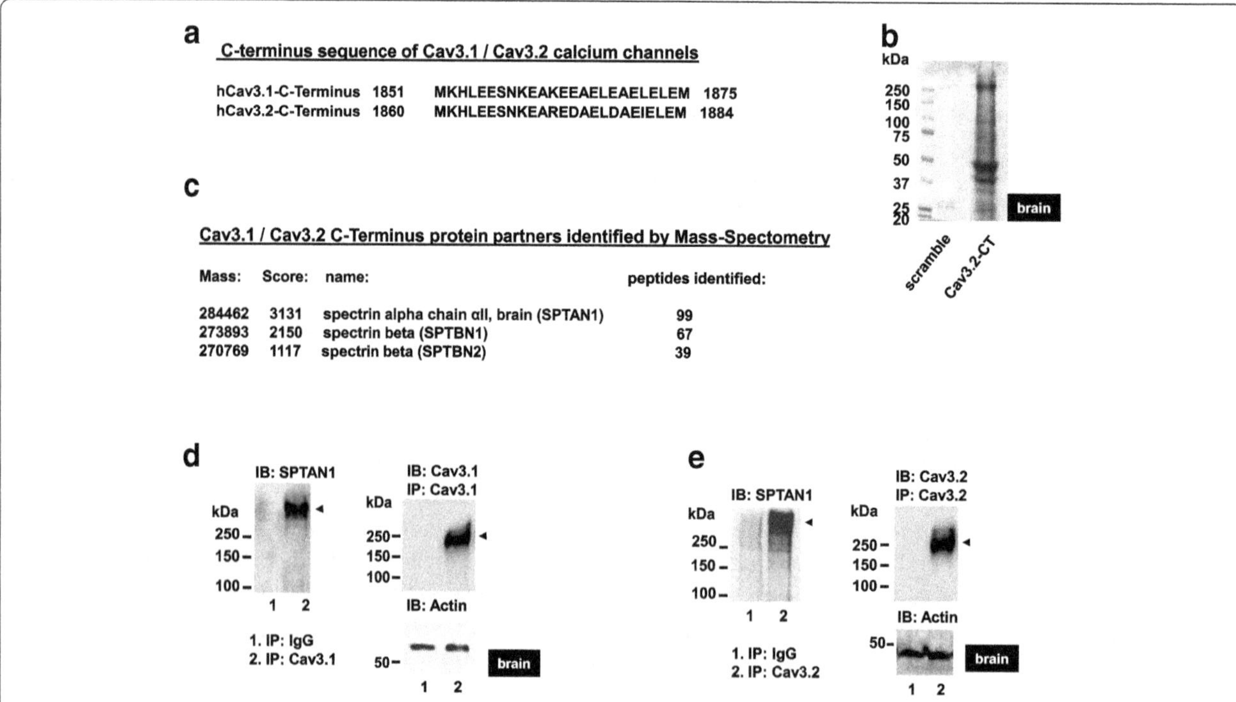

Fig. 1 Identification of spectrin (α/β) as a Cav3.1 / Cav3.2 calcium channel interacting protein. (**a**) Conserved proximal C-terminus region of Cav3.1 and Cav3.2 calcium channels. (**b**) Proteins bound to scramble (lane 1) or Cav3.2 CT 1860–1884 biotinylated peptides (lane 2) from mouse whole brain lysates, as seen by Coomassie staining (**c**) Mass spectrometry analysis of proteins bound to the Cav3.2 CT 1860–1884 biotinylated peptide by affinity precipitation assay using mouse whole brain lysates. (**d**) Cav3.1 or (**e**) Cav3.2 immunoprecipitates from mouse whole brain lysates were probed for spectrin αII (SPTAN1) by Western blot. An actin loading control is shown

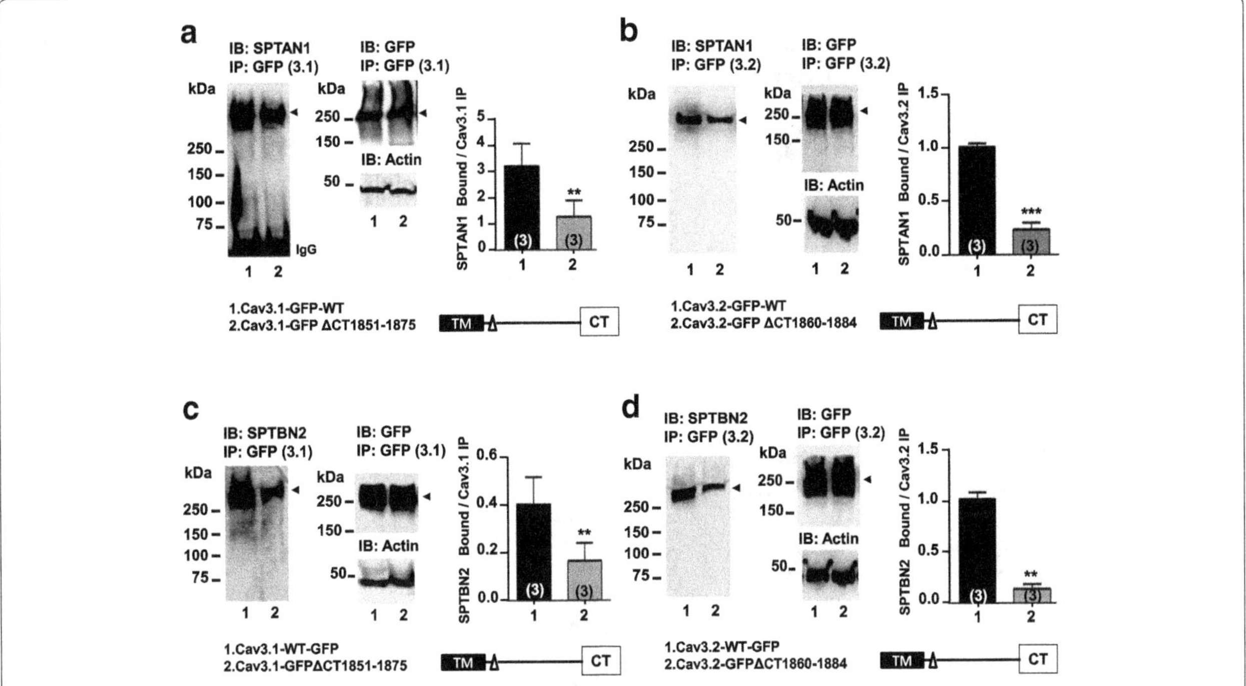

Fig. 2 Effect of Cav3.1-GFP and Cav3.2-GFP C-terminal deletions on SPTAN1 and SPTBN2 binding in tsA-201 cells. (**a**) Cav3.1-GFP ΔCT (1851–1875) and wild type channel immunoprecipitates probed with anti-Spectrin αII (SPTAN1) polyclonal antibody. Densitometry analysis of SPTAN1 bound to Cav3.1-GFP immunoprecipitates is shown. ($P = 0.0051$, $n = 3$). (**b**) Cav3.2-GFP ΔCT (1860–1884) and wild type channel immunoprecipitates probed with anti-Spectrin αII (SPTAN1) polyclonal antibody. Densitometry analysis of SPTAN1 bound to Cav3.2-GFP immunoprecipitates is shown ($P = 0.0005$, n = 3). (**c**) Cav3.1-GFP ΔCT (1851–1875) and wild type channel immunoprecipitates probed with anti-Spectrin βII (SPTBN2) polyclonal antibody. Densitometry analysis of SPTBN2 bound to Cav3.1-GFP immunoprecipitates is shown ($P = 0.0085$, n = 3). (**d**) Cav3.2-GFP ΔCT (1860–1884) and wild type channel immunoprecipitates probed with anti-Spectrin βII (SPTBN2) polyclonal antibody. Densitometry analysis of SPTBN2 bound to Cav3.2-GFP immunoprecipitates is shown. ($P = 0.0047$, n = 3)

(1860–1884)) reduced, but did not completely eliminate binding of SPTAN1 to both channel isoforms (Fig. 2a and b), confirming that this region is involved in spectrin interactions, but also that spectrin may associate with contact sites in other regions of the channels. These putative additional interactions do not appear to involve the distal C-terminus regions, since deletion of residues 1875–2377 in Cav3.1 (Cav3.1-GFP ΔCT (1875–2377)) had no effect on co-immunoprecipitations with SPTAN1 (Additional file 1: Figure S1).

Given that other spectrin isoforms were pulled down with the C-terminal helix bait, we wanted to confirm these interactions in tsA-201 cells. Unfortunately, these cells do not appear to express spectrin-β1, and hence we could not test these interactions with this expression system. However, tsA-201 cells do express spectrin-βII (SPTBN2) which could be co-immunoprecipitated with both Cav3.1-GFP and Cav3.2-GFP (Fig. 2c and d). As with SPTAN1, the SPTBN2 interactions were significantly weakened by deleting the helical regions in the Cav3.1 and Cav3.2 C-termini (Fig. 2c and d). As these data are based upon co-immunoprecipitations and that SPTAN1 and SPTBN2 interact with each other, it is unclear if either the two spectrin isoforms is the primary interaction partner, or whether there may be another intermediate protein(s) involved in linking the channels to the cytoskeleton. Taken together, these data indicate that spectrins physically interact with a putative helical region conserved in the C-terminal domains of Cav3.1 and Cav3.2 calcium channels.

Ankyrin B interacts with T-type calcium channels

Direct interactions with spectrin have been reported for epithelial sodium channels, whereas neuronal voltage-gated sodium channels are reportedly linked to spectrin via ankyrin B or G [22]. We therefore examined binding of ankyrin B to Cav3.1 and Cav3.2 channels. Following expression of Cav3.1-GFP and Cav3.2-GFP constructs in tsA-201 cells immunoprecipitates with GFP were probed with an ankyrin B antibody, revealing interactions with both channel isoforms (Fig. 3a and b). Deletion of the proximal C-terminal alpha helix in the two channels reduced ankyrin B interactions with Cav3.1 and to a lesser extent with Cav3.2 (Fig. 3a and b). These data raise the possibility that, similar to voltage gated sodium channels, spectrin may link to Cav3 channels via ankyrin interactions.

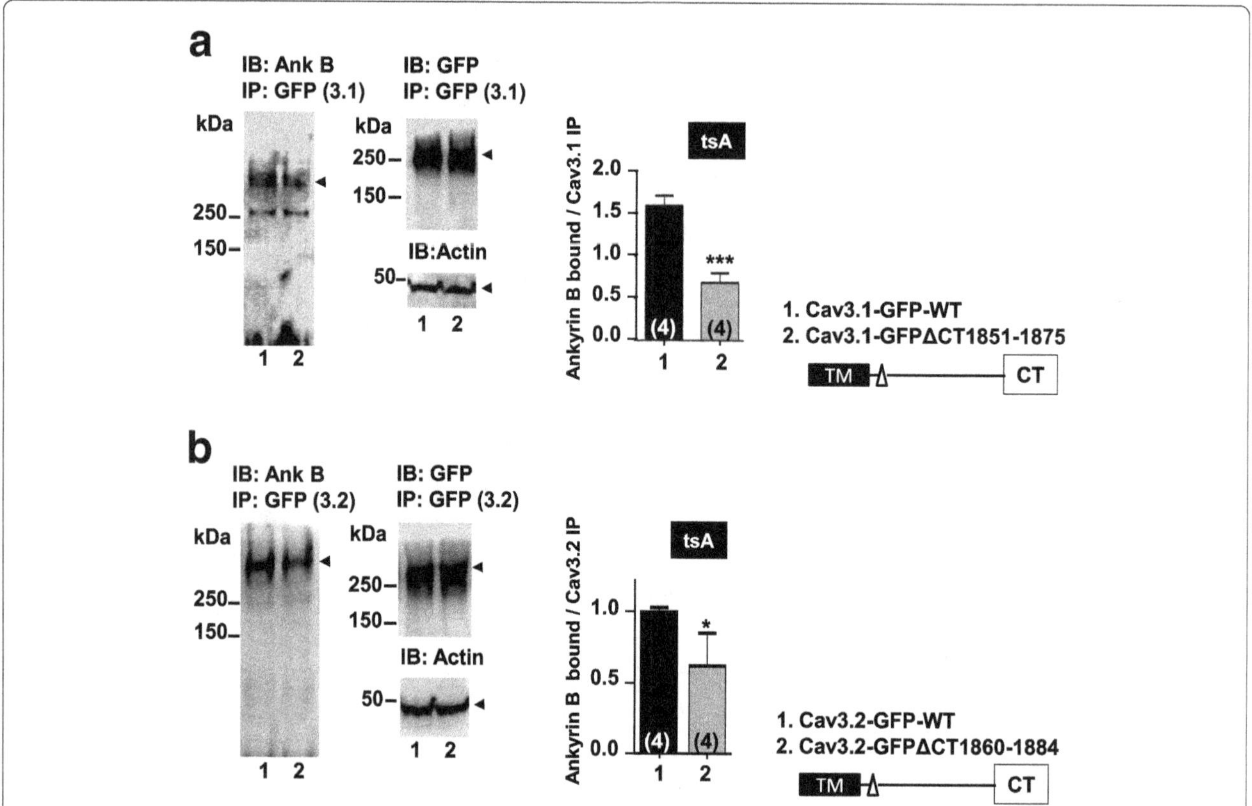

Fig. 3 Effect of Cav3.1-GFP and Cav3.2-GFP C-terminal deletions on ankyrin B binding in tsA-201 cells. (**a**) Cav3.1-GFP ΔCT (1851–1875) and wild type channel immunoprecipitates probed with anti-ankyrin B polyclonal antibody. Densitometry analysis of ankyrin B bound to Cav3.1-GFP immunoprecipitates is shown ($P = 0.0005$, $n = 4$). (**b**) Cav3.2-GFP ΔCT (1860–1884) and wild type channel immunoprecipitates probed with anti-ankyrin B polyclonal antibody. Densitometry analysis of ankyrin B bound to Cav3.2-GFP immunoprecipitates is shown ($P = 0.015$, n = 4)

Functional role of the Cav3 cytoskeletal interacting domain

We next examined whole cell calcium currents from wild type and deletion-mutant Cav3.1 expressed in tsA-201 cells by recording current-voltage relationships for wildtype Cav3.1 (wt) and mutant Cav3.1 (Δ1851–1875). Deletion of (MKHLEESNKEAKEEAE-LEAELELE) reduced Cav3.1 current density by approximately 75% (wt Cav3.1 = – 238.68 ± 20.36 pA/pF at – 20 mV; Cav3.1 Δ1851–1875 = – 60.96 ± 12.71 pA/pF at – 20 mV; $P < 0.001$, $n = 10$); Fig. 4a and b). Similarly, for wt Cav3.2 and mutant Cav3.2 (Δ1860–1884) deletion of conserved sequence (MKHLEESNKEAREDAELDAEIELE) significantly reduced the current density of Cav3.2 (wt = – 95.84 ± 4.45 pA/pF at – 20 mV; Cav3.2 Δ1860–1884 = – 35.67 ± 4.60 pA/pF at – 20 mV; $P < 0.001$, n = 10; Fig. 4c and d). There were no changes in the voltage-dependence of activation of the channels, nor were there any changes in channel kinetics (not shown), suggesting that the reduced current densities might be due to fewer channels in the plasma membrane. This notion is supported by experiments examining the cell surface pool of transiently expressed Cav3.1 channels incubated with a cell permeant (i.e., Tat epitope fused) disruptor peptide corresponding to the putative spectrin interaction site. When compared to a scrambled Tat control peptide, Cav3.1 cell surface expression was diminished by the disruptor peptide (Additional file 1: Figure S2), indicating that the cytoskeletal interactions may regulate the cell surface density of Cav3.1 channels.

Next, we tested whether deletion of the cytoskeleton interaction region in Cav3 channels altered Cav3.x channel trafficking. To address this, we transfected full-length and deletion-mutant Cav3-GFP channels into cultured hippocampal neurons and performed fluorescence recovery after photobleaching (FRAP) experiments. Fluorescence intensity mediated by the full-length Cav3.1-GFP and Cav3.2-GFP channels was found to recover more strongly than signals mediated by the deletion mutants (Fig. 5a-c), suggesting that the reduced ability of the deletion mutants to interact with cytoskeletal proteins affects the lateral mobility or insertion of new Cav3 channels in the plasma membrane.

We then examined the expression of endogenous Cav3 channels in cultured hippocampal neurons in response to knockdown of SPTAN1 and ankyrin B. For these experiments we focused on the Cav3.2 isoform. Western blots

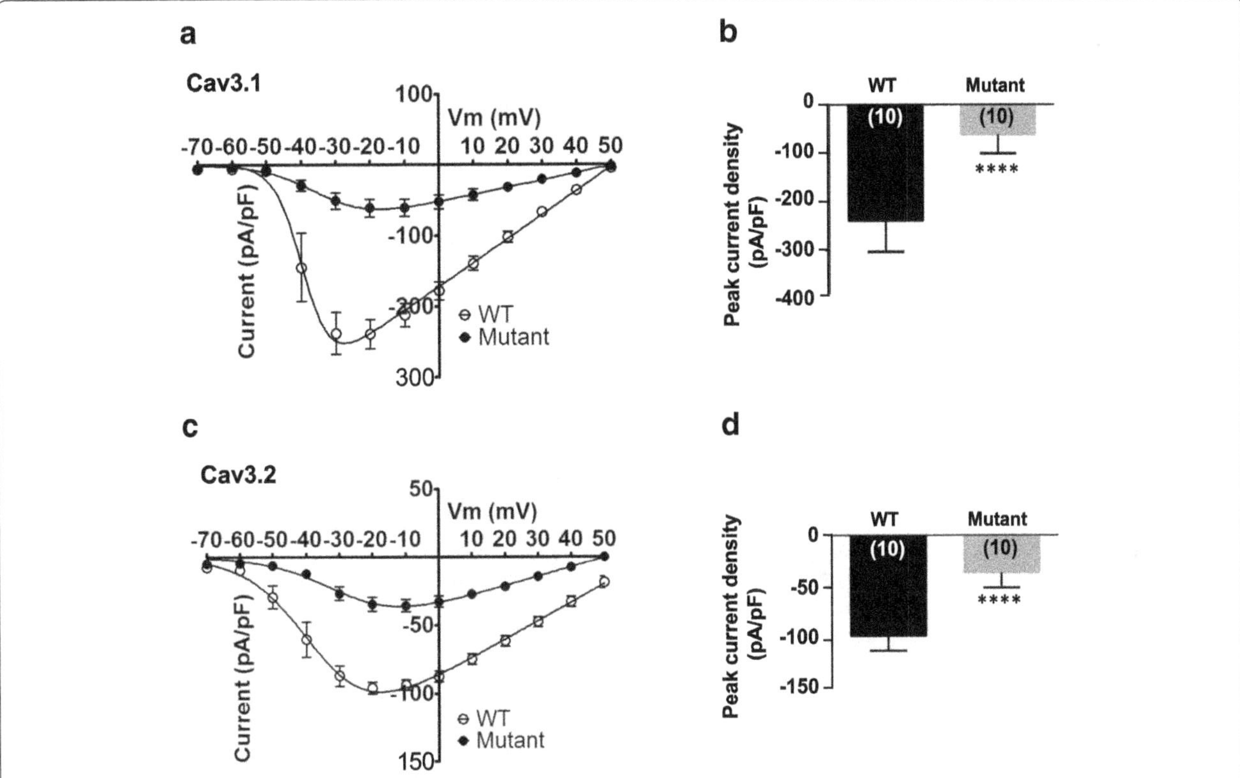

Fig. 4 Calcium currents evoked by wild type and mutant Cav3.1 and Cav3.2 channels in tsA-201 cells. (**a**) Current-voltage (I/V) relationship of wild type or mutant Cav3.1-GFP ΔCT (1851–1875) mutant channels ($n = 10$). Values are represented as means +/− S.E. The solid lines are fits with the Boltzmann equation. (**b**) Mean peak current density representation from wild type or mutant Cav3.1-GFP ΔCT (1851–1875) channels ($P < 0.001$, n = 10). Asterisks denote statistical significance relative to wild type (****$P < 0.0001$, Student's t-test). (**c**) Current-voltage (I/V) relationship of wild type or mutant Cav3.2-GFP ΔCT (1860–1884) channels ($n = 18–19$). Values are represented as means +/− S.E. The solid lines are fits with the Boltzmann equation. (**d**) Mean peak current density representation from wild type or mutant Cav3.2-GFP ΔCT (1860–1884) channels (P < 0.001, n = 10). Asterisks denote statistical significance relative to wild type (****P < 0.0001, Student's t-test)

confirmed the expression and subsequent shRNA-mediated knockdown of endogenous SPTAN1 and ankyrin B in hippocampal neurons (Fig. 6a and d). We performed immunostaining experiments in which endogenous Cav3.2 channels were stained with a Cav3.2 antibody. Cav3.2 channel expression was evident in cell bodies, axons and proximal dendrites (Fig. 6b and e). Upon shRNA-mediated knockdown of SPTAN1, total Cav3.2 fluorescence was consistently diminished (Fig. 6b and c). A similar effect was observed upon knockdown of ankyrin B (Fig. 6e and f). Altogether, these data are consistent with the reduced channel current densities and FRAP signals observed upon depletion of the Cav3 interaction domain, and support an effect of cytoskeletal elements in the expression of native T-type calcium channels.

Discussion

In this study, we used a proteomic approach to identify interacting partners of the proximal Cav3.1 and Cav3.2 C-terminus regions. The screen identified both α and β spectrin as both interacting partner with the first 24 amino acids of the C terminal region. Both spectrin subtypes are membrane cytoskeleton components [23, 24] and there is a growing body of literature implicating spectrins in the clustering of ion channels (e.g., sodium and potassium channels) at specific subcellular loci [25–27], often indirectly via specific ankyrins [22, 28, 29]. We confirmed the spectrin interactions via co-immunoprecipitation from mouse brain tissue and also identified ankyrin B as part of the putative Cav3.2/spectrin binding complex. Deletion of 24 amino acid residues of the proximal Cav3 C-terminus from the full-length channels reduced whole cell current densities in transient expression systems. Furthermore, shRNA depletion of both spectrin α and ankyrin B in hippocampal neurons reduced Cav3.2 type channel expression. Finally, fluorescence recovery experiments using GFP-tagged Cav3 channels in hippocampal neurons revealed that Cav3.1 and Cav3.2 channels lacking the interaction domain display significantly reduced mobility in the plasma membrane and/or trafficking to the membrane compared to wild type channels. Taken together, we conclude that cytoskeleton interactions are important determinants of T-type calcium channel trafficking to and within the plasma membrane.

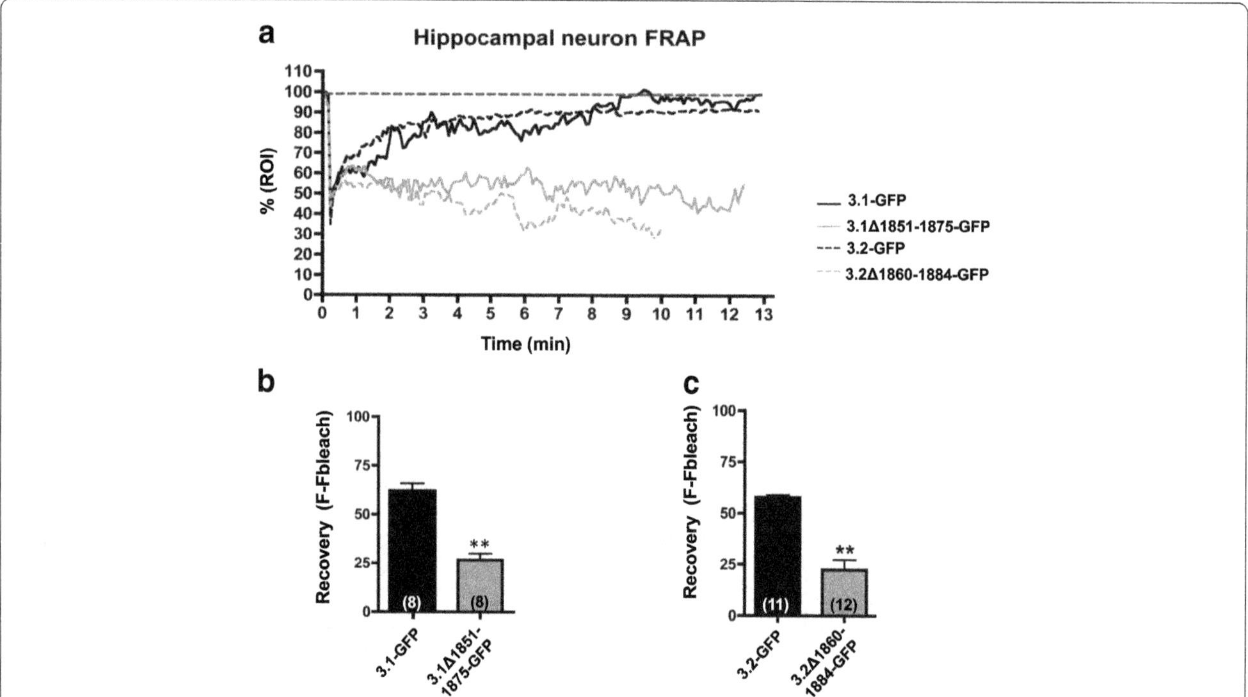

Fig. 5 Mobility of wild type and mutant Cav3.1 and Cav3.2 channels in hippocampal neurons. (**a**) Fluorescence recovery after photobleaching (FRAP) assay of Cav3.1-GFP wild type and ΔCT (1851–1875) mutant channels or Cav3.2-GFP wild type and ΔCT (1860–1884) mutant channels transfected into mouse hippocampal neuron cultures. (**b**) Recovery (Fluorescence-Fluorescence bleach) of Cav3.1-GFP wild type and ΔCT (1851–1875) mutant channels. Recovery values are calculated as F(maximum after photobleach)-F(photobleach) ($n = 8$ WT, $n = 8$ mutant, $P < 0.01$, Student's t-test). (**c**) Recovery (Fluorescence-Fluorescence bleach) of Cav3.2-GFP wild type and ΔCT (1860–1884) mutant channels. Recovery values are calculated as F(maximum after photobleach)-F(photobleach) ($n = 11$ WT, $n = 12$ mutant, $P < 0.01$, Student's t-test)

The molecular mechanisms by which these cytoskeletal interactions affect T-type channel trafficking remain to be determined. Within the plasma membrane, interactions of the channel with the cytoskeleton may facilitate the lateral trafficking due to dynamic cytoskeletal rearrangements. It is also possible that interactions with spectrin facilitate the effective translocation of the channel from the endoplasmic reticulum to the cell surface, either by facilitating transport, or by occluding an ER retention signal.

The data indicate that the proximal carboxy-terminus regions of Cav3.1 and Cav3.2 binds to spectrins (α/β) via a 24 amino acid stretch containing many negatively charged residues located in close proximity to the transmembrane domain of these channels. This interaction may be responsible for promoting binding of ankyrin B to the complex, likely via direct binding to the described α/β spectrin ankyrin binding repeat [18]. In contrast with the previously identified proline rich motif present in other ion channels [30] that binds to the SH3 domain in spectrins, this novel motif conserved across T-type calcium channels is enriched with glutamic and aspartic acids, possibly involved in electrostatic interactions with spectrin (α/β).

Literature from the voltage-gated sodium channel field identifies ankyrin as a key determinant of sodium channel clustering at Nodes of Ranvier [31, 32]. It is thus possible that spectrin/ankyrin interactions with Cav3 mediate a similar clustering/targeting role for localization of T-type channels at specific subcellular loci. The observation that deletion of the putative spectrin/ankyrin interaction motif in both Cav3.1 and Cav3.2 channels greatly impeded fluorescence recovery in FRAP experiments and reduced whole cell current densities is consistent with a role of the cytoskeleton trafficking to and within the plasma membrane. Whether these interactions are involved in targeting the channels to specific membrane compartments such as nodal regions, or synaptic/dendritic sites remains to be determined.

In the nervous system, T-type calcium channels fulfill two major roles. One is to regulate the excitability of neurons, being of particular importance in the corticothalamic circuitry wherein T-type channels are known to mediate rebound bursting [33] and is of particular relevance to the genesis of absence seizures [34]. A second major role that has emerged more recently is their contribution towards low threshold-mediated neurotransmitter release [1]. Indeed, Cav3 channels interact with syntaxin 1A and have been shown to contribute to synaptic release in dorsal horn synapses [7, 35, 36]. This is of particular relevance for conditions such as

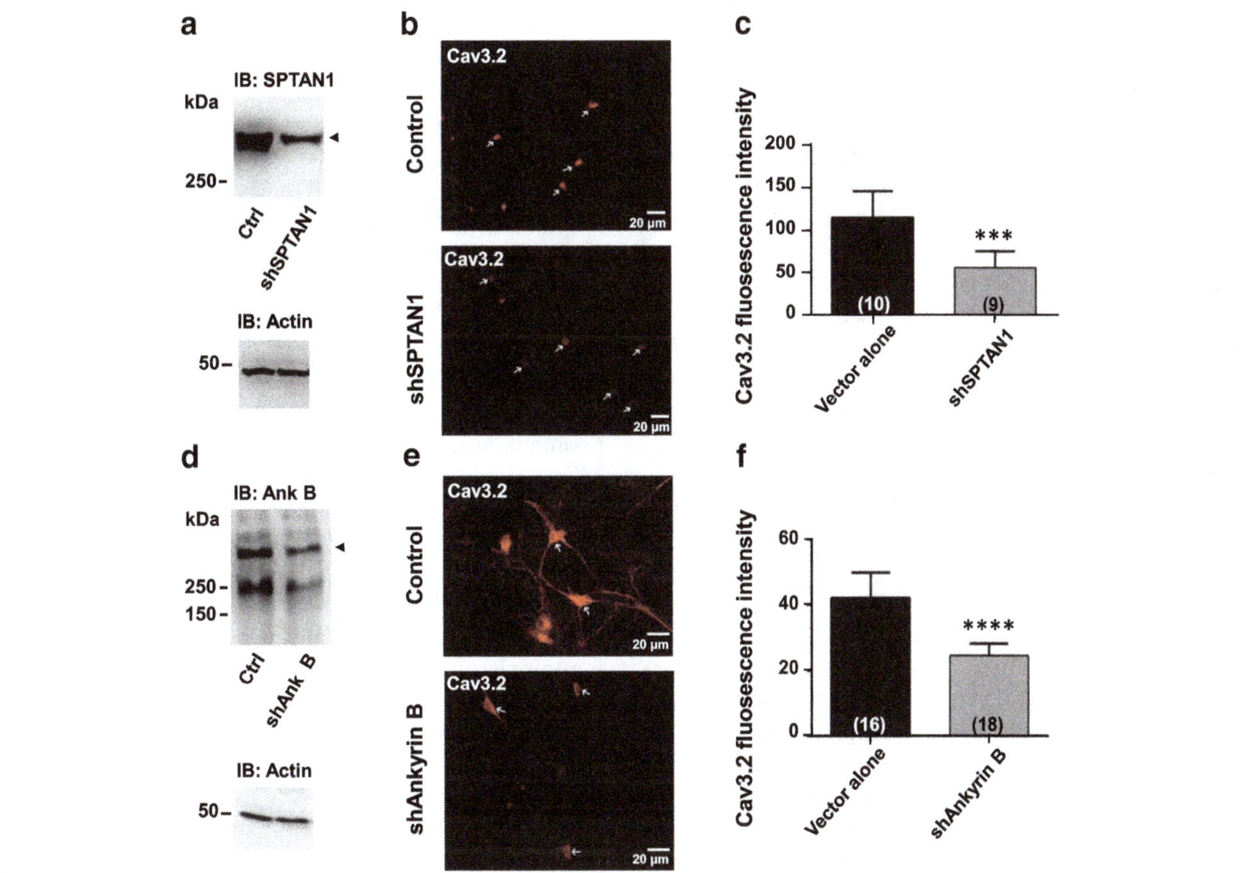

Fig. 6 SPTAN1 and ankyrin B knockdown effect on endogenous Cav3.2 calcium channel density in mouse and rat hippocampal neurons. (**a**) SPTAN1 expression levels in mouse hippocampal neurons treated with shRNA as seen by western blot. (**b**) Mouse hippocampal neurons untreated or treated with shRNA for SPTAN1 were stained for Cav3.2 channels with a specific anti-Cav3.2 polyclonal antibody. (**c**) Cav3.2 channel intensity values from untreated neurons or neurons treated with SPTAN1 shRNA. (**d**) Ankyrin B expression levels in rat hippocampal neurons treated with shRNA as seen by western blot. (**e**) Rat hippocampal neurons untreated or treated with shRNA for ankyrin B were stained for Cav3.2 channels with a specific anti-Cav3.2 polyclonal antibody. (**f**) Cav3.2 channel intensity values from untreated neurons or neurons treated with specific ankyrin B shRNA

neuropathic pain where increases in Cav3 channel current density facilitate neuronal firing and synaptic communications in the afferent pain pathway. Given their potent effects on T-type channel expression, spectrins and ankyrins may act as regulatory elements for controlling nervous system function via T-type channel interactions.

The regulation of T-type calcium channels by cytoskeletal elements is likely to extend beyond the nervous system. For example, ankyrin B is highly expressed in cardiac myocytes where it regulates excitation-contraction coupling in concert with other signaling molecules [37]. Myocytes also express Cav3.1 and Cav3.2 T-type calcium channels, especially during early post-natal development [38]. T-type channel expression is however increased under pathological conditions such as cardiac hypertrophy [39] thus it would be interesting to determine whether T-type channel expression increases are related to cytoskeletal remodeling.

Conclusion

In summary, we have identified cytoskeletal interactions as a molecular mechanism for regulating T-type channel mobility and current density. It is possible that targeting these interactions may offer a means for affecting T-type calcium channel activity in disorders such as chronic pain and epilepsy.

Methods

Drugs and peptides

Human biotin-Cav3.2-CT 1860–1884, biotin-Cav3.2-CT scramble peptides (Genemed synthesis, San Antonio, Tx). SPTAN1 and ankyrin B shRNAs were purchased from Thermo Scientific, Open Biosystems.

Cell culture and transfection

Human embryonic kidney tsA-201 cells were cultured as described [40]. Cells were transfected with Lipofectamine

2000 and used for biochemical and electrophysiological analysis 48–72 h post-transfection.

Hippocampal neuron primary cultures

Mouse or rat hippocampal neurons were dissociated as described before [41] and seeded at low density onto coverslips pretreated with poly-D-lysine (Sigma) followed by Laminin (Sigma) in 24-well plates. At day six of culture, transfection of cDNA was performed using Lipofectamine 2000 (Invitrogen) following the manufacturer's instructions. We used 1.5 μg of cDNA per well with 2 μl of Lipofectamine. cDNA and Lipofectamine solution were mixed together for 30 min at room temperature. Cells were incubated in cDNA–Lipofectamine 2000 complexes for 2 h at 37 °C and coverslips were placed back in their medium. Four days after transfection, immunostaining with GFP antibody (1500) was conducted at 37 °C.

Plasmids

To generate the GFP-tagged Cav3.1 or Cav3.2, the coding sequences of human Cav3.1 or human Cav3.2 was cloned into the pcDNA3.1(+) vector (Invitrogen) with stop codon removed; GFP was amplified by PCR and inserted into the C-terminus of Cav3.1 or Cav3.2. To delete the specific fragment amino acids 1860–1884 from Cav3.1 or Cav3.2, we used two-step PCR. The first round of PCR amplified the upstream and downstream flanking regions of that fragment. Products were purified and used as templates for the second round of PCR, which recombined these two regions together. The final PCR product was used to replace wide type Cav3.1 or Cav3.2 by making use of appropriate restriction sites in the two flanking regions.

Affinity precipitation of Cav3.2 interacting proteins

Mouse brain proteins were solubilized in buffer (in mM; 50 Tris pH 7.6, 150 NaCl, 1% Triton X-100, 1% NP40, 10 EDTA, 10 EGTA and protease inhibitors). Soluble proteins were collected by centrifugation at 16,100 g for 10 min. Supernatant fractions (500 μg) were precleared by incubation with neutravidin beads for 1 h at 4 °C (Thermo Scientific) and then incubated in a modified solubilization buffer (in mM; 50 Tris pH 7.6, 150 NaCl, 0.2% Triton X-100, 0.2% NP40, 10 EDTA, 10 EGTA and protease inhibitors) for 2 h at 4 °C with a human Cav3.2-carboxy-terminal (1860–1884 a.a.(MKHLEESNKEAR EDAELDAEIELEM)) or a scramble (SEMADLEKAENH MDEIMEKAEEREL) biotinylated peptides (5 μg) covalently linked to a C-terminal biotin (Genemed synthesis Inc., San Antonio, Tx). After Cav3.2-interacting proteins were collected, samples were washed three times with modified solubilization buffer. Bound proteins were analyzed by SDS-PAGE and visualized by Coomassie blue staining (Sigma). Visible bands were excised and samples analyzed by MALDI/TOF-MS (Bruker Instruments Co., Bremen, Germany).

Western blotting

Western blot analysis was performed using anti-actin mouse (Sigma), anti-GFP (Abcam) anti-αII-spectrin (Santa Cruz, Biotechnology, Inc.) and anti-ankyrin B (Santa Cruz Biotechnology, Inc.) rabbit antibodies. Western blot quantification was performed using densitometry analysis (Quantity One-BioRad software). Student's t-tests for unpaired data were performed to determine statistical significance.

Co-immunoprecipitation assays

Mouse whole brain tissue or tsA-201 cells were lysed in a modified RIPA buffer (in mM; 50 Tris, 100 NaCl, 0.2% (*v*/v) Triton X-100, 0.2% (v/v) NP-40, 10 EDTA + protease inhibitor cocktail, pH 7.5) that was used to co-immunoprecipitate Cav3.2 channels with spectrin (α/β) or ankyrin B proteins. Lysates were prepared by sonicating samples at 60% pulse for 10 s and by centrifugation at 13,000 rpm for 15 min at 4 °C. Supernatants were transferred to new tubes and solubilized proteins were incubated with 50 μl of Protein G/A beads (Piercenet) and 2 μg of anti-Cav3.2 (H-300, Santa Cruz Biotechnologies, Inc) antibody or anti-GFP antibody (Abcam) overnight while tumbling at 4 °C. Total inputs were taken from whole cell samples representing 4% of total protein and probed for actin. Co-immunoprecipitates were washed twice with (mM) 150 NaCl 50 Tris pH 7.5 buffer, beads were aspirated to dryness. Laemmli buffer was added and samples were incubated at 96 °C for 7 min. Eluted samples were loaded on 7.5% Tris-glycine gel and resolved using SDS-PAGE. Samples were transferred to 0.45 mm polyvinylidenedifluoride (PDVF) membranes by dry transfer using an Iblot machine (Invitrogen).

Electrophysiological recordings

Whole-cell voltage-clamp recordings for tsA-201 cells were performed 72 h after transfection with cDNA (Cav3.1-GFP wild type (2 μg) or Cav3.1-GFP Mutant (2 μg) and Cav3.2-GFP wild type or Cav3.2-GFP Mutant (2 μg)). Recordings were conducted with 10 mM barium as the charge carrier, using internal and external recording solutions; (in mM): 110 CsCl, 3 Mg-ATP, 0.5 Na-GTP, 2.5 MgCl2, 5 D-glucose, 10 EGTA, 10 HEPES (pH 7.3 with CsOH). The external solution contained (in mM): 10 BaCl2, 1 MgCl2, 140 TEACl, 10 D-glucose, 10 HEPES (pH 7.2 with TEAOH). Currents were elicited from a holding potential of − 100 mV and depolarized from − 70 to + 50 mV with 10-mV increments. Data were collected from multiple batches of transfections with similar numbers of cells tested from the different groups. For data analysis, peak currents and cell capacitance were measured and converted into current density.

FRAP assays

Primary hippocampal neurons were transfected at 10 DIV and imaged 48 h afterward. Transfections were done with 2 μg of DNA/ matek dish with 6ul of Lipofectamine 2000 for 2 h.

Photobleaching experiments: FRAP experiments were imaged using a ZEISS 510 LSM. A ROI was selected on an axon proximal to the cell body of a neuron. After 3 baseline images, 10 iterations of 100% laser power was used to bleach the ROI, and recovery imaged for 13 min, with a picture every 5 s. Fluorescence intensity values were normalized to an initial intensity of 100%. Cells were excluded if photobleaching did not decrease fluorescence intensity to more than 50% of initial 100%. Traces: Fluorescence intensity values are normalized to an initial value of 100%. Intensity values were normalized to an initial value of 100%. Recovery values are calculated as F maximum after photobleach- F photobleach.

Immunofluorescence

Briefly, cultured rat hippocampal neurons were washed twice with PBS containing (mM) 1 $MgCl_2$ and 2 $CaCl_2$. Neurons were fixed with 4% paraformaldehyde for 20 min at room temperature (RT) and washed 3 times after fixation. Then neurons were permeabilized with PBS containing 0.1% triton x-100 and 2 mg/ml BSA for 30 min. Neurons were blocked with PBS containing 4% milk and 2 mg/ml BSA for 2 h at RT. Cav3.2 (mouse anti-Cav3.2, 1 μg/ml, Novus Biologicals,CA) primary antibodies were incubated overnight at 4 °C. After washing three times, the secondary antibodies Alexafluor 546 conjugated Donkey anti-mouse (Thermo Fisher Scientific, CA) were incubated 2 h. All images were digitally captured with an 8 bit camera, thus giving grey level (intensity) values of 0–255. Immunostaining was visualized using a 40 × 0.4 NA objective lens on a Zeiss LSM 510 META confocal systems, running Velocity 6.

Data analysis and statistics

For biochemical and electrophysiological analyses, data values are presented as mean ± SEM for n experiments. Statistical significance was determined using Student's t test unless stated otherwise: $^{*}p < 0.05$; $^{**}\ p < 0.01$; $^{***}\ p < 0.001$; NS, statistically not different.

Additional file

Additional file 1: Figure S1. Binding of SPTAN1 to Cav3.1-GFP ΔCT 1875–2377 mutant channels lacking a distal C-terminus region. Cav3.1-GFP ΔCT (1875–2377) and wild type channel immunoprecipitates from transfected tsA-201 cells probed with anti-Spectrin αII (SPTAN1) polyclonal antibody. Densitometry analysis of SPTAN1 bound to Cav3.1-GFP immunoprecipitates is shown. **Figure S2.** Disrupting Cav3.1 SPTAN1 interactions reduces cell surface expression of Cav3.1. Left: Surface biotinylation experiments on Cav3.1 channels transiently expressed in tsA-201 cells in the presence of a cell permeant Tat peptide corresponding to the putative spectrin interaction site (Tat-Cav3.1-CT) on the channel, or a scrambled peptide sequence. Right: Densitometry analysis of Cav3.1 surface pool normalized to the actin control. Note that the Tat- Cav3.1-CT peptide reduces the cell surface expression of the channel by ~40%. (DOC 118 kb)

Abbreviations

FRAP: Fluorescence recovery after photobleaching; GFP: Green fluorescent protein; PCR: Polymerase chain reaction; shRNA: Short hairpin ribonucleic acid, wt: wild type

Funding

This work was supported by a Discovery grant to GWZ from the Natural Sciences and Engineering Research Council. GWZ is a Canada Research Chair in Molecular Neuroscience. Work in the laboratory of TPS is supported by an operating grant from the Canadian Institutes of Health Research (#10677) and the Canada Research Chair in Biotechnology and Genomics-Neurobiology.

Authors' contributions

AG-C-performed biochemistry experiments, and with GWZ designed the study and co-wrote the manuscript, FXZ, VH, IAS, SC, SA, JK and JH performed experiments, LC harvested and cultured tissue, TS and GWZ supervised experiments, and GZ and TPS edited the manuscript. All authors read and approved the final manuscript.

Competing interests

The authors declare that they have no competing interests.

Author details

[1]Department of Physiology and Pharmacology, Hotchkiss Brain Institute and Alberta Children's Hospital Research Institute, Cumming School of Medicine, University of Calgary, 3330 Hospital Dr. NW, Calgary T2N 4N1, Canada. [2]Michael Smith Laboratories and Djavad Mowafaghian Centre for Brain Health, University of British Colombia, Vancouver, BC, Canada.

References

1. Weiss N, Hameed S, Fernandez-Fernandez JM, et al. A ca(v)3.2/syntaxin-1A signaling complex controls T-type channel activity and low-threshold exocytosis. J Biol Chem. 2012;287(4):2810–8.
2. Weiss N, Zamponi GW, De Waard M. How do T-type calcium channels control low-threshold exocytosis? Commun Integr Biol. 2012;5(4):377–80.
3. Perez-Reyes E. Molecular physiology of low-voltage-activated t-type calcium channels. Physiol Rev. 2003;83(1):117–61.
4. McKay BE, McRory JE, Molineux ML, et al. Ca(V)3 T-type calcium channel isoforms differentially distribute to somatic and dendritic compartments in rat central neurons. Eur J Neurosci. 2006;24(9):2581–94.
5. Zamponi GW, Lory P, Perez-Reyes E. Role of voltage-gated calcium channels in epilepsy. Pflugers Arch. 2010;460(2):395–403.
6. Miwa H, Kondo T. T-type calcium channel as a new therapeutic target for tremor. Cerebellum. 2011;10(3):563–9.

7. Garcia-Caballero A, Gadotti VM, Stemkowski P, et al. The deubiquitinating enzyme USP5 modulates neuropathic and inflammatory pain by enhancing Cav3.2 channel activity. Neuron. 2014;83(5):1144–58.
8. Tringham E, Powell KL, Cain SM, et al. T-type calcium channel blockers that attenuate thalamic burst firing and suppress absence seizures. Sci Transl Med. 2012;4(121):121ra19.
9. M'Dahoma S, Gadotti VM, Zhang FX, et al. Effect of the T-type channel blocker KYS-05090S in mouse models of acute and neuropathic pain. Pflugers Arch. 2016;468(2):193–9.
10. Lu HK, Fern RJ, Nee JJ, Barrett PQ. Ca(2+)-dependent activation of T-type Ca2+ channels by calmodulin-dependent protein kinase II. Am J Phys. 1994; 267(1 Pt 2):F183–9.
11. Lu HK, Fern RJ, Luthin D, et al. Angiotensin II stimulates T-type Ca2+ channel currents via activation of a G protein, Gi. Am J Phys. 1996;271(4 Pt 1):C1340–9.
12. Huang CH, Chen YC, Chen CC. Physical interaction between calcineurin and C.
13. Asmara H, Micu I, Rizwan AP, et al. A T-type channel-calmodulin complex triggers alphaCaMKII activation. Mol Brain. 2017;10(1):37.
14. Proft J, Rzhepetskyy Y, Lazniewska J, et al. The Cacna1h mutation in the GAERS model of absence epilepsy enhances T-type ca(2+) currents by altering calnexin-dependent trafficking of Cav3.2 channels. Sci Rep. 2017;7(1):11513.
15. Anderson D, Mehaffey WH, Iftinca M, et al. Regulation of neuronal activity by Cav3-Kv4 channel signaling complexes. Nat Neurosci. 2010;13(3):333–7.
16. Turner RW, Kruskic M, Teves M, Scheidl-Yee T, Hameed S, Zamponi GW. Neuronal expression of the intermediate conductance calcium-activated potassium channel KCa3.1 in the mammalian central nervous system. Pflugers Arch. 2015;467(2):311–28.
17. Rehak R, Bartoletti TM, Engbers JD, Berecki G, Turner RW, Zamponi GW. Low voltage activation of KCa1.1 current by Cav3-KCa1.1 complexes. PLoS One. 2013;8(4):e61844.
18. Zhang R, Zhang C, Zhao Q, Li D. Spectrin: structure, function and disease. Sci China Life Sci. 2013;56(12):1076–85.
19. Grum VL, Li D, MacDonald RI, Mondragon A. Structures of two repeats of spectrin suggest models of flexibility. Cell. 1999;98(4):523–35.
20. Goodman SR. Discovery of nonerythroid spectrin to the demonstration of its key role in synaptic transmission. Brain Res Bull. 1999;50(5–6):345–6.
21. Featherstone DE, Davis WS, Dubreuil RR, Broadie K. Drosophila alpha- and beta-spectrin mutations disrupt presynaptic neurotransmitter release. J Neurosci. 2001;21(12):4215–24.
22. Bennett V, Healy J. Membrane domains based on ankyrin and spectrin associated with cell-cell interactions. Cold Spring Harb Perspect Biol. 2009; 1(6):a003012.
23. Machnicka B, Czogalla A, Hryniewicz-Jankowska A, et al. Spectrins: a structural platform for stabilization and activation of membrane channels, receptors and transporters. Biochim Biophys Acta. 2014;1838(2):620–34.
24. Dubreuil RR. Functional links between membrane transport and the spectrin cytoskeleton. J Membr Biol. 2006;211(3):151–61.
25. Hund TJ, Snyder JS, Wu X, et al. Beta(IV)-Spectrin regulates TREK-1 membrane targeting in the heart. Cardiovasc Res. 2014;102(1):166–75.
26. Kosaka T, Komada M, Kosaka K. Sodium channel cluster, betaIV-spectrin and ankyrinG positive "hot spots" on dendritic segments of parvalbumin-containing neurons and some other neurons in the mouse and rat main olfactory bulbs. Neurosci Res. 2008;62(3):176–86.
27. Devaux JJ. The C-terminal domain of ssIV-spectrin is crucial for KCNQ2 aggregation and excitability at nodes of Ranvier. J Physiol. 2010;588(Pt 23):4719–30.
28. Makara MA, Curran J, Little SC, et al. Ankyrin-G coordinates intercalated disc signaling platform to regulate cardiac excitability in vivo. Circ Res. 2014; 115(11):929–38.
29. Clarkson YL, Perkins EM, Cairncross CJ, Lyndon AR, Skehel PA, Jackson M. Beta-III spectrin underpins ankyrin R function in Purkinje cell dendritic trees: protein complex critical for sodium channel activity is impaired by SCA5-associated mutations. Hum Mol Genet. 2014;23(14):3875–82.
30. Rotin D, Bar-Sagi D, O'Brodovich H, et al. An SH3 binding region in the epithelial Na+ channel (alpha rENaC) mediates its localization at the apical membrane. EMBO J. 1994;13(19):4440–50.
31. Buffington SA, Rasband MN. Na+ channel-dependent recruitment of Navbeta4 to axon initial segments and nodes of Ranvier. J Neurosci. 2013; 33(14):6191–202.
32. Ho TS, Zollinger DR, Chang KJ, et al. A hierarchy of ankyrin-spectrin complexes clusters sodium channels at nodes of Ranvier. Nat Neurosci. 2014;17(12):1664–72.
33. Huguenard JR, Prince DA. A novel T-type current underlies prolonged ca(2 +)-dependent burst firing in GABAergic neurons of rat thalamic reticular nucleus. J Neurosci. 1992;12(10):3804–17.
34. Khosravani H, Zamponi GW. Voltage-gated calcium channels and idiopathic generalized epilepsies. Physiol Rev. 2006;86(3):941–66. https://doi.org/10.1152/physrev.00002.2006.
35. Jacus MO, Uebele VN, Renger JJ, Todorovic SM. Presynaptic Cav3.2 channels regulate excitatory neurotransmission in nociceptive dorsal horn neurons. J Neurosci. 2012;32(27):9374–82.
36. Stemkowski P, Garcia-Caballero A, De Maria GV, et al. TRPV1 nociceptor activity initiates USP5/T-type channel-mediated plasticity. Cell Rep. 2017; 18(9):2289–90.
37. Koenig SN, Mohler PJ. The evolving role of ankyrin-B in cardiovascular disease. Heart Rhythm. 2017;14(12):1884–9.
38. Ono K, Iijima T. Cardiac T-type ca(2+) channels in the heart. J Mol Cell Cardiol. 2010;48(1):65–70.
39. Cribbs L. T-type calcium channel expression and function in the diseased heart. Channels (Austin). 2010;4(6):447–52.
40. Altier C, Garcia-Caballero A, Simms B, et al. The Cavbeta subunit prevents RFP2-mediated ubiquitination and proteasomal degradation of L-type channels. Nat Neurosci. 14(2):173–80.
41. Khosravani H, Altier C, Zamponi GW, Colicos MA. The Arg473Cys-neuroligin-1 mutation modulates NMDA mediated synaptic transmission and receptor distribution in hippocampal neurons. FEBS Lett. 2005;579(29):6587–94.

16

Mechanistic target of rapamycin is necessary for changes in dendritic spine morphology associated with long-term potentiation

Fredrick E. Henry[1,2,3†], William Hockeimer[2,3†], Alex Chen[1,2,3], Shreesh P. Mysore[4] and Michael A. Sutton[1,2,3,5*]

Abstract

Alterations in the strength of excitatory synapses in the hippocampus is believed to serve a vital function in the storage and recall of new information in the mammalian brain. These alterations involve the regulation of both functional and morphological features of dendritic spines, the principal sites of excitatory synaptic contact. New protein synthesis has been implicated extensively in the functional changes observed following long-term potentiation (LTP), and changes to spine morphology have similarly been documented extensively following synaptic potentiation. However, mechanistic links between de novo translation and the structural changes of potentiated spines are less clear. Here, we assess explicitly the potential contribution of new protein translation under control of the mechanistic target of rapamycin (mTOR) to LTP-associated changes in spine morphology. Utilizing genetic and pharmacological manipulations of mTORC1 function in combination with confocal microscopy in live dissociated hippocampal cultures, we demonstrate that chemically-induced LTP (cLTP) requires *do novo* protein synthesis and intact mTORC1 signaling. We observed a striking diversity in response properties across morphological classes, with mushroom spines displaying a particular sensitivity to altered mTORC1 signaling across varied levels of synaptic activity. Notably, while pharmacological inhibition of mTORC1 signaling significantly diminished glycine-induced changes in spine morphology, transient genetic upregulation of mTORC1 signaling was insufficient to produce spine enlargements on its own. In contrast, genetic upregulation of mTORC1 signaling promoted rapid expansion in spine head diameter when combined with otherwise sub-threshold synaptic stimulation. These results suggest that synaptic activity-derived signaling pathways act in combination with mTORC1-dependent translational control mechanisms to ultimately regulate changes in spine morphology. As several monogenic neurodevelopmental disorders with links to Autism and Intellectual Disability share a common feature of dysregulated mTORC1 signaling, further understanding of the role of this signaling pathway in regulating synapse function and morphology will be essential in the development of novel therapeutic interventions.

Introduction

Dendritic spines comprise the primary sites of excitatory synaptic contact in the mammalian central nervous system. At mature synapses, these actin-rich protrusions are typically composed of a large head compartment densely packed with proteins of numerous types [48], and a thin neck region that attaches the head to the dendritic shaft. The high resistance of the neck can significantly boost synaptically-driven depolarization of the associated spine head [17]. The distinct structural characteristics of spines are believed to provide both chemical and electrical compartmentalization of incoming synaptic signals [5, 14].

In mature networks, synaptic connections at dendritic spines can be quite stable, as newly emergent spines generated after motor learning have been shown to persist for

* Correspondence: masutton@med.umich.edu
†Equal contributors
1Neuroscience Graduate Program, University of Michigan, Ann Arbor, MI 48109, USA
2Molecular and Behavioral Neuroscience Institute, University of Michigan, Ann Arbor, MI 48109, USA
Full list of author information is available at the end of the article

months [62]. Yet, individual spines have long been known to be highly dynamic structures [21]. While the distribution of spine size across the dendritic arbor of a single neuron can be quite variable [30], spine size generally correlates with excitatory synapse strength both in vitro [37] and in vivo [41]. Though clear mechanistic explanations for this correlation are just beginning to be understood [45], it is generally accepted that spine head diameter and synapse strength co-vary during the expression of long term potentiation (LTP), for example, because additional volume is required in the spine head to accommodate the insertion of additional AMPA receptors into the postsynaptic density [31, 38, 42].

The molecular mechanisms involved in the regulation of spine size and shape largely involve remodeling of the actin cytoskeleton [10]. Cytoskeletal rearrangement is necessary for the expression of long lasting plasticity at excitatory synapses, as inhibitors of actin polymerization impair LTP in the CA1 region of the hippocampus [25, 26]. The Rho family of small GTPases has been shown to play pivotal roles in the induction and maintenance of altered spine morphology, particularly in the context of long lasting synaptic plasticity [60]. An emerging model of the signaling dynamics involved in spine enlargement during LTP suggests that calcium influx through NMDARs activates CaMKIIα, leading to the subsequent recruitment of multiple RhoGTPases, wherein RhoA is critical for the initial enlargement of spine size and Cdc42 is necessary for sustaining these structural changes over time [29, 39, 40].

In addition to cytoskeletal remodeling, there is also a well-established role for new protein synthesis in the expression of long lasting plasticity at excitatory synapses. While early work focused on the contribution of cell-wide changes in gene expression via altered transcription [36], more recent evidence has established a role for de novo protein translation operating locally in dendrites during the expression of long term plasticity and memory formation [54]. Despite a clear requirement for actin remodeling as well as new protein synthesis during LTP, relatively little is known about whether these processes influence each other or are otherwise co-regulated for the expression of long lasting changes in synaptic strength.

Insofar as alterations in spine morphology during LTP are indeed bolstered by or are dependent on de novo protein synthesis, it is currently an open question as to the specific signaling pathways that may be involved in linking these processes. Given the previously demonstrated importance of BDNF signaling and protein synthesis in spine enlargement driven by local glutamate uncaging [13, 19, 58], one system of particular interest is the mechanistic target of rapamycin complex 1 (mTORC1) pathway. The mTORC1 pathway is known to be activated by BDNF signaling at excitatory synapses [49, 57] and is a well-characterized regulator of new protein synthesis, operating at the level of translation initiation [34]. mTORC1 signaling is necessary for the induction of LTP in the CA1 region of the hippocampus, where it has been demonstrated to act locally in dendrites to orchestrate the synthesis of new proteins which are crucial for long lasting changes in synaptic strength [8, 56, 61]. mTORC1 has also been shown to play a role in dendritic spine morphology as chronic pharmacological blockade of mTORC1 results in a decrease in spine density in dissociated hippocampal neurons [27]. In addition, animal models which harbor mutations leading to dysregulated mTORC1 signaling display deficits in long term potentiation [11, 53], and commonly exhibit abnormal spine morphology [28, 55]. Collectively, these results suggest that mTORC1 may play an active role in regulating new spine structure, though whether it contributes to morphological changes during long term potentiation remains an open question.

Here, we use a live cell imaging approach to demonstrate a requirement for mTORC1-dependent protein synthesis in the emergence of altered spine morphology after chemically induced LTP. We find that mTORC1 activation is not sufficient for changes in spine morphology, as transient genetic enhancement of mTORC1 activity via overexpression of a constitutively active mutant version of the upstream mTORC1 effector Rheb does not induce increases in spine head volume on its own. However, when paired with a subthreshold dose of glycine, mTORC1 activation results in robust increases in spine volume, suggesting that the combined action of mTORC1 signaling and other synaptically driven signals are required for activity-dependent changes in spine morphology. As dysregulation in spine morphology is a common feature of many neuropsychiatric disorders including autism spectrum disorders (ASD) and schizophrenia [43], a more precise understanding of the mechanisms that regulate their properties in response to changes in activity will be essential for the development of future therapeutic advances.

Methods

Cell culture and transfection

Dissociated postnatal hippocampal neuron cultures, prepared from postnatal day 1–2 rat pups of either sex, were plated at a density of 230–460 mm^2 in poly-D-lysine-coated glass bottom Petri dishes (Mattek), as previously described [24]. Cultures were maintained for at least 21 DIV at 37 °C in growth medium [Neurobasal A supplemented with B27 and Glutamax-1 (Invitrogen)] before use. To achieve sparse expression, neurons were transfected with 0.5 μg of total DNA using the Ca^{2+} phosphate CalPhos Transfection kit (ClonTech) according to the manufacturer's protocol. Unless otherwise indicated, all experiments were performed 24 h post-transfection.

Chemically-induced LTP

Under baseline conditions, neurons were incubated in HEPES-buffered saline (HBS) containing (in mM) the following: 119 NaCl, 5 KCl, 2 $CaCl_2$, 2 $MgCl_2$, 30 Glucose, 10 HEPES, pH 7.4. Pharmacological induction of LTP in cultured hippocampal neurons was achieved via brief (5 min) exposure to a Mg^{2+} –free HBS solution supplemented with (in mM): 0.4 Glycine (Fisher, Waltham, MA), 0.02 Bicuculline (Tocris), and 0.003 Strychnine (Tocris, Bristol, UK) Neurons were immediately washed with warm HBS after glycine stimulation and imaged.

Live-imaging

Neurons were imaged 1–3 days post-transfection. All imaging was performed on an inverted Olympus FV1000 laser-scanning confocal microscope using a Plan-Apochromat 63×/1.4 oil objective with 1× or 2× digital zoom. GFP was excited with the 488 nm line of an argon ion laser and emitted light was typically collected between 500 and 530 nm with a tunable emission filter. Z-stack images of eGFP signal were obtained at 10 min intervals, beginning with a pre-stimulus series of baseline measures, immediately after completion of the 5 min glycine stimulus, then regularly until 45 min post-treatment. During the imaging session, cells were perfused with HBS using a closed-loop perfusion system (Ismatec, Wertheim, Germany) and maintained at 37 °C using an in-line heater (Warner Instrument Corporation, Hamden CT). The perfusion loop was opened after stimulation to empty the system of glycine. During experiments involving treatment with anisomycin or rapamycin, these reagents were added to the HBS and perfused over the cells for the duration of the experiment.

Analysis

Maximum projected Z-stack images (6 per cell) were first preprocessed in ImageJ (NIH, Bethesda, MD). Series of z-stacks obtained over the course of a 45 min imaging session were registered using the StackReg plugin (EPFL, Lausanne, Switzerland). Images were adjusted for size (1500 × 1500 pixels) and type (8-bit) before further processing. Automated analysis of spine morphology was performed using a custom package ('SpineZap') developed in the MATLAB computing environment (Mathworks, Natick, MA). Neurons were imaged so that their cell body was positioned to one corner slightly out of frame, to maximize the length of primary dendrite captured. ROI's were defined over all visible spines on primary, secondary, and tertiary dendrites beginning immediately adjacent to the cell soma and extending progressively along the length of the primary dendrite. We did not detect obvious differences in the behavior of proximal and distal spines and those spines emanating from primary dendrites vs secondary or tertiary dendrites. The following parameters were automatically generated for each spine: head width, length, neck width and morphological class. Spines were grouped into the following morphological classes based on previously published anatomical studies using electron microscopy [15, 44]: filopodial, mushroom, flat (or "cup-shaped") thin, and stubby. Filopodia are defined as protrusions with a length greater than or equal to 5 μm. Mushroom spines are defined as having a head to neck ratio greater than or equal to 2.5. Flat spines are defined as having a head width to length ratio greater than or equal to 1. Thin spines are defined as having a length to neck width ratio greater than or equal to 3. A spine that does not satisfy any of these conditions is classified as a stubby spine. The class of each spine is determined by checking against these conditions sequentially (in the order described above). Data analysis was performed in Origin (OriginLab, Northhampton, MA) and MATLAB. Statistical differences between multiple groups were assessed by ANOVA, followed by Tuckey's HSD post hoc tests. For comparisons of probability distribution using the Kolmogorov–Smirnov test, alpha was set at 0.001. Ideal number of clusters for the dataset in Fig. 2e-i was determined using the NbClust package for R [9].

Results

To study the role of mTORC1 in spine morphological plasticity, we imaged mature cultured hippocampal neurons (> 21 DIV) transiently transfected with eGFP following cLTP induction using a glycine-induced stimulus protocol (5-min exposure to 400 μM glycine in a low Mg^{2+}, HBS-based, stimulus solution). As previously reported [31, 42], we find that this induction protocol produces reliable, long-lasting increases in postsynaptic strength as assessed via changes in mEPSC amplitude and frequency in whole-cell voltage-clamp recordings (Fig. 1a-d). In cells expressing GFP to mark the extent of dendritic protrusions (Fig. 1e), we found that cLTP induction elicited a strong, time-dependent increase in spine head width, with population averages showing significant differences as early as 15 min after stimulation (Fig. 1e, Glycine group: 1538 spines across 19 neurons). Glycine treatment induced a significant rightward shift in the cumulative distribution of spine head widths in the population of assessed spines (Fig. 1g). Cells treated with HBS alone as a control group displayed no significant change from baseline levels over the course of the imaging period (Fig. 1f, Control group: 1320 spines across 24 neurons). Though we observed an average change in spine head width of +28.85% when assessed 45 min post-stimulation, the population as a whole exhibited a diverse set of responses, in terms of both valence and intensity (Fig. 1h-i). Roughly 35% of spines

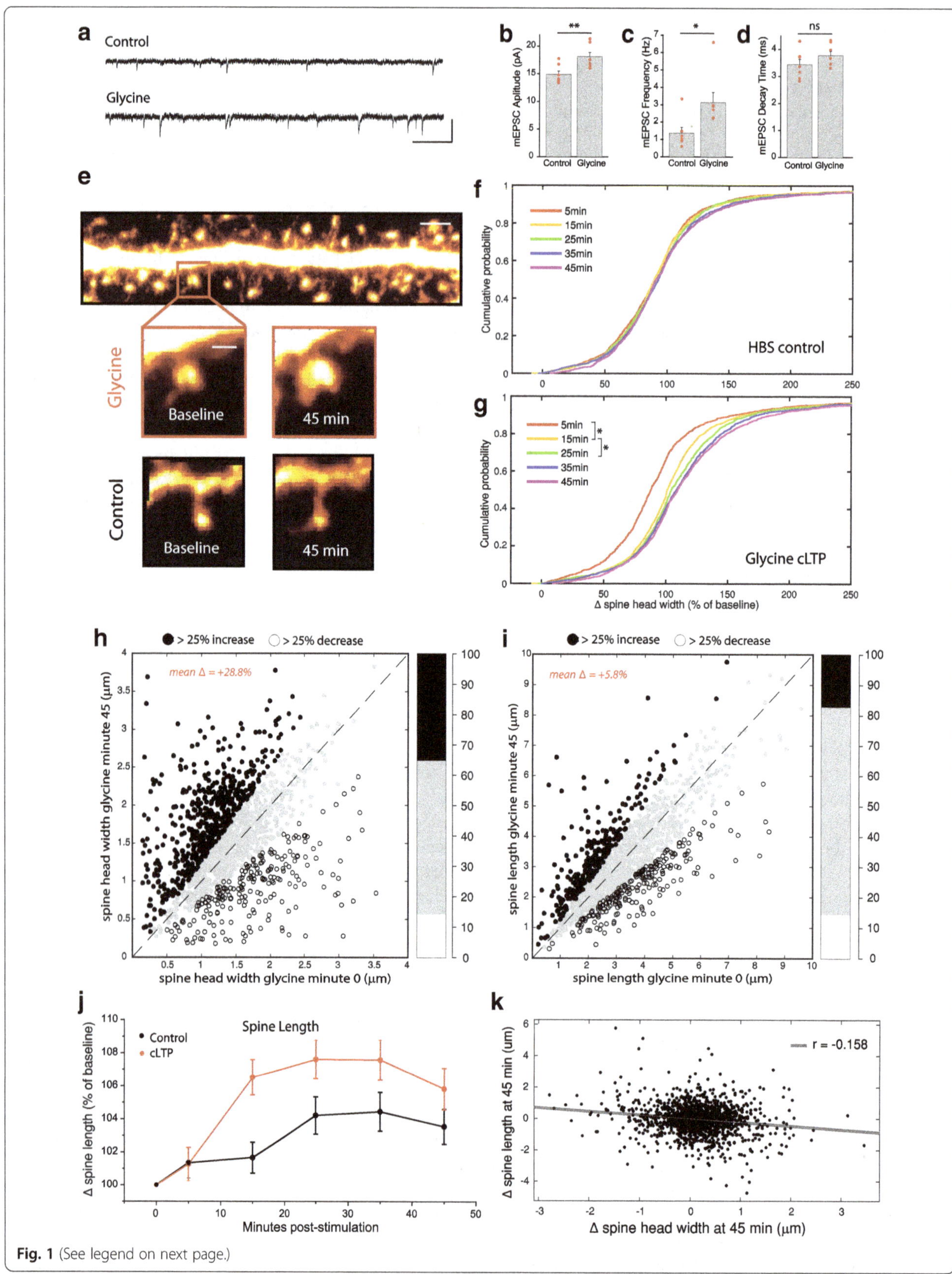

Fig. 1 (See legend on next page.)

(See figure on previous page.)
Fig. 1 Long lasting changes in dendritic spine morphology induced by cLTP in vitro. (**a-d**) Example traces and mean (+SEM) mEPSC amplitude (**b**), frequency (**c**), and decay time (**d**) for cultured rat hippocampal neurons recorded after treatment with glycine-based cLTP (400 μM) stimulus or HBS alone as a control ($n = 7$ recordings in each condition). Glycine cLTP induces a strong increase in the strength of excitatory inputs in culture. (**e**) Example images of dendritic spines from hippocampal neurons expressing eGFP in dissociated culture under conditions of cLTP (glycine 400 μM) or HBS control. cLTP induces robust increases in dendritic spine head width. Scale bar = 2.5 μm in upper panel 1 μm in enlarged close up image. (**f-g**) Cumulative probability distributions of change in spine head diameter quantified as percent of baseline value for all spines imaged under conditions of cLTP (**g**, $n = 1538$ spines across 20 cells) or HBS alone (**f**, $n = 1320$ spines across 21 cells) at time-points 5, 15, 25, 35, and 45 m post stimulation. Glycine treatment elicits a time-dependent expansion of dendritic spine heads, * denotes significant difference in a given population from the distribution obtained in the proceeding timepoint via ks test. (**h**) Scatter plot comparing raw values of head diameter for all spines imaged before vs 45 m after treatment with 400 μM glycine during the cLTP protocol. Black symbols denote spines with head diameter increases over 25%, while white symbols mark spines that shrink by 25%. Gray symbols along the line of equality indicate spines with less extreme alterations. Bar graph on right hand side represents distribution of these groups (black = increase, white = decrease, gray = no change) as percent of total. (**i**) Comparison of pre and 45 m post stimulation values for spine length, as reported for the same set of cells in (**h**). (**j**) Timecourse of changes in spine length (represented as % of baseline values). Degree of length change was not significantly different between HBS treated controls and the glycine cLTP groups when assessed 45 m post stimulation. (**k**) Scatter plot of individual changes in protrusion length (pre vs 45 m post glycine stimulation) vs changes in head diameter for the same group of spines

exhibited increases in head width over 25% of their baseline value ($n = 543/1538$), whereas 14% ($n = 218/1538$) exhibited a 25% or greater diminishment in head width. By contrast to alterations in spine head width, the changes we observed in spine length following cLTP were more subtle. While there is a trend towards spine lengthening following cLTP, the magnitude of this change is small (< 10%), and by 45 min, is not significantly different from spine length changes observed under control conditions (Fig. 1j). We also asked whether changes in spine head width and length following LTP might be related, but found no significant correlation between these morphological changes in response to glycine-induced potentiation (Fig. 1k). For these reasons, we focused our analysis primarily on spine head width in subsequent experiments.

Having shown that structural remodeling can be reliably induced using a glycine-based stimulus protocol in mature hippocampal cultures, we next examined the role of protein synthesis in structural remodeling after chemically induced LTP (Fig. 2). As a group, glycine-treated spines exhibited a rapid enlargement in head diameter after stimulus onset, increasing roughly 17% over baseline levels by 15 min post-stimulation. Average head width in glycine-treated neurons steadily increased for the duration of the imaging session to a final value of roughly 28% larger than baseline values at 45 min post stimulation (Fig. 2a). Pre-treatment with the protein-synthesis inhibitor anisomycin (40 μM, 30 min) significantly diminished glycine-mediated increases in spine head width (Fig. 2a). This difference in mean head diameter is reflective of an overall change across the population of imaged cells, as the cumulative probability distribution of altered head diameter for spines treated with glycine + anisomycin was significantly different from the distribution of size changes in spines treated with glycine alone (Fig. 2b).

Recent work has indicated that mTORC1-mediated phosphorylation of 4E–BP is an indispensable step in the process by which this pathway controls cap-dependent translation [59]. As such, we next addressed whether our previously observed protein synthesis-dependent increases in spine head width were also dependent on mTORC1 activity. Similar to our results using anisomycin, pretreatment with the mTORC1 inhibitor rapamycin (100 nM, administered 30 min prior to glycine treatment), resulted in significantly less pronounced head enlargements than spines treated with glycine alone (Fig. 2a). By 45 min post stimulation, cells treated with glycine + rapamycin displayed a net gain in spine head width of 8.6%, which was not significantly different from HBS-treated controls (Fig. 2a). Like the effects of co-treatment with anisomycin, the cumulative probability distribution of altered head diameter for spines treated with glycine + rapamycin was significantly different from the distribution of size changes in spines treated with glycine alone (Fig. 2b). The finding that both anisomycin and rapamycin attenuate persistent increases in spine head width after glycine treatment collectively support the hypothesis that morphological plasticity after LTP relies on mTORC1-dependent protein synthesis.

We next considered the possibility that starting differences in spine size might contribute to the magnitude of relative changes in spine head area among the various treatment groups assessed above. Figure 2d shows the full distribution of spine head areas at baseline in each of the six relevant treatment conditions. Overall, the distribution of spine head widths is similar among treatments, though the proportion of large- and small-diameter spines is not uniform in all cases, which gives rise to significant differences in mean spine head widths among the conditions (ANOVA, $F_{5,5061} = 18.13$, $p = 7.00e^{-18}$, Fig. 2d). These differences were not systematic according to pre-treatment condition, however, with only one group receiving pretreatment with anisomycin ("Control + aniso") and one group later receiving glycine ("Glycine alone") showing significant differences

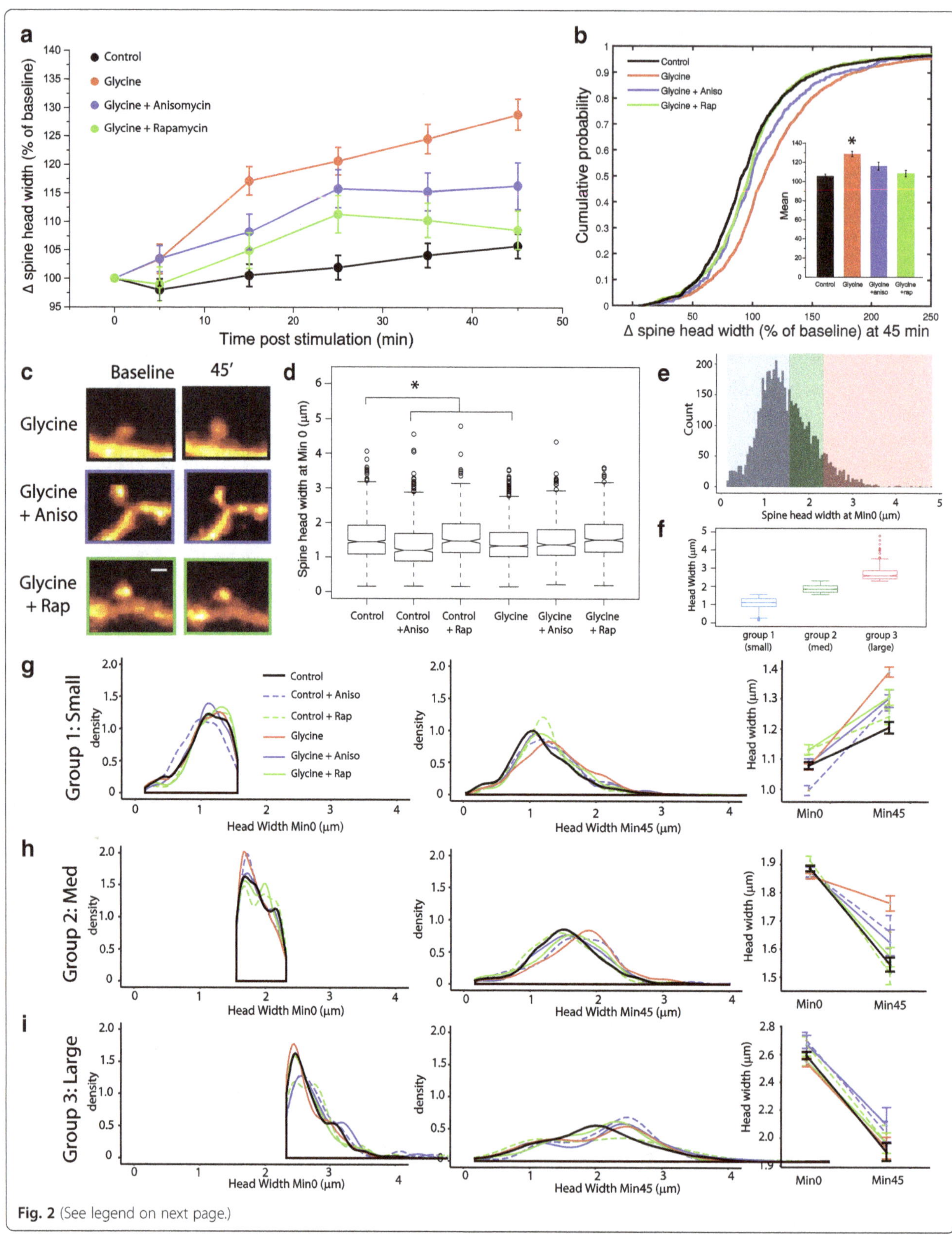

Fig. 2 (See legend on next page.)

(See figure on previous page.)

Fig. 2 Glycine induced spine head enlargement is protein synthesis and mTORC1 dependent. (**a**) Time-course of relative changes in spine head diameter (represented as percentage of baseline value) for neurons treated with glycine (400 μM) either alone (red, n = 1538 spines across 20 cells) or after pretreatment with anisomycin (blue, $n = 494$ spines across 8 cells) or rapamycn (green, $n = 684$ spines across 9 cells). Control cells were treated with HBS alone. (**b**) Cumulative probability distribution and mean (+/−SEM) change in spine head width for cells treated with glycine with or without anisomycin, or rapamycin assessed 45 min post-stimulation. *$p < 0.05$ relative to control cells treated with HBS alone. (**c**) Example images taken from neurons treated with 400 μM glycine and either 40 μM anisomycin (blue) or 200 nM rapamycin (green). Scale bar = 1 μm. (**d**) Box plots showing distribution of values for spine head width across each group at baseline (recorded at min 0). One way ANOVA and post Hoc measures reveal significant variation of two groups from control values. (**e**) Frequency histogram of all spines in groups down in **d**, ($n = 5061$), colored according to groups determined by kmeans clustering. (**f**) Box plot showing range of spine head values represented in each of the three groups determined by k means cluster (Group 1 "small", $n = 3068$; Group 2 "medium", $n = 1504$; Group 3 "large", $n = 438$ spines). (**g-i**) Kernel density estimates of spine head width for each cluster group as identified in 2E–F at baseline (minute 0) and 45 min post stimulus onset (middle panel). Right, direct comparison of mean values for spine head width at min0 vs min45

from HBS treated control values by Tukey HSD post hoc tests. Given that these baseline differences exist before treatments were initiated, it is unlikely that they reflect any specific treatment effect. However, in principle, the starting size of spines can impact the assessment of relative changes in spine size over time, as smaller spines are closer to a measurement floor and larger spines closer to a measurement ceiling. Small spines, for example, are limited in the range where they can shrink further, but there is a large dynamic range for these spines to increase in size. Accordingly, mean spine head width will tend to increase across repeated measurements even if an equal number of spines grow and shrink within a group. Likewise, for initially large diameter spines, mean spine head width will adopt a negative trajectory over time given equal proportions of spines that grow and shrink. To account for this potential issue, it was necessary to compare treatment effects on spines of different sizes separately.

To determine ideal threshold values to separate spines in our dataset according to size, we used the 'NbClust' package in R which compares multiple indices to determine the ideal number of naturally occurring clusters in a dataset [9]. Out of 5061 total spines across all 6 experimental conditions, we found that our data was best represented by a separation into three groups (Fig. 2e-f). Kmeans clustering revealed groups as follows: group 1 $n = 3068$ spines, range = 0.15–1.558um; group 2 $n = 1504$ spines, range = 1.559–2.317um, group 3 $n = 489$ spines, range = 2.319–4.795um (Fig. 2e-f). When partitioned into these clusters, we observed that the sampling from each group across experimental conditions was non-uniform (Control = 55.757% group 1, 32.575% group 2, and 11.666% group 3; Control + Aniso = 71.374% group 1, 17.748% group 2, and 10.877% group 3; Control + Rap = 56.28% group 1, 32.534% group 2, 11.1776% group 3; Glycine = 65.669% group 1, 27.828% group 2, 6.5019% group 3; Glycine + Aniso = 61.336% group 1, 29.959% group 2, 8.7044% group 3; Glycine + Rap = 53.070% group 1, 35.380% group 2, 11.5497% group 3). A comparison of these populations separated out by group at baseline (minute 0) or 45 min post stimulus are shown in Fig. 2g-i. We find that after clustering, within a particular spine group, mean spine head widths are now highly similar across treatment conditions at baseline (Fig. 2g-i, rightmost panels). For group 1 spines (the most represented in all treatment conditions), the glycine treatment condition exhibits an increase in spine head width that is substantively higher than in controls, despite similar spine head width in the two conditions at baseline. Likewise, for group 2 spines (the next most represented in all treatment conditions) where mean spine head width tends to decrease, the drop is noticeably less in the glycine treatment condition than in the controls. Anisomycin or rapamycin pre-treatment eliminates this effect in both cases, while having little impact when administered alone. Of note, no apparent treatment effects are evident in group 3 spines (the least represented in the data set), likely due to a measurement ceiling effect. Together, this analysis reveals that relative changes in spine head diameter are influenced by basal differences in spine head size. For the majority of spines (groups 1 and 2), glycine stimulation positively regulates spine head area relative to control conditions, an effect that is both protein synthesis- and mTORC1-dependent.

Given previous research showing unique relationships between morphological classes of dendritic spines and functional plasticity at excitatory synapses [12], we next investigated whether particular spine types display unique responsiveness to chemically-induced LTP or requirements for mTORC1 activity. Using custom Matlab analysis routines for automated morphological classification (see methods), we divided all spines from previous data sets into the following classes: mushroom (Fig. 3a-c), stubby (Fig. 3d-f), flat (Fig. 3g-i), thin (Fig. 3j-l), or filopodial (Fig. 3m-o). When parceled into these defined morphological classes, we found striking differences between spine type that were not immediately apparent from analysis of the combined group data. While we examine changes in spine width at various times following cLTP induction, we specifically focused on the 45-

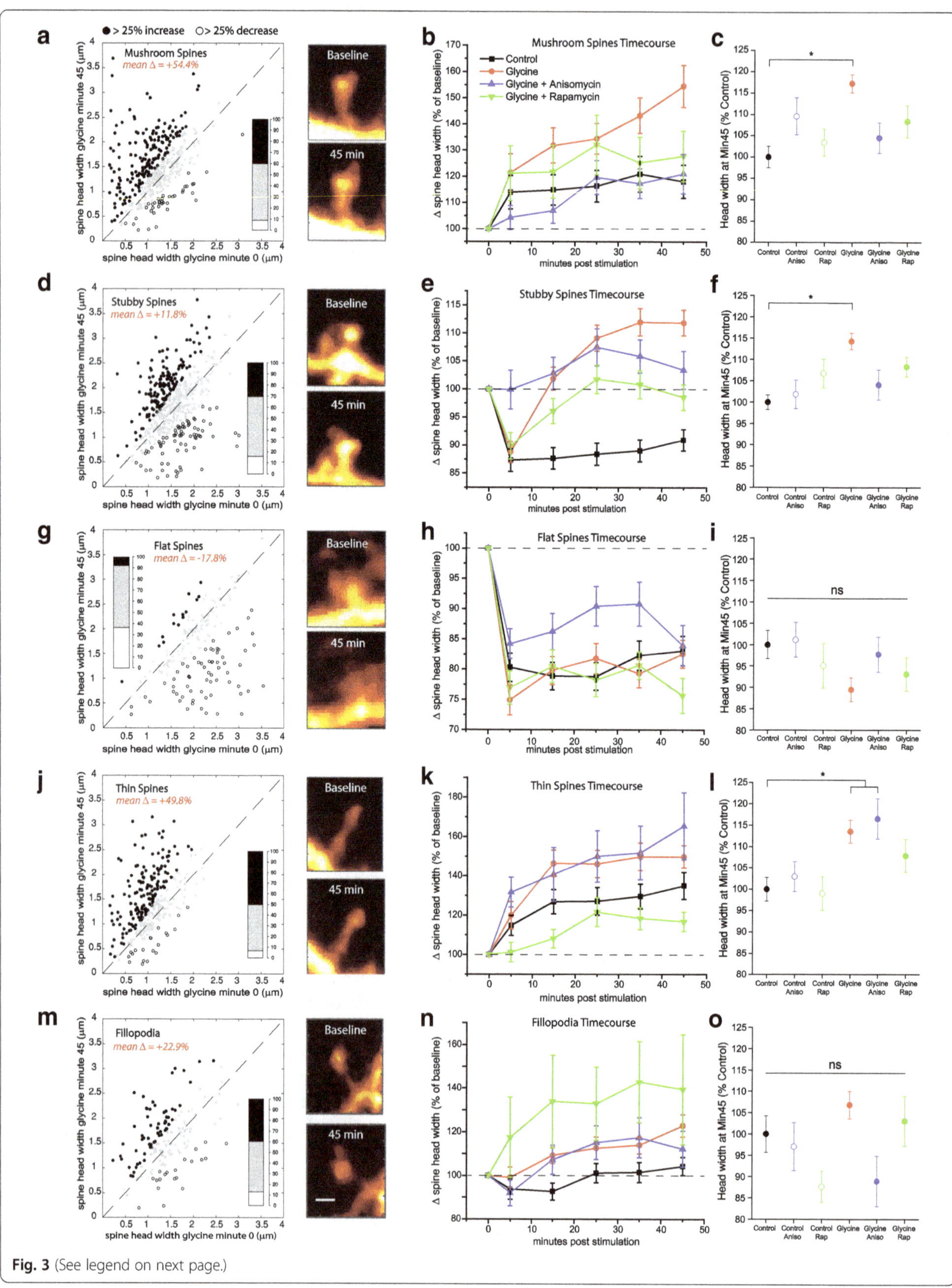

Fig. 3 (See legend on next page.)

(See figure on previous page.)
Fig. 3 Diversity of response properties across different morphological categories during cLTP. (**a**) Scatter plot (left) and representative example images (right) of mushroom type spines (*n* = 432) comparing raw value of head diameter measured before vs 45 min after treatment with 400 μM glycine. Black symbols = > 25% increase, white symbols = >25% decrease, gray symbols = changes outside this range. Bar graph inset represents distribution of these groups as percent of total (where black = increase, white = decrease, gray = no change). (**b**) Timecourse of changes in head diameter for mushroom spines represented as percentage of baseline values after glycine treatment alone (n = 432) or in combination with anisomycin (40 μM, *n* = 119) or rapamycin (200 nM, *n* = 129), compared to HBS treated controls (*n* = 261). (**c**) Mean (+SEM) head width of mushroom spines assessed 45 min after glycine-induced potentiation with or without pretreatment from anisomycin or rapamycin. Here, all values were normalized to the average spine head width of HBS treated controls at the 45 min time point only. *p < 0.05 relative to HBS treated controls. Remaining panels as indicated above, for stubby spines (**d-f**; control stubby *n* = 487, glycine stubby *n* = 467, glycine + aniso stubby *n* = 152, glycine + rap stubby *n* = 272), flat spines (**g-i**; control flat *n* = 169, glycine flat *n* = 184, glycine + aniso flat *n* = 92, glycine + rap flat *n* = 85), thin spines (**j-l**; control thin *n* = 273, glycine thin *n* = 301, glycine + aniso thin n = 92, glycine + rap thin n = 129), and filopodia (**m-o**; control fil *n* = 125, glycine fil n = 152, glycine + aniso fil *n* = 34, glycine + rap *n* = 64). Scale bar = 1 μm

min post-treatment time-point for comparison between spine types. At this time-point, mushroom spines (432 of 1538 total in the glycine treatment group), exhibited an average increase in head width of 54.47% over baseline values, with 174 exhibiting increases over 25%, and 38 showing a greater than 25% decrease (Fig. 3a). Stubby spines showed a somewhat similar response pattern at this time-point, though lesser in magnitude with an average change in spine head width of 11.8% greater than baseline. Of the 468 stubby spines assessed in the glycine group, 142 displayed a > 25% increase, while 73 had >25% decrease (Fig. 3d). While thin spines (Fig. 3j) and filopodia (Fig. 3m) displayed general increases in head diameter in response to glycine treatment (Thin spines: mean 49.88% over baseline with 152/302 increasing, and 20/302 decreasing; Filopodia: mean 22.91% over baseline with 61/153 increasing and 20/153 decreasing), it should be noted that thin spines also showed a large increase in head diameter over the course of the 45 min imaging experiment under HBS control conditions as well (Fig. 3k). Flat (aka "cup-shaped") spines showed a strikingly divergent response pattern from the other morphological classes assessed. Of the 183 total flat spines imaged in the glycine alone group, only 14 had a final change in head width over 25% of baseline values, while 67 decreased by over 25%, resulting an average change of −17.843% (Fig. 3g). However, this gradual decrease in head width was also seen in thin spines subject to HBS control solution alone (Fig. 3h), indicating that this decrement was unlikely to be due to glycine stimulation specifically.

We next assessed the requirements for protein synthesis and mTORC1 signaling during glycine-induced potentiation for each morphological sub-class. In most cases, blocking either protein synthesis (40 μM anisomycin,30 min pretreatment) or mTORC1 kinase activity (100 nM rapamycin, 30 min pre-treatment) tended to produce similar effects on changes in spine head width following cLTP induction within each sub-group. For mushroom spines (Fig. 3b-c, pre-treatment with either anisomycin or rapamycin resulted in a significant decrease in head width compared to spines treated with glycine alone (normalized control mushroom head width 45 min post stim = 100 +/−40.68%, Control plus anisomycin = 109.59+/−45.4%, Control plus rapamycin = 103.39+/−36.06%, glycine = 117.27 +/−43.59%, glycine + anisomycin = 104.49+/−38.77%, glycine + rapamycin = 108.32+/−43.01%; ANOVA, $F_{5,1181}$ = 6.54, p = 5.22e^{-6}). A similar effect was observed for stubby spines (Fig. 3e-f); normalized control stubby head width 45 min post stim = 100+/−37.42% Control + Aniso = 101.86+/−40.39%, Control + Rap = 106.74 +/−41.27%, glycine = 114.29+/−41.08, glycine + anisomycin = 104.11+/−43.35%, glycine + rapamycin = 108.28 +/−37.48%; ANOVA, $F_{5,1679}$ = 6.86, p = 2.40e^{-6}). Glycine-induced head width changes in thin spines (Fig. 3k-l) were not sensitive to protein synthesis inhibition with anisomycin (normalized control thin head width 45 min post stim = 100+/−45.71%, Control plus aniso = 102.96 +/−41.77% of HBA treated controls, Control + Rapamycin = 98.97+/−41.77%, glycine = 113.56+/−47.01%, glycine + anisomycin = 116.55+/−45.49%, glycine + rapamycin = 107.86+/−44.13; ANOVA, $F_{5,1020}$ = 4.26, p = 7.62e^{-4}) and neither flat spines nor filopodia showed significant differences between any of the groups assessed at 45 min post-glycine stimulation (Fig. 3h-i, n-o).

Collectively, these data suggest that mTORC1-dependent protein synthesis may play an important role in the maintenance of glycine-induced increases in spine head width, particularly in spines with a mushroom type morphology. In particular, it is possible that strong excitatory glutamatergic inputs interact with mTORC1 signaling to maintain altered spine morphology during long-term potentiation. As such, artificially enhanced mTORC1 signaling would predispose dendritic spines to display an enhanced response to what would otherwise be a subthreshold excitatory stimulus. To test this directly, we transfected dissociated hippocampal neurons with RhebQ64L, a constitutively active mutant version of the GTPase that positively regulates mTORC1, to drive this signaling pathway over a period of 24 h. We have previously utilized this strategy to activate mTORC1 signaling during a similar time period, and have verified that expression of this Rheb point mutant elicits profound increases in levels of phosphorylated ribosomal protein S6, a commonly used marker of mTORC1 activity [20]. Within a population of hippocampal neurons fixed and imaged following 24 h expression of eGFP alone or alongside either RhebQ64L or the upstream mTORC1 inhibitors TSC1/2 as a basis of comparison (Fig. 4a), we observed that either genetic upregulation (RhebQ64L) or downregulation (TSC1/2) of mTORC1 activity each resulted in a slight decrease in spine head size compared to control neurons expressing eGFP alone (Fig. 4b; eGFP alone = 1.12 +/−0.55um, RhebQ64L = 1.06+/−0.41um, TSC1/2 = 1.03 +/−0.40um; ANOVA, $F_{2,2375} = 7.16$, $p = 7.95e^{-4}$). This finding is perhaps surprising given previous reports of increased spine head diameter after genetic deletion of the mTORC1 inhibitor TSC1 [55], and likely reflects differences in the duration of mTORC1 activation (10–20 days in previous experiments vs 24 Hrs here). This reduction in head diameter appeared to be restricted to stubby and flat spines, as none of the other morphological subtypes displayed significant differences according to mTORC1 activation status when analyzed separately (Fig. 4c). In control neurons expressing eGFP alone, there was a small negative correlation between spine head width and overall length (Fig. 4d); this trend was unaltered following 24 Hrs of enhanced mTORC1 activity via RhebQ64L expression or down-regulation via TSC1/2, suggesting no overall change in gross spine morphology as a result of this short-term alteration in mTORC1 signaling (Fig. 4d). Taken together, these data suggest that the more broad-scale malformation in spine structure commonly associated with prolonged

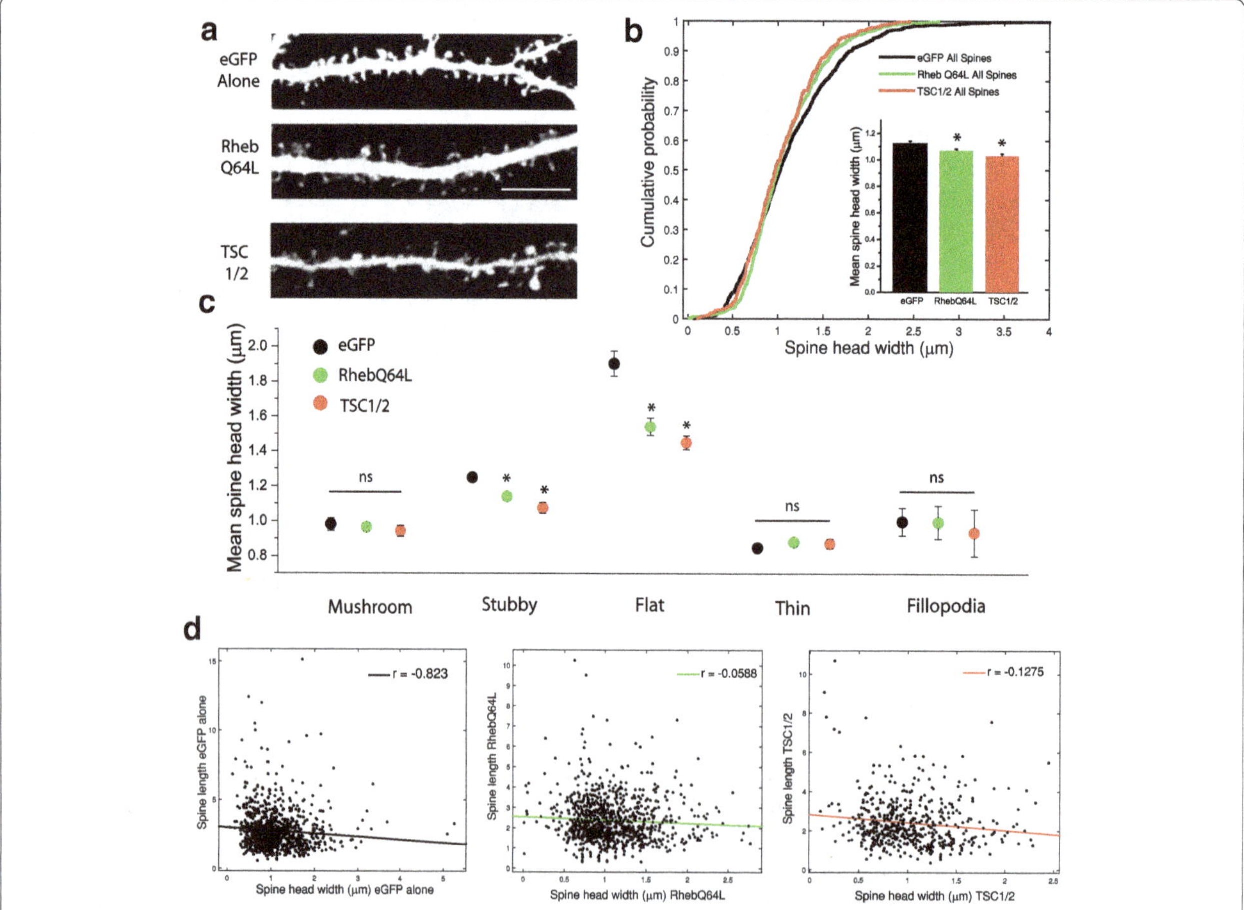

Fig. 4 Genetic up- or down-regulation of mTORC1 activity is not sufficient to increase spine head size on its own. (**a**) Representative images of dendritic regions from hippocampal neurons 24Hrs after expression of either eGFP alone (*n* = 940 spines across 12 cells) or alongside either a constitutively active version of the positive upstream regulator RhebQ64L (*n* = 929 spines across 15 cells) or the complex of inhibitory mTORC1 effectors TSC1/2 (*n* = 509 spines across 10 cells). Scale bar =10 μm. (**b**) Cumulative probability distribution and mean (+SEM) values (inset) for spine head width in neurons with genetic alterations in mTORC1 signaling as indicated. *p < 0.05 relative to control cells expressing eGFP alone. (**c**) Mean (+/−SEM) values of spine head width in groups as indication, broken up according to morphological subtype. 24 h of genetically-mediate up- down-regulation of mTORC1 activity produced a moderate but significant decrease in dendritic head width, primarily observed in stubby and flat morphological types. *p < 0.05 relative to control cells expressing eGFP alone. (**d**) Scatter plots comparing spine head width and protrusion length for cells expression eGFP (left), RhebQ64L (middle) or TSC1/2 (right)

mTORC1 dysregulation [18, 55] does not emerge over the acute 24 h time scale used in our experiments.

We next proceeded to ask whether constitutive mTORC1 activation may predispose spines to potentiation-like growth under conditions of sub-threshold excitatory input. We empirically determined a cLTP regimen (reducing Glycine from 400 μM to 10 μM) that produced no significant change in dendritic spine head width at any time point assessed (Fig. 5a-b). Using this sub-threshold stimulation protocol, we performed time-lapse imaging of cells expressing either RhebQ64L or eGFP alone as a control. Spine heads treated with 10 μM glycine alone (595 spines across 8 neurons) were not significantly different from vehicle treated controls at any time-point assessed after stimulation (Fig. 5c). In contrast, pairing sub-threshold glycine stimulation with persistent mTORC1 activation drove rapid spine growth (Fig. 5c), which at 15 m post-stimulation appeared similar to the increases observed following cLTP induced with 400 μM glycine at 45 m post-stimulation (Fig. 2c). These changes following RhebQ64L + 10 μM glycine persisted for at least 45 min, though the difference with the RhebQ64L alone group diminished slightly at that time-point. While, at 15 min, the mean change in spine head width for the paired RhebQ64L + 10 μM glycine group was significantly elevated compared to either condition separately or HBS controls (Fig. 5d insert; HBS control = 104.4+/−86.98% of baseline value, 10 μM glycine = 103.2+/−63.6% of baseline value, RhebQ64L alone = 106.63+/−84.1% of baseline value, RhebQ64L + 10 μM glycine = 128.75+/−122.88% of baseline value; ANOVA, $F_{3,3149} = 14.09$, $p = 4.03e^{-9}$), a comparison of the probability distributions of the percent head width changes for these groups reveals that strong differences in these populations are carried largely by the top half of the distribution (Fig. 5d). This implies that the large increase in spine head width resulting from concurrent mTORC1 activation and low intensity stimulation with glycine was not uniform across all members of the population. Indeed, a comparison of raw values of spine head width before and 15 min post stimulus initiation reveals a significant degree of response heterogeneity across each treatment condition (Fig. 5e-g). For cells receiving sub-threshold (10 μM) glycine alone ($n = 595$ total), we observed a mean difference in spine head width of +3.203% at 15 mi post stim, with 18.5% of spines (110/595) showing increases in head width 25% over baseline values and 23.8% of spines (142/595) displaying a decrease of similar degree (Fig. 5e). Neurons expressing RhebQ64L, but receiving mock cLTP stimulation with HBS ($n = 1227$ total) showed an average change in spine head width of +6.63% when assessed 15 m after initiation of the experiment, with roughly equal numbers showing spontaneous fluctuations in head width (245 with >25% increase, 282 with >25% decrease, Fig. 5f). When genetic activation of mTORC1 activity was paired with low threshold glycine stimulation (RhebQ64L + 10 μM glycine, 1076 total), the average change in individual spine head width reflected a strong bias for potentiation, as 30% (323/1076) of spines increased in size by 25% or more and an average increase of +28.67% above baseline values was observed for the population as a whole (Fig. 5g). The heterogeneity of response properties within this population indicates that the fast alterations in spine head width might be unique to particular morphological categories. Separated out by class, we observed that spines of mushroom (10 μM glycine mushroom = 11.67+/−67.37% change from baseline, RhebQ64L mushroom = 29.22+/−129.78% change from baseline, RhebQ64L + 10 μM glycine mushroom = 53.95 +/−167.94% change from baseline; ANOVA, $F_{2,778} = 5.73$, $p = 0.003$), thin (10 μM glycine thin = 16.87+/−89.60% change from baseline, RhebQ64L thin = 16.31+/−76.16% change from baseline, RhebQ64L + 10 μM glycine = 53.19 +/−113.31% change from baseline; ANOVA, $F_{2,592} = 10.57$, $p = 3.08e^{-5}$), and filopodial (10 μM glycine fil = −13.17 +/−34.18% change from baseline, RhebQ64L fil = 1.53 +/−67.10% change from baseline, RhebQ64L + 10 μM glycine = 116.12+/−267.71% change from baseline; ANOVA, $F_{2,195} = 13.21$, $p = 4.17e^{-6}$) types were uniquely responsive to the combined effects of mTORC1 activation and low intensity glycine stimulation (Fig. 5h). Notably, we observed a diminishment in head width of flat spines over the course of imaging, in keeping with our previous observations (Fig. 3g).

When assessing individual examples of spine enlargements in the paired Rheb + glycine group, we noticed a number of spines with rapid changes in head width, often changing size to an extreme degree over the course of a single imaging time-point. An example of one of these spines can be seen in Fig. 6a. We observed many such cases, and denote this phenomenon related to sudden large changes in spine head width as "high volatility". This feature may be distinguished from other spines whose head width may also change significantly over the course of an experiment, though at a more gradual rate of transition (denoted as "low volatility", Fig. 6b). To explore this effect further, we examined the relationship between maximum single period (i.e. 0 to 5 min or 5 to 15 min, etc) change in head width (quantified as absolute percent difference from preceding time-point) and initial spine head diameter at min 0 (Fig. 6c). Unsurprisingly, small spines (<0.5um) tend to show the largest relative changes in head diameter compared to medium or larger sized spines. In an effort to eliminate the possibility of these smaller spines biasing our assessment of volatility differences between experimental conditions, we limited our subsequent analyses only to spines with head diameter > 0.5 μm at the start of the experiment (red box in 6C indicates excluded cases). Under these conditions, a comparison of the probability distributions (Fig. 6d) and mean value (inset) of

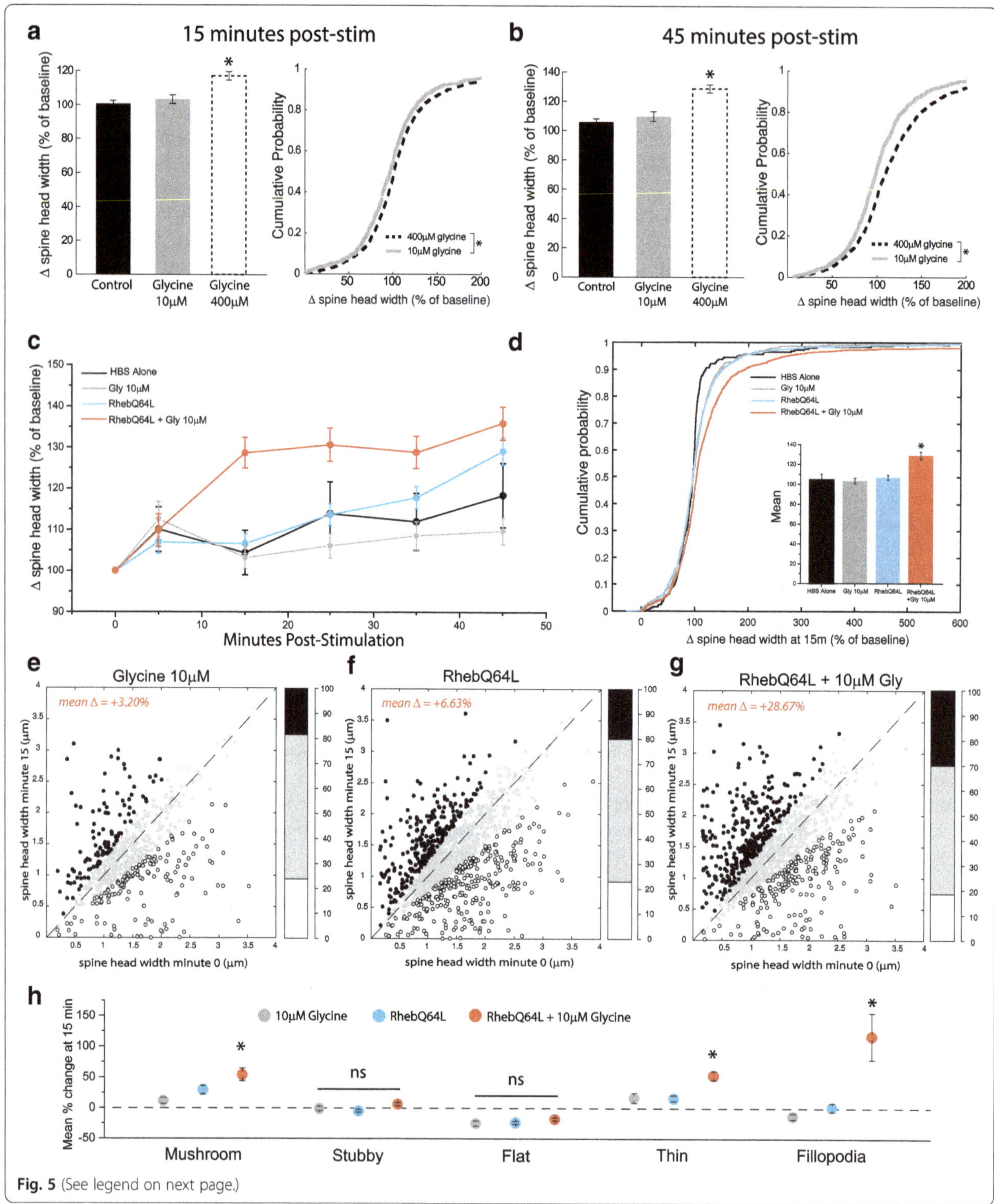

Fig. 5 (See legend on next page.)

(See figure on previous page.)

Fig. 5 mTORC1 acts in combination with synaptically derived signals to enhance spine head diameter. (**a-b**) Mean (+/–SEM) normalized spine head width and cumulative probability distribution and of cells treated with a subthreshold (10 μM) or super-threshold (400 μM) concentration of glycine assessed 15 min (**a**) and 45 min (**b**) post-stimulation. *p < 0.05 relative to vehicle treated controls. Spines treated with a sub-threshold dose of glycine do not exhibit significant changes in head width compared to controls at either time point assessed. (**c**) Timecourse of head expansion in neurons expressing eGFP alone or in combination with genetic upregulation of mTORC1 activity via RhebQ64L expression after sub-threshold (10 μM) glycine treatment. Co-occurrence of increased mTORC1 signaling with synaptic activation elicited a rapid increase in spine head diameter observed 15 m post stimulation. (**d**) Cumulative probability distribution and mean +/–SEM values (inset) of altered spine head diameter at 15 m post stimulation shown as percentage of baseline values. HBS alone, n = 255 across 3 cells; 10 μM glycine, n = 595 across 8 cells; RhebQ64L alone, n = 1227 across 7 cells; RhebQ64L + 10 μM glycine, n = 1076 across 9 cells. (**e-g**) Scatter plots comparing raw spine head values pre vs 15 m post experiment initiation under conditions of sub-threshold glycine stimulation (**e**), expression of RhebQ64L alone (**f**), or both stimuli combined (**g**). Bar graphs on right hand side represent spines that increase (black), decrease (white) or remain stable (gray) as a proportion of total spines in each condition. Spines subject to paired activation RhebQ64L expression with sub-threshold glycine application exhibits increases in head growth well above either condition alone. (**h**) Mean (+/– SEM) of altered head diameter 15 min post stim, represented a percent change from baseline values separated according to morphological category as indicated. Rapid spine expansion after 15 m under conditions of paired synaptic stimulation and mTORC1 activation are specific to mushroom spines (10 μM glycine mushroom n = 185; RhebQ64L alone mushroom n = 336; RhebQ64L + 10 μM glycine mushroom n = 260), thin spines (10 μM glycine thin n = 57; RhebQ64L alone thin n = 169; RhebQ64L + 10 μM glycine thin n = 185), and filopodia (10 μM glycine fil n = 55; RhebQ64L alone fil n = 90; RhebQ64L + 10 μM glycine fil n = 53). Stubby (10 μM glycine stubby n = 186; RhebQ64L alone stubby n = 395; RhebQ64L + 10 μM glycine stubby n = 362) and flat spines (10 μM glycine flat n = 122; RhebQ64L alone flat n = 247; RhebQ64L + 10 μM glycine flat n = 226) show no significant differences across experimental groups

maximum spine head change in a single time-point for each group assessed showed a significant increase in overall volatility for the paired mTORC1 activation + glycine group compared with any other condition, including the stronger glycine stimulus (400 μM) used in earlier experiments. When broken out into specific morphological subtypes, we found that mushroom spines, stubby spines and filopodia exhibited significantly enhanced volatility under conditions of paired mTORC1 upregulation and low intensity synaptic stimulation (RhebQ64L + 10 μM Glycine). We also note an unanticipated increase in volatility for stubby spines when treated with low threshold glycine (10 μM) alone. Thin and flat spine types show no significant changes between any of the groups assessed (Fig. 6e).

Discussion

Here, we examined the role of mTORC1 signaling in structural remodeling of synapses during LTP. We show that cLTP induction caused an expansion in dendritic spine heads in cultured hippocampal neurons (Fig. 1), a specific form of structural plasticity that is widely believed to be necessary for persistent strengthening of excitatory synaptic connections. The maintenance of this altered head diameter at later time points (here, 45 m post-stimulation) is notably dependent on mTORC1-dependent protein synthesis, as it is blocked by concurrent application of anisomycin or rapamycin during glycine-induced cLTP (Fig. 2). This effect appears to be most strongly seen in a subpopulation of dendritic spines with a mature, mushroom type morphology (Fig. 3). Despite being necessary to induce these changes, enhanced mTORC1 activity alone is not sufficient to elicit increased spine head diameter (Fig. 4). However, when active mTORC1 signaling is paired with a sub-threshold level of synaptic stimulation, strong changes in spine morphology rapidly emerge, resulting in significant increases in head width by 15 m post stimulation (Fig. 5). Lastly, we show that glycine-dependent changes in spine morphology occurring in the context of elevated mTORC1 signaling are highly volatile, with strong increases in head diameter often occurring between single imaging periods (Fig. 6). Collectively these results suggest that mTORC1 acts in tandem with additional activity-dependent synaptic signals to produce structural changes, and shed new light on the cellular mechanisms needed to induce structural changes underlying long lasting increases in the strength of excitatory synapses.

A role for mTORC1-mediated protein synthesis in maintaining altered spine morphology

Of general interest was our finding that changes in spine morphology during chemically-induced LTP require cap-dependent translation. We found that pharmacological blockade of protein synthesis using anisomycin significantly diminished the extent of spine head enlargement after glycine treatment, an effect which was much stronger at 45 min post stimulation than at 15 min post stimulation (Fig. 2c). Spine head growth was similarly blocked by the mTORC1 inhibitor rapamycin (Fig. 2c-f). Given the well established role of mTORC1 in regulating translation initiation, the inhibitory effect of anisomycin/rapamycin at later time points could indicate that potentiated spines require new proteins for the maintenance of increased head width, possibly as a compensatory response to concurrent activity-dependent degradation of synaptic proteins mediated by the ubiquitin proteasome system [3, 4].

Contribution of particular morphological types

Dendritic spines are often distinguished by morphological classification. Historically, categories have included stubby,

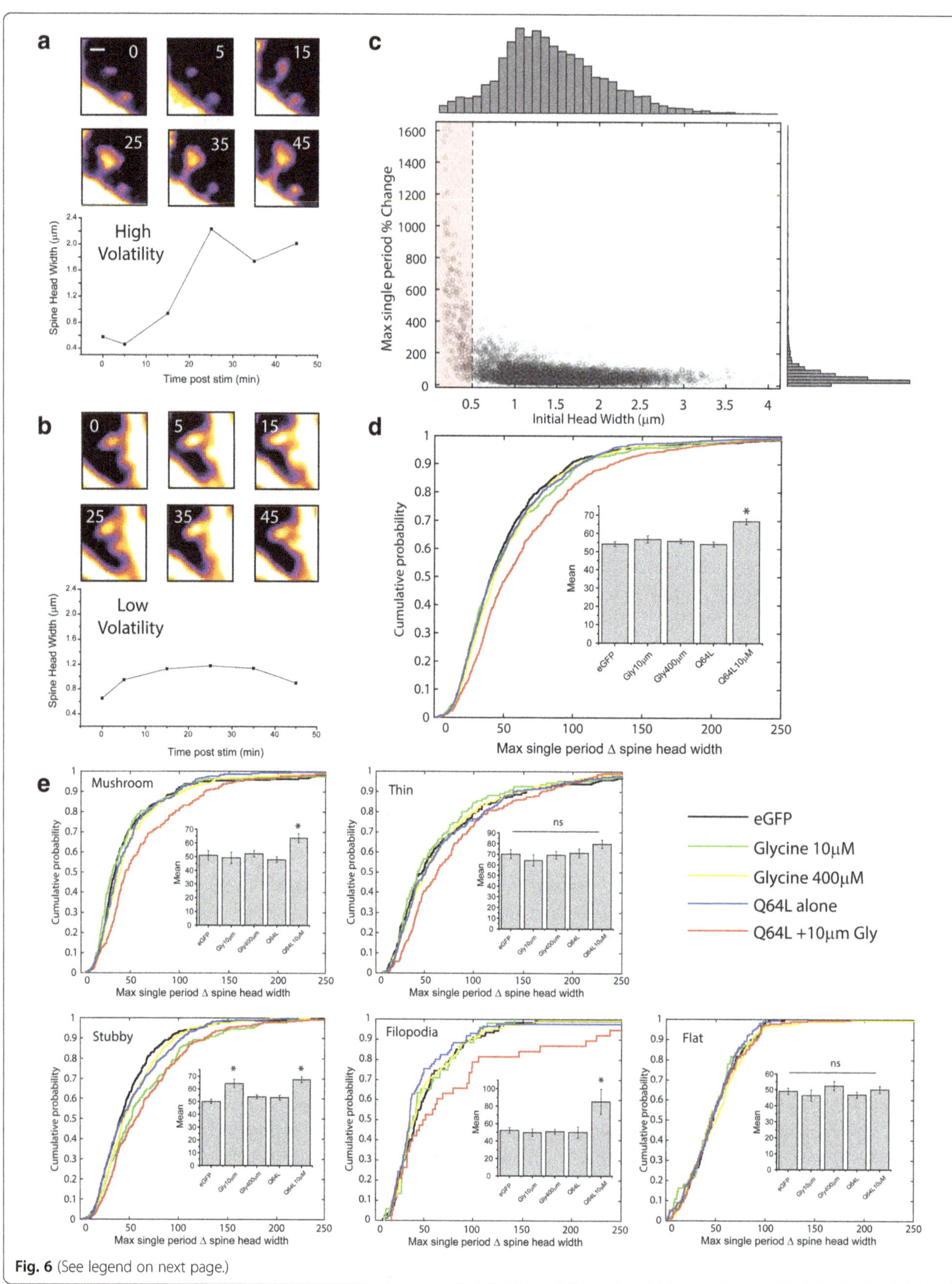

Fig. 6 (See legend on next page.)

(See figure on previous page.)

Fig. 6 Paired mTORC1 and synaptic stimulation increases morphological volatility. (**a-b**) Representative images and example timecourses from spines sorted into categories of (**a**) "high volatility" (i.e. spines with changes spine head diameter > 200% in a single imaging timepoint) or (**b**) "low volatility" (i.e. spines that exhibit more gradual alterations in spine head diameter). Scale bar = 0.5 μm. (**c**) Scatter plot with marginal frequency histograms displaying the relationship between maximum change in head width during entire experiment (quantified as absolute percent difference from preceding timepoint) vs initial spine head diameter in μm. Each dot represents a single spine. Spines across all experimental parameters show in **d-f** included (n = 5756 spines). Excluding spines with head width smaller than 0.5um at minute zero (red shading) resulted in truncated data set with n = 5495 spines. (**d**) Cumulative probability distribution (and mean +/−SEM, inset) of the maximum single period change in head diameter (quantified as absolute percent difference from preceding timepoint) for groups as indicated. Pairing of low threshold synaptic stimulation with mTORC1 upregulation (Q64L+ 10 μM glycine) results in significantly enhanced 'volatility' of spine head diameter compared to all other experimental groups assessed. (ANOVA, $F_{4,5490} = 13.956$, $p = 3.95e^{-11}$; eGFP n = 1267 spines, 10 μM Glycine n = 572 spines, 400 μM Glycine n = 1469 spines, RhebQ64L alone n = 1171 spines, RhebQ64L + 10 μM Glycine n = 1016 spines). * denotes significant difference from eGFP controls by Fisher LSD post hoc. (**e**) Cumulative probability distribution (and mean +/−SEM, inset) of the maximum single period change in head diameter for groups as in (**d**), separated by morphological type. * denotes significant difference from eGFP controls by Fisher LSD post hoc

thin, and mushroom, flat, and filopodial [15, 44], although some schemes include other categories such as bifurcated [21]. Different spine types are thought to be functionally distinct, with larger, mushroom spines widely presumed to harbor stronger synapses. It has been proposed that thin and mushroom spines contribute to learning and memory in different ways, with thin spines believed to be both more transient and plastic than mushroom spines [22]. The head diameter of thin spines is, by definition, smaller than those of mushroom spines and as such theoretically have more room to grow under LTP. For these reasons some hold that thin spines are converted into mushroom-type spines during the stabilization process of a structural engram after learning has occurred [6].

We found remarkable separation between the responsiveness of particular morphological spine classes to a glycine-based stimulation paradigm (Fig. 3). Of all types assessed, mushroom spines display particularly large changes in head diameter in response to glycine, and appear to be particularly reliant on new protein synthesis for this effect to be maintained (Fig. 2a-c). Because of their cardinal role in integrating synaptic transmission, dendritic spines are endowed with a variety of organelles and sub-cellular entities that mediate and modulate their role in synaptic plasticity. The smooth endoplasmic reticulum (SER) plays a known role in regulating calcium levels, an ion centrally implicated in LTP. Roughly half of all spines contain a SER stack [51] and the stack tends to occupy almost 20% of the total spine volume, suggesting a mechanism for regulating the calcium concentration within spines. Additionally, Ca2+ released from the SER can augment stimulus- induced Ca2+ currents [46]. It has also long been known that polyribosomes are capable of localizing to dendritic spines [52]. These dendritic polyribosomes are not uniformly distributed at synapses, but are far more prevalent in mature spines, such as mushroom spines [50], suggesting they play some specific role in mediating changes in synapse form or function during activity-induced plasticity. Furthermore, after LTP there is an increase in the proportion of spines containing polyribosomes, the presence of which can predict which spine will exhibit potentiation [33]. It will be interesting for future experiments to examine the unique mechanisms which support persistent, protein-synthesis dependent morphological changes after potentiating stimuli.

Combinatorial action of mTOR with synaptically derived signals

Our results regarding cell autonomous mTORC1 activation paired with application of otherwise sub-threshold concentration of glycine (Fig. 5) suggest that synaptically evoked signaling mechanisms operate in conjunction with mTORC1 activity to mediate the morphological changes observed after cLTP. Constitutive mTORC1 activation alone appears to be insufficient to induce these changes (Fig. 3), possibly because they depend on synaptically driven signals to direct mTORC1-dependent translation of particular sets of mRNA to maintain altered spine structure. In such a scenario, synaptic activity would not induce a global increase in the synthesis of dendritically localized mRNAs, but might rather elicit the synthesis of specific sets of 'LTP proteins', a scenario that has been previously suggested for mTORC1 signaling at the synapse [1, 2]. Interestingly, we found that a sub-threshold dose of glycine can elicit rapid increases in spine size, provided this stimulus occurs on a background of high mTORC1 signaling (Fig. 5). This result supports the hypothesis that mTORC1 activation provides a context of active translation upon which even slight activity can drive synthesis of the new proteins required for changes in spine morphology. Additionally, the rapid nature of these changes is in agreement with previous reports showing an immediate impact of protein synthesis inhibitors on the extent of initial spine growth after induction of LTP at single spines using 2-photon glutamate uncaging [13, 58].

The question remains, however, as to the nature of the upstream synaptic signals that co-activate mTORC1 signaling alongside signaling pathways involved in actin cytoskeletal rearrangement. Calcium influx after LTP-inducing stimuli at single dendritic spines has been shown to induce a brief, spine-specific increase in the phosphorylation of CaMKII [29], which subsequently activates members of the Rho family of small GTPases including RhoA and Cdc42 [39, 40]. Transiently autophosphoylated CaMKII also activates the small GTPase Ras in the postsynaptic domain [16, 63]. Ras is a known activator of the PI3K/mTOR pathway [7], and it remains an intriguing possibility that Ras acts to stimulate mTORC1 directly or perhaps operates in tandem with Wnt signaling [35] to activate mTORC1 in the context of LTP. Recent work has also highlighted an important role for mTORC2 in directly regulating actin polymerization during LTP in the hippocampus [23]. This molecularly distinct complex of proteins, comprised of mTOR bound to rictor, among other partners, plays a role in regulating the actin cytoskeleton, but is usually insensitive to acute inhibition by rapamycin [32]. However, rapamycin has been shown to exert effects on mTORC2 signaling via disruption of mTOR complex formation with rictor, though only after chronic exposure of 24 h or longer [47]. As such, we find it unlikely that our reported inhibition of spine growth with acute rapamycin pre-treatment (30 min; Fig. 2) is due to an effect on mTORC2-mediated actin polymerization rather than mTORC1-mediated signaling.

Achieving a more detailed understanding of the signaling underlying structural remodeling of dendritic spines provides a window into how information is stored within the mammalian brain. Our results implicate mTORC1 activation as an important combinatorial signal that interacts with other local synaptic events to promote spine enlargement during long-lasting synaptic plasticity. Since dysregulation of mTORC1 has been strongly implicated in neurodevelopmental disorders characterized by disorders of social interaction, intellectual disability, and epileptic seizures, a better understanding of mTORC1's role in structural plasticity may shed insight into novel therapeutic approaches for such disorders.

Acknowledgements
We thank Cindy Carruthers and Christian Althaus for generating the cultured hippocampal neurons used in these studies.

Funding
This work was supported by NIH grants RO1MH085798 and RO1NS097498 to M.A.S.

Authors' contributions
FEH carried out experiments, helped conceive the study, analyzed data, and co-wrote the manuscript. WH carried out experiments, analyzed the data, and participated in the design of the study. AC carried out experiments and analyzed data. SPM designed the automated spine analysis and provided input on interpretation of the results. MAS conceived the study, designed the experiments, and co-wrote the manuscript. All authors read and approved the final manuscript.

Competing interests
The authors declare that they have no competing interests.

Author details
[1]Neuroscience Graduate Program, University of Michigan, Ann Arbor, MI 48109, USA. [2]Molecular and Behavioral Neuroscience Institute, University of Michigan, Ann Arbor, MI 48109, USA. [3]Department of Molecular and Integrative Physiology, University of Michigan, Ann Arbor, MI 48109, USA. [4]Department of Pyschological and Brain Sciences, Johns Hopkins University, Baltimore, MD 21218, USA. [5]Molecular and Behavioral Neuroscience Institute, Department of Molecular and Integrative Physiology, University of Michigan, 5067 BSRB, 109 Zina Pitcher Place, Ann Arbor, MI 48109-2200, USA.

References

1. Auerbach BD, Osterweil EK, Bear MF. Mutations causing syndromic autism define an axis of synaptic pathophysiology. Nature. 2011;480(7375):63–8.
2. Bhakar AL, Dölen G, Bear MF. The pathophysiology of fragile X (and what it teaches us about synapses). Annu Rev Neurosci. 2012;35:417–43.
3. Bingol B, Schuman EM. Activity-dependent dynamics and sequestration of proteasomes in dendritic spines. Nature. 2006;441(7097):1144–8.
4. Bingol B, Wang CF, Arnott D, Cheng D, Peng J, Sheng M. Autophosphorylated CaMKIIalpha acts as a scaffold to recruit proteasomes to dendritic spines. Cell. 2010;140(4):567–78.
5. Bloodgood BL, Giessel AJ, Sabatini BL. Biphasic synaptic ca influx arising from compartmentalized electrical signals in dendritic spines. PLoS Biol. 2009;7(9):e1000190.
6. Bourne J, Harris KM. Do thin spines learn to be mushroom spines that remember? Curr Opin Neurobiol. 2007;17(3):381–6.
7. Castellano E, Downward J. Role of RAS in the regulation of PI 3-kinase. Curr Top Microbiol Immunol. 2010;346:143–69.
8. Cammalleri M, Lütjens R, Berton F, King AR, Simpson C, Francesconi W, Sanna PP. Time-restricted role for dendritic activation of the mTOR-p70S6K pathway in the induction of late-phase long-term potentiation in the CA1. Proc Natl Acad Sci U S A. 2003;100(24):14368–73.
9. Charrad M, Ghazzali, Boiteau V, Niknafs A. NbClust: An R Package for Determining the Relevant Number of Clusters in a Data Set. J Stat Softw. 2014;61(6):1–36.
10. Cingolani LA, Goda Y. Actin in action: the interplay between the actin cytoskeleton and synaptic efficacy. Nat Rev Neurosci. 2008;9(5):344–56.
11. Fraser MM, Bayazitov IT, Zakharenko SS, Baker SJ. Phosphatase and tensin homolog, deleted on chromosome 10 deficiency in brain causes defects in synaptic structure, transmission and plasticity, and myelination abnormalities. Neuroscience. 2008;151(2):476–88.
12. Gipson CD, Olive MF. Structural and functional plasticity of dendritic spines - root or result of behavior? Genes Brain Behav. 2017;16(1):101–17.
13. Govindarajan A, Israely I, Huang SY, Tonegawa S. The dendritic branch is the preferred integrative unit for protein synthesis-dependent LTP. Neuron. 2011;69(1):132–46.
14. Grunditz A, Holbro N, Tian L, Zuo Y, Oertner TG. Spine neck plasticity controls postsynaptic calcium signals through electrical compartmentalization. J Neurosci. 2008;28(50):13457–66.
15. Harris KM, Jensen FE, Tsao B. Three-dimensional structure of dendritic spines and synapses in rat hippocampus (CA1) at post-natal day 15 and adult ages: implications for the maturation of synaptic physiology and long-term potentiation. J Neurosci. 1992;12:2685–705.
16. Harvey CD, Yasuda R, Zhong H, Svoboda K. The spread of Ras activity triggered by activation of a single dendritic spine. Science. 2008;321(5885):136–40.

17. Harnett MT, Makara JK, Spruston N, Kath WL, Magee JC. Synaptic amplification by dendritic spines enhances input cooperativity. Nature. 2012; 491(7425):599–602.
18. Haws ME, Jaramillo TC, Espinosa F, Widman AJ, Stuber GD, Sparta DR, Tye KM, Russo SJ, Parada LF, Stavarache M, Kaplitt M, Bonci A, Powell CM. PTEN knockdown alters dendritic spine/protrusion morphology, not density. J Comp Neurol. 2014;522(5):1171–90.
19. Hedrick NG, Harward SC, Hall CE, Murakoshi H, McNamara JO, Yasuda R. Rho GTPase complementation underlies BDNF-dependent homo- and heterosynaptic plasticity. Nature. 2016;538(7623):104–8.
20. Henry FE, McCartney AJ, Neely R, Perez AS, Carruthers CJ, Stuenkel EL, Inoki K, Sutton MA. Retrograde changes in presynaptic function driven by dendritic mTORC1. J Neurosci. 2012;32(48):17128–42.
21. Hering H, Sheng M. Dendritic spines: structure, dynamics and regulation. Nat Rev Neurosci. 2001;2(12):880–8.
22. Holtmaat AJ, Trachtenberg JT, Wilbrecht L, Shepherd GM, Zhang X, Knott GW, Svoboda K. Transient and persistent dendritic spines in the neocortex in vivo. Neuron. 2005;45(2):279–91.
23. Huang W, Zhu PJ, Zhang S, Zhou H, Stoica L, Galiano M, Krnjević K, Roman G, Costa-Mattioli M. mTORC2 controls actin polymerization required for consolidation of long-term memory. Nat Neurosci. 2013;16(4):441–8.
24. Jakawich SK, Nasser HB, Strong MJ, McCartney AJ, Perez AS, Rakesh N, Carruthers CJ, Sutton MA. Local presynaptic activity gates homeostatic changes in presynaptic function driven by dendritic BDNF synthesis. Neuron. 2010;68(6):1143–58.
25. Kim CH, Lisman JE. A role of actin filament in synaptic transmission and long-term potentiation. J Neurosci. 1999;19(11):4314–24.
26. Krucker T, Siggins GR, Halpain S. Dynamic actin filaments are required for stable long-term potentiation (LTP) in area CA1 of the hippocampus. Proc Natl Acad Sci U S A. 2000;97(12):6856–61.
27. Kumar V, Zhang MX, Swank MW, Kunz J, Wu GY. Regulation of dendritic morphogenesis by Ras-PI3K-Akt-mTOR and Ras-MAPK signaling pathways. J Neurosci. 2005;25(49):11288–99.
28. Kwon CH, Luikart BW, Powell CM, Zhou J, Matheny SA, Zhang W, Li Y, Baker SJ, Parada LF. Pten regulates neuronal arborization and social interaction in mice. Neuron. 2006;50(3):377–88.
29. Lee SJ, Escobedo-Lozoya Y, Szatmari EM, Yasuda R. Activation of CaMKII in single dendritic spines during long-term potentiation. Nature. 2009; 458(7236):299–304.
30. Lisman JE, Harris KM. Quantal analysis and synaptic anatomy–integrating two views of hippocampal plasticity. Trends Neurosci. 1993;16(4):141–7.
31. Lu W, Man H, Ju W, Trimble WS, MacDonald JF, Wang YT. Activation of synaptic NMDA receptors induces membrane insertion of new AMPA receptors and LTP in cultured hippocampal neurons. Neuron. 2001;29(1):243–54.
32. Oh WJ, Jacinto E. mTOR complex 2 signaling and functions. Cell Cycle. 2011; 10(14):2305–16.
33. Ostroff LE, Fiala JC, Allwardt B, Harris KM. Polyribosomes redistribute from dendritic shafts into spines with enlarged synapses during LTP in developing rat hippocampal slices. Neuron. 2002;35(3):535–45.
34. Ma XM, Blenis J. Molecular mechanisms of mTOR-mediated translational control. Nat Rev Mol Cell Biol. 2009;10(5):307–18.
35. Ma T, Tzavaras N, Tsokas P, Landau EM, Blitzer RD. Synaptic stimulation of mTOR is mediated by Wnt signaling and regulation of glycogen synthetase kinase-3. J Neurosci. 2011;31(48):17537–46.
36. Nguyen PV, Abel T, Kandel ER. Requirement of a critical period of transcription for induction of a late phase of LTP. Science. 1994;265(5175):1104–7.
37. Matsuzaki M, Ellis-Davies GC, Nemoto T, Miyashita Y, Iino M, Kasai H. Dendritic spine geometry is critical for AMPA receptor expression in hippocampal CA1 pyramidal neurons. Nat Neurosci. 2001;4(11):1086–92.
38. Matsuzaki M, Honkura N, Ellis-Davies GC, Kasai H. Structural basis of long-term potentiation in single dendritic spines. Nature. 2004; 429(6993):761–6.
39. Murakoshi H, Wang H, Yasuda R. Local, persistent activation of rho GTPases during plasticity of single dendritic spines. Nature. 2011;472(7341):100–4.
40. Murakoshi H, Yasuda R. Postsynaptic signaling during plasticity of dendritic spines. Trends Neurosci. 2012;35(2):135–43.
41. Noguchi J, Nagaoka A, Watanabe S, Ellis-Davies GC, Kitamura K, Kano M, Matsuzaki M, Kasai H. In vivo two-photon uncaging of glutamate revealing the structure-function relationships of dendritic spines in the neocortex of adult mice. J Physiol. 2011;589(Pt 10):2447–57.
42. Park M, Penick EC, Edwards JG, Kauer JA, Ehlers MD. Recycling endosomes supply AMPA receptors for LTP. Science. 2004;305(5692):1972–5.
43. Penzes P, Cahill ME, Jones KA, VanLeeuwen JE, Woolfrey KM. Dendritic spine pathology in neuropsychiatric disorders. Nat Neurosci. 2011;14(3):285–93.
44. Peters A, Kaiserman-Abramof IR. The small pyramidal neuron of the rat cerebral cortex. The perikaryon, dendrites and spines. Am J Anat. 1970;127:321–55.
45. Pi HJ, Otmakhov N, El Gaamouch F, Lemelin D, De Koninck P, Lisman J. CaMKII control of spine size and synaptic strength: role of phosphorylation states and nonenzymatic action. Proc Natl Acad Sci U S A. 2010;107(32):14437–42.
46. Rose CR, Konnerth A. Stores not just for storage. Intracellular calcium release and synaptic plasticity. Neuron. 2001;31(4):519–22.
47. Sarbassov DD, Ali SM, Sengupta S, Sheen JH, Hsu PP, Bagley AF, Markhard AL, Sabatini DM. Prolonged rapamycin treatment inhibits mTORC2 assembly and Akt/PKB. Mol Cell. 2006;22(2):159–68.
48. Sheng M, Hoogenraad CC. The postsynaptic architecture of excitatory synapses: a more quantitative view. Annu Rev Biochem. 2007;76:823–47.
49. Slipczuk L, Bekinschtein P, Katche C, Cammarota M, Izquierdo I, Medina JH. BDNF activates mTOR to regulate GluR1 expression required for memory formation. PLoS One. 2009;4(6):e6007.
50. Spacek J. Three-dimensional analysis of dendritic spines. II. Spine apparatus and other cytoplasmic components. Anat Embryol (Berl). 1985;171(2):235–43.
51. Spacek J, Harris KM. Three-dimensional organization of smooth endoplasmic reticulum in hippocampal CA1 dendrites and dendritic spines of the immature and mature rat. J Neurosci. 1997;17(1):190–203.
52. Steward O, Levy WB. Preferential localization of polyribosomes under the base of dendritic spines in granule cells of the dentate gyrus. J Neurosci. 1982;2(3):284–91.
53. Stoica L, Zhu PJ, Huang W, Zhou H, Kozma SC, Costa-Mattioli M. Selective pharmacogenetic inhibition of mammalian target of Rapamycin complex I (mTORC1) blocks long-term synaptic plasticity and memory storage. Proc Natl Acad Sci U S A. 2011;108(9):3791–6.
54. Sutton MA, Schuman EM. Dendritic protein synthesis, synaptic plasticity, and memory. Cell. 2006;127(1):49–58.
55. Tavazoie SF, Alvarez VA, Ridenour DA, Kwiatkowski DJ, Sabatini BL. Regulation of neuronal morphology and function by the tumor suppressors Tsc1 and Tsc2. Nat Neurosci. 2005;8(12):1727–34.
56. Tang SJ, Reis G, Kang H, Gingras AC, Sonenberg N, Schuman EM. A rapamycin-sensitive signaling pathway contributes to long-term synaptic plasticity in the hippocampus. Proc Natl Acad Sci U S A. 2002;99(1):467–72.
57. Takei N, Inamura N, Kawamura M, Namba H, Hara K, Yonezawa K, Nawa H. Brain-derived neurotrophic factor induces mammalian target of rapamycin-dependent local activation of translation machinery and protein synthesis in neuronal dendrites. J Neurosci. 2004;24(44):9760–9.
58. Tanaka J, Horiike Y, Matsuzaki M, Miyazaki T, Ellis-Davies GC, Kasai H. Protein synthesis and neurotrophin-dependent structural plasticity of single dendritic spines. Science. 2008;319(5870):1683–7.
59. Thoreen CC, Chantranupong L, Keys HR, Wang T, Gray NS, Sabatini DM. A unifying model for mTORC1-mediated regulation of mRNA translation. Nature. 2012;485(7396):109–13.
60. Tolias KF, Duman JG, Um K. Control of synapse development and plasticity by rho GTPase regulatory proteins. Prog Neurobiol. 2011;94(2):133–48.
61. Vickers CA, Dickson KS, Wyllie DJ. Induction and maintenance of late-phase long-term potentiation in isolated dendrites of rat hippocampal CA1 pyramidal neurones. J Physiol. 2005;568(Pt 3):803–13.
62. Yang G, Pan F, Gan WB. Stably maintained dendritic spines are associated with lifelong memories. Nature. 2009;462(7275):920–4.
63. Zhu JJ, Qin Y, Zhao M, Van Aelst L, Malinow R. Ras and rap control AMPA receptor trafficking during synaptic plasticity. Cell. 2002;110(4):443–55.

17

Novel and *de novo* mutations in pediatric refractory epilepsy

Jing Liu[1,2], Lili Tong[1,2], Shuangshuang Song[3], Yue Niu[1,2], Jun Li[1,2], Xiu Wu[1,2], Jie Zhang[4], Clement C. Zai[5], Fang Luo[4], Jian Wu[4], Haiyin Li[5], Albert H. C. Wong[5], Ruopeng Sun[1,2], Fang Liu[2,5] and Baomin Li[1,2*]

Abstract

Pediatric refractory epilepsy is a broad phenotypic spectrum with great genetic heterogeneity. Next-generation sequencing (NGS) combined with Sanger sequencing could help to understand the genetic diversity and underlying disease mechanisms in pediatric epilepsy. Here, we report sequencing results from a cohort of 172 refractory epilepsy patients aged 0–14 years. The pathogenicity of identified variants was evaluated in accordance with the American College of Medical Genetics and Genomics (ACMG) criteria. We identified 43 pathogenic or likely pathogenic variants in 40 patients (23.3%). Among these variants, 74.4% mutations (32/43) were *de novo* and 60.5% mutations (26/43) were novel. Patients with onset age of seizures ≤12 months had higher yields of deleterious variants compared to those with onset age of seizures > 12 months ($P = 0.006$). Variants in ion channel genes accounted for the greatest functional gene category (55.8%), with *SCN1A* coming first (16/43). 81.25% (13/16) of *SCN1A* mutations were *de novo* and 68.8% (11/16) were novel in Dravet syndrome. Pathogenic or likely pathogenic variants were found in the *KCNQ2, STXBP1, SCN2A* genes in Ohtahara syndrome. Novel deleterious variants were also found in West syndrome, Doose syndrome and glucose transporter type 1 deficiency syndrome patients. One *de novo MECP2* mutation were found in a Rett syndrome patient. *TSC1/TSC2* variants were found in 60% patients with tuberous sclerosis complex patients. Other novel mutations detected in unclassified epilepsy patients involve the *SCN8A, CACNA1A, GABRB3, GABRA1, IQSEC2, TSC1, VRK2, ATP1A2, PCDH19, SLC9A6* and *CHD2* genes. Our study provides novel insights into the genetic origins of pediatric epilepsy and represents a starting-point for further investigations into the molecular pathophysiology of pediatric epilepsy that could eventually lead to better treatments.

Keywords: Refractory epilepsy, Next-generation sequencing, ACMG scoring

Introduction

Epilepsy is a complex group of chronic brain disorders that are characterized by recurrent spontaneous seizures, and these can often begin in childhood. Repeated and refractory seizures can cause long-term cognitive impairment, decreased social participation and significantly lower quality of life [1, 2]. Epilepsy is one of the most common neurological disorders with 50 to 100 million affected worldwide, and 2 to 4 million new cases diagnosed each year [3].

Epilepsy is a heterogeneous disease with diverse clinical manifestations and causes, including altered ion channel expression, neurotransmitter signaling, synaptic structure, gliosis, and inflammation [1]. Estimates of heritability from twin studies range from 25% to 70% [4, 5]. Although the range of heritability estimates is quite large, disparate studies using varied methods and studying divergent populations are all consistent in concluding that there is a substantial inherited component to epilepsy [6]. Because of this, we sought to investigate the genome in a heterogeneous set of patients with epilepsy and their parents, with the hope that we would identify novel mutations and confirm existing reports of genetic associations with epilepsy. This type of genetic information can provide an entry point into the biology of epilepsy that could eventually lead to new molecular treatment targets.

With the rapid progress of next-generation sequencing (NGS) techniques, our knowledge of the genetic etiology in many brain disorders such as epilepsy, autism and

* Correspondence: 198962000693@sdu.edu.cn
[1]Department of Pediatrics, Qilu Hospital of Shandong University, Jinan, Shandong, People's Republic of China
[2]Shandong University, Jinan, Shandong, People's Republic of China
Full list of author information is available at the end of the article

intellectual disability has expanded greatly [7, 8]. NGS is now capable of efficient and accurate sequencing of entire genomes with small amounts of tissue at ever decreasing costs and has required new approaches to analysing the very large amount of data obtained. For this study, our priority was to separate common and benign genetic variants from those that are likely to be related to the cause of epilepsy, and we chose to apply the American College of Medical Genetics and Genomics (ACMG) guidelines [9–11]. The ACMG guidelines classify variants into pathogenic, likely pathogenic, uncertain significance, likely benign, and benign categories based on genetic information that includes population, functional, computational and segregation data. In this study, we investigated 153 epilepsy candidate genes in a cohort of 172 refractory epilepsy pediatric patients. We aimed to provide genetic diagnoses of this patient cohort and explore the genetic etiology of pediatric refractory epilepsy.

Method

Participants

We retrospectively collected and analyzed 172 cases of pediatric refractory epilepsy patients between the ages of 1 day to 14 years old in the Department of Pediatrics of Qilu Hospital, China. The program adhered to guidelines of patients' consent for participation and research was supported by the Ethics Committee of Qilu hospital, Shandong University (No. 2016(027)).

All patients were examined and diagnosed at the Pediatric Department in Qilu Hospital using a combination of patients' illness history, previous history, family history, physical examinations, developmental evaluation, hematological examination, ambulatory or video electroencephalography (AEEG/VEEG) monitoring, magnetic resonance imaging (MRI) or computed tomography (CT), and genetic sequencing. Developmental evaluation included gross motor, fine motor, language, and personal-social skills. The above information was reviewed by two qualified pediatric epileptologists. Seizure types and epilepsy syndromes were diagnosed and classified according to the guidelines of International League Against Epilepsy (2014, 2017) [12, 13].

Next-generation sequencing

Targeted gene capture and sequencing

Blood samples of the patients and their biological parents were collected to test if the mutations were *de novo* or inherited. Genomic DNA was extracted from peripheral blood using the QIAamp DNA Mini Kit (Qiagen, China).

One hundred fifty-three genes (Table 1) associated with epilepsy were selected by a gene capture strategy, using the GenCap custom enrichment kit (MyGenostics, China) following the manufacturer's protocol. The biotinylated capture probes were designed to tile all of the exons without repeated regions. The captured DNAs were eluted, amplified and then their polymerase chain reaction (PCR) products were purified with SPRI beads (Beckman, USA). The enriched libraries were sequenced for paired-end reads of 150 bp by Illumina HiSeq X Ten.

Data analysis and pathogenicity of candidate variants

After sequencing, raw data were saved in FASTQ format. Illumina sequencing adapters and low quality reads (< 80 bp) were filtered by Cutadapt [14]. Clean reads were aligned to UCSC hg19 human reference genome using the Burrows-Wheeler Alignment [15] tool. Duplicated reads were removed using Picard (http://broadinstitute.github.io/picard). Insertions, deletions and SNP variants were detected and filtered using the Genome Analysis Toolkit [16]. Then the identified variants were annotated using ANNOVAR [17] and associated with the following databases: 1000 genomes, Exome Aggregation Consortium, The Human Gene Mutation Database, and predicted by Mutation Taster (MT) [18], Sorting Intolerant From Tolerant (SIFT) [19], PolyPhen-2 (PP2) [20] and Genomic Evolutionary Rate Profiling (GERP++) [21, 22]. Splice-site were predicted by Human Splicing Finder [23]. All variants identified by the Illumina HiSeq X Ten sequencer were confirmed by Sanger sequencing. The pathogenicity of mutations was assessed in accordance with American College of Medical Genetics and Genomics guideline (ACMG) [9–11].

Statistical analysis

Statistical analysis was performed using SPSS19. The yields of deleterious variants in patients with different onset age or family history were compared using the chi-squared test.

Results

In the current study, we recruited 172 epilepsy pediatric patients, including 23 with Dravet syndrome, ten with Ohtahara syndrome, two with Ohtahara syndrome evolving to West syndrome, ten with West syndrome, two with West syndrome evolving to Lennox-Gastaut syndrome, five with Lennox-Gastaut syndrome, four with Doose syndrome, two with epilepsy of infancy with migrating focal seizures, two with epileptic encephalopathy with continuous spike and wave during sleep, and one each with temporal lobe epilepsy, early myoclonic encephalopathy, Landau-Kleffner syndrome, and glucose transporter type 1 deficiency syndrome. Three patients had Rett syndrome, five had tuberous sclerosis complex, and one had Sturge-Weber syndrome. Forty-two patients were diagnosed as unclassified epileptic encephalopathy and 57 patients were diagnosed as unclassified

Table 1 One hundred fifty-three epilepsy genes tested in this study by NGS

ADSL	*CHD2*	*DHFR*	*GLB1*	*MAGI2*	*PNPO*	*SLC9A6*
ALDH7A1	*CHRNA2*	*DIAPH3*	*GLRA1*	*MAPK10*	*POLG*	*SPTAN1*
ALG13	*CHRNA4*	*DNAJC6*	*GPR56*	*MBD5*	*PPT1*	*SRPX2*
ARG1	*CHRNA7*	*DNM1*	*GPR98*	*MDGA2*	*PROC*	*ST3GAL2*
ARHGEF15	*CHRNB2*	*DOCK7*	*GRIN1*	*ME2*	*PRRT2*	*ST3GAL5*
ARHGEF9	*CLCN2*	*EEF1A2*	*GRIN2A*	*MECP2*	*RBFOX1*	*STRADA*
ARX	*CLCN4*	*EFHC1*	*GRIN2B*	*MEF2C*	*RBFOX2*	*STXBP1*
ASAH1	*CLN3*	*ELP4*	*HAX1*	*MFSD8*	*RBFOX3*	*SYNGAP1*
ATP13A4	*CLN5*	*EPHB2*	*HDAC4*	*MTHFR*	*RELN*	*SYNJ1*
ATP1A2	*CLN6*	*ERBB4*	*HEXA*	*MTOR*	*RYR3*	*SZT2*
ATP1A3	*CLN8*	*FASN*	*HEXB*	*NDE1*	*SCN1A*	*TBC1D24*
ATP6AP2	*CNTN5*	*FLNA*	*HNRNPH1*	*NEDD4L*	*SCN1B*	*TCF4*
ATP7A	*CNTNAP2*	*FOLR1*	*HNRNPU*	*NID2*	*SCN2A*	*TNK2*
BRAF	*COX6B1*	*FOXG1*	*IQSEC2*	*NRXN1*	*SCN8A*	*TPP1*
BSN	*CSTB*	*FOXP2*	*KCNB1*	*PAFAH1B1*	*SHANK3*	*TSC1*
CACNA1A	*CTNNA3*	*GABBR2*	*KCNH5*	*PCDH19*	*SLC13A5*	*TSC2*
CACNA1H	*CTSD*	*GABRA1*	*KCNMA1*	*PDHA1*	*SLC19A3*	*TUBA1A*
CACNB4	*CYB5R3*	*GABRA6*	*KCNQ2*	*PIGA*	*SLC1A3*	*UBE3A*
CASR	*DBH*	*GABRB2*	*KCNQ3*	*PIGV*	*SLC25A22*	*VRK2*
CDH13	*DCX*	*GABRB3*	*KCNT1*	*PLCB1*	*SLC2A1*	*WDR45*
CDH9	*DEPDC5*	*GABRD*	*LGI1*	*PNKD*	*SLC35A2*	*ZEB2*
CDKL5	*DGKD*	*GABRG2*	*LIAS*	*PNKP*	*SLC46A1*	

refractory epilepsy due to nonspecific manifestations (Table 2).

One hundred fifty-three epilepsy-related genes were selected for sequencing in all patients. The expression pattern of the targeted 153 genes across tissues were analyzed and classified according to the National Center for Biotechnology Information (NCBI, https://www.ncbi.nlm.nih.gov) and The Human Protein Atlas (https://www.proteinatlas.org) database (Additional file 1: Table S1). In our 153-gene panel, 51 genes show elevated expression, 14 genes have low expression, and 88 of them exhibit medium levels of expression in brain. The 14 low-expression genes have been associated with epilepsy, including: *ARG1* [24–27], *ARHGEF15* [28], *CASR* [29, 30], *CHRNA2* [31], *DBH* [32–34], *DIAPH3* [35], *FOLR1* [36, 37], *GABRA6* [38, 39], *GLRA1* [40, 41], *NID2* [42, 43], *PROC* [44], *SLC13A5* [45, 46], *SLC19A3* [47], *SRPX2* [48]. Specifically, among 51 elevated genes in brain, 4 genes (*GABRG2, GABBR2, GABRA1, GRIN1*) show restricted brain expression.

The DNA samples of patients were analyzed by using NGS and the variants were validated by Sanger Sequencing. For the samples subjected to targeted sequencing, the quality assurance (QA) /quality control (QC) file are provided in Additional file 1: Table S2.

After sequencing the 153 epilepsy genes, we identified 43 deleterious variants in 23.3% patients (40 of 172), with three children harbouring more than one deleterious variant. Our results were similar to previous reports, with diagnostic yields ranging between 10% and 48.5% [49–56]. There were 60.5% (26/43) novel deleterious variants found in our study. A total of 43 variants in 22 genes were scored as pathogenic or likely pathogenic, including *SCN1A* (16), *TSC2* (5), *STXBP1* (2), *SCN8A* (2), *TSC1*(1), *MECP2* (1), *CHD2* (1), *PCDH19* (1), *GABRA1* (1), *GABRB3* (1), *SLC2A1* (1), *SLC9A6* (1), *IQSEC2* (1), *KCNQ2* (1), *SCN2A* (1), *CACNA1A* (1), *KCNT1* (1), *SYNGAP1* (1), *ATP1A2* (1), *CDKL5* (1), *ADSL* (1), *VRK2* (1) (Fig. 1a). Among these 43 pathogenic or likely pathogenic variants, there were 18 (41.9%) missense mutations, 3 (7%) splice site mutations, 11 (25.6%) nonsense mutations, 10 (23.3%) frame-shifts, and 1 (2.3%) deletion mutations (Fig. 1a, Table 3).

More recent studies suggest that many severe epilepsy types begin in infancy or childhood, especially those with psychomotor retardation and epileptic encephalopathies are often due to *de novo* mutations [30, 31]. In our study, 32/43 (74.4%) pathogenic or likely pathogenic variants were *de novo*, five (11.6%) were paternal, one (2.3%) was maternal, and five (11.6%) were unknown due to blood samples from parents were unavailable (Table 3).

To further explore the genetic pathogenesis of epilepsy, we subdivided the mutated genes into nine groups according to

Table 2 Clinical diagnosis in 172 refractory epilepsy and their pathogenic or likely pathogenic mutations

Clinical diagnosis	Cases	P/LP mutations	P/LP gene(recurrent no.)
DS	23	16	*SCN1A* (16)
OS	10	2	*KCNQ2* (1), *SCN2A* (1)
OS-WS	2	1	*STXBP1* (1)
WS	10	4	*STXBP1* (1), *KCNT1* (1), *CDKL5* (1), *ADSL* (1)
WS-LGS	2	–	–
LGS	5	–	–
EIMFS	2	–	–
ECSWS	2	–	–
EME	1	–	–
LKS	1	–	–
UEE	42	8	*CACNA1A* (1), *GABRA1* (1), *GABRB3* (1), *SCN8A* (2), *IQSEC2* (1), *PCDH19* (1), *CHD2* (1)
Doose	4	1	*SYNGAP1* (1)
TLE	1	–	–
GLUT1-DS	1	1	*SLC2A1* (1)
Rett	3	1	*MECP2* (1)
TSC	5	5	*TSC2* (5)
SWS	1	–	–
UE	57	4	*VRK2* (1), *ATP1A2* (1), *TSC* (1), *SLC9A6* (1)
Total	172	43	–

P pathogenic, *LP* likely pathogenic, *DS* Dravet syndrome, *OS* Ohtahara syndrome, *OS-WS* Ohtahara syndrome evolves to West syndrome, *WS* West syndrome, *WS-LGS* West syndrome evolves to Lennox-Gastaut syndrome, *LGS* Lennox-Gastaut syndrome, *Doose* Doose syndrome, *ECSWS* epileptic encephalopathy with continuous spike and wave during sleep, *EIMFS* epilepsy of infancy with migrating focal seizures, *TLE* temporal lobe epilepsy, *EME* early myoclonic encephalopathy, *LKS* Landau-Kleffner syndromes, *UEE* unclassified epileptic encephalopathy, *GLUT1-DS* glucose transporter type 1 deficiency syndrome. *Rett* Rett syndrome, *TSC* tuberous sclerosis complex, *SWS* Sturge-Weber syndrome, *UE* unclassified refractory epilepsy

the molecular and biological function of the gene produce. These functional groups included voltage-gated ion channels, enzyme/enzyme modulators, membrane trafficking, ligand-gated ion channels, DNA/RNA binding, cell-adhesion proteins, glucose transporter, proton antiporter, and GTP/GDP exchanges. Variants in ion channel genes (*SCN1A, SCN2A, SCN8A, CACNA1A, KCNT1, KCNQ2*) accounted for 51.2% (22/43) of the pathogenic or likely pathogenic variants. Variants in enzyme/enzyme modulator genes (*TSC1, TSC2, SYNGAP1, ATP1A2, CDKL5, ADSL, VRK2*) accounted for 25.6% (11/43) of pathogenic or likely pathogenic variants. Variants in genes encoded membrane trafficking (*STXBP1*), ligand-gated ion channels (*GABRA1, GABRB3*), DNA/RNA binding proteins (*MECP2, CHD2*) each accounted for 4.7% (2/43) (Fig. 1b). Ion channels (voltage-gated and ligand-gated) accounted for 55.8% in total, suggesting that dysfunction of ion channels plays critical roles in the pathogenesis of epilepsy.

We then analyzed the yield of the epilepsy gene panel testing based on electroclinical syndrome (Fig. 1c). The yield of deleterious variants in Dravet syndrome (69.6%, 16/23) and glucose transporter type 1 deficiency syndrome (100%, 1/1) patients was higher than that in others. Patients with onset age of seizures ≤12 months had higher yields of deleterious variants compared to those with onset age of seizures > 12 months (31/101 vs 9/71; $\chi 2 = 7.583$, df = 1, $P = 0.006$). The family history did not affect whether or not a deleterious genetic variant was identified (7/27 vs 33/145; $\chi 2 = 0.128$, df = 1, $P = 0.804$).

There were 16 mutations in *SCN1A* gene, of which six (37.5%) were missense mutations, one (6.25%) was a splice site mutation, four (25%) were nonsense mutations, four (25%) were frame-shifts, and one (6.25%) was deletion mutation. Thirteen of the 16 (81.3%) *SCN1A* mutations were *de novo* and 11 (68.8%) were novel. We further analysed the positions of the mutations in the affected proteins corresponding to gene mutations and found that 43.8% (7/16) of protein changes are in the intracellular loop of sodium channel protein type 1 subunit alpha, 31.3% (5/16) are in the extracellular loop, 18.8% (3/16) are in the transmembrane region, and 6.25% (1/16) are in the pore forming area (Fig. 2).

There has been a marked increase in genetic diagnoses of a number of key childhood-onset epilepsy syndromes, such as Dravet syndrome, which has been mainly linked to *SCN1A* [17]. In our 16 patients diagnosed as Dravet syndrome with pathogenic or likely pathogenic variants, all identified mutations were in the *SCN1A* gene. These 16 Dravet syndrome patients had typical manifestations: onset between 3 to 8 months of age, fever-sensitive, multiple seizure types, and developmental delay after seizure onset. 81.25% (13/16) *SCN1A* mutations were *de novo* in Dravet syndrome patients and one was inherited from the father who had a history of febrile seizures (FS). 12.5% (2/16) *SCN1A* mutations were unknown. Pathogenic and likely pathogenic mutations each accounted for 50% (Table 4). 50% (8/16) of the Dravet syndrome variants cause nonsense or frameshift mutations that result in truncated proteins, which was consistent with a previous study [57]. We evaluated whether different seizure types, family history, abnormal brain MRI, or developmental delay were associated with specific *SCN1A* mutation types or locations within the gene. We did not detect any bias towards particular regions of the gene or in the type of mutation, although our small sample size did not provide substantial power (Additional file 1: Tables S3 and S4).

Twelve patients presented typical manifestation of Ohtahara syndrome: onset age within postnatal 30 days, tonic spasms, burst suppression EEG and developmental delay. Pathogenic or likely pathogenic variants in Ohtahara syndrome were in the *KCNQ2* (1), *STXBP1* (1),

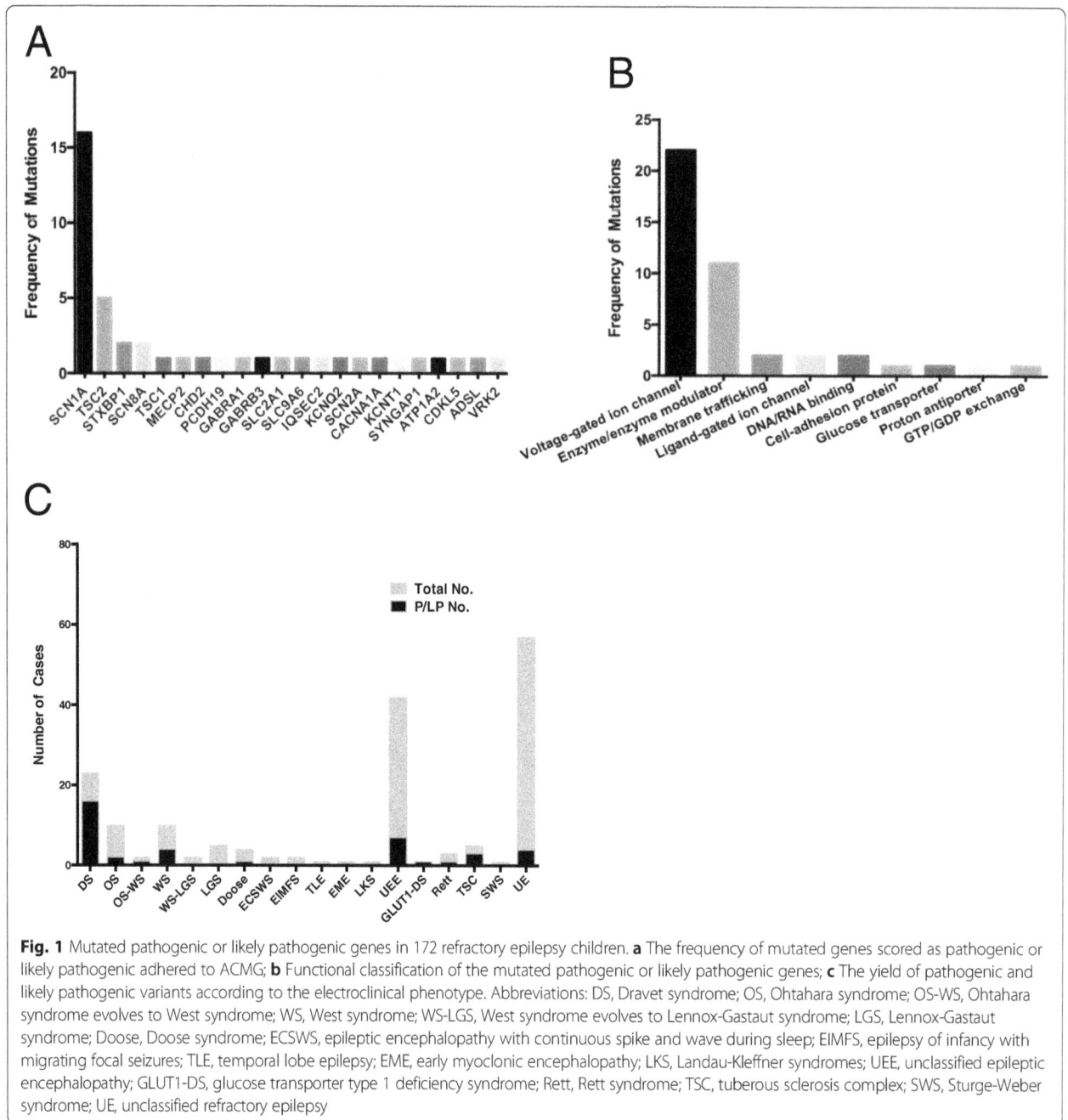

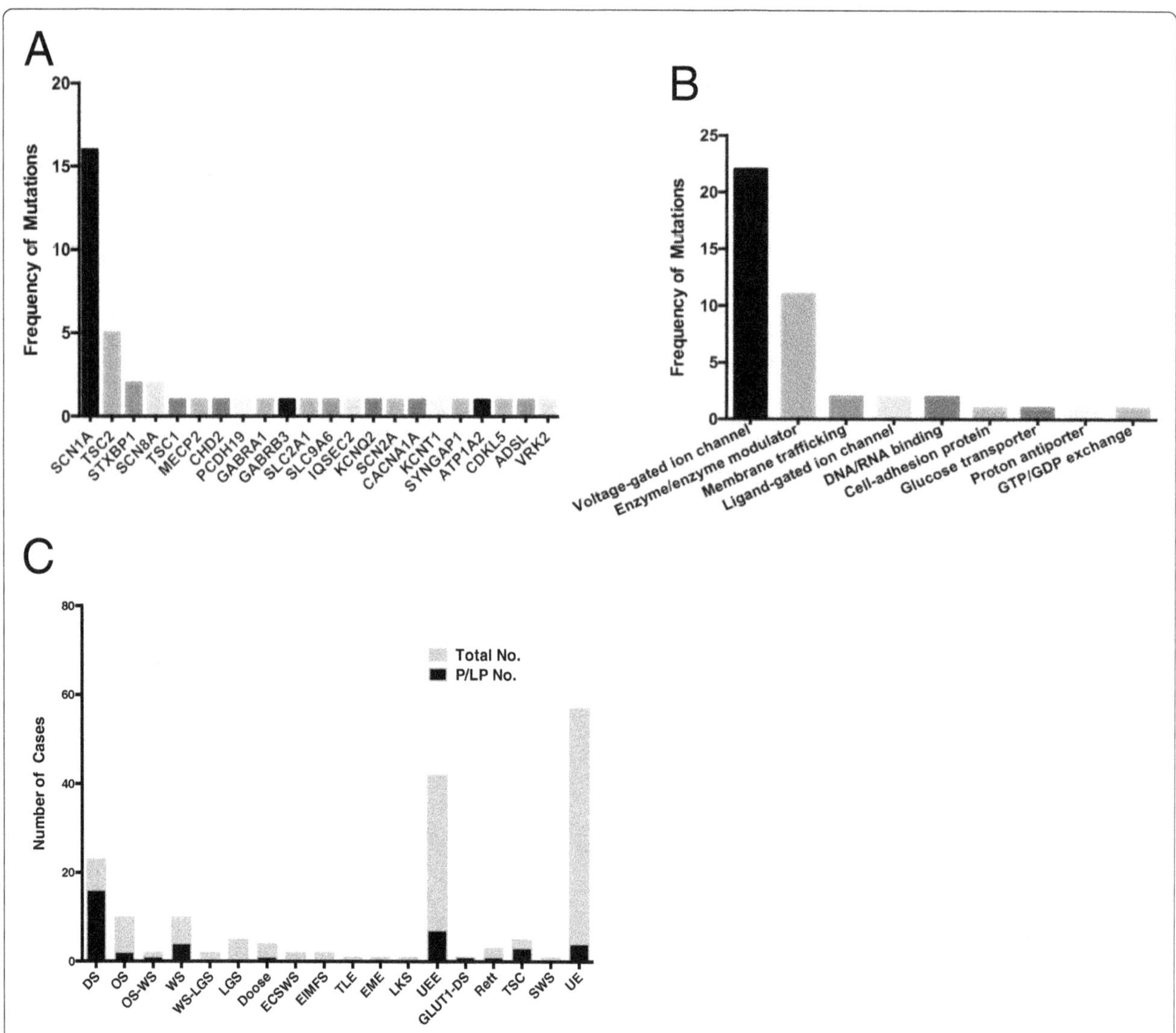

Fig. 1 Mutated pathogenic or likely pathogenic genes in 172 refractory epilepsy children. **a** The frequency of mutated genes scored as pathogenic or likely pathogenic adhered to ACMG; **b** Functional classification of the mutated pathogenic or likely pathogenic genes; **c** The yield of pathogenic and likely pathogenic variants according to the electroclinical phenotype. Abbreviations: DS, Dravet syndrome; OS, Ohtahara syndrome; OS-WS, Ohtahara syndrome evolves to West syndrome; WS, West syndrome; WS-LGS, West syndrome evolves to Lennox-Gastaut syndrome; LGS, Lennox-Gastaut syndrome; Doose, Doose syndrome; ECSWS, epileptic encephalopathy with continuous spike and wave during sleep; EIMFS, epilepsy of infancy with migrating focal seizures; TLE, temporal lobe epilepsy; EME, early myoclonic encephalopathy; LKS, Landau-Kleffner syndromes; UEE, unclassified epileptic encephalopathy; GLUT1-DS, glucose transporter type 1 deficiency syndrome; Rett, Rett syndrome; TSC, tuberous sclerosis complex; SWS, Sturge-Weber syndrome; UE, unclassified refractory epilepsy

SCN2A (1) genes. The nonsense mutation in *STXBP1* (c.364C > T, p.R122X) was detected in one Ohtahara syndrome patients that evolved to West syndrome. This patient had an onset age of postnatal 17 day, spasms, and burst-suppression EEG at postnatal 22 day and hypsarrhythmia EEG at 4 months (Table 5).

West syndrome patients in our study had onset ages of seizures ranging from postnatal 19 days to 6 months. Typical clinical manifestations were all observed, including spasms, hypsarrhythmia EEG, and developmental delay. 16.7% (2/12) of the West syndrome children evolves to Lennox-Gastaut syndrome. After sequencing, we identified 4 pathogenic or likely pathogenic mutations in the following genes: *STXBP1* (1), *KCNT1* (1), *CDKL5* (1), *ADSL* (1). 75% (3/4) of these variants were *de novo*.

One of the West syndrome patients were found to carry two mutations: a nonsense *ADSL* (c.253C > T, p.R85X) mutation was scored as likely pathogenic and was inherited from her unaffected mother. Another reported missense *ADSL* (c.71C > T, p.P24L) [58] mutation which was inherited from her unaffected father were scored as uncertain pathogenicity. *ADSL* has been reported to be related

Table 3 Pathogenic and likely pathogenic mutations adhered to ACMG guidelines in 172 refractory epilepsy children

Case code	Gene	Gene location	Transcript	cDNA change	Protein change	SIFT	PP2	MT	HSF	GERP ++	MAF-ExAC	MAF-KG	Parental Origin	ACMG scoring	ACMG pathogenicity	Diagosis
13	*SCN1A*	chr2–166,901,702	NM_006920	c.1513A > T	p.K505X	–	–	A	–	6.17 (C)	–	–	*De novo*	PVS1 + PS2 + PM2	LP	DS
23	*SCN1A*	chr2–166,854,657 166,854,660 [a] [101]	NM_006920	c.4331_4334del	p.E1444fs	–	–	–	–	–	–	–	*De novo*	PVS1 + PS1 + PS2 + PM2	P	DS
26	*SCN1A*	chr2–166,870,270	NM_001165963	c.3689T>C	p.L1230P	D	D	D	–	5.28 (C)	–	–	*De novo*	PS2 + PM1 + PM2 + PP3	LP	DS
35	*SCN1A*	chr2–166,900,287 166,900,288	NM_001165963	c.1934_1935del	p.V645fs	–	–	–	–	–	–	–	*De novo*	PVS1 + PS2 + PM2	P	DS
38	*SCN1A*	chr2–166,859,121	NM_006920	c.G4112T	p.G1371V	D	P	D	–	5.54 (C)	–	–	*De novo*	PS2 + PM2	LP	DS
53	*SCN1A*	chr2–166,894,306 166,894,337	NM_001165963	c.2895_2926del	p.Q965fs	–	–	–	–	–	–	–	Unknown	PVS1 + PM2	LP	DS
56	*SCN1A*	chr2–166,908,355 [a] [102]	NM_006920	c.838T > C	p.W280R	D	D	D	–	5.41 (C)	–	–	*De novo*	PS1 + PS2 + PM2 + PP3	P	DS
65	*SCN1A*	chr2–166,850,927	NM_006920	c.4549-1G > C	splicing	–	–	D	+	5.76 (C)	–	–	*De novo*	PVS1 + PS2 + PM2	P	DS
115	*SCN1A*	chr2–166,848,614	NM_006920	c.5138C > A	p.A1713D	D	D	D	–	5.8 (C)	–	–	*De novo*	PS2 + PM2 + PP3	LP	DS
124	*SCN1A*	chr2–166,848,438 [a] [103]	NM_006920	c.5314G > A	p.A1772T	D	D	D	–	5.69 (C)	–	–	*De novo*	PS1 + PS2 + PM2 + PP3	P	DS
130	*SCN1A*	chr2–166,854,634 166,854,639 [a] [101]	NM_006920	c.4352_4356del	p.Y1451Cfs*22	–	–	–	–	–	–	–	*De novo*	PVS1 + PS1 + PS2 + PM2	P	DS
140	*SCN1A*	chr2–166,911,210 166,911,211	NM_006920	c.539delT	p.L180X	–	–	–	–	–	–	–	*De novo*	PVS1 + PS2 + PM2	P	DS
148	*SCN1A*	chr2–166,901,579	NM_001165963	c.1636G > T	p.E546X	–	–	A	–	6.17 (C)	–	–	Unknown	PVS1 + PM2	LP	DS
149	*SCN1A*	chr2–166,894,430 [a] [104]	NM_006920	c.2769G > A	p.M923I	D	D	D	–	5.18 (C)	–	–	Paternal	PS1 + PM2 + PP3	LP	DS
162	*SCN1A*	chr2–166,848,043 166,848,045	NM_001165963	c.5740_5742del	p.1914_1914del	–	–	–	–	–	–	–	*De novo*	PS2 + PM2 + PM4	LP	DS
172	*SCN1A*	chr2–166,903,330	NM_006920	c.1327G > T	p.E443X	–	–	A	–	5.31 (C)	–	–	*De novo*	PVS1 + PS2 + PM2	P	DS
93	*SCN2A*	chr2–166,243,416	NM_001040142	c.4712T > C	p.I1571T	D	D	D	–	5.17 (C)	–	–	*De novo*	PS2 + PM1 + PM2 + PP3	LP	OS
55	*KCNQ2*	chr20–62,073,781 [a] [105]	NM_172107	c.794C > T	p.A265V	D	P	D	–	3.38 (C)	–	–	*De novo*	PS1 + PS2 + PM2	P	OS
90	*STXBP1*	chr9–130,423,419 [a] [53]	NM_003165	c.364C > T	p.R122X	–	–	A	–	4.92 (C)	–	–	Unknown	PVS1 + PS1 + PM2	P	OS-WS
52	*ADSL*	chr22–40,745,935	NM_000026	c.253C > T	p.R85X	–	–	A	–	5.59	–	–	Maternal	PVS1 + PM2	LP	WS

Table 3 Pathogenic and likely pathogenic mutations adhered to ACMG guidelines in 172 refractory epilepsy children *(Continued)*

Case code	Gene	Gene location	Transcript	cDNA change	Protein change	SIFT	PP2	MT	HSF	GERP ++	MAF-ExAC	MAF-KG	Parental Origin	ACMG scoring	ACMG pathogenicity	Diagosis
										(C)						
		chr22–40,742,633 [58]	NM_000026	c.71C > T	p.P24L	T	B	D	–	0.153 (N)	–	–	Paternal	PM2	UC	
89	*KCNT1*	chr9–138,651,532 [a] [106]	NM_020822	c.862G > A	p.G288S	T	D	D	–	5.05 (C)	–	–	*De novo*	PS1 + PS2 + PM1 + PM2	P	WS
104	*CDKL5*	chrX-18,593,592 18,593,593	NM_003159	c.265delT	p.F89Lfs*24	–	–	–	–	–	–	–	*De novo*	PVS1 + PS2 + PM2	P	WS
151	*STXBP1*	chr9–130,428,529	NM_003165	c.748C > T	p.Q250X	–	–	A	–	5.72 (C)	–	–	*De novo*	PVS1 + PS2 + PM2	P	WS
29	*SYNGAP1*	chr6–33,393,659 33,393,662	NM_006772	c.274_277del	p.G92fs	–	–	–	–	–	–	–	*De novo*	PVS1 + PS2 + PM2	P	Doose
164	*SLC2A1*	chr1–43,396,517	NM_006516	c.296T > G	p.M99R	D	B	D	–	5.51 (C)	–	–	*De novo*	PS2 + PM2	LP	GLUT1-DS
30	*MECP2*	chrX-153,296,516 [a] [63]	NM_001110792	c.799C > T	p.R267X	–	–	A	–	3.55 (C)	–	–	*De novo*	PVS1 + PS1 + PS2 + PM2	P	Rett
32	*TSC2*	chr16–2,126,095 [a] [91]	NM_000548	c.2666C > T	p.A889V	D	D	D	–	5.09 (C)	–	–	Paternal	PS1 + PM2 + PP3	LP	TSC
94	*TSC2*	chr16–2,130,180 [a] [107]	NM_000548	c.3412C > T	p.R1138X	–	–	A	–	4.74 (C)	–	–	*De novo*	PVS1 + PS1 + PS2 + PM2	P	TSC
	TSC2	chr16–2,130,366 [a] [66]	NM_000548	c.3598C > T	p.R1200W	D	D	D	–	4.74 (C)	–	–	*De novo*	PS1 + PS2 + PM2 + PP3	P	
98	*TSC2*	chr16–2,138,467	NM_001077183	c.5079C > G	p.Y1693X	–	–	D	–	0.137 (N)	–	–	Paternal	PVS1 + PM2	LP	TSC
	TSC2	chr16–2,138,465 2,138,466	NM_001077183	c.5077delT	p.Y1693fs	–	–	–	–	–	–	–	Paternal	PVS1 + PM2	LP	
7	*SCN8A*	chr12–52,184,209 [a] [108]	NM_001177984	c.4324G > A	p.E1442K	D	D	D	–	4.68 (C)	–	–	Paternal	PS1 + PM2 + PP3	LP	UEE
	IQSEC2	chrX-53,263,621 53,263,622	NM_001111125	c.4246_4247insG	p.S1416fs	–	–	–	–	–	–	–	*De novo*	PVS1 + PS2 + PM2	P	
63	*CACNA1A*	chr19–13,566,019 [a] [109]	NM_001127221	c.301G > C	p.E101Q	D	D	D	–	5.01 (C)	–	–	*De novo*	PS1 + PS2 + PM1 + PM2 + PP3	P	UEE
66	*SCN8A*	chr12–52,200,885 [a] [110]	NM_001177984	c.5492G > A	p.R1831Q	D	D	D	–	4.91 (C)	–	–	*De novo*	PS1 + PS2 + PM2 + PP3	P	UEE
69	*PCDH19*	chrX-99,551,873 99,551,874	NM_001184880	c.2849-1G > –	splicing	–	–	–	+	–	–	–	Unknown	PVS1 + PM2	LP	UEE
157	*GABRB3*	chr15–26,812,802 [a] [111]	NM_021912	c.761C > T	p.S254F	D	D	D	–	6.06 (C)	–	–	*De novo*	PS1 + PS2 + PM1 + PM2 + PP3	P	UEE
160	*GABRA1*	chr5–161,309,645 [a] [112]	NM_001127648	c.641G > A	p.R214H	D	D	D	–	5.34 (C)	–	–	*De novo*	PS1 + PS2 + PM1 + PM2 + PP3	P	UEE

Table 3 Pathogenic and likely pathogenic mutations adhered to ACMG guidelines in 172 refractory epilepsy children *(Continued)*

Case code	Gene	Gene location	Transcript	cDNA change	Protein change	SIFT	PP2	MT	HSF	GERP ++	MAF-ExAC	MAF-KG	Parental Origin	ACMG scoring	ACMG pathogenicity	Diagosis
54	*CHD2*	chr15–93,540,231	NM_001271	c.3640G > T	p.G1214X	–	–	A	–	5.64 (C)	–	–	*De novo*	PVS1 + PS2 + PM2	P	UEE
40	*VRK2*	chr2–58,312,086	NM_001130483	c.C256 + 1G > A	splicing	–	–	D	+	5.86 (C)	–	–	Unknown	PVS1 + PM2	LP	UE
44	*ATP1A2*	chr1–160,098,521	NM_000702	c.1097G > T	p.G366V	D	D	D	–	4.77 (C)	–	–	*De novo*	PS2 + PM1 + PM2 + PP3	LP	UE
68	*TSC1*	chr9–135,772,854	NM_000368	c.2768_2769insC	p.L924Ffs*26	–	–	–	–	–	–	–	*De novo*	PVS1 + PS2 + PM2	P	UE
79	*SLC9A6*	chrX-135,080,322 135,080,336	NM_001042537	c.582_595del	p.Y194fs	–	–	–	–	–	–	–	*De novo*	PVS1 + PS2 + PM2	P	UE

Abbreviations: *M* male, *F* female, *m* month, *y* year, *SIFT* Sorts intolerant from tolerant (D, damaging; T, tolerant), *PP2*, polymorphism phenotyping v2 (D, damaging; P, possible damaging; B, benign), *MT* mutation taster (D, disease causing; A, disease causing automatic), *HSF* human splicing finder (+, altering splicing), *GERP++* genomic evolutionary rate profiling (C, conserved; N, nonconserved), *KG* 1000 Genomes project, *LP* likely pathogenic, *P* pathogenic, *DS* Dravet syndrome, *OS* Ohtahara syndrome, *OS-WS* OS syndrome evolves to West syndrome, *WS* West syndrome, *Doose* Doose syndrome, *GLUT1-DS* glucose transporter type 1 deficiency syndrome, *Rett* Rett syndrome, *TSC* tuberous sclerosis complex, *UEE* unclassified epileptic encephalopathy, *UE* unclassified refractory epilepsy

[a] Mutations have been reported in HGMD database

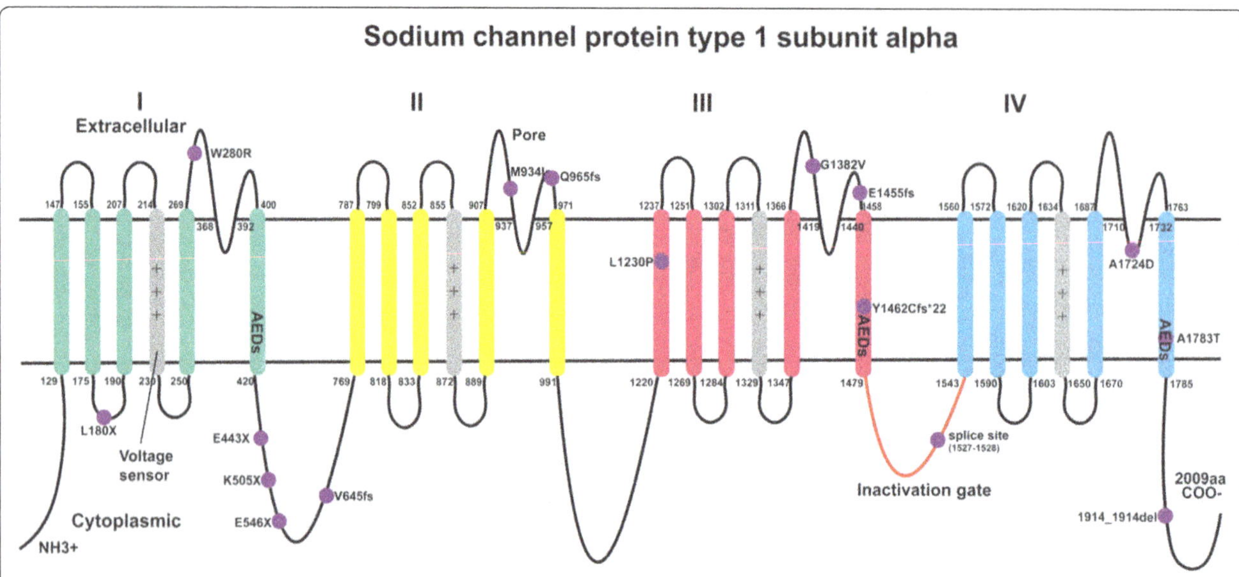

Fig. 2 Schematic representation of the mutations in subunit alpha of sodium channel type 1 (SCN1A) in our study. SCN1A alpha unit has four domains (I–IV), each domain includes 6 transmembrane segments (S1–S6). Purple circle = mutation; AEDs, anti-epileptic drugs. The position of mutations in SCN1A is approximate and is according to reference transcript NM_001165963.

to adenylosuccinate lyase deficiency, which is an autosomal recessive defect of purine metabolism [59, 60]. The patient presented with spasms 2 months after birth. Brain MRI showed cerebral dysplasia and EEG showed hypsarrhythmia and multifocal discharges. The patient also had developmental delay and lack of eye contact. A definitive diagnosis can be made with high performance liquid chromatography examination of the urine to detect the ratio of succinyladenosine and succinyl-aminoimidazole carboximide riboside, but this was not available for the patient in question. Thus, this patient was diagnosed clinically as having West syndrome.

A novel frame-shift mutation in *SYNGAP5* (c.274_277del, p.G92fs) was detected in a patient with Doose syndrome. This patient presented with myoclonic and myoclonic-astatic seizures, as well as having atypical absence seizures. *SYNGAP5* had been reported to be associated with Doose syndrome and mental retardation, autosomal dominant 5 (MRD5) [51, 61, 62]. This mutation, which is very rare, was *de novo*, and caused frameshift changes in Ras/Rap GTPase-activating protein SynGAP, was therefore scored as pathogenic (Table 5).

One glucose transporter type 1 deficiency syndrome patient presented with seizures at age 28 months. The patient has alopecia and was almost bald at 4 years old. The child did not have other abnormalities in blood tests, brain MRI, or neurological exam. Her cerebrospinal fluid glucose value was 2.04 mmol/L (blood glucose value was 7.2 mmol/L before lumbar puncture; fasting blood glucose value was 5.2 mmol/L). NGS identified a missense mutation in *SLC2A1* (c.296T > G, p.M99R). The mutation was *de novo* and novel. The patient's parents and sister were normal, which is consistent with the sequencing results. Symptoms improved with a ketogenic diet, with seizures controlled for more than 6 months.

One *MECP2* mutation (c.799C > T, p.R267X) was detected in a girl diagnosed as Rett syndrome. The girl developed normally for the first 18 months, gradually lost speech ability while developing repetitive hand-wringing. Seizures began at age 3 years. The *MECP2* gene is located on the X-chromosome, and Rett syndrome is inherited through this gene in a dominant fashion [63]. This patient had a *de novo MECP2* nonsense mutation, consistent with her parents being unaffected.

40% (2/5) of tuberous sclerosis complex patients were diagnosed with West syndrome associated with tuberous sclerosis complex in our study. Tuberous sclerosis complex is closely related to the *TSC1/TSC2* genes [64–67].

In our study, all of the tuberous sclerosis complex patients' initial presentations were seizures, of which 80% (4/5) presented in the first year of life. 60% (3/5) had hypomelanotic macules and 40% (2/5) had multi nodules. One patient's only clinical manifestation was seizures and three (60%) patients with seizures had only one major feature of tuberous sclerosis complex. After sequencing, 60% (3/5) patients were found to have deleterious *TSC1* or *TSC2* mutations.

We identified more than one *TSC1/2* mutations in 2 patients. One patient has two *TSC2* mutations inherited from his affected father. Facial angiofibromas appeared by age 3–4 years in 60% (3/5) patients in the follow-up period. Gilboa et al. [68] reported four patients with the same *TSC1* genomic deletion (9q34.13q34.2) in a family

Table 4 Clinical features in DS patients

Case code	Gender/ age	Diagosis	Age of onset	Seizure types	EEG	Brain MRI/CT	Developmental delay	Gene	cDNA change	Protein change	Parental Origin	ACMG pathogenicity
13	F/2y6m	DS	3m	FS, FoS, Myo	FSW	Normal	Yes	*SCN1A*	c.1513A > T	p.K505X	*De novo*	LP
23	F/3y	DS	7m	FS, FoS (A), Myo, FBTC	Multi. FD	Underdeveloped myelin	Yes	*SCN1A*	c.4331_4334del	p.E1444fs	*De novo*	P
26	F/ 5y11m	DS	5m	FS, SE, FoS (A), Myo, FBTC	FSW	Normal	Yes	*SCN1A*	c.3689T>C	p.L1230P	*De novo*	LP
35	M/4y	DS	3m	FS, SE, GTCS, aAb	Multi. FD	Normal	Yes	*SCN1A*	c.1934_1935del	p.V645fs	*De novo*	P
38	F/1y6m	DS	4m	FS, SE, Myo	FSW	Nonspecific	Yes	*SCN1A*	c.G4112T	p.G1371V	*De novo*	LP
53	M/5y	DS	7m	FS, aAb, Myo, Fos (I)	Multi. FD	Normal	Yes	*SCN1A*	c.2895_2926del	p.Q965fs	Unknown	LP
56	F/3y6m	DS	5m	FS, Myo, GTCS, SE, FoS (A), aAb	Multi. FD	Nonspecific	Yes	*SCN1A*	c.838T > C	p.W280R	*De novo*	P
65	M/2y4m	DS	5m	FS, SE, FoS (A)	FSW	Normal	Yes	*SCN1A*	c.4549-1G > C	splicing	*De novo*	P
115	M/2y1m	DS	8m	FS, FoS (I), FoS (hemi clonic), GTCS	FSW	Enlargement of the subarachnoid space in front of left temporal lobe	Yes	*SCN1A*	c.5138C > A	p.A1713D	*De novo*	LP
124	M/3y	DS	5m	FS, FoS (A), FBTC	FSW	Nonspecific	Yes	*SCN1A*	c.5314G > A	p.A1772T	*De novo*	P
130	F/11y	DS	6m	FS, FoS (A), aAb, Myo, GTCS	Multi. FD	Normal	Yes	*SCN1A*	c.4352_4356del	p.Y1451Cfs*22	*De novo*	P
140	F/1y9m	DS	3m	FS, GTCS, C, FoS (I)	FSW	Normal	Yes	*SCN1A*	c.539delT	p.L180X	*De novo*	P
148	F/6y8m	DS	4m	FS, GTCS, FoS, aAb	Multi. FD	Normal	Yes	*SCN1A*	c.1636G > T	p.E546X	Unknown	LP
149	M/3y6m	DS	4m	FS, FoS (A), Myo, GTCS	Multi. FD, GSW	Normal	Yes	*SCN1A*	c.2769G > A	p.M923I	Paternal (FS)	LP
162	M/4y	DS	5m	FS, FoS (A), Myo, FBTC	Multi. FD	Normal	Yes	*SCN1A*	c.5740_5742del	p.1914_1914del	*De novo*	LP
172	F/8y	DS	5m	FS, aAb, Myo, FBTC	Multi. FD, GSW, GPSW	Normal	Yes	*SCN1A*	c.1327G > T	p.E443X	*De novo*	P

Abbreviations: *M* male, *F* female, *m* month, *y* year, *P* pathogenic, *LP* likely pathogenic, *UC* uncertain, *DS* Dravet syndrome, *FS* febrile seizures, *SE* status epilepticus, *FoS* focal seizures, *FoS (I)* focal seizures (impaired awareness), *FoS (A)* focal seizures (aware), *FBTC* focal to bilateral tonic-clonic, *Myo* myoclonic, *aAb* atypical absence, *GTCS* generalized tonic-clonic seizures, *FSW* focal spike wave, *Multi. FD* multifocal discharges, *GSW* generalized spike-wave, *GPSW* generalized polyspike-wave

Table 5 Clinical features in OS, WS, LGS, Doose, GLUT1-DS, Rett, TSC, UEE and UE patients

Case code	Gender/ age	Diagosis	Age of onset	Seizure types	EEG	Brain MRI/CT	Developmental delay	Gene	cDNA change	Protein change	Parental Origin	ACMG pathogenicity
55	M/54d	OS	1d	FoS, Tonic spasms	BS, FSW	Normal	Yes	*KCNQ2*	c.794C > T	p.A265V	*De novo*	P
93	M/40d	OS	3d	Tonic spasms	BS	Normal	Yes	*SCN2A*	c.4712T > C	p.I1571T	*De novo*	LP
90	M/ 2y11m	OS-WS	17d	Tonic spasms, Spa.	BS, Hypsarrhy.	Normal	Yes	*STXBP1*	c.364C > T	p.R122X	Unknown	P
52	F/1y8m	WS	2m	Spa.	Multi. FD, Hypsarrhy.	Cerebral dysplasia	Yes	*ADSL*	c.253C > T	p.R85X	Maternal	LP
								ADSL	c.71C > T	p.P24L	Paternal	UC
89	F/1y11m	WS	19d	FoS, Spa.	Multi. FD, Hypsarrhy.	Subdural hemorrhage	Yes	*KCNT1*	c.862G > A	p.G288S	*De novo*	P
104	F/2y10m	WS	3m7d	Spa.	Hypsarrhy., Multi.FD	Normal	Yes	*CDKL5*	c.265delT	p.F89Lfs*24	*De novo*	P
151	F/9m	WS	3m	Spa.	Hypsarrhy., Multi. FD	Enlargement of the subarachnoid space	Yes	*STXBP1*	c.748C > T	p.Q250X	*De novo*	P
29	M/5y6m	Doose	1y3m	Myo-At., Myo, aAb	Abnormal background theta, GSW, GPSW	Normal	No	*SYNGAP1*	c.274_277del	p.G92fs	*De novo*	P
164	F/6y	GLUT1-DS	2y4m	GTCS	FSW, Multi. FD	Nonspecific (Hair loss leads to bald)	No	*SLC2A1*	c.296T > G	p.M99R	*De novo*	LP
30	F/4y4m	Rett	3y2m	Fos (I), FBTC	Multi. FD	Normal	Yes	*MECP2*	c.799C > T	p.R267X	*De novo*	P
32	M/8y	TSC	1y6m	FoS (I), FBTC	Multi. FD	Multi nodules	No	*TSC2*	c.2666C > T	p.A889V	Paternal	LP
94	F/9m	TSC (WS)	3m	Spa.	Multi. FD, Hypsarrhy.	Multi nodules	Yes	*TSC2*	c.3412C > T	p.R1138X	*De novo*	P
								TSC2	c.3598C > T	p.R1200W	*De novo*	P
98	M/3y	TSC (WS)	4m	Spa., aAb	Multi. FD, Hypsarrhy.	Nonspecific	Yes	*TSC2*	c.5079C > G	p.Y1693X	Paternal	LP
								TSC2	c.5077delT	p.Y1693fs	Paternal	LP
7	M/2y	UEE (EIEE13)	6m	FoS (I), FBTC	Multi. FD	Enlargement of the subarachnoid space	Yes	*SCN8A*	c.4324G > A	p.E1442K	Paternal	LP
								IQSEC2	c.4246_4247insG	p.S1416fs	*De novo*	P
63	M/4y	UEE (EIEE42)	5m	FoS, GTCS	Multi. FD	Normal	Yes	*CACNA1A*	c.301G > C	p.E101Q	*De novo*	P
66	M/1y9m	UEE (EIEE13)	4m	FBTC, FoS	Multi. FD	Enlargement of the subarachnoid space	Yes	*SCN8A*	c.5492G > A	p.R1831Q	*De novo*	P
69	F/2y1m	UEE (EIEE9)	1y3m	FBTC, C, T	Multi. FD	Normal	Yes	*PCDH19*	c.2849-1G > –	splicing	Unknown	LP
157	F/2y	UEE (EIEE43)	2m	C, FoS (I)	FSW	Normal	Yes	*GABRB3*	c.761C > T	p.S254F	*De novo*	P
160	M/6y	UEE (EIEE19)	6m	FoS (I), GTCS	FSW	Normal	Yes	*GABRA1*	c.641G > A	p.R214H	*De novo*	P
54	F/7y	UEE (EEOC)	4y2m	SE, GTCS, FoS (I)	Mult. FD	Normal	Yes	*CHD2*	c.3640G > T	p.G1214X	*De novo*	P

Table 5 Clinical features in OS, WS, LGS, Doose, GLUT1-DS, Rett, TSC, UEE and UE patients *(Continued)*

Case code	Gender/ age	Diagosis	Age of onset	Seizure types	EEG	Brain MRI/CT	Developmental delay	Gene	cDNA change	Protein change	Parental Origin	ACMG pathogenicity
40	F/2y11m	UE	4m	FoS	FSW	Normal	No	*VRK2*	c.C256 + 1G > A	splicing	Unknown	LP
44	F/5y6m	UE	4y	FoS (automatisms, emotional)	Multi. FD	Nodules in internal side of left anterior limb of internal capsule; caput of caudate nucleus or heterotopic gray matter	Yes	*ATP1A2*	c.1097G > T	p.G366V	*De novo*	LP
68	M/6y	UE	4y	FoS (A)	FSW	Normal	No	*TSC1*	c.2768_2769insC	p.L924Ffs*26	*De novo*	P
79	M/3y	UE	1y2m	FoS (I), FBTC	Multi. FD	Normal	Yes	*SLC9A6*	c.582_595del	p.Y194fs	*De novo*	P

Abbreviations: *M* male, *F* female, *m* month, *y* year, *P* pathogenic, *LP* likely pathogenic, *UC* uncertain, *OS* Ohtahara syndrome, *OS-WS* Ohtahara syndrome evolves to West syndrome, *WS* West syndrome, *Doose* Doose syndrome, *GLUT1-DS* glucose transporter type 1 deficiency syndrome, *Rett* Rett syndrome, *TSC* tuberous sclerosis complex, *UEE* unclassified epileptic encephalopathy, *UE* unclassified refractory epilepsy, *EEIE* early-infantile epileptic encephalopathies, *EEOC* childhood-onset epileptic encephalopathy, *Spa.* Spasms, *FoS* focal seizures, *FoS (I)* focal seizures (impaired awareness), *FoS (A)* focal seizures (aware), *FBTC* focal to bilateral tonic-clonic, *T* tonic, *C* clonic, *Myo* myoclonic, *aAb* atypical absence, *At.* atonic, *GTCS* generalized tonic-clonic seizures, *SE* status epilepticus, *BS burst suppression*, *Hypsarrhy.* hypsarrhythmia, *Multi. FD* multifocal discharges, *FSW* focal spike-wave, *GSW* generalized spike-wave, *GPSW* generalized polyspike-wave and none of them fulfilled the clinical criteria for tuberous sclerosis complex. In our study, one patient with pathogenic *TSC1* (c.2768_2769insC, p.L924Ffs*26) mutation presented with focal seizures beginning at age four. There were two hypopigmented macules on the patient's abdomen. The brain MRI results were normal and there are no other features of tuberous sclerosis complex. This *de novo* mutation causes a frame-shift in hamartin and has not been reported previously. Thus, this patient was considered to have unclassified refractory epilepsy.

One unclassified epileptic encephalopathy patient had two deleterious mutations: *SCN8A* inherited from his affected father (c.4324G > A, p.E1442K) and *IQSEC2* (c.4246_4247insG, p.S1416fs). Early-infantile epileptic encephalopathies (EIEE) caused by *SCN8A* mutations are designated as EIEE13 (OMIM #614558) [69]. The missense mutation in *SCN8A* is very rare in the general population, and had been previously predicted to be damaging by SIFT, MT and PP2. *IQSEC2* is an X-linked gene that has been reported to be related to intellectual disability and epilepsy, and it encodes the IQ motif and SEC7 domain-containing protein 2 [70]. The identified novel *IQSEC2* mutation was *de novo* and was scored as being pathogenic.

Other pathogenic or likely pathogenic mutations found in patients with unclassified epileptic encephalopathy included *CACNA1A, GABRA1, GABRB3, PCDH19,* and *CHD2.* Epileptic encephalopathies with the above mutations had been designated as EIEE42, EIEE19, EIEE43, EIEE9 and EEOC (childhood-onset epileptic encephalopathy) according to Online Mendelian Inheritance in Man (OMIM). Other deleterious variants found in patients with unclassified refractory epilepsy were in *VRK2, ATP1A2,* and *SLC9A6.* Taking these unclassified epileptic encephalopathies and unclassified refractory epilepsy patients' clinical manifestations into consideration, we found that all patients with deleterious mutations in genes encoding ion channels (*SCN8A, CACNA1A, GABRB3, GABRA1*) had similar clinical symptoms: onset age of seizures within the first year, epileptic encephalopathy and developmental delay. In contrast, patients with mutations in *VRK2, ATP1A2,* and *SLC9A6,* had relatively later onset age of seizures.

We then assessed the clinical benefit of genetic testing in those patients with identified deleterious variants. NGS helped with the diagnosis ($n = 8$), medication selection ($n = 18$), reproductive planning ($n = 4$), and treatment planning ($n = 1$). The finding of the *SLC2A1* variant in Case 164 prompted other tests such as cerebrospinal fluid (CSF) glucose that were clinically useful. Identification of deleterious *SCN1A* mutations in five young infants with clinically suspected Dravet syndrome helped early diagnosis (Case 13, 38, 65, 115, 140) and led to the discontinuation of oxcarbazepine (Case 13) that exacerbated seizures. Identification of *SCN1A* mutations in other Dravet syndrome patients helped to avoid sodium channel blockers such as oxcarbazepine, carbamazepine and lamotrigine. Among the four Dravet syndrome patients who responded to anticonvulsants (Case 13, 26, 149, 172), 75% (3/4) of them were prescribed sodium valproate or clonazepam suggesting that these medications may be effective in Dravet syndrome. The finding of the *TSC2* variants in Cases 94 and 98 helped early diagnosis and Case 32 experienced remission with administration of rapamune. Identification of *TSC1* prompted clinical surveillance for tuberous sclerosis complex in Case 68. The findings of patients with deleterious variants in *TSC2* (Case 32, 98), *SCN8A* (Case 7), *SCN1A* (Case 149), *ADSL* (Case 52) which were inherited, helped in prenatal counselling (Table 6).

Discussion

Epilepsy is highly heterogeneous and can be primarily genetic in origin, or be secondary to structural or metabolic disorders of the central nervous system [71, 72]. To date, over 500 genes have been implicated in epilepsy [73–76]. However, the overlapping clinical features of different epilepsy syndromes and non-specific phenotypes can hamper clinical and genetic diagnosis [53]. The correct genetic diagnosis can help to guide treatment and prognosis. In addition to genetic origins, pediatric epilepsy may also arise from epigenetic mechanisms mediating gene-environment interactions during neurodevelopment. In this study, we used NGS to investigate 153 epilepsy related genes in a cohort of 172 refractory epilepsy children.

Approximately one quarter of genes identified in epilepsy encode ion channel proteins, including voltage-gated channels (Na^+, K^+, $Ca2^+$ channels and hyperpolarization-activated cyclic nucleotide-gated channels) and ligand-gated ion channels (N-Methyl-D-Aspartate receptors, Gamma-aminobutyric acid receptors and Nicotinic Acetylcholine receptors) [77]. The genes that encode ion channels and are relevant to epilepsy include *SCN1A, SCN1B, SCN2A, SCN8A, KCNA1, KCNA2, KCNB1, KCNC1, KCNMA1, KCNQ2, KCNQ3, KCNT1, KCTD7, HCN1, CACAN1A, CACNA1H, GRIN1, GRIN2A, GRIN2B, GRIN2D, GABRA1, GABRB3, GABRG2, CHRNA2, CHRNA4, CHRNB2.* In our study, 51.2% pathogenic or likely pathogenic variants were found in voltage-gated ion channels and 4.7% were found in ligand-gated ion channels. Thus, we further confirmed that ion channels play an important role in the pathogenesis of epilepsy.

An *SCN1A* mutation was first discovered in epilepsy in 2000 [72], and now hundreds of new *SCN1A* mutations have been described in epilepsy patients, making it the most common epilepsy-related gene [78]. In our study, we found *SCN1A* mutations in 16/44 deleterious variants, making it the most common gene to show variation in

Table 6 Clinical benefits after molecular diagnosis

Clinical benefits		Effects (Case details)
Diagnosis	*SLC2A1* (GLUT1-DS)	Definitive diagnosis (Case 164)
	SCN1A (DS)	Definitive diagnosis (Case 13, 38, 65, 115, 140)
	TSC2 (TSC)	Definitive diagnosis (Case 94, 98)
Management implications	*SLC2A1*, using KD	Controlled (Case 164, KD)
	SCN1A, stopping OXC	Remitted (Case 13, VPA, TPM,10–20 / month)
	SCN1A, avoiding OXC, CBZ, and LTG	Remitted (Case 23, VPA, TPM, seizure-free for 5 months; Case 26, LEV, TPM, CZP, seizure-free for 6 months; Case 149, VPA, TPM, LEV, CZP, seizure-free for 4 months; Case 172, VPA, TPM, CZP, seizure-free for 1 year)
		Uncontrolled (Case 35, 38, 53, 56, 65, 115, 124, 130, 140, 148, 162)
	TSC2, using rapamune	Remitted (Case 32, seizure-free for 7 months)
Long-term follow up	*TSC1* (risk of TSC)	Case 68
Reproductive planning	Suggesting the family conduct genetic counseling	*TSC2* (Case 32, 98), *SCN8A* (Case 7), *SCN1A* (Case 149), *ADSL* (Case 52)

Abbreviations: *DS* Dravet syndrome, *GLUT1-DS* glucose transporter type 1 deficiency syndrome, *Rett* Rett syndrome, *TSC* tuberous sclerosis complex, *KD* ketogenic diet, *OXC* oxcarbazepine, *CBZ* carbamazepine, *LTG* lamotrigine, *VPA* sodium valproate, *TPM* topiramate, *LEV* levetiracetam, *CZP* clonazepam

our study. *SCN1A* encodes the Nav1.1 pore-forming α-subunit, expressed mainly in inhibitory GABAergic neurons. The α-subunit comprises four homologous domains (I–IV), forming a tetrameric structure. Each domain is composed of six transmembrane segments (S1–S6) [77]. The S4, voltage-sensing segment has multiple positively charged amino acids. The intracellular loop between III and IV domain functions as the inactivation gate. The α-subunit is usually associated with two β-subunits that influence α-subunit localization and function [77]. Among α-subunit of sodium channel genetic variants in our study, 43.8% (7/16) are within the intracellular loop, 31.3% (5/16) in the extracellular loop, 18.8% (3/16) in the transmembrane area, and 6.25% (1/16) in the pore forming area. All the extracellular mutations are between S5 and S6, which is very close to the pore forming area. These variants may influence the initiation and propagation of action potentials, making these inhibitory GABAergic neurons less excitable. Some antiepileptic drugs (AEDs) bind to the inner cavity of the pore of the sodium channel (IS6, IIIS6 and IVS6) [77, 79]. The pore forming area or internal/external loop could be promising targets for new seizure prophylaxis medications.

Patients harboring *SCN1A* mutations can have with Dravet syndrome or generalized epilepsy with febrile seizures plus. One Dravet syndrome patient inherited the *SCN1A* mutations from his father only had febrile seizures. This could be due to somatic mosaicism [72, 80, 81]. A Dravet syndrome mouse model (Nav1.1 knockout-based) responded well to stiripentol and clobazam, which are commonly used to treat Dravet syndrome [82–85]. One of the patients in our study was treated with oxcarbazepine, which blocks sodium channels and worsened seizures, before the diagnosis of Dravet syndrome was made. This case illustrates the importance of correct molecular diagnosis in selecting the best anticonvulsant.

Approximately half of Ohtahara syndrome patients with *STXBP1* mutations evolve to West syndrome [86]. In our study, there was one such patient with a nonsense mutation in *STXBP1*, suggesting that this gene could play a role in the etiology of West syndrome. Our findings also suggest that *STXBP1* is related to both Ohtahara syndrome and West syndrome.

KCNT1 is associated with epilepsy of infancy with migrating focal seizures, autosomal dominant nocturnal frontal lobe epilepsy, and other types of early onset epileptic encephalopathies [87–89]. Ohba et al. [88] found 11 *KCNT1* mutations in a total of 362 epilepsy patients: 9/18 epilepsy of infancy with migrating focal seizures cases (50%), 1/180 West syndrome cases (0.56%), and 1/66 unclassified early onset epileptic encephalopathy cases (1.52%), suggesting that *KCNT1* may be a causal gene for West syndrome. In our study, one *KCNT1* (c.862G > A, p.G288S) mutation was found in a patient diagnosed as West syndrome.

Genetic studies of neuropsychiatric disease have led to the discovery of molecular etiology and pathophysiology. For example, most cases of Rett syndrome are now known to arise from mutations in the *MECP2* gene, which codes for a methyl-CpG-binding protein 2 [90]. Another example is glucose transporter type 1 deficiency syndrome, which has been attributed to variants in *SLC2A1*, *SLC2A2*, and *GLUT1*. In our study, the glucose transporter type 1 deficiency syndrome patient did not have cerebrospinal fluid analysis as part of their diagnostic work-up until the genetic data suggested the diagnosis. This example illustrates the utility of NGS in clinical scenarios, and in time this may become an important part of the evaluation of pediatric patients with epilepsy. In some epilepsy syndromes, crucial interventions such as diet modification can have dramatic beneficial effects, so early diagnosis is vital [91, 92].

In our study, *SCN1A* was the main deleterious variant in Dravet syndrome and *KCNQ2, STXBP1, SCN2A* were found in Ohtahara syndrome. Deleterious variants in *STXBP1, KCNT1, CDKL5, ADSL* genes were found in West syndrome. Novel mutations in *SYNGAP1* were found in Doose syndrome, a *SLC2A1* mutation was found in GLUT1-DS and a *de novo MECP2* mutation were found in Rett syndrome. *TSC1/TSC2* variants were found in 60% of patients with tuberous sclerosis complex. Mutations found in unclassified epileptic encephalopathy were mainly in ion-channel genes. Thus, our study reinforces previous observations that the clinical syndrome and genetic etiology do not always match.

We tested 153 epilepsy genes and found 43 pathogenic and likely pathogenic variants in this study. Considering that over 500 epilepsy genes have been reported [73–76], our work was not comprehensive, which is a limitation of this study. With the decreasing cost of whole genome sequencing, the interrogation of the entire genome is now feasible for larger samples of epilepsy patients, and this approach has already been fruitful in other neuropsychiatric disorders such as autism, Kabuki syndrome, Bohring-Opitz syndrome and others [93, 94].

For genetic testing, it is proposed to conduct the strong candidate gene sequencing first (*SCN1A* for Dravet syndrome, *MECP2* for Rett syndrome and *TSC1/2* for tuberous sclerosis complex) before a NGS multi-gene panel testing [95–97]. In our study, we conducted targeted panel sequencing on Dravet syndrome and Rett syndrome patients before screening the strongest candidate gene for the following reasons. First, the correct clinical diagnosis of these syndromes can be difficult, especially in some of the younger patients in our sample, and often requires longitudinal assessment, which delays the correct diagnosis. Thus, we elected to perform NGS on our subjects before knowing the clinical diagnosis in some cases, such as these syndromes. Since our NGS panel that contains 153 epilepsy genes, our approach could facilitate the correct diagnosis in some cases. Second, it is now apparent that while 70–80% Dravet syndrome patients have *SCN1A* mutations, mutations in other genes such as *SCN1B, SCN2A, SCN8A, PCDH19, GABRA1, GABRG2, STXBP1, CHD2* genes can cause Dravet syndrome like phenotypes [98], which would be missed if only *SCN1A* was sequenced. Similarly, *CDKL5* and *FOXG1* have been associated with atypical Rett syndrome [99], in addition to *MECP2*.

In tuberous sclerosis complex patients, we have a similar clinical scenario in which most features of tuberous sclerosis complex become evident only after 3 years of age, limiting their usefulness for early diagnosis [100]. In our study, all of the tuberous sclerosis complex patients' initial presentations were seizures, of which 80% presented in the first year of life. 60% had hypomelanotic macules and 40% had multi nodules. 20% patient's only clinical manifestation was seizures and 60% patients with seizures had only one major feature of tuberous sclerosis complex. 60% patients were found to have deleterious *TSC1* or *TSC2* mutations by NGS sequencing. Facial angiofibromas appeared by age 3–4 years in 60% patients in the follow-up period.

In summary, we identified 43 pathogenic or likely pathogenic variants, of which 26 mutations were novel and 32 were *de novo*. Variants in ion channel genes accounted for the largest category of gene in children with refractory epilepsy. Dravet syndrome is closely related to the *SCN1A* gene, which was the most frequently-appearing gene showing variants in our study. Novel and *de novo* mutations were found in Ohtahara syndrome, West syndrome, Doose syndrome and tuberous sclerosis complex pediatric patients. We also found a novel mutation in glucose transporter type 1 deficiency. Our results reinforce the importance and feasibility of precise genetic diagnosis for epilepsy, with the hope that in future, this will both aid in understanding the molecular pathophysiology and lead to new treatment targets.

Additional file

Additional file 1: Table S1. The expression levels of the 153 targeted genes in brain. **Table S2.** The quality assurance (QA) /quality control (QC) of targeted sequencing. **Table S3.** The frequencies of different mutation locations in *SCN1A* gene and their corresponding phenotypes in Dravet syndrome patients. **Table S4.** The frequencies of different mutation types in *SCN1A* gene and their corresponding phenotypes in Dravet syndrome patients. (DOCX 98 kb)

Abbreviations

ACMG: American College of Medical Genetics and Genomics; AEDs: antiepileptic drugs; EEOC: childhood-onset epileptic encephalopathy; EIEE: early-infantile epileptic encephalopathies; MT: Mutation Taster; NGS: next-generation sequencing; OMIM: Online Mendelian Inheritance in Man; PP2: PolyPhen-2; SCN1A: subunit alpha of sodium channel type 1; SIFT: Sorting Intolerant From Tolerant

Acknowledgements

All authors greatly appreciate to the families that take part in this research.

Funding

The project was funded by National Key Research and Development Program of China (NO. 2016YFC1306202), Key Research and Development Plan in Shandong Province (NO. 2016GSF201073), and General program of Qilu hospital, Shandong University (NO.2015QLMS08).

Authors' contributions

BML and JL were responsible for the original concept and the overall design of the research. JL, LLT, BML, RPS analyzed the EEG results and diagnosed patients. JL, SSS, YN, JL, XW, FL collected the clinical data and sample. JL, LLT,

SSS, YN, XW, JL, JZ, FL, JW carried the experiments and analysed the sequencing data. JL, HYL performed structural and functional analysis experiments. JL, BML, CZ, AW, FL wrote and revised the manuscript. All authors read and approved the final manuscript.

Competing interests

The authors declare that they have no competing interests.

Author details

[1]Department of Pediatrics, Qilu Hospital of Shandong University, Jinan, Shandong, People's Republic of China. [2]Shandong University, Jinan, Shandong, People's Republic of China. [3]Qilu Children's hospital of Shandong University, Jinan, Shandong, People's Republic of China. [4]MyGenostics Inc., Beijing, People's Republic of China. [5]Campbell Family Mental Health Research Institute, Centre for Addiction and Mental Health, University of Toronto, Toronto, ON, Canada.

References

1. Henshall DC, Hamer HM, Pasterkamp RJ, Goldstein DB, Kjems J, Prehn JHM, et al. MicroRNAs in epilepsy: pathophysiology and clinical utility. Lancet Neurol. 2016;15(13):1368–76.
2. Nickels KC, Zaccariello MJ, Hamiwka LD, Wirrell EC. Cognitive and neurodevelopmental comorbidities in paediatric epilepsy. Nat Rev Neurol. 2016;12(8):465–76.
3. Pitkanen A, Loscher W, Vezzani A, Becker AJ, Simonato M, Lukasiuk K, et al. Advances in the development of biomarkers for epilepsy. Lancet Neurol. 2016;15(8):843–56.
4. Miller LL, Pellock JM, DeLorenzo RJ, Meyer JM, Corey LA. Univariate genetic analyses of epilepsy and seizures in a population-based twin study: the Virginia Twin Registry. Genet Epidemiol. 1998;15(1):33–49.
5. Kjeldsen MJ, Kyvik KO, Christensen K, Friis ML. Genetic and environmental factors in epilepsy: a population-based study of 11900 Danish twin pairs. Epilepsy Res. 2001;44(2–3):167–78.
6. Speed D, O'Brien TJ, Palotie A, Shkura K, Marson AG, Balding DJ, et al. Describing the genetic architecture of epilepsy through heritability analysis. Brain. 2014;137:2680–9.
7. Brandler WM, Sebat J. From de novo mutations to personalized therapeutic interventions in autism. Annu Rev Med. 2015;66:487–507.
8. Hoischen A, Krumm N, Eichler EE. Prioritization of neurodevelopmental disease genes by discovery of new mutations. Nat Neurosci. 2014;17(6):764–72.
9. Directors ABo. ACMG policy statement: updated recommendations regarding analysis and reporting of secondary findings in clinical genome-scale sequencing. Genet Med. 2015;17(1):68–9.
10. Richards S, Aziz N, Bale S, Bick D, Das S, Gastier-Foster J, et al. Standards and guidelines for the interpretation of sequence variants: a joint consensus recommendation of the American College of Medical Genetics and Genomics and the Association for Molecular Pathology. Genet Med. 2015; 17(5):405–24.
11. Green RC, Berg JS, Grody WW, Kalia SS, Korf BR, Martin CL, et al. ACMG recommendations for reporting of incidental findings in clinical exome and genome sequencing. Genet Med. 2013;15(7):565–74.
12. Fisher RS, Acevedo C, Arzimanoglou A, Bogacz A, Cross JH, Elger CE, et al. ILAE official report: a practical clinical definition of epilepsy. Epilepsia. 2014; 55(4):475–82.
13. Fisher RS, Cross JH, D'Souza C, French JA, Haut SR, Higurashi N, et al. Instruction manual for the ILAE 2017 operational classification of seizure types. Epilepsia. 2017;58(4):531–42.
14. Martin M. Cutadapt removes adapter sequences from high-throughput sequencing reads. EMBnet J. 2011; https://doi.org/10.14806/ej.17.1.200.
15. Li H, Durbin R. Fast and accurate short read alignment with burrows-wheeler transform. Bioinformatics. 2009;25(14):1754–60.
16. Van der Auwera GA, Carneiro MO, Hartl C, Poplin R, Del Angel G, Levy-Moonshine A, et al. From FastQ data to high confidence variant calls: the Genome Analysis Toolkit best practices pipeline. Curr Protoc Bioinformatics. 2013;43:11.10.1–33.
17. Wang K, Li M, Hakonarson H. ANNOVAR: functional annotation of genetic variants from high-throughput sequencing data. Nucleic Acids Res. 2010; 38(16):e164.
18. Schwarz JM, Cooper DN, Schuelke M, Seelow D. MutationTaster2: mutation prediction for the deep-sequencing age. Nat Methods. 2014;11(4):361–2.
19. Kumar P, Henikoff S, Ng PC. Predicting the effects of coding non-synonymous variants on protein function using the SIFT algorithm. Nat Protoc. 2009;4(7):1073–81.
20. Adzhubei IA, Schmidt S, Peshkin L, Ramensky VE, Gerasimova A, Bork P, et al. A method and server for predicting damaging missense mutations. Nat Methods. 2010;7(4):248–9.
21. Cooper GM, Stone EA, Asimenos G, Program NCS, Green ED, Batzoglou S, et al. Distribution and intensity of constraint in mammalian genomic sequence. Genome Res. 2005;15(7):901–13.
22. Davydov EV, Goode DL, Sirota M, Cooper GM, Sidow A, Batzoglou S. Identifying a high fraction of the human genome to be under selective constraint using GERP++. PLoS Comput Biol. 2010;6(12):e1001025.
23. Desmet FO, Hamroun D, Lalande M, Collod-Beroud G, Claustres M, Beroud C. Human splicing finder: an online bioinformatics tool to predict splicing signals. Nucleic Acids Res. 2009;37(9):e67.
24. Uchino T, Haraguchi Y, Aparicio JM, Mizutani N, Higashikawa M, Naitoh H, et al. Three novel mutations in the liver-type arginase gene in three unrelated Japanese patients with argininemia. Am J Hum Genet. 1992; 51(6):1406–12.
25. Carvalho DR, Brand GD, Brum JM, Takata RI, Speck-Martins CE, Pratesi R. Analysis of novel ARG1 mutations causing hyperargininemia and correlation with arginase I activity in erythrocytes. Gene. 2012;509(1):124–30.
26. Uchino T, Snyderman SE, Lambert M, Qureshi IA, Shapira SK, Sansaricq C, et al. Molecular basis of phenotypic variation in patients with argininemia. Hum Genet. 1995;96(3):255–60.
27. Wu TF, Liu YP, Li XY, Wang Q, Ding Y, Ma YY, et al. Five novel mutations in ARG1 gene in Chinese patients of argininemia. Pediatr Neurol. 2013;49(2):119–23.
28. Veeramah KR, Johnstone L, Karafet TM, Wolf D, Sprissler R, Salogiannis J, et al. Exome sequencing reveals new causal mutations in children with epileptic encephalopathies. Epilepsia. 2013;54(7):1270–81.
29. Kapoor A, Satishchandra P, Ratnapriya R, Reddy R, Kadandale J, Shankar SK, et al. An idiopathic epilepsy syndrome linked to 3q13.3-q21 and missense mutations in the extracellular calcium sensing receptor gene. Ann Neurol. 2008;64(2):158–67.
30. Sato K, Hasegawa Y, Nakae J, Nanao K, Takahashi I, Tajima T, et al. Hydrochlorothiazide effectively reduces urinary calcium excretion in two Japanese patients with gain-of-function mutations of the calcium-sensing receptor gene. J Clin Endocrinol Metab. 2002;87(7):3068–73.
31. Kurahashi H, Hirose S. Autosomal Dominant Nocturnal Frontal Lobe Epilepsy. In: Adam MP, Ardinger HH, Pagon RA, Wallace SE, Bean LJH, Stephens K, et al., editors. GeneReviews((R)). Seattle (WA): University of Washington, Seattle; 1993–2018.
32. Lauterborn JC, Ribak CE. Differences in dopamine beta-hydroxylase immunoreactivity between the brains of genetically epilepsy-prone and Sprague-Dawley rats. Epilepsy Res. 1989;4(3):161–76.
33. Schank JR, Liles LC, Weinshenker D. Reduced anticonvulsant efficacy of valproic acid in dopamine beta-hydroxylase knockout mice. Epilepsy Res. 2005;65(1–2):23–31.
34. Warter JM, Coquillat G, Kurtz D. Human circulating dopamine-beta-hydroxylase and epilepsy. Psychopharmacologia. 1975;41(1):75–9.
35. Lesca G, Rudolf G, Labalme A, Hirsch E, Arzimanoglou A, Genton P, et al. Epileptic encephalopathies of the Landau-Kleffner and continuous spike and waves during slow-wave sleep types: genomic dissection makes the link with autism. Epilepsia. 2012;53(9):1526–38.

36. Steele SU, Cheah SM, Veerapandiyan A, Gallentine W, Smith EC, Mikati MA. Electroencephalographic and seizure manifestations in two patients with folate receptor autoimmune antibody-mediated primary cerebral folate deficiency. Epilepsy Behav. 2012;24(4):507–12.
37. Perez-Duenas B, Toma C, Ormazabal A, Muchart J, Sanmarti F, Bombau G, et al. Progressive ataxia and myoclonic epilepsy in a patient with a homozygous mutation in the FOLR1 gene. J Inherit Metab Dis. 2010;33(6):795–802.
38. Kumari R, Lakhan R, Kalita J, Garg RK, Misra UK, Mittal B. Potential role of GABAA receptor subunit; GABRA6, GABRB2 and GABRR2 gene polymorphisms in epilepsy susceptibility and pharmacotherapy in North Indian population. Clin Chim Acta. 2011;412(13–14):1244–8.
39. Hernandez CC, Gurba KN, Hu N, Macdonald RL. The GABRA6 mutation, R46W, associated with childhood absence epilepsy, alters 6beta22 and 6beta2 GABA(A) receptor channel gating and expression. J Physiol. 2011; 589(Pt 23):5857–78.
40. Elmslie F, Gardiner M. Genetics of the epilepsies. Curr Opin Neurol. 1995;8(2):126–9.
41. Bakker MJ, van Dijk JG, van den Maagdenberg AMJM, Tijssen MAJ. Startle syndromes. Lancet Neurol. 2006;5(6):513–24.
42. Conroy J, McGettigan PA, McCreary D, Shah N, Collins K, Parry-Fielder B, et al. Towards the identification of a genetic basis for Landau-Kleffner syndrome. Epilepsia. 2014;55(6):858–65.
43. Dong L, Chen Y, Lewis M, Hsieh JC, Reing J, Chaillet JR, et al. Neurologic defects and selective disruption of basement membranes in mice lacking entactin-1/nidogen-1. Lab Investig. 2002;82(12):1617–30.
44. Fong CY, Mumford AD, Likeman MJ, Jardine PE. Cerebral palsy in siblings caused by compound heterozygous mutations in the gene encoding protein C. Dev Med Child Neurol. 2010;52(5):489–93.
45. Thevenon J, Milh M, Feillet F, St-Onge J, Duffourd Y, Juge C, et al. Mutations in SLC13A5 cause autosomal-recessive epileptic encephalopathy with seizure onset in the first days of life. Am J Hum Genet. 2014;95(1):113–20.
46. Hardies K, de Kovel CG, Weckhuysen S, Asselbergh B, Geuens T, Deconinck T, et al. Recessive mutations in SLC13A5 result in a loss of citrate transport and cause neonatal epilepsy, developmental delay and teeth hypoplasia. Brain. 2015;138(Pt 11):3238–50.
47. Zeng WQ, Al-Yamani E, Acierno JS Jr, Slaugenhaupt S, Gillis T, MacDonald ME, et al. Biotin-responsive basal ganglia disease maps to 2q36.3 and is due to mutations in SLC19A3. Am J Hum Genet. 2005;77(1):16–26.
48. Roll P, Rudolf G, Pereira S, Royer B, Scheffer IE, Massacrier A, et al. SRPX2 mutations in disorders of language cortex and cognition. Hum Mol Genet. 2006;15(7):1195–207.
49. Hildebrand MS, Myers CT, Carvill GL, Regan BM, Damiano JA, Mullen SA, et al. A targeted resequencing gene panel for focal epilepsy. Nerology. 2016; 86(17):1605–12.
50. Parrini E, Marini C, Mei D, Galuppi A, Cellini E, Pucatti D, et al. Diagnostic targeted resequencing in 349 patients with drug-resistant pediatric epilepsies identifies causative mutations in 30 different genes. Hum Mutat. 2017;38(2):216–25.
51. Carvill GL, Heavin SB, Yendle SC, McMahon JM, O'Roak BJ, Cook J, et al. Targeted resequencing in epileptic encephalopathies identifies de novo mutations in CHD2 and SYNGAP1. Nat Genet. 2013;45(7):825–30.
52. Trump N, McTague A, Brittain H, Papandreou A, Meyer E, Ngoh A, et al. Improving diagnosis and broadening the phenotypes in early-onset seizure and severe developmental delay disorders through gene panel analysis. J Med Genet. 2016;53(5):310–7.
53. Lemke JR, Riesch E, Scheurenbrand T, Schubach M, Wilhelm C, Steiner I, et al. Targeted next generation sequencing as a diagnostic tool in epileptic disorders. Epilepsia. 2012;53(8):1387–98.
54. Møller RS, Larsen LH, Johannesen KM, Talvik I, Talvik T, Vaher U, et al. Gene panel testing in epileptic encephalopathies and familial epilepsies. Mol Syndromol. 2016;7(4):210–9.
55. Kodera H, Kato M, Nord AS, Walsh T, Lee M, Yamanaka G, et al. Targeted capture and sequencing for detection of mutations causing early onset epileptic encephalopathy. Epilepsia. 2013;54(7):1262–9.
56. Ortega-Moreno L, Giráldez BG, Soto-Insuga V, Losada-Del Pozo R, Rodrigo-Moreno M, Alarcón-Morcillo C, et al. Molecular diagnosis of patients with epilepsy and developmental delay using a customized panel of epilepsy genes. PLoS One. 2017;12(11):e0188978. https://doi.org/10.1371/journal.pone.0188978.
57. Meisler MH, Kearney JA. Sodium channel mutations in epilepsy and other neurological disorders. J Clin Invest. 2005;115(8):2010–7.
58. Mao X, Li K, Tang B, Luo Y, Ding D, Zhao Y, et al. Novel mutations in ADSL for Adenylosuccinate Lyase deficiency identified by the combination of trio-WES and constantly updated guidelines. Sci Rep. 2017;7(1):1625.
59. Jurecka A, Zikanova M, Kmoch S, Tylki-Szymańska A. Adenylosuccinate lyase deficiency. J Inherit Metab Dis. 2015;38(2):231–42.
60. Chen BC, McGown IN, Thong MK, Pitt J, Yunus ZM, Khoo TB, et al. Adenylosuccinate lyase deficiency in a Malaysian patient, with novel adenylosuccinate lyase gene mutations. J Inherit Metab Dis. 2010;33(Suppl 3):S159–62.
61. Hamdan FF, Gauthier J, Spiegelman D, Noreau A, Yang Y, Pellerin S, et al. Mutations in SYNGAP1 in autosomal nonsyndromic mental retardation. N Engl J Med. 2009;360(6):599–605.
62. Berryer MH, Hamdan FF, Klitten LL, Møller RS, Carmant L, Schwartzentruber J, et al. Mutations in SYNGAP1 cause intellectual disability, autism, and a specific form of epilepsy by inducing haploinsufficiency. Hum Mutat. 2013; 34(2):385–94.
63. Amir RE, Van den Veyver IB, Wan M, Tran CQ, Francke U, Zoghbi HY. Rett syndrome is caused by mutations in X-linked MECP2, encoding methyl-CpG-binding protein 2. Nat Genet. 1999;23:185–8.
64. Hasbani DM, Crino PB. Tuberous sclerosis complex. Handb Clin Neurol. 2018; 148:813–22.
65. Zhang H, Nanba E, Yamamoto T, Ninomiya H, Ohno K, Mizuguchi M, et al. Mutational analysis of TSC1 and TSC2 genes in Japanese patients with tuberous sclerosis complex. J Hum Genet. 1999;44(6):391–6.
66. Wilson PJ, Ramesh V, Kristiansen A, Bove C, Jozwiak S, Kwiatkowski DJ, et al. Novel mutations detected in the TSC2 gene from both sporadic and familial TSC patients. Hum Mol Genet. 1996;5(2):249–56.
67. Hoogeveen-Westerveld M, Wentink M, van den Heuvel D, Mozaffari M, Ekong R, Povey S, et al. Functional assessment of variants in the TSC1 and TSC2 genes identified in individuals with tuberous sclerosis complex. Hum Mutat. 2011;32(4):424–35.
68. Gilboa T, Segel R, Zeligson S, Alterescu G, Ben-Pazi H. Ganglioglioma, epilepsy, and intellectual impairment due to familial TSC1 deletion. J Child Neurol. 2018;33(7):482–6.
69. Wagnon JL, Meisler MH. Recurrent and non-recurrent mutations of SCN8A in epileptic encephalopathy. Front Neurol. 2015;6(104) https://doi.org/10.3389/fneur.2015.00104.
70. Zerem A, Haginoya K, Lev D, Blumkin L, Kivity S, Linder I, et al. The molecular and phenotypic spectrum of IQSEC2-related epilepsy. Epilepsia. 2016;57(11):1858–69.
71. Wilmshurst JM, Berg AT, Lagae L, Newton CR, Cross JH. The challenges and innovations for therapy in children with epilepsy. Nat Rev Neurol. 2014; 10(5):249–60.
72. Oyrer J, Maljevic S, Scheffer IE, Berkovic SF, Petrou S, Reid CA. Ion channels in genetic epilepsy: from genes and mechanisms to disease-targeted therapies. Pharmacol Rev. 2018;70(1):142–73.
73. Orsini A, Zara F, Striano P. Recent advances in epilepsy genetics. Neurosci Lett. 2018;667:4–9.
74. Weber YG, Biskup S, Helbig KL, Von Spiczak S, Lerche H. The role of genetic testing in epilepsy diagnosis and management. Expert Rev Mol Diagn. 2017; 17(8):739–50.
75. Wang J, Lin ZJ, Liu L, Xu HQ, Shi YW, Yi YH, et al. Epilepsy-associated genes. Seizure. 2017;44:11–20.
76. Samarasinghe TD, Sands SA, Skuza EM, Joshi MS, Nold-Petry CA, Berger PJ. The effect of prenatal maternal infection on respiratory function in mouse offspring: evidence for enhanced chemosensitivity. J Appl Physiol (1985). 2015;119(3):299–307.
77. Catterall WA, Goldin AL, Waxman SG. International Union of Pharmacology. XLVII. Nomenclature and structure-function relationships of voltage-gated sodium channels. Pharmacol Rev. 2005;57(4):397–409.
78. Oliva M, Berkovic SF, Petrou S. Sodium channels and the neurobiology of epilepsy. Epilepsia. 2012;53(11):1849–59.
79. McDonald CL, Saneto RP, Carmant L, Sotero de Menezes MA. Focal seizures in patients with SCN1A mutations. J Child Neurol. 2017;32(2):170–6.
80. Depienne C, Trouillard O, Gourfinkel-An I, Saint-Martin C, Bouteiller D, Graber D, et al. Mechanisms for variable expressivity of inherited SCN1A mutations causing Dravet syndrome. J Med Genet. 2010;47(6):404–10.
81. Poduri A, Evrony GD, Cai X, Elhosary PC, Beroukhim R, Lehtinen MK, et al. Somatic activation of AKT3 causes hemispheric developmental brain malformations. Neuron. 2012;74(1):41–8.
82. Hawkins NA, Anderson LL, Gertler TS, Laux L, George AL Jr, Kearney JA. Screening of conventional anticonvulsants in a genetic mouse model of epilepsy. Ann Clin Transl Neurol. 2017;4(5):326–39.
83. Chiron C, Dulac O. The pharmacologic treatment of Dravet syndrome. Epilepsia. 2011;52(Suppl 2):72–5.

84. Cao D, Ohtani H, Ogiwara I, Ohtani S, Takahashi Y, Yamakawa K, et al. Efficacy of stiripentol in hyperthermia-induced seizures in a mouse model of Dravet syndrome. Epilepsia. 2012;53(7):1140–5.
85. Oakley JC, Cho AR, Cheah CS, Scheuer T, Catterall WA. Synergistic GABA-enhancing therapy against seizures in a mouse model of Dravet syndrome. J Pharmacol Exp Ther. 2013;345(2):215–24.
86. Di Meglio C, Lesca G, Villeneuve N, Lacoste C, Abidi A, Cacciagli P, et al. Epileptic patients with de novo STXBP1 mutations: key clinical features based on 24 cases. Epilepsia. 2015;56(12):1931–40.
87. Ko A, Youn SE, Kim SH, Lee JS, Kim S, Choi JR, et al. Targeted gene panel and genotype-phenotype correlation in children with developmental and epileptic encephalopathy. Epilepsy Res. 2018;141:48–55.
88. Ohba C, Kato M, Takahashi N, Osaka H, Shiihara T, Tohyama J, et al. De novo KCNT1 mutations in early-onset epileptic encephalopathy. Epilepsia. 2015; 56(9):e121–8.
89. Fukuoka M, Kuki I, Kawawaki H, Okazaki S, Kim K, Hattori Y, et al. Quinidine therapy for West syndrome with KCNTI mutation: a case report. Brain Dev. 2017;39(1):80–3.
90. Leonard H, Cobb S, Downs J. Clinical and biological progress over 50 years in Rett syndrome. Nat Rev Neurol. 2017;13(1):37–51.
91. Zhou P, He N, Zhang JW, Lin ZJ, Wang J, Yan LM, et al. Novel mutations and phenotypes of epilepsy-associated genes in epileptic encephalopathies. Genes Brain Behav. 2018. https://doi.org/10.1111/gbb.12456
92. Daci A, Bozalija A, Jashari F, Krasniqi S. Individualizing treatment approaches for epileptic patients with glucose transporter type1 (GLUT-1) deficiency. Int J Mol Sci. 2018;19(1):122.
93. Ku CS, Polychronakos C, Tan EK, Naidoo N, Pawitan Y, Roukos DH, et al. A new paradigm emerges from the study of de novo mutations in the context of neurodevelopmental disease. Mol Psychiatry. 2013;18(2):141–53.
94. Veltman JA, Brunner HG. De novo mutations in human genetic disease. Nat Rev Genet. 2012;13(8):565–75.
95. Hirose S, Scheffer IE, Marini C, De Jonghe P, Andermann E, Goldman AM, et al. SCN1A testing for epilepsy: application in clinical practice. Epilepsia. 2013; 54(5):946–52.
96. Kammoun F. Screening of MECP2 coding sequence in patients with phenotypes of decreasing likelihood for Rett syndrome: a cohort of 171 cases. J Med Genet. 2004;41(6):e85.
97. Avgeris S, Fostira F, Vagena A, Ninios Y, Delimitsou A, Vodicka R, et al. Mutational analysis of TSC1 and TSC2 genes in tuberous sclerosis complex patients from Greece. Sci Rep. 2017;7(1):16697.
98. Steel D, Symonds JD, Zuberi SM, Brunklaus A. Dravet syndrome and its mimics: beyond SCN1A. Epilepsia. 2017;58(11):1807–16.
99. Guerrini R, Parrini E. Epilepsy in Rett syndrome, and CDKL5- and FOXG1-gene-related encephalopathies. Epilepsia. 2012;53(12):2067–78.
100. Curatolo P, Bombardieri R, Jozwiak S. Tuberous sclerosis. Lancet. 2008; 372(9639):657–68.
101. Depienne C, Trouillard O, Saint-Martin C, Gourfinkel-An I, Bouteiller D, Carpentier W, et al. Spectrum of SCN1A gene mutations associated with Dravet syndrome: analysis of 333 patients. J Med Genet. 2009;46(3):183–91.
102. Nabbout R, Gennaro E, Dalla Bernardina B, Dulac O, Madia F, Bertini E, et al. Spectrum of SCN1A mutations in severe myoclonic epilepsy of infancy. Neurology. 2003;60(12):1961–7.
103. Harkin LA, McMahon JM, Iona X, Dibbens L, Pelekanos JT, Zuberi SM, et al. The spectrum of SCN1A-related infantile epileptic encephalopathies. Brain. 2007;130(Pt 3):843–52.
104. Fukuma G, Oguni H, Shirasaka Y, Watanabe K, Miyajima T, Yasumoto S, et al. Mutations of neuronal voltage-gated Na+ channel alpha 1 subunit gene SCN1A in core severe myoclonic epilepsy in infancy (SMEI) and in borderline SMEI (SMEB). Epilepsia. 2004;45(2):140–8.
105. Saitsu H, Kato M, Koide A, Goto T, Fujita T, Nishiyama K, et al. Whole exome sequencing identifies KCNQ2 mutations in Ohtahara syndrome. Ann Neurol. 2012;72(2):298–300.
106. Ishii A, Shioda M, Okumura A, Kidokoro H, Sakauchi M, Shimada S, et al. A recurrent KCNT1 mutation in two sporadic cases with malignant migrating partial seizures in infancy. Gene. 2013;531(2):467–71.
107. Mayer K, Ballhausen W, Rott HD. Mutation screening of the entire coding regions of the TSC1 and the TSC2 gene with the protein truncation test (PTT) identifies frequent splicing defects. Hum Mutat. 1999;14:401–11.
108. Gardella E, Becker F, Møller RS, Schubert J, Lemke JR, Larsen LH, et al. Benign infantile seizures and paroxysmal dyskinesia caused by an SCN8A mutation. Ann Neurol. 2016;79(3):428–36.
109. Epi4K Consortium. De novo mutations in SLC1A2 and CACNA1A are important causes of epileptic encephalopathies. Am J Hum Genet. 2016; 99(2):287–98.
110. Larsen J, Carvill GL, Gardella E, Kluger G, Schmiedel G, Barisic N, et al. The phenotypic spectrum of SCN8A encephalopathy. Neurology. 2015;84(5):480–9.
111. Hirouchi M, Suzuki H, Itoda M, Ozawa S, Sawada J-i, Ieiri I, et al. Characterization of the cellular localization, expression level, and function of SNP variants of MRP2/ABCC2. Pharm Res. 2004;21(5):742–8.
112. Fokstuen S, Makrythanasis P, Hammar E, Guipponi M, Ranza E, Varvagiannis K, et al. Experience of a multidisciplinary task force with exome sequencing for Mendelian disorders. Hum Genomics. 2016;10(1):24.

Permissions

All chapters in this book were first published in MB, by BioMed Central; hereby published with permission under the Creative Commons Attribution License or equivalent. Every chapter published in this book has been scrutinized by our experts. Their significance has been extensively debated. The topics covered herein carry significant findings which will fuel the growth of the discipline. They may even be implemented as practical applications or may be referred to as a beginning point for another development.

The contributors of this book come from diverse backgrounds, making this book a truly international effort. This book will bring forth new frontiers with its revolutionizing research information and detailed analysis of the nascent developments around the world.

We would like to thank all the contributing authors for lending their expertise to make the book truly unique. They have played a crucial role in the development of this book. Without their invaluable contributions this book wouldn't have been possible. They have made vital efforts to compile up to date information on the varied aspects of this subject to make this book a valuable addition to the collection of many professionals and students.

This book was conceptualized with the vision of imparting up-to-date information and advanced data in this field. To ensure the same, a matchless editorial board was set up. Every individual on the board went through rigorous rounds of assessment to prove their worth. After which they invested a large part of their time researching and compiling the most relevant data for our readers.

The editorial board has been involved in producing this book since its inception. They have spent rigorous hours researching and exploring the diverse topics which have resulted in the successful publishing of this book. They have passed on their knowledge of decades through this book. To expedite this challenging task, the publisher supported the team at every step. A small team of assistant editors was also appointed to further simplify the editing procedure and attain best results for the readers.

Apart from the editorial board, the designing team has also invested a significant amount of their time in understanding the subject and creating the most relevant covers. They scrutinized every image to scout for the most suitable representation of the subject and create an appropriate cover for the book.

The publishing team has been an ardent support to the editorial, designing and production team. Their endless efforts to recruit the best for this project, has resulted in the accomplishment of this book. They are a veteran in the field of academics and their pool of knowledge is as vast as their experience in printing. Their expertise and guidance has proved useful at every step. Their uncompromising quality standards have made this book an exceptional effort. Their encouragement from time to time has been an inspiration for everyone.

The publisher and the editorial board hope that this book will prove to be a valuable piece of knowledge for researchers, students, practitioners and scholars across the globe.

List of Contributors

Qi-xin Shi, Liu-kun Yang, Lu Wang, Shi-meng Zhou, Shao-yu Guan and Ming-gao Zhao
1Department of Pharmacology, School of Pharmacy, Fourth Military Medical University, Xi'an, China

Qi Yang
Department of Pharmacology, School of Pharmacy, Fourth Military Medical University, Xi'an, China
Department of Neurobiology and Collaborative Innovation Center for Brain Science, Fourth Military Medical University, Xi'an, China

Wen-long Shi
Department of Pharmacy, The 155th Central Hospital of PLA, Kaifeng, China

Dong-Yun Jiang, Zheng Wu, Cody Tieu Forsyth, Yi Hu and Gong Chen
Department of Biology, Huck Institutes of Life Sciences, Pennsylvania State University, University Park, PA 16802, USA

Siu-Pok Yee
Department of Cell Biology, University of Connecticut Health center, Farmington, CT 06030, USA

Xu-Hui Li, Qian Song, Qi-Yu Chen and Jing-Shan Lu
Center for Neuron and Disease, Frontier Institutes of Science and Technology, Xi'an Jiaotong University, Xi'an 710049, China

Tao Chen
Center for Neuron and Disease, Frontier Institutes of Science and Technology, Xi'an Jiaotong University, Xi'an 710049, China
Department of Anatomy and K.K. Leung Brain Research Center, Fourth Military Medical University, Xi'an, ShaanXi 710032, China

Min Zhuo
Center for Neuron and Disease, Frontier Institutes of Science and Technology, Xi'an Jiaotong University, Xi'an 710049, China
Department of Physiology, Faculty of Medicine, University of Toronto, Medical Science Building, Room #3342, 1 King's College Circle, Toronto, ON M5S 1A8, Canada

Bin Liu, Kaixing Zhou and Xiaojing Wu
Key Laboratory of Developmental Genes and Human Diseases, MOE, School of Medicine, Southeast University, Nanjing 210009, People's Republic of China

Chunjie Zhao
Key Laboratory of Developmental Genes and Human Diseases, MOE, School of Medicine, Southeast University, Nanjing 210009, People's Republic of China
Depression Center, Institute for Brain Disorders, Beijing 100069, China

Qiu Jing Wu
Krembil Research Institute, University Health Network, 60 Leonard St, Toronto, ON M5T2S8, Canada
Department of Physiology, University of Toronto, Toronto, ON, Canada

Michael Tymianski
Krembil Research Institute, University Health Network, 60 Leonard St, Toronto, ON M5T2S8, Canada
Department of Physiology, University of Toronto, Toronto, ON, Canada
Division of Neurosurgery, University of Toronto, Toronto, ON, Canada

Andreas H. Rasmussen and Asli Silahtaroglu
Department of Cellular and Molecular Medicine, Faculty of Medical and Health Sciences, University of Copenhagen, DK-2200 Copenhagen, Denmark

Hanne B. Rasmussen
Department of Biomedical Sciences, Faculty of Medical and Health Sciences, University of Copenhagen, DK-2200 Copenhagen, Denmark

Dale B. Bosco, Jiaying Zheng, Jiyun Peng and Ukpong B. Eyo
Department of Neurology, Mayo Clinic, 200 First Street SW, Rochester, MN 55905, USA

Long-Jun Wu
Department of Neurology, Mayo Clinic, 200 First Street SW, Rochester, MN 55905, USA
Department of Neuroscience, Mayo Clinic, Jacksonville, FL 32224, USA

Zhiyan Xu
Department of Pharmacology, School of Pharmacy, Nantong University, 19 Qixiu Road, Nantong 226001, Jiangsu, China

Hui Wang
Department of Pharmacology, School of Pharmacy, Nantong University, 19 Qixiu Road, Nantong 226001, Jiangsu, China

Department of Neuroscience and Cell Biology, Rutgers-Robert Wood Johnson Medical School, Piscataway, NJ 08854, USA

Ke Tang, Cheng Yan and Jun Huang
Admera Health LLC, South Plainfield, NJ 07080, USA

Lijie Feng
Department of Histology and Embryology, School of Basic Medical Sciences, Anhui Medical University, Hefei 230032, Anhui, China

Gongxiong Wu
One Harvard Street Institute of Health, Brookline, MA 02446, USA

Jason R. Richardson
Department of Pharmaceutical Sciences and Center for Neurodegenerative Disease and Aging, Northeast Ohio Medical University, Rootstown, OH 44272, USA

Yibo Piao
Department of Plastic and Reconstructive Surgery, Department of Pediatrics, Department of Anesthesiology and Pain Medicine, Chungnam National University Hospital, Daejeon 35015, Republic of Korea

Nara Shin, Hyeok Hee Kwon, Yuhua Yin and Sang-Ha Oh
Department of Plastic and Reconstructive Surgery, Department of Pediatrics, Department of Anesthesiology and Pain Medicine, Chungnam National University Hospital, Daejeon 35015, Republic of Korea
Department of Medical Science, Department of Physiology, Department of Anatomy, Brain Research Institute, Chungnam National University School of Medicine, Daejeon 35015, Republic of Korea

Do Hyeong Gwon, Dong-Wook Kang, Tae Woong Hwang, Hyo Jung Shin, Jinpyo Hong, Hyun-Woo Kim and Dong Woon Kim
Department of Medical Science, Department of Physiology, Department of Anatomy, Brain Research Institute, Chungnam National University School of Medicine, Daejeon 35015, Republic of Korea

Jwa-Jin Kim
Department of Medical Science, Department of Physiology, Department of Anatomy, Brain Research Institute, Chungnam National University School of Medicine, Daejeon 35015, Republic of Korea
LES Corporation Inc., Gung-Dong 465-16, Yuseong-Gu, Daejeon 305-335, Republic of Korea

Yonghyun Kim
Department of Chemical and Biological Engineering, The University of Alabama, Tuscaloosa, AL 35487, USA

Sang Ryong Kim
School of Life Sciences, BK21 plus KNU Creative BioResearch Group, Institute of Life Science and Biotechnology, Kyungpook National University, Daegu 41566, South Korea

Jung-Hwa Tao-Cheng
NINDS Electron Microscopy Facility, National Institute of Neurological Disorders and Stroke, National Institutes of Health, Bethesda, MD 20892, USA

Taikai Nagayoshi, Kiichiro Isoda and Nori Mamiya
Department of Bioscience, Faculty of Applied Bioscience, Tokyo University of Agriculture, Tokyo, Japan

Satoshi Kida
Department of Bioscience, Faculty of Applied Bioscience, Tokyo University of Agriculture, Tokyo, Japan
Core Research for Evolutional Science and Technology, Japan Science and Technology Agency, Saitama, Japan

Patrick S. Freymuth and Helen L. Fitzsimons
Institute of Fundamental Sciences, Massey University, Palmerston North, New Zealand

Bhagirathi Dash, Sulayman D. Dib-Hajj and Stephen G. Waxman
Department of Neurology, Yale University Schoolof Medicine, New Haven, CT 06510, USA
Center for Neuroscience and Regeneration Research, Yale University School of Medicine, New Haven, CT 06510, USA
Rehabilitation Research center, VA Connecticut Healthcare System, 950 Campbell Avenue, Bldg. 34, West Haven, CT 06516, USA

Bruce G. Mockett, Shane M. Ohline and Wickliffe C. Abraham
Department of Psychology, University of Otago, Dunedin 9054, New Zealand

Valerie T. Y. Tan and Mohamad Fairuz bin Yahaya
Department of Psychology, University of Otago, Box 56, Dunedin 9054, New Zealand
Department of Biochemistry, Brain Health Research Centre, Brain Research New Zealand, University of Otago, Dunedin 9054, New Zealand

Hollie E. Wicky, Katie Peppercorn, Lucia Schoderboeck, Warren P. Tate and Stephanie M. Hughes
Department of Biochemistry, Brain Health Research Centre, Brain Research New Zealand, University of Otago, Dunedin 9054, New Zealand

Karen D. Parfitt
Department of Neuroscience, Pomona College, Claremont, California 91711, USA

Zachary C. E. Hawley and Danae Campos-Melo
Molecular Medicine Group, Robarts Research Institute, Schulich School of Medicine and Dentistry, Western University, London, Ontario, Canada

Michael J. Strong
Molecular Medicine Group, Robarts Research Institute, Schulich School of Medicine and Dentistry, Western University, London, Ontario, Canada
Department of Clinical Neurological Sciences, Schulich School of Medicine and Dentistry, Western University, London, Ontario, Canada
Department of Pathology, Schulich School of Medicine and Dentistry, Western University, London, Ontario, Canada
Rm C7-120 LHSC, University Hospital, 339 Windermere Road, London, Ontario N6A 5A5, Canada

Agustin Garcia-Caballero, Fang-Xiong Zhang, Victoria Hodgkinson, Junting Huang, Lina Chen, Ivana A. Souza and Gerald W. Zamponi
Department of Physiology and Pharmacology, Hotchkiss Brain Institute and Alberta Children's Hospital Research Institute, Cumming School of Medicine, University of Calgary, 3330 Hospital Dr. NW, Calgary T2N 4N1, Canada

Stuart Cain, Jennifer Kass, Sascha Alles and Terrance P. Snutch
Michael Smith Laboratories and Djavad Mowafaghian Centre for Brain Health, University of British Colombia, Vancouver, BC, Canada

Fredrick E. Henry and Alex Chen
Neuroscience Graduate Program, University of Michigan, Ann Arbor, MI 48109, USA
Molecular and Behavioral Neuroscience Institute, University of Michigan, Ann Arbor, MI 48109, USA
Department of Molecular and Integrative Physiology, University of Michigan, Ann Arbor, MI 48109, USA

Michael A. Sutton
Neuroscience Graduate Program, University of Michigan, Ann Arbor, MI 48109, USA
Molecular and Behavioral Neuroscience Institute, University of Michigan, Ann Arbor, MI 48109, USA
Department of Molecular and Integrative Physiology, University of Michigan, Ann Arbor, MI 48109, USA
Molecular and Behavioral Neuroscience Institute, Department of Molecular and Integrative Physiology, University of Michigan, 5067 BSRB, 109 Zina Pitcher Place, Ann Arbor, MI 48109-2200, USA

William Hockeimer
Molecular and Behavioral Neuroscience Institute, University of Michigan, Ann Arbor, MI 48109, USA
Department of Molecular and Integrative Physiology, University of Michigan, Ann Arbor, MI 48109, USA

Shreesh P. Mysore
Department of Pyschological and Brain Sciences, Johns Hopkins University, Baltimore, MD 21218, USA

Jing Liu, Lili Tong, Yue Niu, Jun Li, Xiu Wu, Ruopeng Sun and Baomin Li
Department of Pediatrics, Qilu Hospital of Shandong University, Jinan, Shandong, People's Republic of China. Shandong University, Jinan, Shandong, People's Republic of China

Fang Liu
Shandong University, Jinan, Shandong, People's Republic of China
Campbell Family Mental Health Research Institute, Centre for Addiction and Mental Health, University of Toronto, Toronto, ON, Canada

Shuangshuang Song
Qilu Children's hospital of Shandong University, Jinan, Shandong, People's Republic of China

Fang Luo, Jian Wu and Jie Zhang
My Genostics Inc., Beijing, People's Republic of China

Clement C. Zai, Haiyin Li and Albert H. C. Wong
Campbell Family Mental Health Research Institute, Centre for Addiction and Mental Health, University of Toronto, Toronto, ON, Canada

Index

www.ingramcontent.com/pod-product-compliance
Lightning Source LLC
Chambersburg PA
CBHW080524200326
41458CB00012B/4330
9781632416766